Laboratory Tests and Diagnostic Procedures with Nursing Diagnoses

Second Edition

Laboratory Tests and Diagnostic Procedures with Nursing Diagnoses

Second Edition

Jane Vincent Corbett, R.N., Ed.D.
Associate Professor
University of San Francisco
San Francisco, California

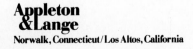
Appleton & Lange
Norwalk, Connecticut/Los Altos, California

0-8385-5592-6

Copyright © 1987 by Appleton & Lange
A Publishing Division of Prentice-Hall

89 90 91 / 10 9 8 7 6 5

Prentice-Hall of Australia, Pty. Ltd., Sydney
Prentice-Hall Canada, Inc.
Prentice-Hall Hispanoamericana, S.A., Mexico
Prentice-Hall of India Private Limited, New Delhi
Prentice-Hall International (UK) Limited, London
Prentice-Hall of Japan, Inc., Tokyo
Prentice-Hall of Southeast Asia (Pte.) Ltd., Singapore
Whitehall Books Ltd., Wellington, New Zealand
Editora Prentice-Hall do Brasil Ltda., Rio de Janeiro

Library of Congress Cataloging-in-Publication Data

Corbett, Jane Vincent.
  Laboratory tests and diagnostic procedures with nursing diagnoses.

  "This book is a combination second edition of Laboratory tests in nursing practice . . . and Diagnostic procedures in nursing practice, a companion volume published in 1983"—Pref.
  Includes bibliographies and indexes.
  1. Diagnosis, Laboratory. 2. Diagnosis. 3. Nursing. I. Corbett, Jane Vincent. Laboratory tests in nursing practice. II. Corbett, Jane Vincent. Diagnostic procedures in nursing practice. III. Title. [DNLM: 1. Diagnosis, Laboratory—nurses' instruction.
  2. Diagnostic Tests, Routine—nurses instruction. QY 4 C789La]
RT48.5.C67 1987   616.07'5   86-22211
ISBN 0-8385-5592-6

Design: M. Chandler Martylewski

PRINTED IN THE UNITED STATES OF AMERICA

To Rod and Rhonda Jane,
who gave me the space and time
to make this book a reality and
whose contributions were invaluable.

CONTENTS

PREFACE TO THE SECOND EDITION

This book is a combination second edition of *Laboratory Tests in Nursing Practice* (an American Journal of Nursing Book of the Year for 1982) and *Diagnostic Procedures in Nursing Practice,* a companion volume published in 1983. The combination of Laboratory Tests as Part I and Diagnostic Procedures as Part III has allowed extensive cross referencing which should help the reader gain a more comprehensive picture of the role of the nurse for clients undergoing tests of all kind. As before, examples used include all age groups (newborn to the aged), from a variety of practice settings.

Outdated tests and procedures have been deleted and many new ones included, such as urine tests for leukocyte esterase and PEP; blood tests for AIDS, 5'N, GGTP, LAP, CEA, C_1 esterase inhibitor, lactic acid, prolactin, osmole gap, A_{1c}, plasminogen, RDW, MPV, and fibrin split products; and diagnostic procedures such as chorionic villa biopsy and magnetic resonance imaging. The extensive reference list for each chapter has been updated with an even stronger emphasis on current nursing literature that emphasizes research. Reference values for the laboratory tests have been updated by using the Normal Reference Values printed in the January, 1986, *New England Journal of Medicine.*

The use of the nursing process was implicit in the first edition books although specific nursing diagnosis terminology was not used. In this edition, possible nursing diagnoses for each test and procedure are clearly identified. Related tests or procedures are grouped so that common nursing diagnoses can be highlighted. The nursing diagnoses presented in this book are not meant to be used in cookbook form. The nurse can read about the test and *possible* nursing diagnoses, but then must evaluate the actual clinical situation and apply what seems appropriate. The major purpose of this book is to make nurses think more, not less. The case studies in Part II give the reader an opportunity to practice interpreting lab data to formulate nursing diagnoses.

As health care becomes more and more technical, the multitude of diagnostic procedures and laboratory tests continues to grow. Nurses can become dazzled by the technical details and discouraged about keeping pace with these advances. This book is based on the belief that the nurse's role in relationship to diagnostic testing should continue to focus on the human element. Professional nurses are involved in health teaching, client preparation, and assessment for adverse reactions to diagnostic procedures. Thus, from a nursing point of view, detailed technical information on diagnostic procedures, using a disease or systems model, may not be the most helpful. Witness the difference in nursing care needed for a client having a liver biopsy compared to a client having a liver scan. Although both tests are used to diagnose potential disease in the same organ, there is no similarity in the nursing care. Yet, for some tests the disease state is an important focus. The pathophysiology that causes altered laboratory values is explained in an easy-to-understand format. Medical diagnoses and medical interventions are discussed when that information is pertinent to the nurse who may be assisting with treatment. A discussion of usual medical intervention for a particular set of circumstances is included to show how nursing use is related to and yet different from medical use of laboratory data. The independent role of the nurse is stressed.

Each chapter of this book is organized as an independent study unit complete with objectives, an organizing theme with background information (called an expository organizer), and test questions. The organization of the chapters is based on educational research recently conducted by the author.* This book, meant to be both scholarly and practical, is intended for use in both the academic and clinical setting. For example:

1. Undergraduate and graduate nursing students can use the book as a textbook in theory classes that integrate laboratory data as one aspect of nursing care.
2. Practicing nurses can use the book to update themselves in specific areas. The content in this book has been used extensively for continuing education courses for RNs.
3. Nurses in clinical settings can use the book as a quick reference. By consulting the index or the listing for each chapter, the nurse can retrieve information about one specific test.

It is intellectually challenging to broaden one's knowledge in a field, and in nursing we often have the added benefit of seeing that our increased knowlege is of direct benefit to the client. My enthusiasm and sense of purpose in writing this book stem from my belief that students and practicing nurses will be able to use the practical information in the book to improve the care of many clients. I hope the reader finds the book informative, interesting, and useful in the practice of nursing.

---

*Corbett, J. V. (1985). *The effects of two types of preinstructional strategies on two levels of cognitive learning from a written study unit.* Dissertation for School of Education, University of San Francisco. Reprints available from University Microfilms International, Ann Arbor, MI.

ACKNOWLEDGMENTS

The writing of this second edition was done while I was on sabbatical from the University of San Francisco. My thanks to all my colleagues who have always been willing to share their expertise with me.

The students at the University of San Francisco, particularly the class of 1986 who were involved in my research project, have given me many helpful suggestions for the second edition.

The format for this book was based on work I did for my doctoral dissertation. I am grateful to S. Alan Cohen, Ed.D., Joan Hyman, Ed.D., and William Schwarz, Ed.D., who helped me gain an indepth knowledge about how written strategies such as behavioral objectives and expository organizers can influence cognitive learning from study units. Eleanor Hein, R.N., Ed.D., Jean Nicholson, R.N., M.S., Mae Paulfrey, R.N., M.S., and Ginny Jones, R.N., B.S., also helped a great deal by their careful critiques of Chapter 13 used as the prototype chapter.

A large number of nurses from various clinical settings have participated in my continuing education classes and a senior elective class. I am particularly indebted to them for the discussion on the case studies included in this edition.

Also, many practicing nurses have participated in my surveys about laboratory tests. The data from the surveys were useful for updating and refining the content for this second edition.

Carol Bailey, R.N., M.S., Kaiser Hospital, San Francisco, has been most helpful in obtaining information for this edition. Other people at Kaiser, such as Sunny Holland, R.N., Cardiac Catheterization Lab, and Elaine Vaughn, Nuclear Medicine and Ultrasound, have also been helpful in answering many of my questions and allowing me to observe many types of diagnostic procedures. The University of California at San Francisco (UCSF) provided me with excellent library resources and also the opportunity to observe some clinical tests and consult with various experts.

And finally, a thank you to my editor, Marion Kalstein-Welch, whose ideas on revision were most helpful to me and to Michael Mollerus who typed my sometimes rather messy first drafts.

Laboratory Tests and Diagnostic Procedures with Nursing Diagnoses

Second Edition

Part I

LABORATORY TESTS

1

Using Laboratory Data

- Laboratory Reports and the Nursing Process
- Nursing Functions in Laboratory Testing
- "Normal" Reference Values and the Variability of Test Results
- False-Positive Tests and False-Negative Tests
- Establishing the "Normal" Value
- Measurements in Laboratory Reports
- Screening Tests for Asymptomatic Adult Populations
- Laboratory Personnel

OBJECTIVES

1. Describe how laboratory data can be used in the framework of the nursing process and how nursing use differs from the medical use of data.
2. Describe the traditional functions of nurses in relation to laboratory tests, including peripheral testing.
3. Identify the two nondisease factors that cause the greatest variations in normal reference values for laboratory tests.
4. Compare the meanings of the terms *specificity* and *sensitivity* in relation to diagnostic tests.
5. Explain in general terms how the normal curve and percentiles are used to establish normal reference ranges for laboratory tests.
6. Explain the meaning of the measurement symbols in the conventional laboratory system and in the SI system.
7. Describe the purpose of each of the basic diagnostic screening tests recommended for asymptomatic adult populations.
8. Define how nurses can foster smooth working relationships with personnel in the laboratory department.

In discussing several issues that are pertinent to the nurse's utilization of laboratory data, this chapter touches briefly on the nursing process, on the differences between nursing care and medical care, and on the traditional roles of the nurse in relation to diagnostic tests. Emphasis is given to the many factors that influence test results, such as physiology, drug interference, and the statistical methods used to determine "normal" ranges. A comparison of conventional measurements and SI is included, and the purpose of screening tests is explored. The last section in the chapter discusses ways that the nurse can effectively work with personnel in other departments.

LABORATORY REPORTS AND THE NURSING PROCESS

Up to the early seventies, problem solving was emphasized as a way of thinking about the needs of clients. About that time, most nursing educators started turning to the nursing process, which is an elaboration of the problem-solving technique used by all disciplines. In essence, the *nursing process* is a way of systematically identifying the needs of patients or clients, and then logically planning the appropriate nursing actions to meet those needs. (The term client is used in this book but "patient" may be substituted if one wishes.) Most practicing nurses use the nursing process even though they may be unsure about how to describe it step-by-step in writing. On the other hand, nursing students learn to develop care plans based on the nursing process in a very systematic manner (Rezler & Tichy, 1985). Yet, whether written out or not, the nursing process, as a way of thinking, helps the nurse to provide nursing care that is based on more than guesswork or generalizations about clients. This process is a deliberate way of using data to make the assessments and to identify the problems that are under the jurisdiction of the nurse. The evaluation and the modification of care are also essential components of the nursing process. The format for a written nursing care plan is shown in Table 1-1. Most hospitals have similar formats for use on the kardex, but the collection of data is not written out.

Collection of Data (Assessment)
Nurses use of a variety of ways to collect data, including physical assessment skills and interviewing techniques; laboratory data constitutes only one small part of the entire clinical picture. Consequently one can never use the laboratory data apart from other clinical data. For example, although an increased specific gravity is one objective sign of dehydration or a fluid volume deficit, the nurse must collect other data that may be relevant to this client's situation. If the client has just had diagnostic tests with radiopaque dye (Chapter 20), the specific gravity is not a meaningful contribution to data collection.

Nursing Diagnosis (Analysis)
Taking all the collected data, nurses must then formulate a *nursing diagnosis,* which is a problem within the scope of nursing practice. In a national conference, held in 1972, nurses identified a list of nursing diagnoses that were generally agreed to be under the control of the nurse. Since then the list has been periodically updated by national meetings of nurses called the North American Nursing Diagnosis Association (NANDA). Research is continuing to test each diagnosis in the clinical setting and to refine the characteristics (Dalton, 1985). While many nurses use this official and quite specific list of nursing diagnoses, others may prefer to use their own words to describe client problems. The important point is that nurses must make sure the diagnosis or problem is truly within the scope of nursing and that other health care

TABLE 1-1. USE OF LABORATORY DATA IN NURSING PROCESS

Collection of Data (Assessment)	Nursing Diagnosis or Statement of Problem (Analysis)	Client/Nurse Goals (Planning)	Interventions (Nurse-to-Nurse Orders Implementation)	Evaluation and Modification Needed (Evaluation)
Cannot use left arm to hold glass; mouth is dry; skin turgor poor; I&O for last 24 hours I = 800 O = 600 s.g. = 1.036 Hct 50% BUN 35 mg	Fluid volume deficit due to inability to feed self	Client will remain hydrated with a s.g. no higher than 1.020 *Short-term:* client will drink at least 1000 cc on the day shift and 600 cc on the evening shift	Give mouth care at least once a shift Ask client what type of fluids are wanted— does not like *water* Assist client to drink out of glass—likes straw In addition to meals, offer 250 ml fluids at: 10 A.M. 2 P.M. 4 P.M. 8 P.M.	Intake for 2–10: 7–3 P.M. 1,000 cc 3–11 P.M. 650 cc Client's s.g. now 1.015 on 2–11 2–11: Continue with plan

Note: Although a nursing diagnosis may arise from the use of one or two laboratory tests, more often there are many tests and much clinical data needed to fashion an individualized care plan. This text helps the reader by suggesting *potential* nursing diagnoses related to specific abnormal test results. The nurse must then gather relevant clinical data to validate the use of those diagnoses in a given situation.

workers understand the terminology. Carnevali (1984) notes that one of the things required for the process and products of nursing diagnosis to become fully established in the health care field would be for nursing textbooks to take a nursing perspective.

A nursing diagnosis is not the same as a medical diagnosis. While medicine is focused on the diagnosis and treatment of disease, nursing has to do primarily with the care, comfort, and support of people whose patterns of daily life are in some way threatened (Gordon, 1979). Nursing focuses on restorative support, nurturance, comfort measures, and health teaching.

Many client problems can be identified by using the nursing process. For example, through assessment, the nurse may discover that Mr. Smith's urine has become concentrated because he cannot feed himself and no one has been offering him any fluids between meals. Thus the nursing diagnosis would be a fluid volume deficit due to an inability to obtain fluids. On the other hand, dehydration, or a fluid volume deficit may be due to a serious medical problem such as ketoacidosis. The second case warrants medical interventions such as insulin administration and intravenous fluids. (See Chapter 8 on medical interventions for ketoacidosis.) As other examples:

1. An elevated direct bilirubin often causes itching in clients. What *comfort* measures by the nurse may be effective? (Alteration in comfort)
2. A client has a low serum potassium level. What *health teaching* does the client need about foods rich in potassium? (Knowledge deficit)
3. A woman is to have hormone tests as part of an infertility workup. The nurse

observes that the client is very anxious. What can the nurse do to prepare the woman and to give her *nurturance?* (Moderate anxiety)

4. A young child has a low hemoglobin reading. What can the nurse teach the parents that would be *restorative support?* (Alteration in nutritional requirements)

The nursing process, however, is effective only if one knows the answers to go with the questions raised by the process. Hence the subsequent chapters provide the information necessary for planning individualized client care. Only potential nursing diagnoses are listed for each test. The nurse must decide if the diagnosis is really appropriate for a particular setting.

Writing Goals for Client Outcomes

With the nursing diagnosis, the nurse can write client/nurse goals in behavioral terms. The goal should be acceptable to the client and compatible with medical goals. For example, in Mr. Smith's case, an immediate short-term goal is to have him drink so many milliliters of fluid during each shift. The long-term goal is that he will not show any signs of dehydration, that is, his specific gravity will remain in a normal range.

Nursing Interventions (Implementation)

The nurse then plans what nursing actions or interventions are needed to reach the goals. She or he may consult with the client about how to best achieve a mutually acceptable goal. Maybe Mr. Smith needs to be fed completely. Maybe he could feed himself and drink fluids if he were properly positioned. Maybe the client would drink juice better than water. Collaboration with the physician and with other health team members (such as the dietician) is also necessary if medical interventions are needed too.

Nurses write goals and interventions in various ways. These interventions, called "nurse-to-nurse" orders, need to be written on the kardex. The important point is to distinguish between actions that depend on physicians' orders and those that are independent nursing actions. Too often nurses do their own orders only by word of mouth from shift to shift. While nursing as a profession becomes more assured of its uniqueness, as something separate from medical care, one hopes that nurse-to-nurse orders will become more common a practice.

Evaluation of Goals

Evaluation is necessary to see if the goals were met. If goals are not achieved, what needs to be modified? For example, a specific gravity measurement can be considered evidence that the client has regained a normal fluid balance. "Responsibility" and "accountability" in nursing mean that nurses do take responsibility for the quality of client care and that they are accountable if the care does not meet certain standards. Hence evaluation is an integral part of accountability.

NURSING FUNCTIONS IN LABORATORY TESTING

Gathering Information from Charts

In collecting data from a chart, nurses should always look at the latest laboratory data first to see the current status of the client and to note trends in the data. One of the hardest things for novices to figure out is the meaning of the abbreviations used for many of the laboratory tests and diagnostic procedures. "ANA" on a chart, for example, has nothing to do with the American Nurses Association! It stands for antinuclear antibody test, which is a test done for systemic lupus erythematosus (SLE). The standard abbreviations used to denote laboratory tests are listed in Appendix E. Learning them makes reading charts and collecting data much easier.

Transcribing Orders and Ordering Laboratory Tests

Generally, because the procedures for transcribing orders and making out laboratory requisitions vary from institution to institution, this skill is best learned by in-service or on-the-job training. In this book, the essential points to include on the laboratory requisitions are discussed in relation to each specific test. Ordering laboratory tests is a skill usually reserved for experienced nurse clinicians in special situations. In some clinical settings, however, nurses may order certain laboratory tests in accordance with the hospital's standardized orders. For example, the regulations for nursing practice in California note that ordering routine laboratory tests, such as urinalysis, occult blood tests, or wound cultures, may be part of basic health care given by the nurse (Chow, 1986). See the later discussion on interpretation of laboratory results.

Peripheral Testing by Nurses

Peripheral testing refers to testing that is done by nonlaboratory personnel, and it is often done by nurses whenever there is a need for quick results. Several simple tests require only a drop or two of blood or urine and no special equipment. Some of these tests include the dipsticks for urine chemistry, slide tests for occult blood, and simple procedures such as specific gravity reading by refractometers (Table 1-2). In special care units, such as intensive care units or emergency rooms, nurses may also operate automated equipment that measures blood gases or hematocrits.

Nurses must be aware of the potential problems with administering such tests. For instance, the diagnostic test kits are reliable only if the nurses follow the instructions. Another problem is that test materials may not be properly cared for. Bottles are left open, materials get wet or hot, and the issue date of the test is unknown. Aides, inexperienced nurses, or interns may not do the test accurately, or the people doing the test may be color-blind. (All laboratory people are tested for color-blindness as a requirement for their job.) Too often the results of the test are recorded haphazardly on the chart.

Another interesting objection to peripheral testing is the cost to the hospital. Muschenheim & Przada (1979) make the point that, right or wrong, many hospitals depend on the laboratory as one of the key services to generate income. So if laboratory tests are done outside the laboratory, the client is not billed properly.

Quality control is another point of concern. The inspection standards of both the Joint Commission for Accreditation of Hospitals (JCAH) and the College of American Pathologists (CAP) state that the laboratory and the pathologist are charged with the responsibility for all clinical testing, inside and outside of the laboratory. Usually, with peripheral tests, control by the laboratory is not very evident, although some institutions have required that all nurses take a "wet lab" session so that they can do the tests correctly (Spark & Kundert, 1979). Only a few states have comprehensive regulation of laboratories in clinics or physicians' offices (Crawley et al., 1986).

The reader may be interested in finding out how a local hospital or clinic handles peripheral testing. If nurses are not comfortable with the procedures used for peripheral testing, they should request in-service. Many of the manufacturers of diagnostic kits give free in-service to nurses and other health care workers. Also, many teaching aides about products may be obtained by writing directly to the manufac-

TABLE 1-2. EXAMPLES OF COMMON TYPES OF PERIPHERAL TESTINGS

Specimen	Test for	Product Example[a]	Discussed in
Urine	Glucose	Tes-Tape (3)	Chaps. 2, 9
Serum	Glucose	Dextrostix (1) Visodex II (1) Chem Strip bG (2)	Chap. 9
Urine	Glucose and other sugars	Clinitest (1)	Chaps. 2, 9
Serum and urine	Ketone bodies	Ketostix (1) Acetone tablets (1)	Chaps. 2, 9
Body secretions	pH of urine, vaginal secretions, nasogastric contents	Nitrazine (1)	Chap. 2
Urine	Protein	Dipsticks Refractometer	Chap. 3
Urine	Specific gravity	Refractometer Urinometer	Chap. 3
Stool or other secretions	Occult blood	Guaiac tests Hematest (1) Hemoccult (5)	Chap. 13
Capillary blood	Hypothyroidism, galactesemia, and PKU in newborn	Heel stick on filter papers, various brands	Chap. 18
Urine	Phenylketonuria	Phenestix (1)	Chap. 18
Urine	Bilirubin	Icotest (1)	Chap. 11
Urine	Pregnancy	Various home kits	Chap. 18
Urine	Infection	Microstix (1) Unibac (2) Clinicult (5)	Chap. 16
Serum	Sickle cell screening	Sickledex (4)	Chap. 18

[a]Manufacturers
 (1) Ames Laboratory, Elkhart, Indiana 46514
 (2) Bio-Dynamics, Indianapolis, Indiana 46250
 (3) Eli Lilly Co., Indianapolis, Indiana 46206
 (4) Ortho Diagnostics, Raritan, New Jersey 08869
 (5) Smith Kline Diagnostics, Philadelphia, Pennsylvania 19101

Note that these major companies and many smaller companies have printed information to send to professionals.

turer or by talking to the local sales representatives. Table 1–2 includes the addresses of some of the major manufacturers of products for peripheral testing.

Preparation of the Client for the Laboratory Test

The nurse's role includes preparing the client physically and psychologically. As a client advocate, the nurse can make sure that the client has adequate knowledge of what is to be done. As information giver or health teacher, the nurse can also seek additional input from other members of the health team so that the client gives an informed consent. The responsibilities of nurses in effecting the implementation of a doctrine of informed consent are related to her/his role within the health team, the facility wherein which health care is given, and the current law. In the past few years, there has been more emphasis on clients' rights as states have enacted laws to enforce the doctrine of informed consent.

Collection and Transportation of Specimens

Venous Samples. Experienced nurses often draw venous blood for blood work. When they do, they must avoid the following possible causes of hemolysis, which particularly invalidates tests such as potassium or LDH (Strand & Elmer, 1980).

1. Skin too wet with antiseptic
2. Moisture in the syringe or collection tube
3. Prolonged use of a tourniquet
4. Use of a small gauge needle to withdraw a large volume of blood
5. Use of suction on the syringe
6. Vigorous shaking of the blood specimen
7. Not removing the needle from the syringe before expelling the blood into the collection tube
8. Vigorous expulsion of blood from the syringe into the collection tube

Other tips include not drawing blood on the arm where there is an intravenous because the values will be changed by the solution being infused. Intracath or scalp vein needles used for blood samples should be inserted 30 minutes prior to obtaining fasting samples, which could be affected by stress (Tallman, 1982). Reker and Webb (1986) stress the usefulness of a serial sampling technique to avoid multiple vein punctures for the client. Appendix A includes notes for specific tests in relation to collection methods. The meanings of the various colors for tubes are also explained in Table 1-3. For example, a red top tube means "no additives." (Most venous blood samples for chemistry are collected without additives or in the red and black tube that separates the serum; see Chapter 13 for techniques for *arterial* blood samples.)

Finger and Heel Sticks. For some tests, such as hematocrits and blood sugars, finger sticks may be used rather than a venipuncture. Earlobes are used, too. The usual

TABLE 1-3. MEANING OF COLOR CODE FOR BLOOD SPECIMENS

Color of Tube Top	Contents	Use
Red	No Additives No Separator	Most chemistry, serology, and blood banking
Red and black	Silicone gel to separate serum from cells[a]	Most chemistry and serology
Green	Heparin	Special tests such as ammonia levels, blood gases
Lavender	EDTA	Hematology, some chemistry and blood banking
Blue	Sodium citrate	PT, PTT, and other coagulation tests
Gray	Glycolytic inhibitor such as oxalate and fluoride	Glucose

[a]The use of the silicone gel, which separates the cells from the plasma, makes it easier for the laboratory worker to obtain the serum. The gel is more costly, however. Tubes should be rotated if additive is present so it will mix with the specimen.

See Appendix A for type of specimen needed for each blood test.

procedure is to cleanse with 70% alcohol, dry with a gauze sponge, and puncture with a sterile blade deep enough to get a free flow of blood. The first drop of blood is discarded, and enough blood is collected to fill a capillary tube supplied by the laboratory. Or a drop of blood may be put onto special filter paper. It is important not to squeeze to get capillary blood because the squeezing causes tissue fluids to dilute the sample. (If clients need to do finger sticks at home, they can buy from most surgical supply houses a small apparatus that automatically punctures the finger to the right depth.) In the infant, heel sticks are used for capillary blood. The foot is warmed for 5 minutes to dilate the capillaries and arterioles. The lateral aspects of the heel are used to avoid the plantar artery. A small adhesive Band-Aid is placed over the puncture site.

Urine and Other Specimens. The procedure for urine collection, including 24-hour testing, is detailed in Chapter 3. Chapter 16 gives explicit details on all the types of specimens collected for cultures.

   After a specimen is collected, the way it is stored and transported to the laboratory can affect the test values. Some specimens, such as the serum for cold agglutinins must be carried to the laboratory in a 37 °C bath. Other specimens, such as blood gases or anaerobic cultures, must not be exposed to the air. The nurse must check with the laboratory to determine if there are any special requirements about the transportation of specimens.

Seeing That Stat Tests Are Stat

The word "stat" means "at once." Because a stat request interrupts the normal laboratory routine, a test should be marked "stat" only when the results really do need to be known as soon as possible. In most stat situations, someone should hand-carry the specimen to the laboratory. The nurse should be familiar with the preparation needed and with the expected results of stat tests because these tests are done in emergency situations when there is little time to do reviews. Barnett et al. (1978) did a study to find out which laboratory tests are most commonly done as stats in different hospitals. Table 1–4 lists 22 tests done as stats by at least 90% of the hospitals in that survey.

Action in the Event of Abnormal Test Results

Often the nurse is the first one to see the results of a laboratory report. In one study of 60 laboratories, 17 called the doctor to give the results of stats, 32 called the floor, and 11 carried the results to the floor (Barnett et al., 1978). So nurses need to determine if a physician should be notified immediately or if the report is not urgent. The nurse may also need to alert other people to watch for symptoms or to take certain precautions. Although it is usually an abnormal report that requires immediate attention, a normal report may also have great diagnostic importance. For example, the clinician uses normal results to rule out the probability of certain disease entities (Gorry, 1978). The significance of abnormal and normal results is discussed in detail with each specific test.

   Interpreting laboratory data is becoming more expected of nurses. An Appeals Court upheld a judge's decision to allow a nurse to testify that the nursing duty of care increased as a client's partial thromboplastin time (PTT) increased. The defendant nurse's attorney had objected, contending that relating a nurse's duty to the client's laboratory values went beyond the field of nursing and invaded that of the physician (Cushing, 1985).

TABLE 1-4. TESTS MOST COMMONLY DONE AS STAT PROCEDURES

Name of Test	Discussed in
Complete blood count (CBC)	Chap. 2
Urinalysis (UA)	Chap. 3
Blood urea nitrogen (BUN)	Chap. 4
Electrolytes (Na, K, Cl, Bicarb)	Chap. 5
Blood gases	Chap. 6
Calcium	Chap. 7
Glucose	Chap. 8
Acetone (serum)	Chap. 8
Bilirubin	Chap. 11
Amylase	Chap. 12
Prothrombin time (PT)	Chap. 13
Partial thromboplastin time (PTT)	Chap. 13
Platelet Count	Chap. 13
Fibrinogen	Chap. 13
Type and cross match	Chap. 14
Direct Coombs	Chap. 14
Transfusion reaction investigation	Chap. 14
Innoculate media for cultures	Chap. 16
Gram stains	Chap. 16
Alcohol	Chap. 17
Salicylates	Chap. 17
Cerebrospinal fluid (CSF)	Chap. 16

Based on studies reported in Barnett et al. (1978).

"NORMAL" REFERENCE VALUES AND THE VARIABILITY OF TEST RESULTS

Laboratory values in the literature are referred to as *normal reference values* or *reference values* and not as *normal values,* because each laboratory must determine what is "normal" for a test done in a specific laboratory. *The use of any of the reference values in this book may be hazardous to the well-being of clients unless values are verified by the local laboratory. No book can be the authority on what is normal for a specific laboratory.*

For the most part, the reference values used throughout this book are those periodically published in the *New England Journal of Medicine.* (See Appendix A for the address to write to obtain reprints of all the printed values.) These values, based on the ones used at Massachusetts General Hospital, have been periodically published since 1946 (Scully, 1986). The reprint is of particular interest because it documents the source in the literature for each method of testing used. Reference values for some tests were gained from other literature and from Kaiser Hospital and Children's Hospital in San Francisco, California. Other sources for reference values are listed in each chapter and with the tables in the appendices.

Variables That Affect Test Results

Besides the obvious differences of technique and method, many other variables can influence laboratory reference values. Age and sex (gender) are the chief physiological factors that change the "norms." Pregnancy alters the normal reference values. (See the tables in Appendices A, B, C, and D for examples of changes in values in different populations.) Reference values for adults are often better documented than those for children (Cherjan & Hill, 1978; Wallach, 1983).

Other physiological factors, such as diet, the time of day, activity level, and stress, may also alter what is "normal" for a test. For example, hormones (Chapter 15) have a diurnal variation; so the time of day must be noted when the specimen is drawn. Geographical location, including the altitude, temperature, and humidity, may also affect the results. Racial or ethnic variation can also cause different reference values for different groups, but usually ethnic or racial differences are not of much importance for most tests (Galen, 1979).

Drug Interferences

Drugs can change laboratory tests in two ways (Galen, 1978):

1. They can change the client's physiology. For example, birth control pills (Appendix D) cause changes in many of the laboratory tests by altering the woman's hormonal balance.
2. Drugs may have a direct interference with the method of chemical analysis. For example, the urine test for phenylketonuria (PKU) is not reliable if the infant has had salicylates or phenothiazines, either of which also cause a reaction to the dipstick (Chapter 18).

Often the reports in the literature on drug effects are in conflict. How significantly a drug alters a laboratory value may depend on the dosage, timing, physiology of the client, and other variables such as the mixture of drugs. So the reader must consult pharmacology references or other more specialized texts than this for details on drug interactions, both from the physiological effects and the chemical effects on laboratory results. Wallach (1986) has extensive lists of these effects. Only the more common drug interferences are included in this text.

FALSE-POSITIVE TESTS AND FALSE-NEGATIVE TESTS

Specificity

If a test is 100% *specific,* it reacts positively only when the client actually has the condition being tested. No laboratory test is 100% specific because there is always some factor, such as drugs, that can effect a false positive. For example, the radioimmunoassay (RIA) test for pregnancy is a very specific test because almost all women who have a positive result for the test are indeed pregnant. Still, other factors, such as the elevation of other hormones, can make the test a false positive. On the other hand, the VDRL, a test for syphilis, is not a highly specific test; that is, a significant number of people can have a positive VDRL even though they do not have syphilis. The danger of false positives is that the client may receive additional tests and treatments that are unnecessary.

Sensitivity

The *sensitivity* of a test is the degree to which a test detects disease without yielding false negatives. No test is 100% sensitive, because there is always some possibility that the test will not reveal the abnormality even though it is present. For example, the direct agglutination technique of detecting pregnancy is not as sensitive as indirect agglutination methods, and neither is it as sensitive as the radioimmunoassay method (Chapter 18). So with the direct agglutination method, there are more false negatives than with the radioimmunoassay method; that is, the client is pregnant, but the agglutination method does not reveal it.

In disease states, false negative tests mean that clients are misclassified as not needing treatment or care when actually they *do* need treatment. For example, the electrocardiogram is not a sensitive test for coronary disease prior to a myocardial infarction. In other words, coronary disease is not detected by this particular test. Thus a person may have a "normal" electrocardiogram (EKG) one day and a myocardial infarction the next. Larson (1986) describes several quantitative methods used to evaluate the validity of screening tests used in nursing research.

New Tests

Specificity and sensitivity are important criteria when a new test is introduced into practice. Balint (1978, p. 291) has suggested five questions to decide whether a new test or a diagnostic procedure is worthwhile:

1. Does the new procedure provide a greater specificity and sensitivity than current methods?
2. Is the new information valuable in client management?
3. Is the new approach as effective in routine clinical practice as it is in selected populations of a university center?
4. Would it provide answers not provided by clinical findings and established diagnostic procedures?
5. In light of the other four factors, is it cost effective?

ESTABLISHING THE "NORMAL" VALUE

It should be increasingly apparent that "blind faith" in the validity of laboratory tests is simply not realistic. In addition to the problems already discussed, even the so-called normal value can be misleading. The normal ranges are determined by testing a large sample of healthy individuals and then analyzing the results by statistical methods.

The Normal Curve

One such method is the so-called *normal curve* or *Gaussian distribution*. In this method a cutoff point, which usually consists of two standard deviations from the mean or average, is determined for each side of the curve. In other words, the lowest 2.5% and the highest 2.5% are outside the "normal" range. Even without a statistical background, the reader should be able to appreciate that any system with cutoff points automatically mean that some *healthy* people in the sample do not fall within the "normal" range. Also, if the distribution is not normal, the curve will be skewed. (Most students who have been exposed to grading by the bell curve know the situation where students who do exceptionally well are called "curve wreckers" by those on the other end of the curve.) Most physiological parameters do not fall in normal distributions, and so it is usually incorrect to speak of averages and normal curves in relationship to laboratory data (Elrebach et al., 1970).

The Percentile Ranking System

The percentile ranking system is usually a better method than the curve because data that do not have a normal distribution can still be ranked. *All* the values are ranked, and a percentage is given for each value in relation to the other values. The value in the middle (the median) is at the 50th percentile. This means 50% of the scores are higher and 50% are lower. When laboratory data is ranked by percentiles, a cutoff point must be established to indicate an abnormality. For example, values above the 95th percentile are usually considered beyond the "normal" reference values. Thus 5% of *healthy* people are *unhealthy* according to this statistical determination of "normalcy" (Harwood, 1978).

   Obviously nurses do not have to determine normal ranges or even understand the underlying statistics. They do, however, need to realize that a significant margin of error arises from the arbitrary setting of limits. In effect, with each laboratory test, the results *may* be outside the normal range due entirely to mathematical probability. It should be stated again, if a laboratory test is considered normal up to the 95th percentile, then five times out of 100 a test will show an abnormality *even though the client is not ill.* If the person has two tests done, the probability that both will be within the normal range is 0.95 times 0.95 or 90.25%. With three tests, the probability is 0.95 times 0.95 times 0.95 or 85.7375%. The point is that, if a client has a battery of tests, such as the SMA discussed at the end of this chapter, the possibility is great that some of the tests will be abnormal due purely to chance (Casscells et al., 1978; Sox, 1986).

MEASUREMENTS IN LABORATORY REPORTS

Conventional Measurements
Probably most of the measurements used in laboratory reports, such as "ml" (milliliter) or "mg" (milligram), are already very familiar. A list of the common abbreviations used for metric measurements is included in Table 1–5, and a more complete list is included as Appendix G. Note that "mg/dl" means so many "milligrams in a deciliter," which is 1/10 of a liter, or 100 milliliters. In other words, a blood sugar report of 90 mg/dl is the same as 90 mg per 100 ml.

TABLE 1–5. METRIC MEASUREMENTS USED IN LABORATORY REPORTS[a]

Nonmetric Equivalent

Length
   Meter (m) —————————————————————→ 39.37 in
   Centimeter (cm) = 1/100 m ————————————→ 2.5 cm = 1 in
   Millimeter (mm) = 1/1000 m

Weight
   Kilogram (kg) ————————————————————→ 2.2 lb
   Gram (g) ——————————————————————→ 453 g = 1 lb
   Milligram (mg) = 1/1000 of a kg
   Microgram (mcg or μg) = 1/1000 of a mg
   Nanogram (ng) = 1/1000 of a mcg
   Picogram (pg) = 1/1000 of a ng
   Femtogram (fg) = 1/1000 of a pg

Volume
   Liter (L) = 1000 ml (or 1000 cc[b] or 1.05/qt)
   Deciliter (dl) = 100 ml or 1/10 of a L
   Milliliter (ml) = 1 ml or 1/1000 of a L

[a]See Appendix G for an expanded list of measurement terms used in laboratory reports.
[b]Note that "ml" and "cc" are interchangeable, but "ml" is preferred because it is in the metric system.

The term *picogram* (pg) and *nanogram* (ng) are also becoming commonly used, now that radioimmunoassay (RIA) has made it possible to detect trace amounts of substances such as hormones or drugs in the serum (Chapter 15).

The measurement used for electrolytes is *milliequivalent* (mEq). This term's exact meaning, as well as how mg can be converted to mEq, is explained in Chapter 5. *Milliosmoles* (mOsm) are used to express the concentration of body fluids. (See Chapter 3 for a definition of milliosmoles in relation to urinary osmolality.) Note that m*Os*m is different from m*m*ol discussed next.

SI: A New Measurement System

SI units are based on a comprehensive modern form of the metric system called *Le Systeme Internationale* (hence "SI"). The rationale for the adoption of this international system is to provide a common language for all the various disciplines all over the world (Young, 1974). Used not just for the biological sciences but for all sciences, SI utilizes *moles* as the basic unit for the amount of a substance and *kilograms* for its mass. Length is still by *meter*.

The most profound change in laboratory reports effected by SI is that concentration is expressed as an amount per volume (moles or millimoles per liter) rather than as a mass per volume (grams or milligrams per 100 ml or dl). For some laboratory tests, the numbers stay the same even though the unit is new. For example, the normal range for potassium (K) in the conventional system is 3.5 to 5.0 *mEq/L* and 3.5 to 5.0 *mmol/L* in the new SI. Some of the other tests involve a radical change in numbers, so health workers must totally relearn the reference values. For example, the conventional reference value for glucose of *70 to 110 mg/dl* becomes *3.9 to 5.6 mmol/L* in the new SI.

Due to the drastic change in many of the laboratory reports, the conversion is taking place slowly in our country. Plans are underway for a gradual change to this new system (Powsner, 1984; Wallach, 1986). At present, many laboratories report results in both conventional and SI units. Appendix A gives the reference values in both conventional and SI units.

SCREENING TESTS FOR ASYMPTOMATIC ADULT POPULATIONS

Biochemical profiles (BCPs) consist of a battery of tests, usually six or twelve, in which the client's individual results are compared against the normals. BCP tests are provided by automatic analyzers from a number of manufacturers. The battery of tests is often called "SMA" because this was the first brand name commonly used: SMAC, for sequential multiple analysis computer by Technicon Corporation. More correctly, the test should be called a *biochemical profile* (BCP). The usual tests done by an automatic analyzer are listed in Table 1-6.

Many years ago, Reece and Hobbie (1972) developed a computer program that compared the client's biochemical pattern of low and high test values with known patterns for at least 70 different pathological conditions. The computer was programmed to account for age and sex (gender) variations. The information that has been gained from studies with computer analysis have helped the physician focus on the most likely diagnoses of the client and today many charts and decision trees are available to help with differential diagnosis.

Because such tests as the biochemical profile have become very easy to do in mass volume, screening tests have been used widely for many populations. The use

TABLE 1–6. USUAL TESTS DONE BY AN AUTOMATIC ANALYZER

Name of Test	Described in
	Chap. 10
Total protein (TP)	Chap. 10
Albumin (Alb)	Chap. 7
Calcium (Ca)	Chap. 7
Phosphate (P)	Chap. 8
Glucose (RBS)	Chap. 4
Blood Urea Nitrogen (BUN) (creatinine can be substituted)	Chap. 4
Uric acid (optional)	Chap. 11
Total bilirubin	Chap. 12
Alkaline phosphatase	Chap. 12
LDH (optional)	Chap. 12
SGOT or AST	Chap. 9
Cholesterol (optional)	Chap. 5
Sodium (Na^+)	Chap. 5
Potassium (K^+)	Chap. 5
Chloride (Cl^-)	Chap. 6
Bicarbonate (HCO_3^-) or CO_2 content	

Automated measurement of 6 or 12 tests at once using a single sample of a few ml of serum. Check the brand of automatic analyzer for the exact amount needed. Laboratories may vary in the number of tests chosen. See text for discussion on abuse of screening tests.

of multiscreening tests for apparently healthy people was undertaken with the belief that many diseases could be detected early. However, the wide use of nondiscriminatory laboratory testing has not proven as valuable as once thought. The majority of such studies have concluded that it is seldom justified to do mass screening on asymptomatic populations (Schaefer & Dickman, 1978). Kaiser Foundation had a multiphasic screening program for two decades (Kaiser Foundation Health Plan, 1981). Over the years, all the screening tests were evaluated to see if each specific test was valuable in detecting a disease before the client has symptoms. The study's conclusion at Kaiser and at other facilities is that only a few tests should be routinely done for all adults.

Blue Cross and Blue Shield (1979) recommended the phasing out of *routine* admission test panels. Biochemical profiles were to be done only on the order of the physician. The introduction of diagnostic related grouping (DRG) led to more curtailing. The emphasis is now that laboratory tests and other diagnostic procedures should be determined by the nature of the client's problem, which must be discovered by careful history taking and physical examination. Blue Cross and Blue Shield have commissioned a series of articles to help physicians become more aware of appropriate diagnostic testing (Sox, 1986). These articles appear in the *Annals of Internal Medicine*.

The cost of testing compared to its usefulness is an issue that perplexes health care today. Past research (Daniels & Schroder, 1977; Skendzel, 1978) has found little relationship between laboratory use and the outcome of care. Even the usefulness of preoperative laboratory tests is questionable. Kaplan et al. (1985) noted that in the absence of specific indications, routine preoperative tests contributed little to client care decisions. In their study only 1–2% of the tests were abnormal. In summary, the use of a test does not always mean better client care, but it does mean an increased cost. However, Showstack et al. (1985) found that laboratory tests are not a major factor of rising costs. The reader is encouraged to consult recent literature on the usefulness of diagnostic screening tests and on the cost to the individual.

Some health care workers may dispute the medical control of most diagnostic testing. Clients can go directly to private laboratories, where they can get multiphasic screening exams done and sent to the physician or to themselves. Self-help organizations may also encourage the use of some screening tests for preventive medicine.

Publications for lay people have stressed that some critical screening tests and procedures for adults are: blood pressure checks to detect hypertension, tonometry to detect glaucoma, occult blood in stool to detect cancer, and Pap smears and mammograms for women. Cholesterol levels and TB skin tests are also good screening tests. Sobel and Ferguson (1985) list suggested tests for various age groups. The point is that there are only a few routine tests needed for apparently healthy people. Nurses need to help educate the public on practical and cost-effective methods of health screening.

LABORATORY PERSONNEL

Who Works in a Clinical Laboratory?

The Pathologist. The laboratory is directed by a physician with a specialty in pathology, which focuses on the use and interpretation of laboratory tests in the diagnosis and treatment of disease. Many of the books listed as general references for this book were written by pathologists. Because they often interpret the results of laboratory tests to the attending physician, pathologists are often called the "doctor's doctors."

Medical Technologist. The actual management of the laboratory is done by a medical technologist who has had additional training in management and administration. Usually the director of the laboratory sets up the policies and procedures that affect nursing. In most states, medical technologists have a bachelor's degree in a biological science, which includes a year or more study in a school of medical technology. States have their own medical technology examination, but a national examination is also available for certification. Licensing is not mandatory in all states.

Medical technologists typically become specialists in different areas, such as serology, hematology, or bacteriology. Nurses should understand how the laboratory is organized well enough that they do not call the chemistry section, for example, for the results of a culture and sensitivity test.

Laboratory Assistants. The meaning of the commonly used term "lab technician," is not precise. Medical technologists want to be known as medical technologists because any lab assistant may be called a lab technician. Laboratory assistants have a high school diploma, along with some on-the-job experience or training in certain laboratory techniques. Laboratory assistants draw blood, process specimens, and assist in performing some of the more routine tests in the laboratory.

Cooperating with Laboratory Personnel

Too often nursing and laboratory personnel conflict with each other rather than cooperate for the good of the client. Laboratory personnel complain that specimens are not marked correctly—that they are lost or otherwise ineptly handled by the nursing staff. Clients are not always correctly prepared for examinations, or the laboratory personnel are not informed of changes in orders. On the other hand, nurses complain that the laboratory is insensitive to the individual needs of the client, late with stat requests, curt and demanding with nurses, and so forth. Unfortunately, both departments often have legitimate reasons for gripes, but poor communication between the departments often allows small problems to become major frustrations (Stocker, 1985).

For their own part in this ongoing feud, nurses need to perform their own functions as accurately as possible. The information in the rest of this book should enable nurses to function better in preparing the client for laboratory testing, as well as make them sensitive to what the laboratory personnel needs to know about any special problems with clients. For example, if the nurse knows a client is disoriented and potentially combative, the laboratory personnel should be warned about this attitude before they go in to draw blood or to do other procedures. Nurses forget that they are often the only health professional that see the client for more than 15 minutes at a time.

Nurses in hospitals also have to face a fact of hospital life: Although they often complain that they must always plan their care around the visits from physicians, laboratory personnel, X-ray personnel—who drop in for brief contacts with the client—these people must have access to the client. Whereas the emphasis in nursing is on caring and nurturing to meet not only the physical needs but also the psychosocial needs of the client, such is not always the emphasis of other health workers who are trained to do more technical jobs. Hence nurses can foster smoother relationships with other health care workers by making the client available whenever possbile. At the same time, because they spend more time with the client than the others, they can often be advocates for the sick client who must deal with a host of other people in a fragmented way.

In general, nurses need to work in a spirit of cooperation with other health care personnel so that each can function well. If they have specific problems with the laboratory—stats not being done, lost reports, or whatever—nurses should collect written data about the problem and present this to the nursing supervisor so that some changes can be made. A lot of complaining to other nurses during a coffee break accomplishes little, if it goes no further than a gripe session.

QUESTIONS

1. Mrs. Rhoades has a specific gravity of 1.030 and other clinical signs of a fluid volume deficit. In using the nursing process, the nurse should use this information about specific gravity not only to make an assessment of the problem but also to:
   a. Diagnose the pathophysiology or underlying disease
   b. Initiate treatment for the disease
   c. Evaluate the effectiveness of nursing interventions
   d. Determine the intravenous rate

2. The traditional functions of the nurse in relation to laboratory tests include all the following *except:*
   a. Transcribing physicians' orders and making out requisitions for the laboratory
   b. Collecting and transporting specimens to the laboratory
   c. Conducting peripheral testing on the unit
   d. Scheduling the times when tests are done by laboratory personnel on the unit

3. Which of these two factors are generally the most common reasons for variations in normal reference values for laboratory tests?

    a. Genetic factors and drugs
    b. Sex (gender) and age
    c. Activity levels and stress
    d. Geographic location and diet

4. If a test yields too many false positives, the test is described as:

    a. "Not very sensitive"
    b. "Too sensitive"
    c. "Not specific"
    d. "Highly specific"

5. If the normal curve is used to establish normal references for laboratory values, the results of a large sample of healthy individuals are compiled and the normal range is usually designated as:

    a. 37.5% above and 37.5% below the average (75% of all scores)
    b. The lower half of the sample (50% of all scores)
    c. Any value within the range (100% of all scores)
    d. Two standard deviations above and below the average (95% of all scores)

6. In conventional laboratory reports, the smallest amount of a substance would be measured by weight as a:

    a. ng
    b. pg
    c. mcg
    d. mg

7. Laboratory results measured in SI units are reported as amount per volume as expressed by:

    a. Milliequivalents (mEq)
    b. Milliosmoles (mOsm)
    c. Millimoles (mmol)
    d. Milligrams (mg)

8. Which of the following is of questionable value as a *basic* screening test for *asymptomatic* adult populations over age 50?

    a. Biochemical profile (BCP) or SMA-12
    b. Checking stools for occult blood (guaiac tests)
    c. Checking for increased intraocular pressure (tonometry)
    d. Blood pressure checks

9. Nurses can foster smooth working relationships with personnel in laboratory departments by all the following measures *except:*

a. Calling the laboratory to seek information about client preparation for an unfamiliar test

b. Seeing that stat specimens are hand delivered to the laboratory and that only real emergencies are marked stat

c. Making sure that special needs of the client are conveyed to personnel from other departments who must interact with the client

d. Complaining only to other nurses about the mistakes made by the laboratory personnel

REFERENCES

Balint, J. (1978). When is a new test a valid test? *American Journal of Digestive Diseases, 23*, 291–292.

Barnett, R., et al. (1978). Medical usefulness of STAT tests. *American Journal of Clinical Pathology, 69*, 520–523.

Blue Cross/Blue Shield. (1979). Limits of admission test payments. *American Journal of Nursing, 79*(4), 572.

Casscells, W., et al. (1978). Intepretation by physicians of clinical laboratory results. *NEJM, 229*, 999–1000.

Carnevali, D. (1984). Nursing diagnosis: An evolutionary view. *Topics in Clinical Nursing, 5*(4), 10–20.

Cherjan, G., & Hill, G. (1978). Percentile estimates of references values for 14 chemical constituents in sera of child and adolescents. *American Journal of Clinical Pathology, 69*, 24–31.

Chow, M. (1986). *Regulation of nursing practice in California.* San Francisco: California Nurses Association.

Crawley, R., et al. (1986). Regulation of physicians' office laboratories. *JAMA, 255*(3), 374–382.

Cushing, M. (1985). Lessons from history: The picket-guard nurse. *AJN, 85*(10), 1073–1076.

Dalton, J. (1985). A descriptive study: Defining characteristics of the nursing diagnosis, cardiac output, alterations in: Decreased. *Image, 17*(4), 113–117.

Daniels, M., & Schroder, S. (1977). Variations among physicians in use of laboratory tests, relation to clinical productivity and outcomes of care. *Medical Care, 15*, 482–487.

Elrebach, L.R., et al. (1970). Health, normality and the ghost of Gauss. *JAMA, 211*, 69–75.

Galen, R. (1978). True or false? Drugs significantly affect clinical laboratory tests. *Diagnostic Medicine, 1*, 99–100.

Galen, R. (1979). Predictive value of laboratory testing. *Orthopedic Clinics of North America, 10*, 465–494.

Gordon, M. (1979). The concept of nursing diagnosis. *Nursing Clinics of North America, 14*, 487–495.

Gorry, A. (1978). The diagnostic importance of the normal finding. *NEJM, 298*, 486–489.

Harwood, S. (1978). Reference values based on hospital admission laboratory data. *JAMA, 240*, 270–274.

Kaiser Foundation Health Plan. (1981). Adult health screening. *Planning for Health, 23*, 1.

Kaplan, E., et al. (1985). The usefulness of preoperative laboratory screening. *JAMA, 253*(24), 3576–3581.

Larson, E. (1986). Evaluating validity of screening tests. *Nursing Research, 35*(3), 186–188.

Muschenheim, F., & Przada, S. (1979). We banned peripheral testing in our hospital. *Medical Laboratory Observer, 11*, 143–145.

Powsner, E. (1984). SI quantities and units for American medicine. *JAMA, 252*(1), 1737–1741.

Reece, R., & Hobbie, R. (1972). Computer evaluation of chemistry values. *American Journal of Clinical Pathology, 57*, 664–675.

Reken, D., & Webb, E. (1986). Multiple blood samples without multiple blood sticks. *RN, 49*(4), 39–41.

Rezler, A., & Tichy, A. (1985). *Nursing care plan workbook.* Norwalk, CT: Appleton-Century-Crofts.

Schaefer, S., & Dickman, J. (1978). Automated laboratory screening: An analysis of value in a nursing home population. *Wisconsin Medical Journal, 77*(8), 81–82.

Scully, R.E. (Ed.). (1986). Case records of Massachusetts General Hospital. "Normal reference laboratory values." *NEJM, 314*(1), 39–49.

Showstack, J., et al. (1985). The role of changing clinical practice in the rising costs of hospital care. *NEJM, 313*(19), 1201–1206.

Skendzel, L. (1978). How physicians use laboratory tests. *JAMA, 239,* 1077–1980.

Sobel, D., & Ferguson, T. (1985). *People's book of medical tests.* New York: Summit Books.

Sox, H. (1986). Probability theory in the use of diagnostic tests. *Annals of Internal Medicine, 104*(1), 60–65.

Spark, R., & Kundert, L. (1979). Control of peripheral testing by the laboratory. *Medical Laboratory Observer, 11,* 112–129.

Stocker, S. (1985). No more Dracula jokes, please. *Nursing 85, 15*(4), 104.

Strand, M., & Elmer, L. (1980). *Clinical Laboratory Tests: A Manual for Nurses* (2nd ed.). St. Louis, MO: C.V. Mosby.

Tallman, V. (1982). Effect of venipuncture on glucose, insulin, and free fatty acid levels. *Western Journal of Nursing Research, 4*(1), 21–34.

Wallach, J. (1983). *Interpretation of pediatric tests.* Boston: Little, Brown.

Wallach, J. (1986). *Interpretation of diagnostic tests.* Boston: Little, Brown.

Young, D.S. (1974). Standardized reporting of laboratory data: The desirability of using SI units. *NEJM, 290,* 368–373.

2

Hematology Tests

- Red Blood Cell Count (RBC)
- Hematocrit (Hct, PCV, or Crit)
- Hemoglobin (Hb or Hgb)
- Erythrocyte Indices
  Mean Corpuscular Volume (MCV), Mean Corpuscular Hemoglobin (MCH), and Mean Corpuscular Hemoglobin Concentration (MCHC)
- Red Blood Cell Distribution Width (RDW)
- Serum Folic Acid and Vitamin B_{12}
- Serum Iron (Fe) Levels, Total Iron Binding Capacity (TIBC) or Transferrin Saturation, and Serum Ferritin Levels
- Glucose-6-Phosphate-Dehydrogenase (G-6-PD)
- Reticulocyte Count (Retic Count)
- Peripheral Blood Smear
- Erythrocyte Sedimentation Rate (ESR or Sed Rate)
- Total White Blood Cell Count (WBC) and Differential (Diff)
- Nitroblue Tetrazolium Test (NBT)

OBJECTIVES

1. Describe the purpose for each of the different tests done by the Coulter counter.
2. Identify appropriate nursing diagnoses for clients with increased and decreased hemoglobin and RBC levels.
3. Anticipate how a change in the hydration status of a client affects hematocrit (Hct) results.
4. Describe how acute and chronic blood loss, iron deficiency anemia, and pernicious anemia change the erythrocyte indices (MCV, MCH, and MCHC).

5. Prepare teaching plans, which include specific information on drugs and diet, for clients with abnormal serum folic acid, B$_{12}$, iron or G-6-PD levels.
6. Give examples of clinical situations in which an elevated reticulocyte count is an expected physiological response.
7. Plan appropriate nursing interventions for a client who has an increasing erythrocyte sedimentation rate (sed rate or ESR).
8. Compare and contrast reference values for the WBC differential count in children, in adults, and in pregnancy.
9. Define the meaning of the phrase "shift to the left" with regard to the WBC differential count.
10. Identify appropriate nursing diagnoses for clients with increased and decreased levels of the different types of leukocytes.

Routine hematology tests can be done by automatic counters so the results are more reliable than the older method of counting under a microscope. Table 2–1 lists the tests routinely done by an automatic counter, a standard instrument in almost all laboratories. If the WBC is abnormal, it is necessary to know which of the five types of white blood cells are increased or decreased. The test of the five WBC types is called a *differential*. In some laboratories, differentials are still done by hand, but certain machines can also stain and count the various types of normal white blood cells. Abnormal cells must be examined by microscope.

Sometimes only one component of the CBC is needed. For example, if the primary concern is assessing blood loss, a Hct done a few hours after the bleeding gives an index of the severity of the blood loss. With an undiagnosed anemia, it would be important to have RBC, Hb, and Hct readings. These three different measurements of the erythrocytes (red blood cells) are the figures used to compute the erythrocyte indices: (1) mean corpuscular volume (MCV), (2) mean corpuscular hemoglobin (MCH), and (3) mean corpuscular hemoglobin concentration (MCHC).

A reticulocyte count gives an indication of the rate of production of red blood cells. One test that involves erythrocytes and that is discussed in this chapter is the sed rate, or ESR (erythrocyte sedimentation rate), but it really has nothing to do with erythrocyte production or function. The sed rate or ESR is a test for inflammatory reactions. A peripheral smear of blood is done to look for abnormal blood cells. This chapter mentions some of the common terms used on laboratory reports of peripheral smears. Related hematology tests (such as serum iron levels, folic acid, B$_{12}$ levels, and G-6-PD) are also mentioned because they may be needed to assess a persistent and unexplained anemic state. Although platelets are formed by the bone

TABLE 2–1. USUAL TESTS DONE AUTOMATICALLY BY MACHINE (COULTER)

Hct	Hematocrit
Hb	Hemoglobin
WBC	Leukocyte or white blood cells (differential requires separate test)
RBC	Erythrocyte or red blood cells
MCV	Mean corpuscular volume (RDW can also be calculated)
MCH	Mean corpuscular hemoglobin
MCHC	Mean corpuscular hemoglobin concentration

Platelets may also be done by some counters.
Can do all tests on 1 ml of blood. Blood is collected in a Vacutainer with EDTA as anticoagulant (lavender top). See Appendix A, Table 4 for Ortho ELT-800.

marrow, these fragments of tissue are not really blood cells in the true sense of the word. Platelets are covered with tests of clotting factors in Chapter 13.

■ RED BLOOD CELL COUNT (RBC)

The RBC is a count of the number of red blood cells per cubic millimeter (mm^3) of blood. In addition to other less understood mechanisms, a hormone named erythropoietin is secreted by the kidney and stimulates the production of red blood cells by the red bone marrow. Tissue hypoxia causes an increased secretion of erythropoietin.

Preparation of Client and Collection of Sample
There is no special preparation of the client for this test, which requires 1 ml of venous blood. EDTA is used as the anticoagulant (lavender top Vacutainer).

Reference Values for RBC

Adult:	Male	4.6–5.9 million (or 10^6)/mm^3
	Female	4.2–5.4 million/mm^3
Pregnancy		Slightly lower
Newborn		5.5–6, gradually decreases
Children		4.6–4.8, varies with age

Values increase at high altitudes.

Increased RBC (Polycythemia or Erythrocytosis)

Clinical Significance. Physiological increases of RBCs occur with a move to high altitude or after increased physical training. In both instances, the underlying reason is a response to an increased need for oxygen. At high altitude there is less oxygen in the atmosphere, so the bone marrow increases the production of red blood cells. In the event of prolonged physical training, the increased muscle mass requires more oxygen.

The RBC may be elevated also for many pathological reasons. One is a disease of unknown origin called polycythemia vera, whose name implies that it is a true (vera) increase in RBC. The increase in this case is not due to an oxygen need, as it is in all other cases of polycythemia, which are termed *secondary* polycythemia or erythrocytosis. No general agreement has been reached regarding using the term polycythemia to indicate an increase of red blood cells as well as other cells and erythrocytosis to designate an increase of RBCs alone (Bullock and Rosendahl, 1984). Two very common clinical examples of secondary polycythemia, or more specifically erythrocytosis, are clients with chronic lung diseases and children with congenital heart defects that display cyanosis. The increased RBCs are an attempt to compensate for the chronic hypoxia brought on by the disease state.

In care for a client with an elevated RBC, the nurse must differentiate primary from secondary polycythemia. In the event of primary polycythemia, medical treatment is geared to slowing the overactive bone marrow. Radioactive phosphorus has been used for over 40 years (Herring et al., 1986). If the polycythemia or erythrocytosis is secondary to a state of chronic hypoxia, therapeutic measures are geared toward correcting the cause of the hypoxia. For example, when will the child with a congenital heart defect have surgery? In the meantime, how much activity is optimal? What can the nurse do to help improve the lung functioning of a client with chronic lung disease?

POSSIBLE NURSING DIAGNOSIS RELATED TO ELEVATED RBC

Potential for Injury Related to Possible Formation of Venous Thrombi
One of the basic problems that occurs with polycythemia, regardless of the cause, is that the blood becomes more viscous and this increased viscosity makes the client more susceptible to the formation of venous thrombi. A key goal for the client with polycythemia is to maintain adequate hydration. In some cases, it may be desirable to increase fluids to a set level, such as a minimum of 2000 ml a day for an adult. Before assuming that fluids need to be increased, assess the overall status of the client, particularly the cardiovascular status. Both children with congenital heart defects and adults with chronic lung disease may often be on the verge of congestive heart failure. Confer with the physician to determine the optimal hydration state for individual clients. It is important that any client with polycythemia or erythrocytosis not become dehydrated. For example, it may be harmful for the client to be kept n.p.o. for an extended time for tests.

Encouraging Activity. The client with polycythemia needs as much activity as possible so that venous stasis does not contribute to the potential problem of venous thrombosis.

Decreased RBC

Clinical Significance. A low red blood cell count can result from:

1. An abnormal loss of erythrocytes
2. Abnormal destruction of erythrocytes
3. A lack of needed elements or hormones for erythrocyte production
4. Bone marrow suppression

The term anemia is a nonspecific term that can mean a decrease either in the total number of red blood cells, in the hemoglobin level of red blood cells, or in both the number and the hemoglobin content of red blood cells. Thus if the RBC count is low, looking at hemoglobin levels is also important to classify the type of anemia. The classification of different types of anemia is covered under the section on erythrocyte indices.

It is not necessary for an RBC count to be used routinely to check for bleeding because the hematocrit (Hct) can be done more quickly. Refer to the section on hematocrit to see the nursing implications when the low RBC is due to blood loss.

If the low RBC is caused by some condition other than blood loss, then hemoglobin levels and a peripheral smear that identifies the shape and size of erythrocytes may be necessary to identify the type of anemia. Erythropoietin assay is only available as an experimental procedure (Herring et al., 1986). Refer to the sections on hemoglobin and on erythrocyte indices for related nursing diagnoses in different types of anemias.

■ HEMATOCRIT (Hct, PCV, or Crit)

The hematocrit is a fast way to determine the percentage of red blood cells in the plasma. When the serum is centrifuged, the white blood cells and platelets rise to the top in what is called the buffy coat. Because the heavier red blood cells are packed in the bottom, the hematocrit is sometimes also called the PCV or packed cell volume. The hematocrit is reported as a percentage because it is the proportion of red blood cells to the plasma. Note that the results are based on the assumptions that the plasma volume is normal. A hematocrit is useful as a measurement of the red blood cell count *only if the hydration of the client is normal.*

Preparation of Client and Collection of Sample

There is no special preparation of the client. Because the Hct can be done on capillary blood, a client may have a finger stick (or heel stick for infants) rather than a venipuncture. (See Chapter 1 for the procedure for heel and finger sticks.) The first drop of blood is discarded, enough blood is collected to fill a capillary tube supplied by the laboratory, and a small Band-Aid can be placed over the site. The stick method should be noted on the laboratory requisition because capillary values may be 5–10% higher than values by venipuncture. Do *not* squeeze the tissue to get capillary blood because doing so adds tissue fluids, which dilute the sample.

Reference Values for Hct	
Adult: Male	45–52%
Female	37–48%
Pregnancy	Decreases, particularly in last trimester as serum volume increases
Newborn	Up to 60%
Children	Varies with age

Note that capillary blood may be 5–10% higher. Values are increased in high altitudes.

Relation to Hemoglobin Levels

If the RBC and Hb are both normal, the Hct is about three times the Hb. So a client whose Hct is 45% would be expected to have a Hb of about 15 g.

Increased Hematocrit

Clinical Significance. Because the hematocrit is a proportion (or percentage) of red blood cells to volume, any decrease in the volume of plasma causes an increase in the hematocrit, even though the red blood cells have not increased. Any kind of severe dehydration makes the Hct abnormally high. For example, in the client with a burn, plasma can be lost in large amounts through damaged capillaries in the burned area. The loss of fluid from the vascular space makes the blood very concentrated, and hence the Hct may be as high as 60 or 65%.

If the client's hydration status is normal, an elevated hematocrit signifies a true increase of red blood cells. Reasons for an increased red blood cell count (polycythemia) were discussed under the section on RBC.

POSSIBLE NURSING DIAGNOSIS RELATED TO ELEVATED Hct

Fluid Volume Deficit
When caring for a client with an increased hematocrit, it is essential to find out if this is a reflection of (1) decreased plasma volume or (2) a true increase in red blood cells. If all clinical assessments point to lack of volume, measures to increase the plasma volume are needed. Medical orders may include a plan to give fluids intravenously. For example, parenteral fluid replacement is an essential part of the treatment for a client with severe burns. In other, less severe situations, it may be sufficient to increase fluids orally to overcome dehydration.

   If the elevated hematocrit reflects an increased number of red blood cells, some additional fluids may be appropriate to decrease the blood viscosity. The precautions for overhydrating the client with polycythemia were mentioned in the previous section on increased RBC counts as was a nursing diagnosis related to the potential for the development of venous thrombi.

Decreased Hematocrit

Clinical Significance. A decreased hematocrit can be due to either (1) an overhydration of the client, which increases the plasma volume or (2) a true decrease in the number of red blood cells. The second reason for the low hematocrit is much more common. See the previous discussion on RBC for the causes of decreased RBCs.

   One of the major uses for the hematocrit is assessing the magnitude of blood loss. It is important for nurses to realize that a hematocrit drawn immediately after a massive blood loss will probably be normal because both plasma and red cells have been lost in equal proportions. Within a few hours after a bleeding episode, assuming the client has adequate fluid balance, the plasma volume returns to normal by a shift of some interstitial fluid into the plasma. The red blood cells, however, cannot be replaced so quickly. The bone marrow takes about 7 days to make new cells, and those cells need another 4 days to mature. So a few hours after the bleeding episode, the plasma volume is back to normal and the hematocrit becomes low because the red blood cells that were lost in the hemorrhage are still missing. *A hematocrit reading must always be interpreted in relationship to the time drawn and to the probable hydration status of the client at the time.*

POSSIBLE NURSING DIAGNOSES RELATED TO DECREASED Hct

Potential Fluid Volume Excess
In the rare situation where the low hematocrit reflects an increased plasma volume, the client may show some other signs and symptoms of excess fluid. Therapeutic measures may include a decrease in fluid intake. However, the hematocrit test is not a key assessment tool for volume expansion. (See the discussion on low serum sodium levels, Chapter 5, as a test for overhydration; also see Chapter 4 on osmolality.)

Potential Activity Intolerance Related to Loss of Blood

Paleness of the skin and the conjunctiva is a clue that there has been a significant blood loss. Checking for pallor of the conjunctiva is particularly helpful for assessing black clients. Because the plasma volume is usually replaced within a few hours after a bleeding episode, clients with low hematocrits have normal blood pressures. If there is not enough fluid to shift in the vascular space to make up the loss, the blood pressure falls and the client shows signs of shock. However, if the blood loss is not severe enough to create shock, the pulse may still give a clue to the magnitude of blood loss: The pulse increases when the client sits up—the "tilt" test. The pulse may become even more elevated if much exercise is attempted because the oxygen-carrying capacity of the blood is diminished. When the hematocrit is as low as 28%, the cardiac rate may be increased even at rest. Monitoring the pulse before and after activity helps to assess the effect of the low hematocrit on the individual client.

Weakness and fatigue on exertion should be taken into account when planning activities. It may be better not to do the client's bathing, bed-changing, and mobilization all at once. If a low Hct continues to drop, then a key nursing implication is to assess for signs of continued bleeding. A detailed description of nursing assessments for occult (hidden) bleeding is covered in Chapter 13 on clotting factors.

Differences Between Acute and Chronically Low Hematocrits. The effect of the low hematocrit on the client not only depends on how low the hematocrit is, but also on whether the loss is acute or chronic. If the hematocrit is low due to a sudden blood loss, the client may quickly develop signs of shock. A client with a chronically low hematocrit may have only a few symptoms because the body has had time to adjust to the low number of red blood cells. For example, clients on renal dialysis often tolerate a hematocrit as low as 18%. (The low hematocrit in renal failure is partially due to a lack of the hormone erythropoietin that is normally produced by the kidney.) A client with sickle cell anemia is another example of a client who may have a few symptoms related to a hematocrit as low as 18–20%. (In sickle cell anemia the red blood cells have an abnormal type of hemoglobin, which decreases the life of the red blood cells.) The essential point to remember about interpreting low hematocrits is to understand not just the reason for the low hematocrit, but also whether the drop is acute or chronic.

Alteration in Nutritional Requirements of Iron and Protein

The client with a low hematocrit needs adequate iron and protein in the diet so that the bone marrow can manufacture additional red blood cells. The person who has a lack of protein may produce less protein hormones such as erythropoietin. If oral intake is possible, the nurse may help the client choose foods that are high in protein and iron. Foods rich in iron are liver, egg yolk, lean beef, and prune juice (Cerrato, 1985). Iron derived from animal products, called *heme iron*, is readily available for absorption. Iron from all other sources, called *nonheme iron* is often not absorbed well due to dietary inhibitors. Studies have shown that ascorbic acid is one of the most powerful promoters of nonheme iron absorption (Lynch, 1980). A dietician can be useful to help plan optimal meals for the severely malnourished. The prevalence of anemia is highest in teenage girls, young women, infants, and elderly men (Clydesdale, 1985).

Knowledge Deficit Regarding Iron Supplements
Once a client is deficient in iron, as happens with a chronic blood loss, it may be difficult to increase iron intake by diet alone. Sometimes the client is put on iron supplements. Clients need to be aware that iron supplements cause the feces to be a dark greenish-black in color and that iron can be constipating. Iron is better absorbed in a acidic stomach but some iron combinations are better tolerated with food. The client should not take antacids and iron together because the iron is much less soluble in an alkaline medium. Other drugs, such as tetracycline and cholesterol-lowering drugs, also significantly reduce iron absorption (Rodman, 1981). The usual therapeutic plan is to continue iron supplements for about 3 months after the hematocrit is back to normal because the body takes this long to build up a reserve of iron (Wood, 1977). Clients are usually quite interested in knowing the change in hematocrit reading and their inquiry can be a good occasion to explain why iron supplements are needed.

Potential for Infection
Anemia with an accompanying iron deficiency can lessen the immunological defenses of the client. Studies have shown that iron deficiency causes a reduced bacterial killing by white blood cells (Cook, 1983). Thus measures to protect the anemic client from infection are warranted. (See Chapter 16 on infection control in high-risk clients.)

Alteration in Comfort
In addition to the fatigue and weakness discussed earlier, clients with anemia also are easily chilled. Extra blankets and warm clothing should be provided.

Potential Alteration in Breathing Patterns
Dyspnea usually does not develop unless the hematocrit is quite low. When the hematocrit is low, the amount of oxygen to the tissue is reduced, but the arterial blood gases will be normal. Only increasing the percentage of oxygen in the inspired air (FIO_2) does not solve the problem. For example, an anemic person with dyspnea would probably benefit more from a transfusion of red blood cells than from O_2 administration (Maxwell, 1985). (See Chapter 6 on oxygen therapy, which may be needed for the client for symptomatic relief.)

Potential Alteration in Thought Processes
Some investigators believe that iron deficiency in children is accompanied by an impairment of intellectual performance and behavioral changes (Cook, 1983). Decreased work performance may occur in adults. Nurses should be aware of clients who are in high-risk groups for chronic anemia and malnutrition because of the possible socioeconomic consequences of being unable to perform optimally at school or in the work place.

Potential for Injury Related to Use of Blood Transfusions
If the hematocrit is below 25–30%, a physician may order blood, usually in the form of packed cells, to replace the erythrocytes. Packed cells are used when the client needs the red blood cells but not additional plasma. No set figure means the client needs blood. As discussed earlier, some clients have chronically low hematocrits with few symptoms. Depending on the symptoms of the client and on the individual circumstances, blood may be given before clients have hematocrits as low as 25 or 30%. For example, if a client is going to surgery,

it is important that the hematocrit not be too low—"too low" usually meaning under 30%. Because blood transfusions can create additional problems, such as allergic reactions or transmission of viruses the physician may choose to let the body replenish erythrocytes normally whenever this is feasible. (See Chapter 14 for a discussion on transfusion reactions and nursing actions to prevent injury.) As a rough guideline, a unit of whole blood or packed cells raises the hematocrit about 3% in an adult.

■ HEMOGLOBIN (Hb or Hgb)

Hemoglobin is composed of a pigment (*heme*), which contains iron, and a protein part (*globin*). If each erythrocyte has the normal amount of hemoglobin, the hematocrit is roughly three times the hemoglobin level. A hematocrit of 45% would indicate around 15 g of hemoglobin. It is not necessary to do both tests to assess for bleeding. As already discussed, the hematocrit is a simpler test to monitor blood loss. If red blood cells are abnormal in size or shape, or if hemoglobin is not being produced normally, the hemoglobin level cannot be estimated from the hematocrit reading. Hemoglobin levels are necessary as part of the assessment for various types of anemia. See the erythrocyte indices for an explanation of how the hemoglobin level is used with hematocrit and RBC tests to get a clearer picture of erythrocyte abnormalities.

Preparation of Client and Collection of Sample

There is no special preparation of client. Venous blood is used for the test. EDTA (lavender top Vacutainer) is used as the anticoagulant in the collection tube.

Reference Values for Hgb	
Adult: Male	13.0–18.0 g/100 ml
Female	12–16 g/100 ml
Pregnancy	11–12 g/100 ml
Newborn[a]	17–19 g/100 ml
	average % of fetal
	hemoglobin
	1 day 77%
	3 wk 70%
	4 mo 23%
Children	14–17 g/100 ml, depending on age

Values increase in high altitudes.
[a]From Tietz, 1983

Increased Hemoglobin

Clinical Significance. Because a normal red blood cell already contains the optimum amount of hemoglobin, any increase in hemoglobin levels must be looked at in relation to the number and size of the erythrocytes. See the discussion on erythrocyte indices for an explanation of how the hemoglobin level is used with the hematocrit and RBC to determine if the erythrocyte is hypochromic (less color), normochromic, or (very rarely) hyperchromic.

Decreased Hemoglobin

Clinical Significance. Because hemoglobin is a component of the red blood cell, all the conditions that cause a low RBC naturally result in a low hemoglobin level too. Some of the common conditions for a low RBC would be blood loss, hemolytic anemias, and any type of bone marrow suppression.

Hemoglobin levels are low in persons who have abnormal types of hemoglobin or hemoglobinopathies. Red blood cells with abnormal types of hemoglobin tend to be fragile and easily destroyed in the vascular system. The normal hemoglobin in adults is almost all adult hemoglobin (HbA) with only a very small amount (0–2%) of fetal hemoglobin (HbF). A process called *hemoglobin electrophoresis* can identify the specific type of abnormal hemoglobin that is present. Over 200 hemoglobins can be identified, but only a few cause symptoms (McFarlane, 1977).

In thalassemia major, the person has an unusual amount of fetal hemoglobin and abnormalities in the synthesis of hemoglobin. The abnormal red blood cells can be identified by a peripheral blood smear. In sickle cell anemia, the person has an abnormal hemoglobin called *sickle hemoglobin* (HbS). (See Chapter 18 for screening tests for sickle cell anemia and for thalassemia, which are both genetically determined.)

It is possible to have a normal RBC count with a low hemoglobin level. For example, with an iron deficiency anemia, the count may be near normal but each cell has less hemoglobin than normal. This is called a *hypochromic* (less than normal color) anemia. The cells also tend to be *microcytic* (smaller than normal). Women in general need more iron than men due to the loss of iron in the menstrual flow, and women who have heavy menses may be prone to low hemoglobin levels. The demand for iron is increased in pregnancy. If a woman begins pregnancy with low iron reserves, she may become severely anemic as the pregnancy progresses. It is recommended that a pregnant woman be tested for hemoglobin levels at the beginning of pregnancy, about mid-pregnancy, and during the month prior to delivery. Because there is a normal drop in hemoglobin levels in the last trimester, due to the expanded plasma volume, some lowering in hemoglobin levels is "normal." This lowering is sometimes called the *physiological anemia of pregnancy.* If the mother does not have enough stored iron to meet the demands of the fetus, iron supplements may be needed (Aukamp, 1984).

POSSIBLE NURSING DIAGNOSES

Most of the nursing diagnoses for the patient with a low hemoglobin level have already been covered in the section on low Hct. Additional insights about the significance of low hemoglobin levels are covered in the section on erythrocyte indices. See the section on MCH (mean corpuscular hemoglobin) and MCHC (mean corpuscular hemoglobin concentration) for nursing implications for hypochromic and normochromic anemias.

■ ERYTHROCYTE INDICES

To make the nonspecific term anemia more meaningful, it is necessary to see whether the individual red cells are their normal size and whether they have the normal amount of hemoglobin concentration. The determinations can be made by comparing the results of the Hb, Hct, and RBC. In laboratories that use automated counters—and almost all of them do now—the indices are automatically figured as part of the CBC. Nurses never need to figure out the indices, but the formula for each is given, because they make it easy to explain the meaning of the results. In the examples used, the client has a Hct of 40%, a Hb of 13.5 g, and a RBC of 4.5 million/mm³. Note that with these figures all the indices would, of course, be normal.

Preparation of Client and Collection of Sample
There is no need to draw additional blood because the indices are derived from the Hct, Hb, and RBC.

MEAN CORPUSCULAR VOLUME (MCV)

The MCV describes the mean or average size of the individual red blood cell in cubic microns. The hematocrit is divided by the RBC to obtain the MCV. (Some counters measure the MCV to obtain the Hct.)

Reference Values and Example for MCV

Reference values	86–98 cubic microns
Formula	$MCV = \dfrac{Hct \% \times 10}{RBC \ (millions/mm^3)}$
Client example	$\dfrac{Hct \ 40\% \times 10}{RBC \ 4.5} = 89 \ microns$

Newborns and infants have higher values (Wallach, 1986).

Change in the MCV

Clinical Significance. The MCV is an indicator of the size of the red blood cells. If the MCV is lower than 86 cubic microns, the erythrocytes are *microcytic,* or smaller than normal. Red blood cells are microcytic in certain types of anemia such as iron deficiency anemia and lead poisoning. Thalassemia minor and thalassemia major (Cooley's anemia), which are genetic diseases, also cause microcytosis. (See Chapter 18 on screening tests for the thalassemias.) If the MCV is higher than 98 cubic microns, the erythrocytes are *macrocytic*, or larger than normal. Macrocytic red blood cells are characteristic of pernicious anemia and folic acid deficiencies. If the MCV is within normal reference range, the erythrocytes are *normocytic,* or of normal size. Anemia from an acute blood loss would result in a normocytic anemia. Also, sickle cell anemia may have normal size cells.

Obviously the size of the red blood cells is not enough to diagnose the reason for the anemia, but, with other indices (MCH and MCHC), the anemia can be classified by size and color. Other tests, such as the peripheral blood smear, can identify the characteristic cell shapes of various pathologies.

MEAN CORPUSCULAR HEMOGLOBIN (MCH)

The MCH is the amount of hemoglobin present in a single cell. The result is reported by weight in picograms. The weight of hemoglobin in the average cell is obtained by dividing the hemoglobin by the RBC.

Reference Values and Example for MCH

Reference values	MCH 27–32 pg (picogram)
Formula	$MCH = \dfrac{Hb\ (g/100\ ml) \times 10}{RBC\ (in\ millions/ml^3)}$
Client example	$\dfrac{13.5\ g \times 10}{4.5} = 30\ pg$

MEAN CORPUSCULAR HEMOGLOBIN CONCENTRATION (MCHC)

The MCHC is the proportion of each cell occupied by hemoglobin. Because this is a proportion, the results are reported in percentages. To get the percentage, the hemoglobin is divided by the Hct and multiplied by 100.

Reference Values and Example for MCHC

Reference values	32–36%
Formula	$MCHC = \dfrac{Hb\ (g/100\ ml)}{Hct} \times 100$
Client example	$\dfrac{13.5\ g \times 100}{40\ \%} = 33.8\%$

Changes in MCH and MCHC

Clinical Significance. These two parts of the erythrocyte indices are discussed together because both are ways to determine whether the erythrocytes are *normochromic* (normal color), *hypochromic* (less than normal color), or *hyperchromic* (more than normal color). A decreased MCHC below 32% (or a MCH below 17 pg) indicates that the erythrocytes have a decrease in hemoglobin concentration (hypochromic). Iron deficiency anemia is the most common type of hypochromic anemia. Chronic conditions that cause anemia may show some hypochromia, but they are usually not as marked as when there is a true deficiency of iron. Certain genetically caused anemias such as thalassemia (Cooley's anemia) cause hypochromia too. With many types of anemia, the remaining cells have the normal amount of hemoglobin and hence are called normochromic. Hyperchromia (an abnormally high

MCHC) is not seen except for a rare genetic condition called *hereditary spherocytosis*. As a general rule, normal red blood cells can hold only so much hemoglobin so the cells cannot be hyperchromic.

■ RED BLOOD CELL DISTRIBUTION WIDTH (RDW)

The RDW is calculated from the MCV and the red blood cell count. The variation of the width of the cell may help assess types of anemia. Reference values are usually 11.5–14.5. No subnormal values have been reported (Wallach, 1986).

POSSIBLE NURSING IMPLICATIONS RELATED TO DIFFERENT TYPES OF ANEMIA

It is important for the nurse to undertand that abnormal erythrocyte indices are useful in classifying types of anemia, but they are not enough to establish a definite medical diagnosis. The history of the client, physical assessment findings, and other tests are needed to determine the cause for the anemia. Some general nursing diagnoses for clients with anemia were discussed under the sections on RBC, Hb, and Hct. Other general nursing implications can be classified under the three categories of anemia. Table 2–2 lists the three categories and common pathology that could cause each type.

Microcytic, Hypochromic Anemias. Most likely this type of anemia is due to an iron deficiency, if other causes are ruled out (Crosby, 1979). The serum iron level can be measured, as well as the iron binding capacity, ferritin and transferrin levels discussed later. As discussed earlier in the section on Hb, it is hard to correct an iron deficiency with diet alone. (See the section on hemoglobin for what to teach a client about iron therapy.)

Normocytic, Normochromic Anemias. As discussed, the cause could range from acute blood loss to a chronic genetic problem such as sickle cell disease. With a normocytic anemia, iron supplements may not be needed, but the nurse should make sure that the client has adequate protein and iron in the diet because there is a continuing need for an increased production of red blood cells. If the anemia is of genetic origin, the nurse's role centers on helping the client and the family adjust to a chronic disease (see Chapter 18 on genetic screening). Anemia is but one sign of a larger pathological problem.

Macrocytic Anemias. This type of anemia may be hypochromic, normochromic, or very rarely hyperchromic. The two most common reasons for macrocytic anemias are vitamin B_{12} deficiency and folic acid deficiency. These two anemias are also called *megaloblastic anemias.* "Megaloblastic" refers to the appearance of a certain type of red blood cell precursor in the bone marrow and often in the bloodstream. See the following section for two possible nursing diagnoses related to vitamin B_{12} and folic acid deficiencies

TABLE 2-2. CLASSIFICATION OF ANEMIAS BY ERYTHROCYTE INDICES

Laboratory Results	Classification	Example of Common Pathology
MCV, MCH, and MCHC all normal	Normocytic, normochromic anemias	Acute blood loss
Decreased MCV, decreased MCH, and decreased MCHC	Microcytic, hypochromic anemias	Iron deficiency
Increased MCV, variable MCH and MCHC	Macrocytic anemia	Vitamin B_{12} deficiency, folate deficiency

See text for explanation and Crosby (1979), Tietz (1983), Jacobs et al. (1984), and Dallman (1984) for more details.

■ SERUM FOLIC ACID AND VITAMIN B_{12}

Both vitamin B_{12} and folate can be measured in the serum when the initial laboratory results show macrocytosis (elevated MCV), a low reticulocyte count (discussed later), and hypersegmented neutrophils. These tests are used to help in diagnosing a macrocytic anemia that may be due to dietary deficiency or malabsorption.

Preparation of Client and Collection of Sample
Check with the laboratory about food or drug interference. No special preparation of client is necessary. The test for folic acid requires 1 ml of serum. The test for vitamin B_{12} requires 12 ml of serum.

Reference Values for Folic Acid and Vitamin B_{12}

Folic acid	Greater than 3.3 ng/ml (Borderline 2.5–3.2 ng/ml) (Aged may have lower values)
Vitamin B_{12}	205–876 pg/ml (Borderline 140–204 pg/ml) (Aged may have lower values)

Note: Some laboratories may measure the folic acid in red cells rather than in serum. Red cell values should be greater than 200 ng/ml (Pollycove, 1985).

POSSIBLE NURSING DIAGNOSIS RELATED TO VITAMIN B_{12} DEFICIENCY

Knowledge Deficit Regarding Need for Vitamin B_{12} Injections
Because vitamin B_{12} is present in all animal protein a diet deficiency is rare. Pernicious anemia (a type of macrocytic anemia) refers to a pathological inability of the body to absorb vitamin B_{12} due to the lack of the intrinsic factor in the stomach. (The Schilling test is a test for B_{12} absorption, see Chapter 22.)

Nurses can help clients understand that not all types of "tired blood" can be treated with over-the-counter vitamin and iron mixtures. Clients often do not understand that anemia is only a symptom. The underlying pathological reason for the anemia must be determined to ensure its successful treatment. For example, if the macrocytic anemia turns out to be due to pernicious anemia, the client needs vitamin B_{12} shots for the rest of his or her life. So the nurse will probably be involved in helping the client and a member of the family learn to give injections. The importance of lifelong therapy must be emphasized to prevent relapses. Savage and Lindenbaum (1983) found it took about 5 years for pernicious anemia to develop when clients quit taking their vitamin B_{12} injections.

POSSIBLE NURSING DIAGNOSIS RELATED TO FOLIC ACID DEFICIENCY

Increased Nutritional Requirements for Folic Acid

As noted above, vitamin B_{12} is present in all animal protein, rarely do people in this country develop a true deficiency. However, unless vegetables are fresh, folic acid deficiency can develop because most of the folic acid is destroyed by heat.

Pregnancy and the use of oral contraceptives are situations where a macrocytic anemia may occur due to an increased need for folic acid in the diet (Aftergood & Alfin-Slater, 1980). Oral contraceptives may also cause a decrease in vitamin B_{12} (see Appendix D). Folic acid antagonists, such as methotrexate used for cancer treatment, may also deplete the client of folic acid. It may be necessary for some clients to have oral supplemental vitamin preparations that are high in folic acid. Orange juice is a good natural source of folate. Folic acid can also be given subcutaneously if malabsorption is a problem (Govoni & Hayes, 1985).

Alcohol abuse may contribute to the development of a macrocytic anemia due not only to folate and/or B_{12} deficiency, but also to other unknown factors (Crosby, 1979). In such cases, diet teaching is of little avail until other problems are addressed. It is important for the nurse to see abnormal indices in relation to the client's total picture. It is very important that the exact cause of the macrocytic anemia be identified because folic acid replacements can reverse the anemia, but folic acid cannot prevent the degeneration in the spinal cord from a persisting vitamin B_{12} deficiency due to pernicious anemia (Wood, 1977).

■ SERUM IRON (Fe) LEVELS, TOTAL IRON BINDING CAPACITY (TIBC) OR TRANSFERRIN SATURATION, AND SERUM FERRITIN LEVELS

The measurement of serum iron is used to assess the adequacy of iron in the body. A small amount of ferritin, the major iron-storage protein, is normally present in the serum. In healthy adults, serum ferritin concentrations are directly related to iron stores (Jacobs et al., 1984). Transferrin is the iron-transporting plasma protein; normally about one third of this plasma protein transports iron. The TIBC is a measurement of the transferrin available to bind more iron. Transferrin is also measured as a percent of saturation.

These tests are not *routine* for all clients who are put on iron supplements. Rather, they are reserved for further evaluation of clients with microcytic hypochromic anemia who do not respond to iron therapy. (Screening tests are the Hb, Hct, MCV, and MCH discussed earlier.) Transferrin is not as widely used to confirm iron deficiency anemia as are serum iron levels, serum ferritin, and TIBC (Dallman, 1984). Some of these tests may also be used to diagnose iron depletion in renal failure or in iron storage problems of the liver. Transferrin and ferritin, along with serum albumin (Chapter 10), are also used to evaluate severe malnutritional states.

Preparation of Client and Collection of Sample

The tests of iron and TIBC require 5 ml of serum. Special iron-free tubes and needles are required. (Vacutainers with brown tops have minimal lead content.) Check with the laboratory for specific methods for ferritin levels. Serum iron levels are higher in the evening (Wallach, 1986).

Reference Values for Iron, Ferritin, TIBC, and Transferrin

Serum iron	50–150 µg/dl (higher in men)
Serum ferritin	20–400 ng/l
	Values vary depending on techniques. Mean for men is around 120, and 55 for women
Total iron-binding capacity (TIBC)	250–410 µg/dl
Transferrin saturation	20–50%

Clinical Significance. A low serum iron, a high TIBC and/or transferrin, and a low saturation indicate iron deficiency. Jacobs et al. (1984) emphasize that iron deficiency anemia may be due to an adenocarcinoma of the gastrointestinal tract. A high or normal serum iron and a normal TIBC are evidence that the hematological problem is not due to iron deficiency. Pathological conditions such as liver necrosis, leukemia, and Hodgkin's disease all falsely elevate iron levels. Diseases, such as hemochromatosis, can cause elevated iron stores. The measurement of ferritin gives additional information about the adequacy of iron storage. Iron deficiency shows 0–12 ng/L whereas 13–20 mg/ml is borderline. A serum ferritin level above 400 ng/L is a sign of iron excess. Low ferritin and transferrin levels are seen also in severe protein depletion (see Chapter 10 on albumin levels).

■ GLUCOSE-6-PHOSPHATE-DEHYDROGENASE (G-6-PD)

Glucose-6-phosphate-dehydrogenase is one of many enzymes normally present in the erythrocytes. Some people have a lack of this enzyme due to a genetic defect. Such persons may develop hemolytic anemia if exposed to certain drugs, infections, or an acidotic state. Drugs that cause hemolysis of erythrocytes in susceptible people are the sulfas, nitrofurantoin (Furadantin), aspirin, and phenacetin. Several laboratory tests detect a deficiency of this enzyme. Because there are two common types of G-6-PD deficiencies known as African and Mediterranean variance, some drugs may cause hemolysis only in one or the other (Prchal, 1980).

Preparation of Client and Collection of Sample
There is no special preparation of the client. The test requires 9 ml of venous blood collected in a tube with a special anticoagulant (ACD). Note that various laboratories may do other types of testing that require only a few milliliters of blood with other anticoagulants. A screening test may be done before the quantitive measurement.

Reference Values for G-6-PD

All groups	5–15 U/g Hb

G-6-PD Deficiencies

Clinical Significance. The G-6-PD test may be used to determine if a hemolytic anemia is due to a lack of this specific enzyme. Other enzymes, such as pyruvate kinase, may also be deficient in the erythrocytes and cause anemia, but a lack of G-6-PD is more common. The lack of the enzyme is a sex-linked recessive trait carried on the X chromosomes. The effect is more pronounced in men. (See Chapter 18 for a discussion on genetic diseases.) Unless the person either is exposed to drugs that cause the hemolysis or has a severe infection or an acidotic state, he or she is typically unaware of the defect.

POSSIBLE NURSING DIAGNOSIS

Knowledge Deficit Regarding Drugs and Foods to Avoid
The person who has a lack of G-6-PD must not be given any of the drugs that can cause hemolysis. Clients need health teaching about exactly which drugs are to be avoided. For example, many over-the-counter drugs contain aspirin or phenacetin. Certain foods, such as fava beans, are not tolerated if the defect is the Mediterranean variant (Prchal, 1980).

■ RETICULOCYTE COUNT (RETIC COUNT)

Reticulocytes are the less mature type of red blood cells in the bloodstream. They are called reticulocytes because they show a fine network (reticulum) when stained. After about 4 days in the bloodstream, the cell loses this reticulum and becomes a mature red blood cell. The reticulocyte count is valuable because it is a measure of bone marrow function.

Preparation of Client and Collection of Sample

There is no special preparation of the client. Laboratory needs less than a ml of blood.

Reference Values for Retic Count	
Adult	0.5–2.5% of the total RBC
Pregnancy	Slight increase
Newborn	Increased first week 3–5%

Increased Reticulocyte Count

Clinical Significance.   An increase in the percentage of reticulocytes indicates that the release of red blood cells into the bloodstream is occurring more rapidly than usual. Because this is a physiological response to the need for more red blood cells, the retic count may be as high as 10% after an acute blood loss. Such an increase is also expected when the appropriate treatment is begun for a specific type of anemia. For example, when the client with iron deficiency anemia is given iron supplements, the retic count may go as high as 32%. An increase in the retic count after therapy for anemia has begun is an encouraging sign that the bone marrow is responding to the treatment. Clients with sickle cell anemia usually have reticulocyte counts of 5–10% because of the increased destruction of red blood cells (Wallach, 1986).

Decreased Reticulocyte Count

Clinical Significance. In certain macrocytic anemias (see the discussion under erythrocyte indices), cell development is arrested before the reticulocyte stage. For example, in pernicious anemia, the ineffective production of red blood cells leads to a low reticulocyte count. A decrease in reticulocytes, particularly after a bleeding episode, indicates an abnormal response of the bone marrow. The client needs further medical evaluation to determine the reason for this lack of erythrocyte production.

■ PERIPHERAL BLOOD SMEAR

The peripheral blood smear is useful for the identification of abnormalities in erythrocytes, leukocytes, and platelets. If necessary, a bone marrow may be done as a follow-up for abnormal results (see Chapter 25). A review of hematology studies by Silinsky (1984 b,c) includes technical details about red cell and white cell morphology.

Only the more common terms that may appear on laboratory reports are included here:

Descriptive terms for RBC:

1. *Anisocytosis* means that the cells vary in size.
2. *Poikilocytosis* means that the cells are irregular in shape.
3. *Rouleaux formation* is a laboratory phenomenon in which red blood cells stick to one another. (Note that this is the basis for the sedimentation rate.)
4. *Basophilic stipplings*—certain abnormalities of hemoglobin synthesis give a characteristic pattern of dark spots. This phenomenon is seen in lead poisoning and severe anemias.

5. *Howell Jolly bodies* are small remnants of nuclear material found in certain hemolytic and megoblastic anemias and after a splenectomy.

Descriptive terms for WBC:

1. *Atypical lymphocytes* (Downey cells) are characteristic of infectious mononucleosis, hepatitis, and certain other viral and allergic reactions. Also present with certain malignancies of the bone marrow.
2. *Myelocytes* and *Metamyelocytes* are two stages of immature leukocytes that are normally in the bone marrow, not in the bloodstream. Pathological conditions in bone marrow production may cause the release of various immature forms into the bloodstream.
3. *Blasts* are very primitive cells. Found in certain malignancies involving the bone marrow.
4. *Dohle bodies* are small pear-shaped inclusions in the cytoplasm; found in some anemias, malignancies, and after ingestion of toxic substances.

Descriptive term for platelets:

1. *Thrombocytopathy* means abnormal-looking platelets. (See Chapter 13 for a discussion on platelet counts.)

■ ERYTHROCYTE SEDIMENTATION RATE (ESR OR Sed RATE)

The sed rate measures the speed with which red blood cells settle in a tube of anticoagulated blood. The results are expressed as millimeters in an hour (mm/hr). An increase in plasma globulins or fibrinogen causes the cells to stick together (Rouleaux formation) and thus to fall faster than normal. If the cells are smaller than normal (microcytic), they also fall faster than normal. And if they are larger than normal (macrocytic), they fall more slowly than normal. The laboratory takes into account any change in the size of the erythrocyte and corrects for this.

Because so many different conditions can cause an increase in globulins, fibrinogen, or other substances that can cause erythrocytes to clump together, the sed rate is a very nonspecific test. (See the discussion on C-reactive protein, Chapter 14, for another test of inflammation.) Both the sed rate and the C-reactive protein indicate a pathological condition, but they do not identify the source. Sometimes

Reference Values for Sed Rate		
Westergren Method		
Adult: Male	0–13	mm/hr
Female	0–20	mm/hr
Pregnancy	44–114	mm/hr
Aged: Male over 50	0–20	mm/hr
Female over 50	0–30	mm/hr
Child	0–13	mm/hr
Wintrobe Method		
Adult: Male	0–9	mm/hr
Female	0–20	mm/hr

the sed rate is explained as "showing how hot the fire (inflammation) is, but not where it is."

Preparation of Client and Collection of Sample

There is no special preparation of the client. The test requires a minimum of 5 cc of anticoagulated blood. EDTA is used as the anticoagulant (lavender top Vacutainer).

Z-Sed Rate

The Zeta Sed rate, a mechanical technique, uses a centrifuge to cause red cells to clump quickly. The results are obtained in 5 minutes instead of an hour. The Z-Sed rate is not affected by anemia as are the Westergren and Wintrobe methods (Tietz, 1983).

Reference Values for Z-Sed Rate	
Below age 50	41–54%
Age 50–80	40–60%

Increased Sed Rate

Clinical Significance. A marked increase in the sedimentation rate during pregnancy is a normal occurrence because there is an increase in globulins and in the fibrinogen level in pregnancy. A pathological reason for an increased sedimentation rate is usually an inflammation or tissue injury. For sed rates above 100 mm (in the nonpregnant client, of course), the most likely causes are infections, malignancies, or collagen vascular diseases (Wyler, 1977). The sedimentation rate is often used to monitor the course of rheumatoid arthritis or pelvic inflammatory disease (PID).

POSSIBLE NURSING DIAGNOSIS RELATED TO ELEVATED Sed RATE

Activity Intolerance

If the sed rate is used as a screening device, the results may not be very useful in planning nursing care because an abnormal sed rate requires more testing to determine the underlying pathophysiology. If the disease process is known, then the results of the sed rate are helpful in assessing the acuteness of the inflammatory process. For example, a client with rheumatoid arthritis may exhibit an increasing sed rate, which is one clue that the client may need therapeutic interventions to control the inflammation, as well as bed rest to permit inflamed joints to rest.

A decreasing sed rate is indicative of a lessening of the inflammatory response. The change in the sed rate should alert the nurse to confer with the physician about reevaluating limitations placed on the client who has rheumatoid arthritis. As another example, clients on antibiotics for pelvic inflammatory disease (PID) may be evaluated with sed rates to determine if the pelvic inflammation is subsidiary and thus more activity is allowed.

Decreased Sed Rate

Clinical Significance. Because the range of values begins with zero, a low rate is usually not clinically significant. Clients with polycythemia vera, hypoalbuminemia, sickle cell anemia, or a deficiency in blood Factor V have decreased sedimentation rates (Silinsky, 1984a).

■ TOTAL WHITE BLOOD CELL COUNT (WBC) AND DIFFERENTIAL (Diff)

Two measurements of the white blood cells are commonly done. One is the count of the total number of white blood cells in a cubic millimeter of blood (WBC). The other is the determination of the proportion of each of the five types of white blood cells in a sample of 100 white blood cells (differential). The first measurement, the WBC, is an absolute number of so many thousand WBC per cubic millimeter (/mm³). The second measurement, the differential count (diff) is in percentages because it is a report of the proportion of each type cell in a sample of 100.

It is important to understand that the diff is reported in percentages because an increase in the percentage of one type of cell always means a decrease in the percentage of another type *even though* the absolute number for the second type of cell does not decrease. For example, a man has a normal WBC of 10,000/mm³, with a neutrophil count of 60% and a lymphocyte count of 30%. Although the laboratory report does not report the actual number of lymphocytes, one can figure out that the man has 3,000 lymphocytes per cubic millimeter (10,000 total × 30%). If this man gets a severe bacterial infection, his total WBC may rise to 20,000/mm³. In a severe bacterial infection, almost all of the increase in WBC will be due to an increase in neutrophils. The differential count now shows 75% neutrophils and only 15% lymphocytes, but this does not mean the man has fewer lymphocytes. He has 15% of 20,000 or 3,000 lymphocytes per cubic millimeter, just as before. Only the proportions have changed. Absolute numbers may change, and the proportions of each type of WBC may change, but the percentage must always add up to 100%. Neutrophils, lymphocytes, and the three types of WBC that make up the other 10% of the WBC will be discussed in a separate section.

Increase in Neutrophils and Bands (Neutrophilia)

Clinical Significance. Neutrophils, classified as polymorphonuclear leukocytes (PMNs), seem to be the body's first defense against bacterial infection and severe stress. Normally most of the circulating neutrophils are in the mature form, which the laboratory can identify by the way the nucleus of the cell is segmented. Hence some laboratories call mature neutrophils *segs* or segmented neutrophils. In contrast, the nucleus of the less mature neutrophil is not in segments, but still in a band, so the lab calls these immature neutrophils *bands.* Another name for the bands are *stabs,* a name that comes from the German for rod.

Notice that there are at least four names for mature neutrophils (segs, segmented neutrophils, polymorphonuclear leukocytes, or PMNs) and two names for immature neutrophils (bands or stabs). An increased need for neutrophils will cause an increase in both the segs (mature neutrophils) and the bands (immature or young neutrophils).

Reference Values for WBC Differential

Adult: Male and female			
Total WBC	4300–10,800/mm³		(Smokers tend to have higher rates)
Bands or stabs (young neutrophils)	3–5%		
Polymorphonu-clears or Granulocytes			
Neutrophils or segs	51–67%	or	3000–7000/mm³ as absolute
Eosinophils	1–4%		
Basophils	0–1%		
Mononuclear or nongranular leukocytes			
Lymphocytes	25–33%	or	1700–3400/mm³ as absolute
Monocytes	2–6%		
Differential adds up to 100%[a]			
Pregnancy	The leukocytosis of pregnancy (up to 16,000/mm³) is due mostly to an increase in the neutrophils with only a slight increase in lymphocytes		
Newborn	Day of birth 18,000–40,000/mm³. Drops to adult levels within 2 weeks. Reference values for differential have wide ranges depending on time after birth. Neutrophils predominate for first few days, but eventually lymphocyte predominance is seen (Crist & Dearth, 1980)		
Children	Until about age 5–8, lymphocytes are more prominant than neutrophils. WBC up to 14,500/mm³ may be in normal range depending on age. Consult specific laboratory for relative values for the differential at different ages		
Aged	Some sources suggest total WBC may decrease slightly with age (Tietz, 1983)		

[a]Note that if the laboratory uses certain automated instruments to count the WBC, some large cells may not take the stain properly. These large unstained cells (LUC) may make up to 3% of the normal specimen. If there are more than 3% unstained cells, the laboratory will perform a microscopic examination (peripheral smear) to identify the abnormal cells.

The greater the demand for neutrophils, the higher the number of immature neutrophils in the bloodstream.

When a client may possibly have appendicitis, one of the questions is, "Does the client have a shift to the left?" When laboratory reports were written out by hand, the bands or stabs were written first on the left-hand side of the page. Hence, a "shift to the left" means that the bands or stabs have increased. Table 2-3 demonstrates what a shift to the left would look like in comparison to a normal differential in *an adult*.

Although with a shift to the left, the lymphocytes appear to have decreased, as explained earlier, the diff count is only a percentage. The total number of lymphocytes

TABLE 2-3. COMPARISON OF NORMAL DIFFERENTIAL TO A "SHIFT TO THE LEFT" IN AN ADULT WITH AN ACUTE BACTERIAL INFECTION

	Stabs or Bands (%)	Neutrophils or Segs (%)	Eosinophils (%)	Basophils (%)	Lympho-cytes (%)	Monocytes (%)
Normal differential—total WBC 9,400	3	61	4	1	26	5
"Shift to the left"—total WBC 14,300	10↑	65	3	1	17	4

has not changed, but the neutrophils have increased. In bacterial infections the total WBC does increase, and an examination of the differential enables one to determine that the increase is due to an increase in both immature and mature forms of neutrophils.

The slang "shift to the right" is rarely if ever used to describe the alteration toward the other side of the neutrophil differential. A shift to the right is used to imply that there are abnormal hypersegmented neutrophils, seen in certain anemias and in liver disease. Some references may also call an increase in mature neutrophils a shift to the right (McConnell, 1986).

Besides bacterial infections, an increase in neutrophils can be due to various inflammatory processes, physical stress, or tissue necrosis such as that in myocardial infarction or in severe burns. Childbirth, as well as many drugs and toxins, increase the neutrophil count. Neutrophils are increased in granulocytic leukemia and in many other malignancies. Emotional stress can also increase the neutrophil count, but usually not as dramatically as a physical stress.

POSSIBLE NURSING DIAGNOSES RELATED TO ELEVATED NEUTROPHILS

Potential for Infection and Spread to Others

When a client has an elevated neutrophil count, one of the first things to determine is whether the client has an infection. If so, should he or she be isolated to protect others? Although infection is not the only reason for an increased neutrophil count with a "shift to the left," it should always be considered along with other factors (see Chapter 16 for culture collections). In the absence of any signs of infection, the nurse can assess whether there has been some other assault to the body that has caused the bone marrow to increase the number of neutrophils.

Knowledge Deficit Regarding Measures to Promote Recovery

The increase in neutrophils is actually a healthy response—a defense mechanism against an insult to body integrity. The nurse can help clients maximize their defense against assaults by promoting rest, adequate nutrition, and plenty of fluids. As the body successfully overcomes the assault, bacterial or otherwise, the neutrophil count will fall back to normal. This falling neutrophil count is an objective assessment that therapeutic measures have been successful.

Decreased Neutrophil Count (Neutropenia)

Clinical Significance. Although most bacterial infections cause an increase in the neutrophil count, some bacterial infections (such as typhoid, tularemia, or brucelosis) cause a decreased neutrophil count (neutropenia). (See Chapter 14 on the febrile agglutinization tests for these diseases.) Many of the viral diseases such as hepatitis, influenza, measles, mumps, and rubella also cause a decreased neutrophil count. (Most of these viruses cause a lymphocytosis.) An overwhelming infection of any type may completely exhaust the bone marrow and cause a neutropenia. Certain drugs, particularly those used to treat cancer, can cause severe bone marrow depression. Radiation therapy also carries the risk of neutropenia. Antibiotics such as nafcillin, penicillins, and cephalosporins can also induce neutropenia, as can psychotropic drugs such as lithium and the phenothiazines.

The diagnosis of neutropenia in the pediatric population is fairly common. Most neutropenia observed in children is mild and occurs during viral infections. More severe forms of neutropenia may be hereditary or due to serious pathology such as collagen vascular disease (Crist & Dearth, 1980).

POSSIBLE NURSING DIAGNOSES RELATED TO LOW NEUTROPHIL COUNT

High Risk for Infection
There are two major concerns for the client with a low neutrophil count. First, the client must be protected from sources of infection, and, if the etiology is known, the agent that caused the neutropenia must be avoided. Protective measures may need to be as strict as reverse isolation, depending on the circumstances. The problem is that because the client is often infected by organisms that are normally present in the body, preventing infection may be very hard. Most authorities do not stress isolation as much as meticulous hand washing (Pizzo, 1981).

Brandt (1984) has developed an excellent nursing protocol for the client with neutropenia (less than 500 mm³). Scrupulous personal hygiene is maintained and the environment is controlled for bacterial sources, such as from fresh flowers. In addition, a neutropenic diet is served that avoids fresh fruits and raw vegetables.

Mackey and Hopefl (1980) discusses how to use drugs to keep infections down when a client's absolute neutrophil count is very low (1000/mm³). Besides the usual hygiene measures to protect the client from infection, nonabsorbable antibiotics are given as a prophylaxis. The rationale is that this reduces the number of organisms in the client's gastrointestinal tract that are often the source of the infection in the severely neutropenic client. It is very important to recognize the beginning of the drop in neutrophils before the situation becomes critical. An infection needs to be treated immediately with antibiotics. Fever is usually the most reliable sign of an infection. (See Chapter 16 on tips for collecting cultures.)

Potential for Injury Related to Drugs Causing Neutropenia

The nurse has the responsibility of checking the latest WBC before giving drugs that may cause neutropenia. The nurse must confer with the physician and the drug must be withheld if the neutrophil count drops below a certain number. The *nadir* is the point at which the WBC drops to the lowest after chemotherapy. Because in the adult the majority of white blood cells are neutrophils, the change in neutrophils most affects the total count. But neutropenia may be present even with a normal number of other types of white blood cells.

For clients on chemotherapy for cancer, the WBC and diff may be ordered daily. Some nurses become "chemotherapy specialists" and, under the supervision of a physician, take over the functions of cancer drug preparation and administration, client education, and monitoring of side effects including the effects on the hematologic system. These nurses usually specialize in the care of oncology clients (Zehlevitt, 1980).

Increased Eosinophil Count (Eosinophilia)

Clinical Significance. The actual function of the eosinophils is not clearly understood, but they are associated with antigen–antibody reactions. The most common reasons for an increase in eosinophils (eosinophilia) are allergic reactions such as asthma, hay fever, or hypersensitivity to a drug. Parasitic infestations, such as round worms, are another reason for an eosinophil increase. Other conditions where eosinophils increase are certain skin diseases and neoplasms.

POSSIBLE NURSING DIAGNOSES RELATED TO EOSINOPHILIA

Knowledge Deficit Regarding Avoidance of Allergens

If an increased eosinophil count has been attributed to a specific allergen, the nurse may be involved in helping the client learn to avoid the allergen. Otherwise, the eosinophil count may just be useful as an indication that the client is likely to give a history of allergies; this fact should then be taken into account in planning diets and assessing for allergic reactions to new drugs.

Potential for Injury Due to Infestation

If the elevated eosinophil count is due to a possible parasitic infection, the nurse should question whether stool precautions are necessary. (See Chapter 16 for the collection of stool specimens for parasites.)

Decreased Eosinophil Count

Clinical Significance. Increased levels of adrenal steroids decrease the number of circulating eosinophils. For example, a decrease in eosinophils would be expected for an allergic client who is begun on corticosteroid therapy. Before the refinement of tests to measure corticosteroid levels directly, a drop in the eosinophil count after injection of ACTH (Thorn test) was an indirect measure of functioning adrenal glands. (See Chapter 15 for cortisol measurements.)

Changes in the Basophil Count

Clinical Significance of Increase of Basophils. The purpose of basophils in the bloodstream is not well understood. Very few conditions seem to increase this relatively rare type of white blood cell. Leukemia and other pathological alterations in bone marrow production may give rise to an increase in basophils. If a basophil count is elevated, several repeats may be done to determine whether it is a true increase.

Clinical Significance of Decrease in Basophils. Because the normal basophil count is considered to be 0–2%, a decline is not likely to be detected unless absolute counts are done. Corticosteroids, allergic reactions, and acute infections may all lower the basophil rate.

Increased Lymphocyte Count (Lymphocytosis)

Clinical Significance. Lymphocytes are the principal components of the body's immune system, but only a small proportion of them circulate in the bloodstream. The majority of the lymphocytes are T lymphocytes (55–85%) rather than B lymphocytes (5–25%). To help assess immune deficiencies, such as acquired immune deficiency syndrome (AIDS), the laboratory must do a specialized test. (See Chapter 10 for a discussion on the T and B lymphocytes.) In the differential count (diff), T and B lymphocytes are grouped together. In adults, lymphocytes are the second most common type of white blood cell, after neutrophils. In children up to at least the age of 5–8, the lymphocytes are more numerous than the neutrophils. Even in older children, the percentage of lymphocytes nearly equals or even surpasses the percentage of neutrophils.

Lymphocytes increase in many viral infections, such as mumps or infectious hepatitis; they also increase with pertussis, with infectious mononucleosis, and often with tuberculosis. (See Chapter 14 for serological tests for infectious mononucleosis.) *Chronic* bacterial infections cause an increase in lymphocytes. A common reason for a very marked lymphocytosis (80–90%) is lymphocytic leukemia. Ninety percent of all leukemias, both acute and chronic, are lymphocytic. Acute lymphocytic leukemia is much more common in children, whereas chronic lymphocytic leukemia is most common in older adults. Children also have a rather benign disease called infectious lymphocytosis where the lymph count is quite high.

POSSIBLE NURSING DIAGNOSES RELATED TO LYMPHOCYTOSIS

Potential Alteration in Health Maintenance

If the lymphocyte count is extremely high, the physician orders other tests to establish the possible existence of leukemia. The nurse needs to be aware of the specific type of leukemia diagnosed, because treatment measures and prognosis differ for different subcategories of the disease. The peripheral blood smear, maybe along with a bone marrow biopsy, is needed to clearly differentiate the type of abnormal white cells (see Chapter 24). Three potentially lethal complications in the leukemic client are (1) infection due to the lack of normal white blood cells, (2) hemorrhage due to the lack of platelets, and (3) hyper-uricemia due to the increase of uric acid from cell destruction (Pochedly, 1978). (See Chapter 4 for a discussion about high serum uric acid levels in certain malig-nancies such as leukemia. See Chapter 13 for a discussion on low platelet counts, or thrombocytopenia.)

Potential for Injury Related to Infectious Process

If the lymphocyte count is not due to a malignancy, the important question is whether the client has an infection that may be transmitted to others. Other measures, discussed under increased neutrophil counts, also apply because the nurse needs to help the person resist some type of assault that has triggered an immunoresponse. The increased lymphocyte count is needed for a defense against certain viral or chronic bacterial infections.

Decreased Lymphocyte Count (Lymphopenia)

Clinical Significance. Acquired immune deficiency syndrome (AIDS) causes a reduction in the number and type of lymphocytes. (See Chapter 10 on T and B lym-phocytes and Chapter 14 on AIDS test.) Adrenal corticosteroids and other immuno-suppressive drugs also cause some decrease. Severe malnutrition will decrease the absolute number too. Because increases in neutrophils occur for many reasons, de-creased lymphocyte counts may often be explained by changes in the neutrophils. Review the discussion in the beginning of this chapter if it is not clear why a marked increase in the percentage of neutrophils always causes a decrease in the percentage of lymphocytes, even though the absolute number of lymphocytes has not decreased.

POSSIBLE NURSING DIAGNOSIS RELATED TO LYMPHOPENIA

Potential for Infection Due to Lack of Immunological Protection

A client with a true (or absolute or actual) decrease in the number of lympho-cytes is immunodeficient. This client may need very extensive protection from sources of infection. Also, if an immunodeficient client does get an infection, there may be few signs or symptoms that this assault is occurring. So the nurse needs to use very careful assessment techniques to detect early infections in the absence of the classical signs such as fever. For example, clients on chronic steroid therapy may have lower-than-normal levels of lymphocytes, and so it should not be surprising that these clients sometimes develop tuberculosis or other infections. Clients with AIDS are likely to develop infections such as CMV (Chapter 14) or *Pneumocystis carinii* (see Chapter 27 on bronchoscopy).

Nurses can often help clients with chronic lowered resistance to find ways to enhance their health by diet, rest, and all the measures too often overlooked as "simple" health habits. Sometimes the objective sign of a laboratory test can prompt the nurse to evaluate the total health of the client. Smith (1981) recommends a complete metabolic evaluation for clients who have an absolute lymphocyte count of less than 1800/mm^3.

Increased Monocyte Count

Clinical Significance. Like the basophils and eosinophils, the monocytes are but a small percentage of the total WBC. It is thought that monocytes act as phagocytes in certain chronic inflammatory diseases. A significant increase of monocytes, for example, accompanies tuberculosis. Some protozoan infections such as malaria, as well as some rickettsial infections such as Rocky Mountain spotted fever, cause increases in the monocyte count. (See Chapter 14 on tests for rickettsial infections.) Monocytic leukemia, acute or chronic, also causes an increased count, but monocytic leukemia is far less common than the lymphocytic type. Chronic ulcerative colitis and regional enteritis both cause an increased monocyte count, as do some collagen diseases. As a general rule, the condition that causes increased monocytes is more likely to be a chronic condition, but further investigation for a specific pathology is necessary to make the monocytic count useful clinically.

■ NITROBLUE TETRAZOLIUM TEST (NBT)

The NBT is a test of how well leukocytes can reduce a dye. The reduction of the dye correlates with the ability of the leukocytes to kill microorganisms. The test is used to assess for defective leukocytes in conditions such as granulomatous disease. In chronic granulomatous disease (CGD) there is an inherited absence of neutrophil oxidase (Bullock & Rosenthal, 1984). In healthy people the amount of NBT reduction is increased when the neutrophils are fighting a bacterial infection. However, the NBT is not reliable in the definite diagnosis of bacterial infections (Tietz, 1983). Stimulated NBT reduction seems to decline with age.

Preparation of Client and Collection of Sample
Blood is collected in an anticoagulated tube of heparin. The specimen cannot be stored as the test requires live granulocytes.

Reference Values for NBT

Healthy adults 2–8% reduction of dye by granulocytes
Bacterial infections 12–70% reduction of dye

Note: Considerable variation is noted in various studies (Wallach, 1986).

QUESTIONS

1. Mrs. Landy lost a large amount of blood during surgery for a mastectomy. A hematocrit (Hct) drawn in the recovery room was 43%. It is now 12 hours after surgery, and the Hct just done is 37%. Which action by the nurse is appropriate?

   a. Take her blood pressure and call the physician immediately because Mrs. Landy is most likely bleeding again

   b. Slow down the intravenous rate until the physician can be notified because Mrs. Landy is probably overhydrated

    c. Consult the physician for further fluid orders because Mrs. Landy is probably slightly dehydrated

    d. Notify the physician of the lab report when rounds are made in a couple of hours because this drop in Hct is expected due to a fluid shift from the interstitial space

2. The test that is most frequently done to assess for loss of blood is the:

    a. RBC   **b.** Hb   **c.** Hct   **d.** CBC

3. The practice of being n.p.o. for routine tests is likely to be detrimental for an adult female patient who has a:

    a. Hemoglobin (Hb) of 9 g/100 ml

    b. Red blood cell count (RBC) of 7 million/mm^3

    c. Hematocrit (Hct) of 30%

    d. White blood cell count (WBC) of 3000/mm^3

4. As a rough guide, each unit of packed cells given to an adult raises the hematocrit about:

    a. 3%   **b.** 6%   **c.** 9%   **d.** 12%

5. Assuming that the erythrocyte indices are normal, the estimated hemoglobin level (Hb) for a client whose Hct is 30% would be around:

    a. 6 g   **b.** 8 g   **c.** 10 g   **d.** 12 g

6. Mrs. London has a Hb of 11 g due to a continuing blood loss from a heavy menstrual flow. Which of the following nursing actions is the most appropriate?

    a. Encourage additional fluids to prevent thrombus formation

    b. Explain that increased physical activity stimulates increased production of red blood cells

    c. Assess her dietary intake of protein and iron

    d. Prepare the client for the eventual need for blood transfusions to correct the anemia

7. Anemia due to a recent blood loss would most likely be:

    a. Microcytic (↓MCV), hypochromic (↓MCHC)

    b. Macrocytic (↑MCV), normochromic (normal MCHC)

    c. Normocytic (normal MCV), hypochromic (↓MCHC)

    d. Normocytic (normal MCV), normochromic (normal MCHC)

8. A reticulocyte count above 2% would be expected for all the following clients *except:*

    a. Mr. Joseph, who has an untreated macrocytic anemia due to vitamin B$_{12}$ deficiency

    b. Mrs. Lars, who has been receiving iron supplements for iron deficiency anemia

    c. Timmy Logon, who recently moved to a high altitude

d. Ms. Garfield, who had an acute blood loss last week after a miscarriage

9. Mrs. Toby has rheumatoid arthritis that flares up occasionally. Her sedimentation rate (sed rate) is higher than it has been. The visiting nurse is planning a home visit to evaluate the need for a change in care. In regard to this lab test, the nurse should consult with the physician about teaching Mrs. Toby to:

   a. Take additional fluids to prevent dehydration
   b. Decrease fluid intake to prevent circulatory overload
   c. Increase her activity to promote the full range of motion of all joints
   d. Decrease her activity to promote the rest of joints, which are actively inflamed at the present

10. If the *absolute* number of lymphocytes is increased, what is the effect on the lymphocyte and neutrophil counts in the *differential?*

   a. Lymphocytes and neutrophils remain the same in percentages
   b. Neutrophils show a percentage decrease, and lymphocytes show a percentage increase
   c. Lymphocytes show a percentage increase, and neutrophil percentage stays the same
   d. Any of the above can be produced depending on how much the lymphocytes increase

11. Mr. Jelco is receiving chemotherapy for treatment of cancer of the bowel. His last white blood count (WBC) was 3000/mm³. Based on this laboratory report, a nursing care plan must include nursing interventions to:

   a. Protect from infection   **c.** Prevent stasis of circulation
   b. Protect from stressful situations **d.** Prevent dehydration

12. Mrs. Jaboni is receiving an antibiotic that can cause neutropenia. Which of these laboratory reports would be an indication to withhold the antibiotic until the physician can be consulted?

   a. WBC of 15,000/mm³ with a normal diff
   b. WBC of 15,000/mm³ with a marked shift to the left
   c. WBC of 5000/mm³ with a normal diff
   d. WBC of 5000/mm³ with a marked increase in lymphocytes on the diff

13. Eosinophil counts are usually elevated when the client:

   a. Has had an allergic reaction   **c.** Has a viral infection
   b. Is on corticosteroid therapy   **d.** Has a bacterial infection

14. Which of the following tests is used to check for a lack of an enzyme in the RBC?

   a. NBT   **c.** G-6-PD
   b. RDW   **d.** Serum B_{12} or folic acid levels

15. Which of the following laboratory reports gives the strongest indication that the client is likely to be immunodeficient?

a. Increased neutrophils   **c.** Decreased neutrophils

b. Increased lymphocytes   **d.** Decreased lymphocytes

16. Mary Rogers is on antibiotic therapy because of pelvic inflammatory disease (PID). The nurse checks the WBC and differential to assess if Mary has a shift to the left. Characteristic of a shift to the left is a/an:

a. Increase in stabs or bands (immature neutrophils)

b. Decrease in eosinophils

c. Increase in lymphocytes

d. Decrease in monocytes

REFERENCES

Aftergood, L., & Alfin-Slater, R. (1980). Women and nutrition. *Contemporary Nutrition, 5*(3), 1–2.

Aukamp, V. (1984). *Nursing care plans for childbearing families.* Norwalk, CT: Appleton-Century-Crofts.

Brandt, B. (1984). A nursing protocol for the client with neutropenia. *Oncology Nursing Forum, 11*(2), 24–28.

Bullock, B., & Rosendahl, P. (1984). *Pathophysiology.* Boston: Little, Brown.

Cerrato, P. (1985). Hidden malnutrition in geriatric patients. *RN, 48*(7), 60–62.

Clydesdale, F. (1985). Dietary iron—Chemistry and bioavailability. *Contemporary Nutrition, 10*(4), 1–2.

Cook, J. (1983). Nutritional anemia. *Contemporary Nutrition, 8*(4), 1–2.

Crist, W., & Dearth, J. (1980). Neutropenia in childhood. *Continuing Education for the Family Physician, 13*(7), 33–36.

Crosby, W. (1979). Red cell indices. *Archives of Internal Medicine, 139*(1), 23–24.

Dallman, P. (1984). Diagnosis of anemia and iron deficiency: Cerrolytic and biological variations of laboratory tests. *American Journal Clinical Nutrition, 39,* 937–940.

Govoni, L., & Hayes, J. (1985). *Drugs and Nursing Implications.* Norwalk, CT: Appleton-Century-Crofts.

Herring, W., et al. (1986). Why is that hematocrit so high? *Patient Care, 20*(1), 46–75.

Jacobs, D., Kasten, B., DeMott, W., & Wolfson, W. (1984). *Laboratory test handbook with DRG index.* St. Louis: Mosby/Lexi Comp.

Lynch, S. (1980). Ascorbic acid and iron nutrition. *Contemporary Nutrition, 5*(9), 1–2.

McConnell, E. (1986). Leukocyte studies. *Nursing 86, 16*(3), 42–43.

McFarlane, J. (1977). Sickle cell disorders. *AJN, 77*(12), 1948–1954.

Mackey, C., & Hopefl, A. (1980). Keeping infections down when risks go up. *Nursing 80, 10*(6), 69–73.

Maxwell, M. (1985). Dyspnea in advanced cancer. *AJN, 85*(6), 673–677.

Pizzo, P. (1981). The value of protective isolation in preventing nosocomial infections in high-risk patients. *American Journal of Medicine, 70*(3), 631–636.

Pochedly, C. (1978). Acute lymphoid leukemia in children. *AJN, 78*(10), 1714–1716.

Pollycove, M. (1985). *Nuclear Medicine Manual.* San Francisco. General Hospital Medical Center.

Prchal, J. (1980). Red cell enzymes: An overview. *Continuing Education for the Family Physician, 13*(7), 41–50.

Rodman, M. (1981). The drug interactions we all overlook. *RN, 44*(4), 61–65.

Savage, D., & Lindenbaum, J. (1983). Relapses after interruption of cyanocobalamin therapy in patients with pernicious anemia. *American Journal of Medicine, 74*(5), 765–772.

Silinsky, J. (1984a). What an ESR can—and cannot—tell you. *RN, 47*(9), 91–92.

Silinsky, J. (1984b). Understanding red cell morphology. *RN, 47*(10), 99–100.

Silinsky, J. (1984c). Understanding white cell morphology. *RN, 47*(12), 82–84.

Smith, L. (1981). Implications of malnutrition in surgical patient. *Point of View, 18*(7), 6–7.

Tietz, N. (Ed.). (1983). *Clinical guide to laboratory tests.* Philadelphia: Saunders.

Wallach, J. (1986). *Interpretation of diagnostic tests.* Boston: Little, Brown.

Wood, C. (1977). Iron deficiency anemia. *Nurse Practitioner, 2*(5), 24–29.

Wood, C. (1977). Macrocytic megalobastic anemias. *Nurse Practitioner, 2*(6), 33–35.

Wyler, D. (1977). Diagnostic implications of markedly elevated erythrocyte sedimentation rate: A reevaluation. *Southern Medical Journal, 70*(12), 1428–1430.

Zehlevitt, D. (1980). Cancer chemotherapy. *RN, 43*(6), 53–56.

3

Routine Urinalysis and Other Urine Tests

- pH of the Urine
- Specific Gravity of the Urine
- Protein in the Urine (Proteinuria)
- Sugar in the Urine (Glycosuria)
- Ketones in the Urine
- Examination of Urine Sediment
- Addis Count
- Nitrites
- WBC Leukocyte Esterase
- Urinary Porphyrins
- Delta-Aminolevulinic Acid (ΔALA)
- Urinary 5-HIAA (5-Hydroxyindoleacetic Acid)
- Collection of 24-Hour Urine Specimens

OBJECTIVES

1. State three important nursing considerations in obtaining urine for routine urinalysis and for random testing.
2. Recognize findings on a routine urinalysis report that may have pathological significance.
3. Summarize important points about the various types of dipsticks and other reagents used by the nurse for urine testing.
4. Explain when periodic tests of urine pH, specific gravity, protein, sugar, and ketones may be useful in planning and modifying nursing goals.
5. Describe what should be taught to a client about any 24-hour urine collection.
6. Give examples of common tests and the types of preservatives used for 24-hour urine specimens.

TABLE 3-1. N-MULTISTIX C—REAGENT STRIPS FOR URINALYSIS

Substance Tested and Tips on Interpreting	Further Discussion in Addition to Chapter 3
pH — Colors range from orange through yellow and green to blue to cover entire range of urinary pH. Make sure not to let urine remain on test strip or the acid reagent from neighboring protein may run over and make pH acid or more acid.	Chap. 6 on respiratory and metabolic alkalosis and acidosis
Protein — Detects as little as 5–20 mg albumin/dl. May get false positive with alkaline urine. Does not test for Bence-Jones protein.	Chap. 10 on protein electrophoresis
Glucose — Enzyme method specific for glucose only. So need reduction method (Clinitest) for any other types of sugar. May be affected by ascorbic acid. Large quantities of ketone may depress color.	Chap. 8 on tests for galactosemia
Ketone — Provides results as small, moderate, and large. Reacts with acetoacetic acid and acetone but not beta-hydroxybutyric. PKU, BSP, or L-dopa can cause false positive.	Chap. 8 for serum ketone tests
Bilirubin — Sensitive to 0.2–0.4 mg bilirubin/dl. Icotest tablets are more sensitive. May be affected by chlorpromazine (Thorazine), phenazopyridine (Pyridium), ethoxazene (Serenium), or ascorbic acid.	Chap. 11 for tests of bilirubin
Occult blood — More sensitive to hemoglobin and myoglobin than intact erythrocytes. Complements the microscopic exam. Affected by ascorbic acid and some infections that produce peroxidase.	Chap. 13 for detecting occult bleeding
Nitrites — Any pink color suggests urinary infection, but a negative result does not provide sufficient proof of no bacteria as some bacteria do not produce nitrates. Affected by ascorbic acid. High specific gravity may inhibit.	Chap. 16 on urine cultures
Urobilinogen — False positive with porphobilinogen, P-amino-salicylic acid or azo dyes, such as phenazopyridine, found in Azo Gantrisin or Pyridium.	Chap. 11 for more on urobilinogen
Ascorbic acid — If ascorbic acid is as high as 25 mg/dl, the strip turns purple. Alerts that glucose, nitrite, occult blood, and bilirubin may not be accurate due to interference from ascorbic acid.	

Information compiled from Product Profiles, Ames Division, Elkhart, Indiana. Complete information on all testing products is available by contacting Ames. These tests are also available in separate dipsticks or in other combinations such as Keto-Diastixs for glucose and ketone or Uristix for nitrite, glucose, and protein. See Chapter 1 for the addresses of the major companies that make diagnostic kits.

Because a routine urinalysis is indeed routine for almost every client, the nurse needs to fully understand the meaning of each component of the urinalysis. All these tests are screening tests that may indicate the need for a more thorough assessment. Several of the tests can be done quickly with the use of chemically impregnated paper strips that can be dipped into a urine specimen. In some situations, the nurse may do this "dipstick" method as one part of the assessment of the client. It is important to make sure that the materials for testing are fresh (note the date on the container) and that the directions are followed exactly. Some strips must be read within a certain time limit, and specific directions should always be included with the testing equipment. Because color changes are the basis for the results of the dipstick test, a good light is needed and personnel need to be checked for color blindness. Some laboratories have set up special training sessions for nurses so that they can do the tests accurately. (See Chapter 1 on peripheral testing.)

Specific techniques to do each component of the dipstick (glucose, protein, pH, hemoglobin, and ketone) will be covered with each component of the test. Table 3–1 is a summary of reagent strips for urinalysis. Specific tips on the two methods of testing for glucose in the urine will also be covered in regard to the special points to note when nurses are actually doing the tests.

The second part of the chapter includes information on urine tests for nitrites, leukocyte esterase, porphyrins, occult blood, bilirubin, ascorbic acid, delta-amino-levulinic acid, and 5-HIAA. Information on reagent strips for some of these tests is included. This last part of the chapter also presents the correct procedure for collecting 24-hour urine specimens. The final table (Table 3–7) lists the usual substances tested by 24-hour specimens, whether any preservatives are needed, and where the test is covered in detail in later chapters.

COLLECTION OF URINE SPECIMENS

For a routine urinalysis, the laboratory needs at least 10 ml of urine. The perineal area in women or the end of the penis in men should be cleaned before the urine is collected. For a female client, collecting midstream urine lessens the contamination of the urine from vaginal secretions or menstrual flow; use of a vaginal tampon also helps in this respect. For infants, wiping with a sterile wipe may stimulate voiding. Also various collection bags can be attached to the genitalia. A cotton ball in a diaper can be used for quick collection of urine for dipstick testing.

If a *culture and sensitivity* are to be done in addition to the routine urinalysis, the urine has to be in a sterile container. In that case, collecting a clean catch urine sample will necessitate the use of an antiseptic solution as well as cleansing of the area. Urine for culture and sensitivity is discussed in Chapter 16.

If the client is instructed to bring in a urine specimen from home, any small clean jar with a tight-fitting nonrusty lid may be used. The first voided specimen in the morning is the ideal for a routine urinalysis because the urine is concentrated and any abnormalities will be more pronounced in the screening tests.

Urine specimens need to be examined within 2 hours. Urine that is left standing too long becomes alkaline because bacteria begin to split urea into ammonia. Visualization of microscopic casts and the test for protein are inaccurate if the urine has undergone a conversion to a high pH (that is, if it has become alkaline). Urine should be refrigerated if the specimen cannot be sent to the laboratory within 2 hours.

Reference Values for Routine Urinalysis	
pH	4.3–8 with an average of around 6 (depends on diet)
Specific gravity:	
Adult	Range of 1.001–1.040. Random sample usually around 1.015–1.025
Infant to 2 years	Range of 1.001–1.018

(Continued)

Reference Values for Routine Urinalysis *(Continued)*

Aged	May have a lowered range due to decreasing concentrating ability
Protein	Usually negative, a few healthy people may have orthostatic proteinuria
Sugar	Usually negative, may be trace in normal pregnancy. Lactosuria common in last trimester
Ketone	Should be negative
Nitrites and leukocyte esterase	Both should be negative
Microscopic sediment: Crystals	Usually have little significance, see discussion
Casts	Most are pathological, a few hyaline casts are considered normal
WBC	Should be only a few white blood cells in the urine (less than 4–5 per high power field)
RBC	Only an occasional red blood cell is expected (less than 2–3 per high power field)

COLOR OF URINE

Normally the color of the urine, from light yellow to dark amber, depends on its concentration. *Urechrome* is the name of the pigment that gives urine the characteristic yellow color. Any time urine has an unusual color, it is a good idea to save a specimen of it for the physician to see, as well as sending the urine to the laboratory. When the reason for a color abnormality is not known, the laboratory must do a chemical analysis to discover the cause. Usually the nurse or the client first notes that something is wrong with the urine color. Such changes should always be called to the attention of the physician and recorded in the nurse's notes.

A number of things can cause a change in the color of urine. If the client is known to be on a medication that causes color changes in the urine, this information should be written on the laboratory slip. It is also important that clients be told about expected color changes in the urine so they do not become unnecessarily concerned. For example, phenazopyridine (Pyridium) a drug used as a urinary tract analgesic, causes the urine to turn orange. Table 3–2 lists 26 other drugs that can color urine. Certain foods, such as beets or rhubarb, may cause color changes in the urine, as do certain dyes used in food. Purulent matter in the urine gives urine a cloudy appearance. Blood makes the urine dark and "smokey" looking. Pseudomonas infections of the bladder may give the urine a greenish color. Bilirubin turns the urine a dark orange that foams on shaking. (The other reason that urine may foam is the presence of large amounts of protein.)

ODOR OF URINE

Old urine has the very characteristic smell of ammonia because bacteria split the urea molecules into ammonia. If a freshly voided urine specimen has a foul odor, there may be a urinary tract infection; that is, bacteria are converting urea to ammonia in the bladder.

TABLE 3–2. DRUGS THAT CAN COLOR URINE

Generic Name and Brand Name of Drug	Color Produced in Urine
Acetophenetidin	Pink-red
Amitriptyline (multisource)	Blue-green (rare)
Anisindione (Miradon)	Orange in alkaline urine, pink-red-brown in acid urine
Cascara (multisource)	Red in alkaline urine, red-brown in acid urine
Chloroquine (Aralen)	Rusty yellow or brown
Chlorzoxazone (Paraflex)	Orange or purple-red (rare)
Danthron (multisource)	Pink in alkaline urine
Deferoxamine (Desferal)	Red
Ethoxazene (Serenium)	Orange-red
Furazolidone (Furoxone)	Brown
Iron preparations (multisource)	Dark brown or black on standing
Levodopa (multisource)	Dark brown on standing, red or brown in hypochlorite toilet bleach
Methocarbamol (multisource)	Brown, black, or green on standing
Metronidazole (Flagyl)	Dark brown on standing (rare)
Nitrofurantoin (multisource)	Brown, yellow
Phenacetin	Dark brown
Phenazopyridine (Pyridium also in Azo-Gantrisin)	Orange-red
Phenindione (multisource)	Orange-red in alkaline urine
Phenolphthalein (multisource)	Pink-red in alkaline urine
Phenothiazine (multisource)	Pink-red, red-brown
Phensuximide (Milontin)	Pink, red, red-brown
Phenytoin (Dilantin)	Pink, red, red-brown
Primaquine	Rusty yellow (red or dark brown a sign of inherited hemolytic anemia reaction)
Quinacrine (Atabrine)	Intense yellow, especially in acid urine
Quinine and derivatives	Brown to black
Riboflavin	Intense yellow
Rifampin (multisource)	Red-orange
Sulfasalazine (multisource)	Orange-yellow in alkaline urine
Tolonium	Blue, green
Triamterene (Dyrenium)	Pale blue fluorescence

Compiled from Slawson, (1980, p. 4) and Wallach (1986, p. 636).

A foul odor in freshly voided urine, however, may also be due to drugs or food. Asparagus gives a distinct smell to the urine. The unusual odor should be charted and called to the laboratory's attention for any needed further investigations. Note that certain metabolic abnormalities due to genetic defects can cause a peculiar odor in the urine of newborns. (See Chapter 18 on tests for genetic defects.)

■ pH OF THE URINE

A "higher pH" means "toward the alkaline side," and "lower pH" means "toward the acid side." Normally the pH of urine tends to be "lower" or acidic, largely due to diet. Meat and eggs contribute much of the acid metabolic wastes, whereas most fruits and vegetables, including citrus fruits, contribute to an alkaline urine. Thus a meatless diet would be one reason why the pH of the urine may be higher than usual.

Most of the bacteria that cause urinary tract infections, with the exception of *Escherichia coli* (*E. coli*), create alkaline urine because the bacteria split urea into ammonia and other products. The urea-splitting properties of many bacteria also explains why urine left standing at room temperature for a couple of hours usually turns alkaline from bacterial contamination.

The urine pH varies in different types of acidosis and alkalosis. Generally all forms of acidosis cause a strongly acid urine because the body is trying to compensate for the acidotic state by excreting hydrogen ions. If the acidotic problem is renal in origin, however, the kidneys may not be able to secrete those large amounts of hydrogen ions; so the urine will not be strongly acid. One might expect that in alkalosis the urine would become alkaline because the body would tend to retain hydrogen ions to compensate for the alkalotic state. Yet the pH of the urine often remains acid even with severe types of alkalosis because the kidneys are obligated to excrete hydrogen ions if potassium ions are not available. The relationship of potassium levels, acid–base balance, and urine and blood pH levels are discussed in detail in Chapter 6 on blood gases.

POSSIBLE NURSING DIAGNOSIS RELATED TO pH TESTING

Knowledge Deficit Regarding Measures to Control Urine pH

Usually changes in the pH of the urine are not very important because the pH fluctuates with food and with the metabolic state of the person. Sometimes, however, it may be necessary to see that the urine remains alkaline or acid. For example, if the client has a tendency to form uric acid or cystine stones, it may be desirable to keep the urine alkaline or at least as high as 6.5. Sometimes medications are given to achieve an alkaline urine. The nurse may need to teach the client to monitor the pH of the urine to see that it remains alkaline. This teaching is made easy by means of the dipstick method.

In other situations it may be desirable that the urine pH remain strongly acid. The two common clinical justifications for not letting the urine ever be alkaline are:

1. Alkaline urine promotes the growth of certain organisms in the urine
2. Alkaline urine promotes the formation of calcium phosphate renal stones in susceptible clients. Calcium oxalate stones are not affected by urine pH (Metheny, 1982)

For example, quadriplegic clients are very prone to the formation of renal stones due to the higher calcium content in the urine that results from their lack of mobility. Such clients are also very prone to urinary tract infections because of urinary stasis due to loss of bladder control. Increasing the acidity of the urine may help prevent both infections and calcium stones. Often such clients are given cranberry juice several times a day to increase the acidity of their urine (Kinney & Blount, 1979). Milk products may be limited, as well as citrus fruits, which leave an alkaline ash. However, vitamin C tablets help acidify the urine. Of course, the volume of urine is an important consideration, and worrying about the pH is secondary to the concern of making sure that the person receives enough fluid to keep the urine dilute.

Testing the pH of Vaginal Secretions

Note that dipsticks may also be used on vaginal secretions. The vaginal secretions are usually acidic, but the presence of amniotic fluid makes an alkaline reaction. The pH is a test to assess if the amniotic "bag of waters" has broken.

Dipsticks for the pH of Gastric Contents

The pH of the gastric contents is strongly acid, whereas the contents below the pylorus are alkaline. A dipstick test of secretions from a long gastrointestinal tube, such as a Cantor, helps assess if the tube has progressed through the pylorus. Also a pH of gastric secretions is useful in monitoring the effectiveness of medications, such as cimetidine (Tagamet), given to reduce gastric acidity. See Chapter 13 on combination pH and occult blood tests for gastric contents.

■ SPECIFIC GRAVITY OF THE URINE

The specific gravity is a measure of the density of the urine compared with the density of water, which is 1.000: the higher the number, the more concentrated the urine unless there are certain abnormal constituents in the urine. The adult has a wide range from very dilute to very concentrated. In infants, the upper limits for specific gravity are much lower than the adult limits because the immature kidneys are not able to concentrate urine as effectively as mature kidneys. Often nurses may do the specific gravity as part of an assessment of fluid balance, using either the urinometer or the refractometer.

Two Methods for Testing Specific Gravity

Urinometer. An older method to test specific gravity uses a float called a urinometer or hydrometer. The float has been calibrated to the 1.000 mark when floating in distilled water at 20 °C (68 °F).

Each degree above 20 °C will cause an increase of 0.001 of the specific gravity. Thus urine tested should be at 20 °C (68 °F), which is usually about room temperature. Refrigerated urine will have a pseudo low specific gravity when tested by the urinometer. A test tube is filled with 20 ml of urine, and the float is placed into the liquid. The higher the density of the urine, the more the float rises in the urine. The calibrated mark on the float that the urine covers is the specific gravity reading. Reading the marks exactly is sometimes difficult because the numbers are very small and close together. However, a reading of 1.011 or 1.012 would be acceptable as only wide variations are significant.

Refractometer. A newer technique, the refractometer looks like a small telescope. Only a drop of urine is needed. This drop is placed on a slide at the end of the scope, and the refractor is held up to a light. The instrument must be kept level. The density of the particles in the urine determine the direction of the beam of light through the eye of the scope. The refractor is calibrated to translate the refractive index into the standard way of reporting the specific gravity. For example, if the light beam is at the 1.026 mark, this figure is then recorded as the specific gravity of the urine.

The refractor has an added advantage of measuring the protein content in the same drop of urine. The protein measurements are on the right side of the scale. Knowledge about the presence of protein in the urine is important when doing a specific gravity because protein in the urine is one of the things that makes the specific gravity falsely high. The temperature of the urine does not change the results of the refractometer as it does the test for specific gravity with the urinometer.

Reference Values for Specific Gravity	
Adult	Range of 1.001–1.040 with random samples around 1.015–1.025
Infant to 2 years old	1.001–1.018
Aged	May have a decrease in concentrating power so that upper limits are lowered

Increase in Specific Gravity

Clinical Significance. Urine above 20 °C (68 °F) will have a falsely elevated specific gravity. The specific gravity is falsely high if glucose, protein, or a dye used for diagnostic purposes is in the urine. All these abnormal constituents increase the density of the urine. If they are not present, the high specific gravity means the kidneys are putting out very concentrated urine, for which there are two reasons: (1) either the patient is lacking in fluids or (2) there is an increased secretion of antidiuretic hormone (ADH), which causes a decrease in urine volume. Trauma, stress reactions, and many drugs, cause an increased ADH secretion (Sandifer, 1983).

Assuming the urine does not contain protein, glucose, or dyes, a high urine specific gravity most often indicates that the client needs additional fluids. It is much rarer that a high specific gravity would be due to an increased secretion of ADH (antidiuretic hormone).

Nurses should understand, however, the nature of a phenomenon called *surgical diuresis.* In a client who has been under a lot of stress, such as a major surgical procedure, the urine specific gravity is higher than normal because additional fluid is being held in reserve in the vascular system due to the presence of extra ADH and other hormones. As the stress lessens, the ADH and other hormones, such as the glucocorticosteroids, return to normal levels, and the fluid that was held in reserve is then excreted. This excretion of extra urine a few days after surgery is sometimes referred to as "surgical diuresis." It is important for nurses to understand the nature of this kind of fluid retention so that they do not overload clients with fluids because the specific gravity is a little higher than normal.

POSSIBLE NURSING DIAGNOSIS RELATED TO ELEVATED SPECIFIC GRAVITY

Fluid Volume Deficit
A specific gravity that continues to increase or that remains high when stress is not an overriding factor is a very clear indication that the client is not receiving adequate fluid intake. In acutely ill clients, this condition necessitates medical orders for increased intravenous fluids. In the nursing home setting or for clients with chronic problems, it may be up to the nurse to devise ways to get adequate oral fluids into the client. A specific gravity that drops back to normal is an objective evaluation that the client is no longer dehydrated. Specific gravity readings are more objective than just charting "concentrated" urine.

The nurse also needs to be aware of clients who could be dehydrated due to a shift of fluid into a "third space." The normal two spaces are intracellular fluid and extracellular fluid compartments. A third space is any fluid collection that is physiologically useless such as edema or ascites. "Third spacing" creates the potential for hypovolemia and decreased renal output.

Decreased Specific Gravity

Clinical Significance. Refrigerated urine will have a lower than normal specific gravity. Otherwise a low specific gravity is indicative of dilute urine. Dilute urine (a low specific gravity) is normal if the client has had a lot of fluids. Diuretics cause a large urine output with a low specific gravity too. Chapter 4 contains a discussion of tests for serum and urine osmolality. These tests are much more accurate in determining the actual dilution or concentration of the urine as compared to the dilution or concentration of the plasma. Specific gravity readings are only crude indicators of fluid imbalances in serious conditions.

Sometimes a client has a *fixed specific gravity* around 1.010. (This reading is usually pronounced as "ten-ten" because "one-point-zero-one-zero" is much harder to say.) A fixed specific gravity does not change even when the client becomes dehydrated. This continually low specific gravity indicates that the kidneys have lost the ability to concentrate urine. The fixed specific gravity is always around 1.010 because 1.010 is the density of the plasma.

Another rarer reason for a continually low specific gravity is a deficiency of ADH (antidiuretic hormone). If not enough ADH is being secreted by the posterior pituitary gland, the kidneys excrete too much water. This condition is called *diabetes insipidus.*

POSSIBLE NURSING DIAGNOSES RELATED TO LOW SPECIFIC GRAVITY

Potential for Fluid Volume Excess

Often a careful assessment of the client's total fluid intake uncovers the explanation for a low specific gravity. If the intake is larger than normal, it may be necessary to evaluate the possibility that the client is in danger of a fluid overload. For example, clients may be on intravenous fluids in addition to oral intake. Also note whether the client is on diuretics because this could explain the persistently low specific gravity. Intake and output records and daily weights help assess any fluid overload.

Potential Alterations in Urinary Elimination Patterns

A persistently low specific gravity when the fluid intake is not high is a potentially serious sign that needs medical evaluation. A low specific gravity on a routine early morning specimen indicates the need for a thorough assessment of the renal system and an evaluation of ADH secretion, if the physician deems it necessary. Persons with fixed low specific gravities (1.010) may have difficulty getting medical insurance because they are considered high-risk clients for future renal problems.

A client who is known to have a fixed specific gravity of 1.010 needs to be kept well hydrated so that the kidneys can effectively remove the waste products. Keeping this client n.p.o. for tests and the like may cause an increase in the blood urea nitrogen (BUN). A client with a fixed low specific gravity needs to be taught always to maintain an adequate intake. As kidney disease progresses, fluid restrictions and other interventions are needed. The two common tests for renal function, BUN and creatinine, and the possible nursing diagnoses of each are covered in Chapter 4.

■ PROTEIN IN THE URINE (PROTEINURIA)

Qualitative Method

Most often protein in the urine is checked by the dipstick method. This method, which uses bromophenol paper, does not detect the presence of abnormal proteins such as the globulins and the Bence-Jones protein of myelomas. For most screening purposes, however, the dipstick method is adequate (see Table 3–1 for one type of dipstick). Nurses often use it for testing for albumin in the urine of prenatal clients. If there is a need to check the urine for protein other than albumin, the laboratory uses other agents such as sulfosalicyclic acid. The dipsticks are designed to be used with acid urine so there may be a false positive for protein if the urine is highly alkaline. Time is not critical in reading the results. Note the exact color chart for each particular brand. The deepening shades of green indicate increasing amounts of protein. The following results are for the various reagent strips by Ames (1986).

Reference Values (Qualitative Method) for Protein	
Trace	As little as 5–30 mg/dl
1+	30 mg/dl
2+	100 mg/dl
3+	300 mg/dl
4+	Over 2000 mg/dl

Quantitative Method

The finding on one random sample should be negative. For persons who may have orthostatic or postural proteinuria, a second urine sample should be collected before arising from bed. If random samples are persistently positive for protein, a quantitative (24-hour) sample may be done. A 24-hour specimen should show less than 150 mg of protein. See Table 3–7 for the details about collection.

Clinical Significance. Severe stress can cause proteinuria, but this is usually a temporary occurrence. Persistent protein in the urine is a common characteristic of renal dysfunction. Almost all types of kidney disease cause mild (up to 500 mg a day) to moderate (up to 4000 mg a day) protein leakage into the urine. For children more than 25 mg per kg a day should be investigated (Bastl et al, 1986). Some people have proteinuria that is called orthostatic or postural because it occurs only when the person is in the upright position. Usually no renal abnormalities are associated with this apparently benign condition. Preeclampsia and the toxemia of pregnancy cause massive loss of protein in the urine. In what is called the nephrotic syndrome, which may be the end result of many diseases that cause kidney dysfunction, the protein loss is as much as 4000 mg a day. Albumin is the primary protein lost in all these conditions. Myelomas and certain other malignancies cause large protein losses, too, but as these proteins are abnormal it is necessary for the laboratory to use special quantitative methods to determine the presences of these proteins. (See Chapter 10 on urine protein electrophoresis.)

POSSIBLE NURSING DIAGNOSES RELATED TO PROTEINURIA

Potential Alteration in Urinary Elimination Patterns
Persistent protein in the urine is an indication for further assessment of the renal system. The nurse may be the one to explain to the client how to get another specimen that is collected before the client gets out of bed. If the proteinuria is due to renal dysfunction, other laboratory tests should be looked at to assess the degree of impairment. See the section on renal function tests in Chapter 4.

Alteration in Health Management Related to Pregnancy
For the pregnant client, a check for protein in the urine is a routine part of each prenatal visit. Nurses usually perform this test. Ideally the protein should be negative in pregnancy too. In the event that the pregnant client begins to show protein in the urine, it is important to assess carefully for hypertension and edema. Proteinuria, hypertension, and edema are the classical triad for preeclampsia (Aukamp, 1984). The appearance of this triad is an indication for immediate medical assessment and medical intervention.

■ SUGAR IN THE URINE (GLYCOSURIA)

There are two different methods of screening for glucose in the urine.

1. Dipsticks (Tes-Tape, Clinistix, and the like) change color in the presence of glucose due to the reaction of an enzyme, glucose oxidase
2. Tablets (Clinitest) use the reducing properties of cupric oxide to cause a color change in the presence of glucose *and* of other sugars

Because nurses frequently test the urine for sugar it is necessary to understand how the two methods differ.

Dipstick (Enzymatic) Method
The dipstick or enzymatic method is very easy: A tape is just dipped into the urine and read for color changes after 1 minute. With Tes-Tape (Lilly), a yellow color means the urine is glucose-free. If there is a color change on the darkest area, one should wait an additional minute to make the final comparison with the color chart. Clients often use this at home. The enzyme method is also used for multistix testing (Table 3-1).

The tapes should not be used if they are outdated. The activity of the tape or tablet can be checked by doing a mock test of a cola drink, because commercial beverages (except for diet ones!) all contain more than 2% glucose. The tapes should not be stored in a hot or humid room (such as the bathroom).

TABLE 3-3. DRUGS THAT CAN AFFECT GLUCOSE TESTING

Reduction Method

Clinitest (Ames product)
   False-positive

                                         Ascorbic acid
                                         Cephalosporins (Keflin, Ancef, etc.)
                                         Chloramphenicol (Chloromycetin)
                                         Levo-dopa
                                         Methyl-dopa (Aldomet)
                                         Nalidixic acid (Neg Gram)
                                         Probenecid (Benemid)
                                         Penicillin
                                         Salicylates (high dosages)
                                         Sulfonomides
                                         Tetracyclines
                                       Sugars other than glucose, i.e., lactose, fructose,
                                            galactose, and pentoses

Enzyme Methods

Tes-Tape (Lilly product)
Clinistix (Ames product)
   False-positive or negative   Phenazopyridine (Pyridium, Azo-Gantrisin)
   False-negative   Ascorbic acid
                                         Levo-dopa (only Clinistix)
                                         Methyldopa
                                         Salicylates (high dosages) (only Clinistix)
                                       Cancer metabolites

Information compiled from Lundin (1978); Ames Products (1986). See Chapter 1 for the addresses of Ames, Lilly, and other companies that manufacture urine glucose strips.

As the enzyme method is specific for glucose *only,* this method should be used if the client is on any of the drugs that may make a false positive with the reducing method (Clinitest tablets). Such drugs are salicylates, penicillin, cephalosporins, ascorbic acid, and probenecid. Table 3–3 is a summary of drug effects using both methods.

Tablets (Reducing) Method

Sometimes it is necessary to check for the presence of sugars other than glucose. The reducing method detects the presence of fructose, galactose, lactose, or the pentoses. For example, in screening the urine of an infant for potential abnormal sugars in the urine it would be essential to use Clinitest tablets (Ames Products) and not Tes-Tape or other enzyme tests. (See Chapter 8 on galactosemia and lactose intolerances.)

In what is called the *five-drop method,* five drops of urine and ten drops of water are added to a test tube. When the Clinitest tablet is added, a boiling action occurs. This chemical reaction makes the bottom of the test tube hot. After the boiling stops, wait 15 seconds and then gently shake the tube. Then compare the sample with a chart. Urine that is free of sugar remains blue. There may be a whitish sediment in the urine, but this is not significant. Increasing amounts of glucose turn the urine from green to brown to orange.

As the boiling reaction is taking place, it is important to watch because the color may go very quickly to a dark brown color, which signifies more than 2% sugar. If so, this change is called a *pass-through reaction,* and it should be recorded as over 2%. Otherwise the dark color that occurs *after* the initial reading at 15 seconds should be ignored. Only the color change at 15 seconds is compared to the chart.

The *two-drop method* uses the same tablet and amount of water but only two drops of urine. The two drop method, by making the urine more dilute, avoids the "pass through" effect. Use the specific color chart for each method (Ames Products).

TABLE 3-4. THE MEANING OF THE PULSES FOR URINE GLUCOSE TESTING

	No Sugar	1/10%	1/4%	1/2%	3/4%	1%	2%
Tes-Tape (enzyme method)	neg	+	+ +	+ + +			+ + + +
Lab Stick (enzyme method)	neg	trace	+	+ +		+ + +	+ + + +
Clinitest (reducing method)	neg	neg	trace	+	+ +	+ + +	+ + + +

Note: 1/10% = 100 mg/dl; 1/4% = 250 mg/dl; 1/2% = 500 mg/dl; 1% = 1000 mg/dl.

Reporting Test Results

Unfortunately, the same readings on two different scales do not necessarily mean the same thing. For instance, a "1 +" by one method does not mean the same as a "1 +" by another method. Even enzyme methods from two different companies may use different scales (Lundin, 1978). So it is much better to report the amount of sugar as a percentage. To illustrate the differences in the scales, three methods are compared in Table 3-4. This table shows that a urine sugar of 2 + could mean 1/4%, 1/2%, or 3/4% sugar depending on which commercial preparation is used. Obviously reporting the results in a percentage decreases the confusion when more than one method is used in a given situation. Note that for 2% sugar in the urine all methods report this as "4 +." The American Diabetic Association has recommended that all manufacturers change the color charts to percentage readings so clients (and health care workers!) are not confused by the various meanings of sugar reported in so many pluses.

Increased Glucose in the Urine (Glycosuria)

Clinical Significance. Glucose in the urine signifies either (1) hyperglycemia (see Chapter 8 for a detailed discussion of the causes of hyperglycemia) or (2) a decreased renal threshold for glucose.

The *renal threshold* for glucose is usually around 160–190 mg/100 ml of blood; in other words, no sugar is spilled into the urine until the blood sugar rises above this level. Various situations, including diabetes, may cause a blood glucose level higher than 160 mg, as well as alter the renal threshold for glucose. For example, in pregnancy the renal threshold for glucose may be lowered so that small amounts of glycosuria may be present and are usually not considered abnormal. Lactosuria is common in the third trimester. Clients on hyperalimentation have glycosuria if the intravenous solution (which has very concentrated sugar) is going faster than the pancreas can produce insulin. Hereditary defects, such as galactose intolerance, cause a positive Clinitest, because a positive result with the reducing method is capable of also indicating the presence of sugars other than glucose. But such defects do not effect a positive result with Tes-Tape or other enzyme dipsticks.

POSSIBLE NURSING DIAGNOSES RELATED TO GLYCOSURIA

Knowledge Deficit Regarding Urine Testing Techniques

Diabetic clients need instructions on how to monitor glucose levels. Fingersticks for blood glucose are more accurate (see Chapter 8) but sometimes urine tests are easier. The nurse should allow clients to do the testing several times in the hospital so that they completely understand the technique. It is also a good idea to allow diabetic clients to continue testing their urine when they are admitted to the hospital if conditions permit. This is not only an opportunity to assess the level of the client's understanding, but also a way to promote a level of independence. Nurses in clinics or those who make home visits should also watch clients perform the urine testing and help the diabetic use urine testing to manage self-care (Guthrie, 1980). Gray (1985) notes that elderly clients may have visual problems, lack of manual dexterity, and some short-term memory loss, so they need careful assessment of their capabilities.

A double-voided specimen for periodically testing of sugar in urine is desirable. The client empties the bladder and then voids again as soon as possible. With this procedure one is sure that the urine reflects the current status, which is a particularly important condition if insulin is ordered, as is sometimes done, to cover any glycosuria. From a practical point of view, getting two specimens from a client may not be possible; so it is always wise to test the first voiding too. Clients on hyperalimentation at home may also need instruction on urine testing for glucose.

Potential for Fluid Volume Deficit

A high concentration of sugar in the blood acts as an osmotic diuretic; so water is excreted as the sugar spills into the urine. The presence of glycosuria, from any cause, alerts the nurse to the fact that the client needs additional fluid intake and could undergo severe dehydration if the glycosuria is allowed to continue. (See Chapter 8 for a discussion on hyperglycemic hyperosmolar nonketotic coma [HHNK].) If the glycosuria is due to hyperalimentation therapy, the physician may eliminate the spilling of glucose in two different ways: (1) either slow down the rate of the concentrated sugar solution or (2) order insulin to help the body utilize the large load of glucose.

In the diabetic client a continued spilling of sugar leads not only to severe dehydration, but also to ketonuria and eventually to ketoacidosis as the ketone bodies build up in the serum. The nurse needs to be aware that the presence of a positive acetone with a positive sugar indicates a need for immediate medical intervention. See the discussion on ketoacidosis in Chapter 6.

■ KETONES IN THE URINE

Ketones are metabolic end-products of fatty acid metabolism. When the body does not have sufficient glucose to use for energy, the excretion of ketones increases. The three ketone bodies in the urine are acetone, acetoacetic acid, and beta-hydroxybutyric acid. Test strips and tablets check only for acetone and acetoacetic acid, but this is sufficient as a change in the small amount of acetone signifies the same degree of change in the other ketones. Acetoacetate and acetone can also be measured in the serum (see Chapter 8).

The usual procedure is to test for both sugar and acetone in the urine when there is any question about glucose metabolism. As in the tests for sugar, acetone can be tested either by a dipstick or by a tablet. (Refer to the section on glycosuria, on obtaining a double-voided urine specimen.) Both methods show a deepening purple color when acetone is present. The scale indicates small, moderate, or large amounts of acetone. Symptomatic ketosis occurs at levels of about 50 mg/dl or when the client has moderate acetone in urine testing. Urine containing phenylketones (PKU, Chapter 18), or L-dopa metabolites may give false-positive results.

Reference Values for Ketones

Normally urine should not contain enough ketones to give a positive reading.

Small	20 mg/dl
Moderate	30–40 mg/dl
Large	80 mg/dl or above

Clinical Significance. The presence of ketones in the urine signifies that the body is using fat as the major source of energy. Fats are used when glucose is unavailable to the cells. The unavailability of glucose may be because glucose is not being transported to the cells, as in diabetes, or because glucose is lacking in the body due to starvation, vomiting, fasting, or an all-protein diet.

POSSIBLE NURSING DIAGNOSES RELATED TO KETONES IN URINE

Potential for Injury Related to Development of Diabetic Acidosis
If the client is a known diabetic, ketonuria (a positive acetone by testing) indicates that the insulin and glucose balance is not satisfactory. There is an abundance of glucose in the bloodstream, as evidenced by the 2% sugar in the urine, but it is unavailable to the cells. The diabetic client with a positive acetone has switched to using fats as the primary source of energy because the lack of insulin prohibits the transport of glucose to the cells. As the ketones accumulate they use up the bicarbonate buffer (see Chapter 6) and ketoacidosis can develop. The client needs more insulin so that glucose can reach the cells and be used as the primary source of energy. See Chapter 8 for more information about ketoacidosis and the other treatments needed.

Alteration in Nutritional Needs, Less than Body Requirements of Carbohydrates
If the acetone is positive due to a starvation state, the positive ketone is associated with a *negative* glucose in the urine. If the client is not diabetic, a search must be made for other reasons why the cells do not have glucose. Questions to be asked would be:

1. Has the client had a reduced amount of food?
2. Has there been a lot of vomiting?
3. Is the client trying to lose weight by being on an all-protein diet?

Depending on the circumstances, the client needs glucose in some form so that fats and/or proteins do not continue to be the primary source of energy. The person also needs extra fluids so that the ketones can be excreted by the kidneys. Clients on tube feedings that are very high in protein may show ketones in the urine unless they also receive adequate glucose in the feeding, along with plenty of water to rid the bloodstream of the ketones.

A client who goes on an all-protein diet in an attempt to lose weight should be under careful supervision. The client should check the urine for the amount of ketones that build up. Sufficient fluids must be taken to prevent ketone toxicity. All-protein diets are controversial due to the possible danger to the physiological balance of the body.

■ EXAMINATION OF URINE SEDIMENT

As part of a urinalysis, the urine sediment is centrifuged and examined microscopically for crystals, casts, RBC (red blood cells), WBC (white blood cells), and bacteria or yeast. Table 3–5 contains a brief summary of the meaning of each of these findings. Some laboratories only do a microscopic examination on special request unless the routine urinalysis is positive for protein, blood, nitrites, or WBC esterase. If occult blood is suspected the microscopic analysis is better for detection than the dipsticks. If urine is collected with a syringe and needle from the port of a Foley catheter, the needle should be removed before the urine is squirted into the specimen cup. Pushing the urine through the needle may damage cells and casts. Red cell casts dissolve within 20 minutes (Bastl et al., 1986).

■ ADDIS COUNT

The Addis count is a quantitative measurement of the red blood cells, leukocytes, and casts in a 12-hour overnight urine specimen. Protein and specific gravity may also be done. Fluids may be restricted before the test so urine will be concentrated.

TABLE 3–5. A SUMMARY OF URINE SEDIMENT FINDINGS

WBC	Normally there should not be more than a few white blood cells in the urine (4–5 per high power field). Infections or inflammations anywhere along the urinary tract cause an increase of white blood cells in the urine. Urinary tract infections occur in 1–2% of all pregnancies (Connell, 1979).
RBC	Normally there should be only an occasional red blood cell in the urine (2–3 per high power field). An increased number of red blood cells in the urine indicate bleeding somewhere in the urinary system, which may be due to renal disease, trauma, or a bleeding disorder. In women it is important to make sure that the urine was not contaminated by the menstrual flow. Insertion of a tampon and a collection of midstream urine are ways to prevent this contamination.
Crystals	Most crystals have little clinical significance. If the client is on drugs that may cause crystallization in the urine, such as some of the sulfa drugs, this finding may be clinically important.
Casts	A few hyaline casts are considered normal, but all other casts need to be evaluated by the physician. Unlike crystals, casts are suggestive of actual kidney disease. Casts are a compacted collection of protein, cells, and debris that are formed in the tubules of the kidneys. Those that form in the distal tubule have a narrow caliber. Those that form in the collecting tubules tend to be very broad. Broad granular casts are sometimes called *renal failure casts* because they indicate major renal destruction. The width and composition of the cast has great significance in the diagnosis and prognosis of renal diseases (Schuman et al., 1978).
Bacteria or yeast	Often the presence of a few bacteria or yeasts is indicative only of contamination from the perineal area, but a culture and sensitivity may need to be done if a large amount of bacteria is noted on routine screening. Chapter 16 discusses the nursing implications for obtaining a urine specimen for a culture and sensitivity or for a smear. See the test for nitrates and leukocyte esterase discussed in this chapter.

Some laboratories may do a 24-hour specimen with a restriction of 200 ml of fluid for each meal. (See the later discussion on 24-hour urine collection techniques.) The Addis test may be used to evaluate the course of renal disease by comparing results over a period of time.

Reference Values for 12-Hour Urine Specimen for Addis Count

Red blood cells	Not more than 500,000
White blood cells	Not more than one million
Hyaline casts	Not more than 50,000

INDIVIDUAL URINE TESTS

Random urine specimens may be needed for various other tests besides a routine urinalysis; Table 3–6 shows some tests that are done on a single specimen. Two of these, nitrites and leukocyte esterase, may be part of a routine urinalysis. A multitude of tests can be done on one dipstick. Table 3–1 gives some tips about factors that can affect the N-Multistix C (Ames Products), which tests nine substances. Note that these dipsticks are also available in different combinations for specific testing of one or more urine constituents. Information about nitrites, porphyrins, delta-aminolevulinic acid, and 5-HIAA is included next as these tests are not covered in other chapters.

■ NITRITES

Most species of bacteria, such as Enterobacteriaceae, if present in the urine, cause the conversion of nitrates, which are derived from dietary metabolites, to nitrites. Thus a dipstick for nitrites is a check for urinary infections.

Preparation of Client and Collection of Sample
Optimal results are obtained by using a first morning urine sample that has been "incubating" in the bladder for 4 or more hours. The urine should be done by a clean

---

Reference Values for Nitrites

Nitrate reagent	Turns pink if bacteria are present. The pink color is *not* quantitative in relation to the number of bacteria present. Ascorbic acid or a high specific gravity may invalidate the results. Blood or other pigments in the urine can interfere with the color changes.
Cultures	Usually growth of 100,000 per ml is considered evidence of a bacterial infection (see Chapter 16 on culture reports).

Note: A negative nitrite test or negative culture does not provide proof that the urine is free of all bacteria, particularly if there are clinical symptoms to the contrary. Some bacteria, such as streptococci and gonococci, do not produce nitrites. Note that the nitrite test is often combined with the leukocyte esterase test discussed next.

TABLE 3-6. EXAMPLES OF TESTS ON URINE (other than routine urinalysis or 24-hour urine specimens)

Test	Reference Value	Specimen	Information About Test
Bence-Jones protein	Negative	First morning specimen	Chap. 10
Human chorionic gonadotropin (hCG)	Negative (unless pregnant)	First morning specimen	Chap. 18
Tests for occult blood	Negative	Random	Chap. 13 on tests to detect bleeding. Note microscopic exam is more sensitive test
Hematest—Ames			
Hemastix—Ames			
Hemoccult—Smith, Kline, French			
Porphobilinogen	Negative	Freshly voided specimen	This chapter
Bilirubin	Negative	Random	Chap. 11
Urobilinogen	Up to 1.0 Ehrlich units/2 hr	2-hr specimen (1–3 P.M.)	Chap. 11
Nitrites	No pink color	Clean catch or midstream specimen	This chapter and Chap. 16
Leukocyte esterase	Negative	Random, clean catch	This chapter

Reference values from Sculley, 1986. Also see Appendix A, Table 1. Wallach (1986) lists many drugs which may interfere with tests.

72

catch midstream technique (see Chapter 16 on clean catch urine specimens), and it should be tested within an hour of voiding. As an alternative to the clean catch method, the client may wet the strip by holding it in the urinary stream.

A specialized dipstick for nitrites, Microstix-3 (Ames Products) can also be used for a culture. Immediately after the strip is read, it is put into a transparent bag. The dipstick has two miniaturized culture areas that support both gram-positive and gram-negative bacteria. If the dipstick is to be cultured, it must not be touched. The dipstick in the bag is put into an incubator for a minimum of 18 hours. Results are ready within 18–24 hours. Various other companies make diagnostic culture kits (see Chapter 16).

■ WBC LEUKOCYTE ESTERASE

The leukocyte esterase (LE) test for urine identifies enzymes found in granulocytes, histiocytes, and *Trichomonas*. The test detects 5–15 WBC per high power field and thus has an advantage over the microscopic examination because the LE test detects both lysed and intact cells. The combination of LE with the nitrite test (discussed above) provides a sensitive screen for predicting urinary tract infections.

Preparation of Client and Collection of Sample
Dipsticks, such as Leukostix (Ames Products, 1986), are used the same way as other reagent strips for urinalysis. Concentrated urine is most satisfactory for testing. The dipstick for Leukostix is read at 2 minutes by comparing with a color chart and noting trace to + + +. Color changes that occur after 2 minutes have no diagnostic value. Ascorbic acid and some antibiotics may interfere with the test.

Reference Values for WBC LE

A result matching any color block designated by a + sign indicates the presence of increasing amounts of leukocytes in urine. A "trace" reading should be retested with a fresh urine specimen. Positive results for leukocytes esterase may be followed up with a urine culture (see Chapter 16).

■ URINARY PORPHYRINS

Porphobilinogen, coproporphyrins, and uroporphyrins are intermediaries in the synthesis of heme, which is part of hemoglobin and of several enzymes. Delta-aminolevulinic acid ($\triangle$ALA) is an important enzyme for the formation of porphobilinogen. Abnormalities of porphyrin metabolism may be either genetic or due to drug intoxication, usually lead (Free & Free, 1979). Several tests can be done to demonstrate an abnormality in the metabolism of heme. Because the porphyrins are precursors of the pigment (heme), the urine may be burgundy color or pink when exposed to black light.

Special Preparation of Client and Collection of Sample
Coproporphyria and uroporphyrin require a 24-hour urine specimen. Use 5 g of sodium carbonate as the preservative. Porphobilinogen is done on a random urine

specimen, consisting of 10 ml of freshly voided urine. (See instructions at the end of this chapter on collecting 24-hour specimens.) Specimens should be protected from light.

Reference Values for Porphyrins

Coproporphyrin	50–250 µg/d
Uroporphyrin	0
Porphobilinogen	0

Abnormal Porphyrins

Clinical Significance. Elevations of these tests are indications of one of the porphyrias, which are several different diseases that may be acute or chronic. O'Conner (1981) describes in detail the many nursing needs of a client with acute intermittent porphyria. The disease may be very hard to diagnose because it mimics so many other conditions. At the present time treatment is symptomatic. Acute intermittent porphyria, the most common, can be precipitated by barbiturates. Coproporphyrins may document toxicity to lead (see Chapter 17).

■ DELTA-AMINOLEVULINIC ACID (△ALA)

Delta-aminolevulinic acid is an enzyme that is needed for the proper conversion to porphobilinogen in the metabolic formation of heme. △ALA is not present in the urine of healthy persons, but it is present in lead intoxication. △ALA may also be elevated in certain kinds of genetic deficiencies of porphyrin metabolism (the porphyrias). This test is the number one choice for lead exposure and poisoning (Jacobs et al., 1984).

Preparation of Client and Collection of Sample
Collect a 24-hour urine sample. See instructions at the end of this chapter. Specimen should be protected from light. Various methods require different preservatives.

Reference Values for △ALA

1–7 mg/d

Clinical Significance. See Chapter 17 for the use of this test in relation to lead poisoning. O'Conner (1981) discusses the nursing needs for clients with acute intermittent porphyria.

■ URINARY 5-HIAA (5-HYDROXYINDOLEACETIC ACID)

Glands in the gastrointestinal tract secrete the hormone serotonin. Carried in the platelets, serotonin is a vasoconstrictor that is especially important to small arterioles after tissue injury. It is also a regulator of smooth muscle contraction, such as in peristalsis.

The chief metabolite of serotonin, excreted in the urine, is 5-hydroxyindoleacetic acid (5-HIAA). Certain tumors, called carcinoid tumors, of the argentaffin cells in the gastrointestinal tract may begin to secrete abnormal amounts of serotonin. Hence a measurement of the amount of 5-HIAA in the urine is a help in diagnosing carcinoid tumors (Jacobs et al., 1984).

Preparation of Client and Collection of Sample

The client must not eat foods such as bananas, tomatoes, plums, avocados, eggplants, or pineapples as all these foods contain a significant amount of serotonin. Because many drugs may also affect the test results, the client should not take any medication during the test. The nurse must check with the laboratory about specific drug interactions. Except for the foods mentioned, a normal diet can be taken during the test. The urine is collected in a special container with 10 ml of HCl or boric acid. Follow the procedure for a collection of 24-hour specimen (discussed at the end of this chapter).

Reference Values for 5-HIAA	
24-hour screening test	Negative
Quantitative test	2–9 mg/d— women lower than men

Clinical Significance. An elevated level of 5-HIAA in the urine is evidence of increased serotonin, which may be due to carcinoid tumors. These tumors may be either benign or malignant. Note that tumors in other organs may sometimes produce serotonin. (See Chapter 15 on ectopic hormone production by tumors.) The symptoms of serotonin excess may include cyanotic episodes, flushing of the skin, diarrhea, abdominal cramps, and bronchial constriction. The nurse should note and record any type of symptoms that occur during the time the client is being worked up for a possible carcinoid tumor. The major clinical manifestations of the syndrome are due to biologically active agents released by the tumor. In addition to the release of serotonin, bradykinin, histamine, and ACTH, other substances are also released (Taub, 1980). Treatment involves the surgical removal of the tumor.

■ COLLECTION OF 24-HOUR URINE SPECIMENS

These collections are useful only if *all* the urine is collected for 24 hours. Even if "just one specimen" is discarded, the test is not valid. The nurse must make sure that the client fully understands the importance of saving all the urine. Because of the problem with incomplete urine collections, laboratories sometimes check the creatinine present in the urine to validate that the urine is representative of a full 24 hours. Assuming the client does not have renal problems, a creatinine value below the normal range of age and body weight suggests an incomplete collection (Tietz, 1983).

To begin the 24-hour urine collection, the client voids and *discards* the urine so that the urine from the previous night is not included. Then all the urine for the next 24 hours is saved and put into a large collection bottle. If a client voids and discards the urine at, say, 8:20 A.M., the test ends at 8:20 A.M. the next day. The client should do a final voiding as close to 8:20 A.M. as possible so that the last urine

TABLE 3-7. 24-HOUR URINE SPECIMENS

Substance Tested	Reference Values d = 24-Hour Day	Preservative Needed	Information About Test
Aldosterone	5–19 µg = d	Refrigerate	Chap. 15
Amylase	24–76 U/ml	None	Chap. 12—may do for only 2 hours
Calcium	300 mg/d or less	Need 10 ml of HCl	See Sulkowitch test (Chap. 7) for random tests of urine calcium
Catecholamines Epinephrine Norepinephrine	Under 20 µg/d Under 100 µg/d	Need 10 ml of HCl (pH kept 2–3)	Chap. 15
Coproporphyrin	50–250 µg/d Children under 80 lb: 0–75 µg/d	5 g of Na carbonate	See this chapter
Creatinine	15–25 mg/kg of body weight	None	Chap. 4
Creatinine clearance	Male 95–135 ml/min Female 85–125 ml/min	None	Need serum creatinine too (Chap. 4)
Delta-aminolevulinic acid	1–7 mg/d	None	See this chapter and Chap. 17
5-HIAA	2–9 mg/d (women lower than men)	10 ml of HCl	See this chapter
Lead	120 µg or less/d	None	Make sure lead-free container Chap. 17

Substance	Reference Value	Preservative	Reference
Pregnanetriol	Male 1–2 mg/d Female 0.5–2 mg/d Children less than 0.5 mg/dl	Refrigerate	Chap. 15
Phosphorus	1 g/d—varies with intake	10 ml of HCl	Chap. 7
Potassium	25–125 mEq/d	None	Chap. 5
Pregnanediol	Male less than 1 mg/d Female 1–8 mg/d	Refrigerate	Chap. 15
Protein	Less than 150 mg/d	None	See quantitative and qualitative tests in this chapter
Sodium	40–220 mEq/d	None	Chap. 5
17-Ketosteroids	Varies with age and sex	None	Chap. 15
17-Hydroxysteroids	3–8 mg/d (women lower than men)	None	Chap. 15
Urea Nitrogen	6–17 g/d	None	Chap. 4
Uroporphyrin	0–30 µg/d	5 g of Na carbonate	See this chapter
VMA (vanillylmandelic acid)	Up to 9 mg/d	12 ml of HCl	Chap. 15

Reference values from Sculley (1986) and Modern Chemistry (1982). Note that most laboratories prefer all 24-hour urine specimens iced. Check with the laboratory for the specific technique used. Also see Appendix A, Table 2 for urine values in SI units.

in the bladder can be included. The urine specimen should be sent to the laboratory as soon as possible. Some laboratories may want only 25 ml of the total, but this quantity must be verified with the laboratory. The times for beginning and ending the urine collection should be noted on the requisition.

The laboratory will supply the collection bottle, along with any preservative needed (see Table 3–7 for common 24-hour urine specimens and the preparations needed). The laboratory should also notify the nurse or the client if certain drugs or foods invalidate the test. (See the discussions in the various chapters of specific points for each test.) If a preservative is not used, a few specimens, such as those for hormones, must be refrigerated. Usually refrigeration is preferred for most urine tests but the nurse should validate this requirement with the laboratory. The rationale for refrigeration is to inhibit bacterial growth, which may interfere with some tests.

For toddlers, when a diaper is used at night, a 12-hour specimen may have to suffice. For infants, urine may be collected in disposable paste on collection bags. Rarely, it may be necessary to insert a Foley catheter to get a 24-hour urine collection from a child. The danger of a urinary tract infection is a drawback.

QUESTIONS

1. A specimen of urine for a routine urinalysis should be:

   a. At least 60 ml
   b. Put into a sterile container
   c. An early morning specimen, if possible
   d. Sent to the laboratory as a stat procedure

2. Which of the following tends to make the urine pH higher?

   a. Meat   c. Cranberry juice
   b. Eggs   d. Citrus juices

3. Marie Cotton may have a urinary tract infection (UTI). Which of these urinalysis findings are abnormal and thus should be reported to the physician? (Mary is not vegetarian and was not n.p.o. before the urine was collected.)

   a. pH 5.5, few hyaline casts
   b. s.g. 1.010, 2–3 RBC
   c. 20–25 WBC, pH 7.5
   d. Crystals, s.g. 1.025

4. In interpreting the meaning of specific gravity of a urinalysis for a child under two it is important for the nurse to realize that in a child this young, the maximum specific gravity is:

   a. Much lower than for an adult
   b. Higher than for an adult
   c. Essentially the same as the adult range
   d. Fixed at 1.010

5. Which of the following clients demonstrates the concept of a "fixed" specific gravity (s.g.)?

   a. Mrs. Jung, who has an s.g. around 1.025 on three early morning urine specimens
   b. Mr. Louis, who has an s.g. of 1.010 on a random urine specimen
   c. Mr. Tagelino, whose s.g. remains around 1.008 while he is on diuretics
   d. Mrs. Foley whose s.g. was 1.010 during a prolonged period of fluid restriction

6. A client is asked to obtain a urine specimen before arising to rule out orthostatic or postural:

   a. Glycosuria   c. Proteinuria
   b. Ketonuria   d. Hematuria

7. The nurse in a prenatal clinic has just tested Mrs. Ames' urine and found it to be ½% for glucose and 3+ for protein by the dipstick method. There will be a 30- to 40-minute delay before the client sees the doctor. She says she is "feeling okay" so she wishes to have her appointment rescheduled. Which action by the nurse would be the most appropriate?

   a. Reschedule her appointment for another day as glucose and protein in the urine are not uncommon in the third trimester of pregnancy
   b. Say nothing about the urine test but insist that she wait to see the physician because the clinic schedule is always full
   c. Do a nursing history on the client and tell her the glucose in her urine needs investigation by the physician as she may be diabetic
   d. Take her blood pressure, check her ankles, and explain why it is necessary to make these assessments to help the physician evaluate the seriousness of the proteinuria. Insist that she wait to see the physician

8. The reducing method (Clinitest) of testing for sugar in the urine

   a. Uses the same "plus" scale as other methods of glucose urine testing
   b. Tests for glucose and *other* sugars
   c. Is not affected by drugs such as the cephalosporins (Keflin)
   d. Is easier to perform than the enzyme method (Tes-Tape)

9. Marilyn is a 19-year-old college freshman who is quite obese. She has come to the campus health clinic because she feels very tired. A routine CBC and urinalysis were normal except for a trace of acetone. (Urine sugar was negative.) Based on these laboratory findings, which question by the nurse will most likely help to discover the reason for the abnormal ketones?

   a. Have you been eating a lot of fats lately?
   b. Have you been under a lot of stress?
   c. Is there a history of diabetes in your family?
   d. Have you been on a strict reducing diet lately?

10. Mrs. Zorba is in the last trimester of her pregnancy. A dipstick test for nitrites

and leukocyte esterase in the urine were positive. Her specific gravity was normal. These positive reactions are evidence of:

a. Preeclampsia

b. Normal dietary metabolites of protein

c. Possible urinary tract infection

d. Possible lack of ascorbic acid in her diet

11. Mr. Leggins is to collect a 24-hour specimen for urine coproporphyrins for possible lead toxicity. He has been given a container with the necessary preservative. Which of the following instructions by the nurse is correct?

a. Begin the test exactly at 8 A.M. and collect all urine until 8 A.M. the next day

b. Discard the first urine specimen tomorrow morning and then collect all the urine for the next 24 hours

c. Discarding only one specimen will not create a problem if he can estimate the amount lost

d. Force fluids so the urine will be dilute

REFERENCES

Ames. (1986). *Product profiles on reagent strips for urinalysis.* Elkhart, IN: Ames Division, Miles Laboratories.

Aukamp, V. (1984). *Nursing care plans for the childbearing family.* Norwalk, CT: Appleton-Century-Crofts.

Bastl, C., et al. (1986). Diagnosing kidney disease early. *Patient Care, 20*(4), 28–52.

Connell, E. (1979). *Changes in the urinary tract during pregnancy* (Patient Information Booklet). Chicago: American College of Obstetricians and Gynecologists.

Free, A., & Free, H. (1979). *Urodynamics: Concepts relating to routine urine chemistry.* Elkhart, IN: Ames Division, Miles Laboratories.

Gray, D. (1985). Elderly diabetics and urine testing. *Geniatric Nursing, 6*(6), 332–334.

Guthrie, D. (1980). Helping the diabetic manage his self-care. *Nursing 80, 10*(2), 57–65.

Jacobs, D., Kasten, B., DeMott, W., & Wolfson, W. (1984). *Laboratory test handbook with DRG index.* St. Louis: Mosby/Lexi Comp.

Kinney, A., & Blount, M. (1979). Effect of cranberry juice on urinary pH. *Nursing Research, 28*(5), 287–290.

Lundin, D. (1978). Reporting urine test results: Switch from + to %. *AJN, 78*(5), 876–879.

Metheny, N. (1982). Renal stones and urinary calculi. *AJN, 82*(9), 1372–1375.

Modern Urine Chemistry. (1982). *Application of urine chemistry and microscope examination in health and disease* Elkhart, IN: Ames Division, Miles Laboratories.

O'Connor, L. (1981). Acute intermittent porphyria. *AJN, 81*(6), 1184–1186.

Sandifer, M. (1983). Hyponatremia due to psychotropic drugs. *Journal of Clinical Psychiatry, 44*, 301–303.

Schuman, B., et al. (1978). An improved technique for examining urinary casts and a review of their significance. *American Journal of Clinical Pathology, 69*(1), 18–23.

Scully, R. (Ed.). (1986). Normal reference values. *NEJM, 314*,(1), 41–42.

Slawson, M. (1980). Thirty-three drugs that discolor urine and/or stools. *RN, 43*(1), 40–41.

Taub, S. (1980). Identifying malignant carcinoid syndrome. *Hospital Medicine, 16*(7), 53–54.

Tietz, N. (Ed.). (1983). *Clinical guide to laboratory tests.* Philadelphia: W.B. Saunders.

Wallach, J. (1986). *Interpretation of diagnostic tests.* Boston: Little, Brown.

4

Renal Function Tests

- Blood Urea Nitrogen (BUN)
- BUN to Creatinine Ratio
- Urinary Urea Nitrogen and Nitrogen Balance
- Creatinine Levels in Serum
- Creatinine Clearance Test
- Serum and Urine Osmolality
- Uric Acid (Serum and Urine)

OBJECTIVES

1. Compare and contrast the factors that affect the BUN and serum creatinine levels.
2. Explain the rationale for checking BUN and/or serum creatinine levels before administration of certain antibiotics.
3. Describe the nursing diagnoses that are appropriate when a client has markedly elevated BUN and serum creatinine levels.
4. Given the values for urinary urea nitrogen and the client's intake of protein, calculate the nitrogen balance to determine if dietary adjustments are warranted.
5. Compare the usefulness of urine osmolality to the measurement of urine specific gravity.
6. Given various changes in serum and urine osmolality, plan appropriate nursing interventions.
7. Prepare a teaching plan that helps a client with high serum uric acid levels to decrease the possibility of renal stones.
8. Describe the role of the nurse in preparing clients for creatinine clearance tests.

Some of the tests discussed in this chapter are used only for renal assessment, whereas others have several purposes. For example, serum creatinine levels, urine creatinine levels, and the creatinine clearance tests are all used only to evaluate renal function, and only renal dysfunction changes the result. On the other hand, the blood urea nitrogen (BUN), also used primarily to assess renal function, can be affected by other factors and is used to assess fluid volume deficit. The urinary urea nitrogen is used to assess nitrogen balance. Tests for serum and urine osmolality are newer tests that are useful not only in assessing renal function, but also for assessing fluid requirements and fluid imbalances. The discussions on urine osmolality should be read after one has read about specific gravity measurements in the previous chapter. One test covered in this chapter, uric acid, is not really a test for renal dysfunction, but uric acid is likely to be elevated in severe renal dysfunction. Therefore, the discussion on uric acid fits into a general discussion about renal dysfunction, even though it is not used as an assessment tool for the severity of the dysfunction.

■ BLOOD UREA NITROGEN (BUN)

The blood urea nitrogen test measures the amount of urea nitrogen in the blood. Urea, a waste product of protein metabolism, is formed by the liver and carried via the blood to the kidneys for excretion. Because urea is cleared from the bloodstream by the kidneys, the BUN can be used as a test of renal function. However, protein breakdown, dehydration, overhydration, and liver failure all invalidate the BUN as a test for renal dysfunction.

Preparation of Client and Collection of Sample
There is no special preparation of the client. The laboratory needs 1 ml of blood or serum for the test. Certain drugs, such as streptomycin, chloramphenicol, or mercurial diuretics, may interfere with test results.

Reference Values for BUN

Adult	8–25 mg/100 ml
	Men may be slightly higher than women
Pregnancy	Values may decrease about 25%
Newborn	Values tend to be slightly lower than adult ranges
Aged	Values may be slightly increased due to lack of renal concentration

---

Increased BUN

Clinical Significance. Diseased or damaged kidneys cause an elevated BUN because the kidneys are no longer able to rid the blood of the waste product, urea. Even if the kidneys are not diseased or damaged, conditions where renal perfusion is decreased result in an increase of urea in the blood. Thus either a client in shock or one in congestive heart failure may have higher-than-normal BUN levels due to poor circulation to the kidneys. A client who is severely dehydrated may also have an elevated BUN due to the lack of volume for normal urine output. Because urea is an end-product of protein metabolism, a diet that is very high in protein, such as tube feedings, may cause some increase in the BUN level. Bleeding into the gastrointestinal tract will also cause an elevated BUN because digested blood is a source of protein. For example, loss of 1000 ml of blood into the gastrointestinal tract may elevate the BUN to 40 mg/dl.

■ BUN TO CREATININE RATIO

Because creatinine is changed only by renal dysfunction, a comparison of the BUN with the serum creatinine is useful. A client with a BUN of 15 mg might have a serum creatinine level around 1.0 mg. If the client becomes dehydrated or has increased protein (such as with gastrointestinal bleeding), the BUN increases whereas the creatinine does not; so the ratio of 15:1 would be increased in dehydration or in protein breakdown. One the other hand, the ratio of BUN to creatinine would be less than 15:1 in low-protein intake, overhydration, or severe liver failure, which reduces the BUN but not the creatinine level. BUN to creatinine ratios may range from 1:6 to 1:20 (Tietz, 1983). Jacobs et al. (1984) and Wallach (1986) consider 1:10 to be the mean and note that variability in protein intake and mass of voluntary muscle can cause the ratio to be misleading.

Use of BUN and Creatinine to Monitor Nephrotoxic Drugs

BUN and creatinine levels are also used to monitor clients who are receiving drugs known to be potentially nephrotoxic such as antibiotics classified as aminoglycosides. Some of the aminoglycosides are gentamicin (Garamycin), kanamycin (Kantrex), tobramycin, and a newer antibiotic netilmicin (Netromycin). Before administering a drug that is known to be potentially nephrotoxic, nurses should look at the client's BUN and/or creatinine levels. If either level is higher than the reference range, they should withhold the drug until consulting the physician. Because aminoglycosides tend also to be toxic to the eighth cranial nerve, assessments of auditory and vestibular functions are ways to monitor for neurotoxicity. The impaired hearing or dizziness that may occur is more likely if the drug is continued when there is renal dysfunction. Many hospitals now do measurements of the levels of drugs in the serum so that a therapeutic level can be maintained. (See Chapter 17 for a discussion about the measurement of serum levels of aminoglycosides such as gentamicin.) It is important to keep the client well hydrated when aminoglycosides are used because they are excreted almost unchanged in the urine (Langslet & Habel, 1981).

POSSIBLE NURSING DIAGNOSES RELATED TO ELEVATED BUN

Potential Fluid Volume Deficit

Because an increased BUN may be due to anything that causes poor renal perfusion or renal dysfunction, it is important to look at the BUN in relation to the pathophysical process for the individual client. If the BUN is due to poor renal perfusion, the focus is on increasing renal flow. For example, if the client has dehydration, this must be corrected. However, if the elevated BUN reflects actual renal damage, then fluids may have to be restricted. The nurse must monitor the necessary fluid requirements and keep accurate I&O records. Table 4-1 compares BUN and creatinine in various stages of renal disease. Note that the BUN to creatinine ratio discussed above may help identify dehydration rather

TABLE 4-1. POSSIBLE CONTINUUM OF CHRONIC RENAL DISEASE

Reduced or diminished renal reserve	BUN may be slightly high or high-normal, but no problems unless stress (infections, surgery, emotional crisis, etc.) challenges limited reserve. Creatinine levels within normal range
Renal insufficiency	BUN mildly elevated. May not tolerate high-protein intake. Impaired urine concentration (see serum osmolality). Mild anemia. Stress easily impairs renal function. Creatinine level beginning to rise (see Table 4-2)
Renal failure	Both creatinine and BUN are elevated. Levels vary with severity *and* other factors. Other abnormal tests may be hypernatremia, hyperkalemia (Chapter 5), anemia (Chapter 2), hypocalcemia, hyperphosphatemia (Chapter 7)
End-stage renal disease	Serum creatinine above 10 mg/dl. BUN rise somewhat proportionately. Other tests mentioned are increasingly abnormal

See text, Stark (1980), and Oestreich (1979) for more details.

than renal disease. Also see the discussion on serum and urine osmolality for other assessments of a fluid volume deficit.

If the elevated BUN can be traced to a great increase in protein in the diet, a reduction of protein and/or an increase of fluid intake will help the kidneys get rid of the excess urea. For example, increased fluids will be needed with high protein supplements.

Potential Alterations in Nutritional Requirements of the Problem Nutrients: Potassium, Sodium, and Protein

Because urea is not the only substance that is increasing in the bloodstream as renal dysfunction persists, the nurse must be alert to which medications and foods may be contraindicated. Sodium and potassium are excreted by the kidneys. Sodium may need to be restricted and supplemental potassium is contraindicated in the client who has progressive renal dysfunction. See Chapter 5 on hyperkalemia and hypernatremia. Usually protein in the diet is not restricted for mild renal insufficiency, but one would question a high-protein diet, which would tend to increase the BUN even more. The protein level may need to be adjusted to maintain lean body mass and still not cause a high BUN (Luke, 1979). Clients can self-test their BUN by using Azostix (Ames Products). (See Chapter 7 for the discussion on supplemental calcium and the restriction of phosphorus in renal disease.)

The child and adolescent in renal failure present additional nutritional problems due to the needs of their growing bodies. Few infants are placed on fluid restrictions. Yet as with adults, sodium, potassium, and protein are the problem nutrients (Hetrick, 1979). Infants may be undergoing a life-threatening hyperkalemia (high potassium level), even though the BUN is not over 35 (Jones et al., 1979).

Impairment of Skin Integrity

Azotemia means an increase of nitrogenous waste products in the serum. *Uremia* is the broader name given to the toxic condition in which the kidneys are not able to excrete urea and other substances such as potassium, creatinine, and organic acids. In the days before the advent of peritoneal and renal dialysis, clients with high levels of BUN would develop a condition called *uremic frost,* which consisted of urea crystals that were being excreted through the sweat glands. Fortunately urea levels can be lowered now with dialysis before clients develop toxic uremia. Still itching is often a problem and the potential for skin breakdown is always present.

Potential for Injury Related to Weakness and Possible Confusion

Clients with a mild gradual increase in the BUN level may not have many symptoms. The level of BUN that causes symptoms in clients varies tremendously (Oestreich, 1979). As BUN levels continue to rise, the client is likely to experience fatigue, muscle weakness, and some nausea and vomiting. There may be a decline in mental awareness, drowsiness, or confusion. Nurses need to assess the mental and physical capabilities of any client with increased BUN to ensure safe care. Clients who may be slightly confused or unsteady on their feet need careful watching. Also hypertension and arrhythmias may limit activity, so blood pressure and pulse must be closely monitored. See Chapter 2 for other nursing concerns on the low hematocrit that develops with chronic renal disease.

Alterations in Health Maintenance Related to Need for Readjustment of Medications

Clients with elevated BUN and creatinine levels may need modifications in their drug regime. For example, diabetic clients need less insulin as their renal function decreases. Other common drugs that have a prolonged effect in clients with compromised renal function include digoxin, phenothiazines, meperidine, and several of the antibiotics (Orr, 1981). The nurse must be aware of possible overdose and the necessity to explain its possibility to clients so ongoing monitoring is done. The creatinine clearance test, discussed later in this chapter, is an objective evaluation of the actual extent of the renal damage and will help the physician reevaluate the needed dosage changes of maintenance drugs.

Alteration in Bowel Elimination Due to Constipation

Clients with chronic renal disease often have problems with constipation because of restricted fluid intake and lack of exercise. Increasing roughage in the diet may be limited because many of the high fiber foods are high in potassium and phosphorus. Usually, these clients do need stool softeners on a regular basis and the sodium and calcium in these products are not sufficient to warrant concern (Chambers, 1983). (See Chapter 7 for a discussion on high phosphorus and magnesium levels and the danger of some laxatives for clients with renal failure.)

Potential for Disturbance in Self-esteem and Self-concept

As renal function becomes compromised many pathological changes occur (Table 4–1). These changes and the need for major alterations in life-style can be devastating to the individual and significant others. Depression, anxiety, and a feeling of powerlessness may develop as clients consider possible options such as home or hospital hemodialysis, peritoneal dialysis, or an eventual renal transplant. Stark & Hunt (1983) suggest that the nurse find the coping methods previously used by the clients for major life changes and help them use the successful methods for the present crisis. A psychiatric nurse or a social worker may also be used for support.

Decreased BUN

Clinical Significance. Just as dehydration may cause an elevated BUN, overhydration causes a decreased BUN. An increase in antidiuretic hormone is a pathological reason for dilute plasma. Plasma volume increases, such as in pregnancy, reduce the BUN level. A marked decrease in protein breakdown also tends to lower the BUN. Usually a BUN that is slightly lower than the reference values has little clinical significance (Burke et al., 1978). Because urea is synthesized by the liver, severe liver failure causes a reduction of urea in the serum. Yet, the inability of the liver to form urea results in an increase of other nitrogenous products, such as ammonia, so that tests for ammonia levels are much more clinically significant in liver dysfunction than are lowered BUN levels (see Chapter 10 on ammonia levels).

POSSIBLE NURSING DIAGNOSIS RELATED TO DECREASED BUN

Potential Fluid Volume Excess
Because a decreased BUN raises the possibility of expanded plasma fluid volume, some attention should be given to the overall hydration status of the client. Yet the test by itself is not that helpful in identifying plasma dilution. (See the section on serum osmolality in this chapter and Chapter 5 on the serum sodium as tests for plasma dilution.)

■ URINARY UREA NITROGEN AND NITROGEN BALANCE

The urinary urea nitrogen can be measured and compared with the amount of protein ingested to determine the nitrogen balance of the client. There is about 1 g of nitrogen in each 6 g of protein and the loss of nitrogen is about 4 g from stool and insensible loss. Based on these facts a formula has been devised. The formula is:

$$\text{N balance} = \frac{\text{Protein intake (g)}}{6.25} - \left(\begin{array}{l} \text{24-hour urinary} + 4 \\ \text{urea nitrogen} \end{array} \right)$$

A value below 0 indicates a negative nitrogen balance as shown in this example:

$$\text{N balance} = 50/6.25 - (6 + 4) = -2$$

A negative nitrogen balance is an indication that the client needs a greater protein intake (see Chapter 10).

Preparation of Client and Collection of Sample
See Chapter 3 on method for collecting 24-hour urine specimens. No preservation is needed. The dietician usually does the assessment of the protein intake. The nurse must accurately record all food intake.

Reference Values for Urinary Urea

6–17 g of urinary urea nitrogen in 24 hr

Reference Values for Nitrogen Balance	
0 or greater	(See earlier discussion for formula)

■ CREATININE LEVELS IN SERUM

Creatinine is the waste product of creatine phosphate, a high-energy compound found in skeletal muscle tissue. The measurement of serum *creatinine* is useful in evaluating any type of renal dysfunction where a large number of nephrons have been destroyed.

Preparation of Client and Collection of Sample

The laboratory needs 1 ml of venous blood. High doses of ascorbic acid or barbiturates may distort the results. Ketone bodies and cephalosporin antibiotics may elevate the results.

Reference Values for Serum Creatinine	
Adult: Male	0.6–1.5 mg/100 ml
Female	0.6–1.1 mg/100 ml
	Values tend to be slightly higher for men because of their larger muscle mass
Pregnancy	Values are reduced in pregnancy, presumably because creatinine clearance is markedly increased
Newborn	Lower than children
Children	Slight increases with age because values are proportional to body mass
	After puberty, men slightly higher

Increased Creatinine Level

Clinical Significance. The only pathological condition that causes a significant increase in the serum creatinine level is damage to a large number of nephrons (Table 4–2). Unlike the BUN, the serum creatinine level is not affected by protein meta-

TABLE 4–2. RELATIONSHIP OF CREATININE LEVELS TO ESTIMATED AMOUNT OF NEPHRON LOSS

Creatinine Level	Estimated Loss of Nephron Function
Normal creatinine (0.6–1.5 mg/dl)	Up to 50% loss
Creatinine level above 1.5 mg/dl	Over 50% nephron function loss
Creatinine level of 4.8 mg/dl	As much as 75% nephron function loss
Creatinine level of about 10 mg/dl	90% loss of nephron function—end-stage kidney disease

Modified from Stark, 1980, p. 36.

bolism, and less by the hydration state of the client. Certain muscular diseases may cause a slight change in the creatinine, but if muscular disease is suspected, then the creatine kinase is the test used for assessment (see Chapter 12 on enzymes).

As discussed in the section on BUN, a change in the BUN to creatinine ratio may be useful in pinpointing the primary factor that needs correction. Because the creatinine is not increased until at least half of the nephrons are nonfunctioning, it is not elevated in reduced or diminished renal reserve as is the BUN. Thus clients with an increased creatinine are most likely to have potentially severe renal impairment. Like the BUN, serum creatinine is used to detect potential renal damage when nephrotoxic drugs, such as the aminoglyoside antibiotics, are used. Serum creatinine levels are also routinely done for all dialysis clients and for clients who have had renal transplants. Because creatinine levels rise and fall more slowly than BUN levels, creatinine levels are often preferred for long-term assessment of renal function.

**POSSIBLE NURSING DIAGNOSES RELATED
TO ELEVATED CREATININE**
See section on BUN.

Decreased Creatinine Level

Clinical Significance. A decreased serum creatinine level may indicate atrophy of muscle tissue. However, if skeletal muscle problems are suspected, the serum creatine is used. Note also that the creatine kinase (CK) is an important enzyme test for muscular disease. (See Chapter 12 on CPK or CK.)

■ CREATININE CLEARANCE TEST

The creatinine clearance test is used as an indication of the glomerular filtration rate (GFR). The test compares the serum creatinine level with the amount of creatinine excreted in a volume of urine for a specified time period. The time period may be for 2, 12, or 24 hours. A 24-hour collection is most common. At the beginning of the test, the client empties his or her bladder, and this urine is discarded. Thereafter, all the urine voided during the specified time period is collected. (See Chapter 3 on 24-hour urine collections. No preservative is needed.)

Sometime during the test period, a blood sample is drawn to determine the serum creatinine. The rate of creatinine clearance is thus determined by the following formula:

$$\frac{\text{Urine creatinine} \times \text{Urine volume}}{\text{Creatinine in serum}} = \text{Creatinine clearance rate}$$

expressed as so many millimeters per minute per 1.72 m^2 of body surface

Although nurses are never responsible for calculating the creatinine clearance rate, they should have more insight into the laboratory's report if they have a basic understanding of how the reference values are obtained. Age, weight, and height are used to calculate body surface area.

Reference Values for Creatinine Clearance

Adult:	Male	95–135 ml/min
		Varies with the amount of lean body mass; so muscular men are usually in the upper limits of the range
	Female	85–125 ml/min
Pregnancy		May be as high as 150–200 ml/min
Aged		Values diminish with age even if no renal disease exists. Glomerular filtration rate declines about 10% per decade after 50 (Jacobs et al., 1984)

Decreased Creatinine Clearance

Clinical Significance. A decreased creatinine clearance rate is an indication of decreased glomerular function. In preeclampsia, the creatinine clearance drops as it does with renal impairment. The creatinine clearance rate is a more sensitive indication of renal dysfunction than the serum creatinine alone because the serum creatinine may remain normal until the creatinine clearance is less than half than normal. Creatinine clearance is also used to evaluate the progression of renal disease. A minimum creatinine clearance of around 10 ml/minute is necessary to maintain life without the use of renal or peritoneal dialysis.

The results of the creatinine clearance test, together with other assessments of renal dysfunction, help to determine the long-term plans for the client. Clients may have repeated creatinine clearance tests because the changes in the results may be more significant when compared over a period of time.

■ SERUM AND URINE OSMOLALITY

The osmolality of serum, urine, or any other fluid depends on the number of active ions or molecules in a solution. The osmolality of a solution reflects the total *number* of osmotically active particles in the solution, without regard to the size or weight of the particles. In laboratory reports osmolality is expressed as so many milliosmoles per kilogram of water (mOsm/kg water).

Although nurses do not need to know how to calculate milliosmoles, they may find it helpful to conceptually understand the meaning of a milliosmole (mOsm). A milliosmole is 1/1000 of an osmole. *Osmoles* are a standard of measurement based on the freezing point of a solution: As the number of osmotically active particles in a solution increases, the freezing point decreases. For example, a lower temperature is needed to freeze a salt solution than to freeze plain water. As a standard of measurement, one osmole is the amount of a particular solute that lowers the freezing point of 1 kilogram of water by 1.86 °C. With a standard measurement of osmoles and of milliosmoles for clinical studies, the precise concentration of active solutes in the serum and urine can be calculated. Although sodium is the major constituent of serum osmolality, urea nitrogen is one of the major factors in urine osmolality. An estimation of serum osmolality can be obtained from the laboratory values of sodium, potassium, BUN, and blood glucose as shown in Table 4–3.

TABLE 4–3. ESTIMATION OF SERUM OSMOLALITY FROM LABORATORY VALUES FORMULA

2(Na + K) + BUN/2.8 + Blood glucose/18

Example of normal reference values

2(135 + 3.5) + 12/2.8 + 110/18

277 + 4.29 + 6.11 = 287 mOsm[a]

[a]*Osmole gap.* The osmolality calculated from laboratory values is usually about 9 mOsm less than the measured one (Jacobs et al., 1984). Unmeasured substances such as methanol or ethanol will make the gap greater than 9 therefore serum osmolality may be used to screen for alcohol ingestion (see Chapter 17 for direct measurements of blood alcohol levels). The serum osmolality increases 22 mOsm/kg for each 100 mg/dl of ethanol (Wallach, 1986).
Note: Increases in sodium and glucose can markedly increase the osmolality. See Chapter 5 on hypernatremia (hyperosmolar dehydration) and Chapter 8 on hyperosmolar, hyperglycemic, nonketotic (HHNK) dehydration.

Urine osmolality, like specific gravity, is a measurement of the concentration of the urine. (See Chapter 3 on the specific gravity of urine.) Urine osmolality reflects the total number of osmotically active particles in the urine, without regard to the *size* or *weight* of the particles. As a result, high sugar concentrations, proteins, or dyes do not raise the urine osmolality as they do the specific gravity of the urine (Smithline & Gardner, 1976). The urine osmolality test has at least three other advantages over the specific gravity:

1. The temperature variable is controlled with the osmolality determination, so that the results are more accurate.
2. Also, because the osmolality test is a more sensitive measurement, a small change in the amount of solutes is evident with the osmolality test, but not with the specific gravity.
3. The urine osmolality can be compared with the serum osmolality to get a more definitive picture of the fluid balance or imbalance.

The disadvantage of the osmolality test is that it cannot be done immediately by the nurse as can the specific gravity.

Preparation of Client and Collection of Sample
There is no special preparation of the client for the test. Depending on the type of machine used, the laboratory can perform an osmolality on as little as 2–5 ml of serum or urine.

Reference Values for Serum and Urine Osmolality	
Serum osmolality	Range 280–297 mOsm/kg water. Usually around 285 (290 mOsm = 1.010 specific gravity)
Urine osmolality	Extreme range of 50–1400 mOsm/kg water but average is around 500–800 mOsm (800 mOsm = 1.022 specific gravity). Newborns have low urine osmolality
	After an overnight fast (14 hours), the urine osmolality should be at least three times the serum osmolality (Basil et al., 1986)

TABLE 4-4. CLINICAL IMPLICATIONS OF CHANGES IN OSMOLALITY

Serum Osmolality (282–295 mOsm)	Urine Osmolality (500–800 mOsm)	Clinical Significance
Normal or increased	Increased	Fluid volume deficit
Decreased	Decreased	Fluid volume excess
Normal	Decreased	1. Increased fluid intake or 2. Diuretic use
Increased or normal	Decreased (with no increase in fluid intake)	1. Kidneys unable to concentrate urine or 2. Lack of ADH (diabetes insipidus)
Decreased	Increased	Syndrome of inappropriate secretion of ADH (SIADH) can be due to stress, trauma, drugs, or malignancies

Note: See discussion in text under high and lower urine osmolality for more details on clinical significance and possible nursing diagnoses. Note that alcohol can increase serum osmolality. See Table 4–3 for note on osmole gap.

Increased or High Urine Osmolality

Clinical Significance. A high urine osmolality, when the serum osmolality is normal or increased, indicates that the kidneys are conserving water (Table 4-4). As the serum osmolality rises, due to the presence of abnormal solutes or to hemoconcentration, the urine osmolality should also rise: the higher the number of milliosmoles in the urine, the more concentrated the urine. This is the expected physiological response to a lack of fluids for metabolic needs.

A less-than-normal serum osmolality and a high urine osmolality do not constitute a normal physiological response. For some reason the plasma is remaining dilute. An increased level of the antidiuretic hormone (ADH) causes a dilution of the plasma and a more concentrated urine. Certain drugs, trauma, or stress reactions may cause an increased production of ADH, but this reaction is usually transitory. Advanced age may increase susceptibility to an increased secretion of ADH (Goldstein et al., 1983).

POSSIBLE NURSING DIAGNOSES RELATED TO INCREASED URINE OSMOLALITY

Potential Fluid Volume Deficit

A very high urine osmolality means that the client is dehydrated. A moderately high urine osmolality is probably also due to a lack of fluids, as long as it is not due to some fluid retention resulting from an increased ADH. The urine osmolality should be used as only one part of the data base about the fluid balance of the client. Other factors, such as clinical signs of dehydration, total intake and output, weight gain or loss, and the pathological state of the client, must all be taken into account. The serum osmolality, if available, helps to determine the amount of dehydration present. The type and method of fluid replacement depends on the cause and severity of fluid loss.

Potential for Fluid Volume Excess

If the client's retention of fluids is possibly due to an increased level of ADH, then extra fluids may not be warranted even though the urine osmolality is a little high. For example, in the postoperative client, concentrated urine may be normal for 2 or 3 days after surgery, because ADH is holding some extra fluid in the plasma. As the stress level decreases, hormone levels return to normal, and the extra fluid is released. This is sometimes called *surgical diuresis*. A similar diuresis occurs after other kinds of stress such as a major burn. A comparison of serum and urine osmolality may be very helpful in distinguishing a slightly increased urine osmolality that is due to fluid retention from one that continues to increase due to a basic lack of fluids. It is important neither to overload clients with fluids nor to let them become dehydrated. Nurses can use the serum osmolality as one objective measurement to add to their data collection tools. If there is suspected impaired water excretion the client may undergo a water load test. Boh and Van Son (1982) describe how this inexpensive procedure can be done on an outpatient basis.

Low Urine Osmolality

Clinical Significance. Urine osmolality should always be higher than serum osmolality unless there is a known reason for the excretion of dilute urine, such as increased fluid intake or the use of diuretics (Table 4–4). In the case of either, the serum osmolality is expected to be within normal range as the excess fluid is excreted. What is not expected is a continuing low urine osmolality when the serum osmolality begins to increase. With the client in a dehydrated state, the urine osmolality should be quite high. If the serum osmolality is normal and the urine osmolality remains around 280 mOsm/kg water, this set of conditions indicates an inability to concentrate urine, which may be an early sign of renal damage. Or it may be due to a lack of secretion of the ADH, which causes the client to have very dilute urine all the time. This pathological lack of ADH is called *diabetes insipidus*.

POSSIBLE NURSING DIAGNOSES RELATED TO LOW URINE OSMOLALITY

Potential for Fluid Volume Imbalances

Because dilute urine is expected in clients on diuretic therapy, the major nursing concern is to monitor their fluid balance so that not too much fluid is lost. A low urine osmolality is also expected if the goal is to force fluids to make the urine dilute. Urine osmolality can be an objective evaluation that an increased fluid intake is having the desired results. (Recall that a client who is not getting enough fluids has a consistently high urine osmolality.)

Potential Alteration in Urinary Elimination

Eventually with renal dysfunction, the urine osmolality may remain the same as the plasma level, which is around 290 mOsm/kg water. Chapter 3 explained why a "fixed" urine specific gravity is always around 1.010, because this is the specific gravity of the plasma. The comparison of urine and plasma osmolalities is a more sensitive measurement of this same concept. Nursing implications for clients with an inability to concentrate urine include a careful assessment of the amount of fluids they need to excrete waste products. Dehydration must be avoided.

Knowledge Deficit Regarding Replacement of ADH

Much more rarely, a decreased urine osmolality may be related to a lack of ADH, in which case nurses would observe that the client is excreting huge amounts of urine. ADH levels can be measured by immunoassay. Medical treatment includes the prescribing of ADH replacement, either by the intramuscular route or by nasal spray. Treatment is usually by nasal spray (Bullock & Rosendahl, 1984). Nurses may be responsible for teaching the client how to take the drug and how to observe any side effects or complications.

■ URIC ACID (SERUM AND URINE)

Uric acid is the end-product of purine metabolism. Purines, which are in the nucleoproteins of all cells, are obtained from both dietary sources and from the breakdown of body proteins. The kidneys excrete uric acid as a waste product.

The exact level of uric acid that is considered pathological is controversial. In recent years it has been generally recognized that the so-called normal ranges of uric acid are quite wide. In light of this ambiguity, and because uric acid levels show day-to-day and seasonal variations in the same individual, clinicians usually order several uric acid levels over a period of time. Urine uric acid levels may also be used to evaluate gout or determine overexcretion of uric acid.

Special Preparation of Client and Collection of Sample

There is no special preparation of the client. To do the test, the laboratory needs 1 ml of serum which has to be sent immediately to the laboratory. It may be useful to ask about a dietary history of intake of purine-rich foods. Levo-dopa and diuretics lead to distortion in results. For urine specimens the laboratory may require use of an alkali: preservative in the 24-hour bottle. (See Chapter 3 on client instructions for 24-hour collections.)

Reference Values for Serum Uric Acid

Adults: Male	2–7.5 mg/dl
Female	2–6.5 mg/dl
Pregnancy	In early pregnancy, the levels fall by about one third, but rise to nonpregnant levels by term (Wallach, 1986)
Children (ages 10–18): Male	3.6–5.5 mg/dl
Female	3.6–4 mg/dl
	Striking rise in men 12–14 coincides with puberty. Rise in women may be before age 12 (Harlan et al., 1979)
Aged: Male over 40	2–8.5 mg/dl
Female over 40	2–8.0 mg/dl
	Rise in women is related to menopause

Note uric acid levels tend to vary from day to day and from laboratory to laboratory. Range of 3–7 mg/dl is noted by Sculley (1986).

Reference Values for Urine Uric Acid
250–750 mg/24-hr specimen

Increased Uric Acid Level (Hyperuricemia)

Clinical Significance. Although gout, a disease much more common in men than women, is the specific disease associated with consistently high serum uric acid levels, several other conditions commonly cause uricemia.

1. The most common is renal impairment because the kidneys normally excrete uric acid. However, as the level of the uric acid increase does not correlate with the severity of the renal disease, serum uric acid is not used as a test of renal function. (The BUN and creatinine tests are the two basic blood tests for renal function.)
2. A variety of drugs, such as the thiazides and some other diuretics, can cause an abnormal elevation of serum uric acid by impairing uric acid clearance by the kidneys.
3. In preeclampsia and particularly in eclampsia, serum uric acid levels are quite high, partially due to the reduced glomerular filtration rate.
4. Another common reason is abnormal cell destruction, such as that associated with neoplasms. In neoplastic disease, the utilization of chemotherapy or radiation therapy may further elevate serum uric acid levels due to the accelerated destruction of cells. Allopurinol, which prevents uric acid elevations, is sometimes started 24 hours before chemotherapy.
5. With prolonged fasting or chronic malnutrition, uric acid levels are higher than normal, due to the breakdown of cells.

POSSIBLE NURSING DIAGNOSES RELATED TO ELEVATED URIC ACID LEVELS

Alteration in Comfort Related to Joint Pain
Because some clients with hyperuricemia are asymptomatic, the basic nursing assessments for pain are not always a clue that there is a problem with uric acid. The symptoms characteristic of gout are due to deposit of urate crystals in the joint. For gout clients, the warning symptom may be minor discomfort from the bedspread resting on a toe or some swelling and pain in one joint. Usually the pain becomes intense and requires frequent pain medication until the gout is brought under control.

Alteration in Fluid Requirements
Whatever the reason for the high uric acid level, the danger is that uric acid, in the form of urates, will crystallize in an acid urine and form renal stones. In the absence of some contraindication, clients with high serum uric acid levels need a liberal intake of fluids to prevent renal stones. A "liberal intake of fluids" or "force fluids" should be put into specific terms, such as enough fluid to maintain a urine output of 2000 ml/day. The specific gravity test (Chapter 3) or the urine osmolality covered in this chapter are ways to measure whether the urine is dilute enough.

Knowledge Deficit Regarding Any Dietary Modification

Dietary restrictions are usually not emphasized because drugs are used to reduce persistently high serum uric acid levels. However, foods that are high in purines (such as sardines, anchovies, and organ meats) should probably be completely eliminated from the diet (Table 4–5); the nurse can also find out whether other meats, poultry, or fish should be restricted in their total amounts. Alcohol is to be avoided because it inhibits urate excretion. It is important that clients with high serum uric acid levels have adequate nutrition, because fasting or starvation diets cause more of an increase in the serum acid levels. Any needed weight reduction must be done gradually. Maintaining adequate nutrition for a client on chemotherapy may be very difficult; failure to do so may compound the serum uric acid problem.

Knowledge Deficit Regarding Medications

Depending on the level of the serum uric acid level and the underlying pathophysiological condition, the physician may order:

1. Drugs that interfere with the production of uric acid levels, such as allopurinol (Zyloprim)
2. Uricosuric agents, which promote the elimination of urate salts by the kidneys such as probenecid (Benemid)
3. For acute attacks of gout, colchicine, which does not seem to affect uric acid metabolism but which does decrease urate crystal deposition
4. For maintenance therapy, sulfinpyrazone, which may be continued indefinitely although clients need careful monitoring (Govoni & Hayes, 1985)

In addition to hydration and medications, a third factor may be helpful in decreasing the possibility of renal stones from hyperuricemia: an alkaline urine. Normal urine has an acid pH because cheese, eggs, bread, meat, fish, poultry, and some fruits and vegetables contribute to acid waste products. An acidic urine, as low as 5.5, may contribute to urate crystallization (Metheny, 1982). Because one cannot routinely achieve alkalinization of the urine without severe dietary restrictions, medication such as sodium bicarbonate or potassium citrate, may be used to make the urine pH higher or closer to the alkaline side (Spataro et al., 1978).

The effectiveness of either dietary modifications and/or drug treatments should be periodically evaluated by testing the pH of the urine. This is easily done by using the dipstick method described in Chapter 3. Nurses should teach clients to test their own urine.

TABLE 4–5. EXAMPLES OF FOODS HIGH IN PURINES

Liver	Lentils
Sardines	Mushrooms
Anchovies	Spinach
Kidneys	Asparagus
Sweetbreads	

Decreased Serum Uric Acid Level

Clinical Significance. Decreased levels usually reflect some increase in plasma volume such as with the syndrome of inappropriate secretion of antidiuretic hormone (SIADH) or the effect of drugs. Renal tubular defects and liver disease also can decrease serum uric acid levels. Idiopathic hypouricemia commonly is transient (Jacobs et al., 1984). There are no specific clinical symptoms with low uric acid levels.

QUESTIONS

1. Mrs. Balboa is a client with congestive heart failure who has a slightly elevated BUN. What is the most likely explanation for the abnormal BUN?

   a. Plasma dilution due to aldosterone increase
   b. Increased protein breakdown due to stress
   c. Poor renal perfusion
   d. Impaired liver function

2. Because certain antibiotics may be nephrotoxic, BUN and/or creatinine levels should be checked before the administration of antibiotics, which are classified as which of the following?

   a. Aminoglycosides, such as gentamicin
   b. Cephalosporins, such as cephapirin
   c. Penicillins, such as penicillin G
   d. Tetracyclines, such as deoxycycline

3. Mr. Tod's latest laboratory reports show a BUN of 75 mg and a creatinine level of 6.0 mg. (Reference values for the hospital are BUN 8–25 mg/dl and creatinine 0.6–1.5 mg/dl.) Which nursing action would be appropriate based on the laboratory information?

   a. Put the patient on 2-hour vital signs
   b. Question whether potassium should be continued in the IV solution
   c. Encourage the intake of protein foods in the diet
   d. Encourage more active ambulation

4. Mr. Bobbins is to have a 24-hour creatinine clearance test begun this morning. He had just emptied his bladder. For this test, what should he be instructed to do?

   a. Save a urine sample each time he urinates so this can be compared to serum creatinine levels drawn every 4 hours
   b. Save all the urine voided in the next 24 hours after he is given a dose of creatinine intravenously
   c. Not eat any food or drink any fluids while the urine is being collected as a 24-hour specimen
   d. Save all urine for 24 hours and expect to have blood drawn during the middle of the test for a serum creatinine level

5. For testing for renal function and fluid balance, urine osmolality is a superior test to urine specific gravity because urine osmolality:

   a. Can be done faster on the clinical unit
   b. Detects the presence of specific electrolytes
   c. Is not changed much by sugar, protein, or X-ray dyes
   d. Requires less urine

6. When there is an increased level of ADH in response to severe stress, which of the following are the laboratory reports for serum and urine osmolality most likely to reflect?

   a. A slight increase in serum and urine osmolality
   b. A slight decrease in serum osmolality and an increase in urine osmolality
   c. A slight decrease in serum and urine osmolality
   d. A slight increase in serum osmolality and a decrease in urine osmolality

7. Mrs. Regola has a serum osmolality of 290 mOsm/kg and a urine osmolality of 1400 mOsm/kg. Based on this information, the nurse should assess this client for effects of which of the following?

   a. Fluid overload   **c.** Lack of antidiuretic hormone
   b. Fluid volume deficit   **d.** Renal dysfunction

8. A urine osmolality of 300 mOsm/kg or a specific gravity of 1.010 on a first voided morning urine specimen is an indication that the client needs to be further assessed for which of the following?

   a. Fluid volume deficit   **c.** Renal dysfunction
   b. Circulatory overload   **d.** Nothing (this is a normal
                                          finding)

9. Higher-than-normal serum uric acid levels are likely for all these clients *except* which of the following?

   a. Jackie, age 8, who is undergoing chemotherapy for leukemia
   b. Mrs. Dillon, age 63, who has rheumatoid arthritis
   c. Jennifer, age 21, who is on a starvation diet to lose weight
   d. Mrs. Benidito, age 34, who is showing signs of preeclampsia

10. Which of the following foods are highest in purine content?

    a. Dairy products   **c.** Grains
    b. Organ meats   **d.** Citrus fruits

11. What are the two measures, other than drug therapy, that help reduce the possibility of the formation of uric acid renal stones?

    a. Forcing fluids and keeping urine alkaline
    b. Exercise and forcing fluids
    c. Exercise and keeping urine acid
    d. Forcing fluids and keeping urine acid

REFERENCES

Basil, C., et al. (1986). Diagnosing Kidney disease early. *Patient Care, 20*(4), 28–52.

Boh, D., & Van Son, A. (1982). The water load test. *AJN, 82*(1), 112–117.

Bullock, B., & Rosendahl, P. (1984). *Pathophysiology*. Boston: Little, Brown.

Burke, D., et al. (1978). Laboratory studies: When to act on unexpected test results. *Patient Care, 12,* 14–87.

Chambers, J. (1983). Bowel management in dialysis patients. *AJN, 83*(7), 1051–1052.

Harlan, W., et al. (1979). Physiological determinants of serum urate levels in adolescence. *Pediatrics, 63*(4), 564–577.

Goldstein, C., Braunstein, S., & Goldfarb, S. (1983). Idiopathic syndrome of inappropriate antidiuretic hormone secretion possibly related to age. *Annals of Internal Medicine, 99,* 185–188.

Govoni, L., & Hayes, J. (1985). *Drugs and nursing implications* (5th ed.). Norwalk, CT: Appleton-Century-Crofts.

Hetrick, A. (1979). Nutrition in renal disease: When the patient is a child. *AJN, 79*(12), 2152–2154.

Jacobs, D., Kasten, B., DeMott, W., & Wolfson, W. (1984). *Laboratory test handbook with DRG index*. St. Louis: Mosby/Lexi Comp.

Jones, A., et al. (1979). Renal failure in the newborn. *Clinical Pediatrics, 18*(5), 286–291.

Langslet, J., & Habel, M. (1981). The aminoglycoside antibiotics. *AJN, 81*(6), 1144–1146.

Luke, B. (1979). Nutrition in renal disease: The adult on dialysis. *AJN, 79,* 2155–2157.

Metheny, N. (1982). Renal stones and urinary pH. *AJN, 82*(9), 1372–1375.

Oestreich, S. (1979). Rational nursing care in chronic renal disease. *AJN, 79*(6), 1096–1099.

Orr, M. (1981). Drugs and renal disease. *AJN, 81*(5), 969–971.

Sculley, R. (1986). Normal reference values. *NEJM, 314*(1), 41.

Spataro, R., et al. (1978). The use of percutaneous nephrostomy and urinary alkalinization in the dissolution of obstructing uric acid stones. *Radiology, 129*(12), 629–632.

Stark, J. (1980). BUN/Creatinine: Your keys to kidney function. *Nursing 80, 10*(5), 33–38.

Stark, J., & Hunt, V. (1983). Helping your patient with chronic renal failure. *Nursing 83, 13*(9), 59–63.

Smithline, N., & Gardner, K. (1976). Gaps—Anionic and Osmolal. *JAMA, 236,* 1594–1597.

Tietz, N. (Ed.). (1983). Clinical guide to laboratory tests. Philadelphia. W. B. Saunders.

Wallach, J. (1986). *Interpretation of diagnostic tests*. Boston: Little, Brown.

5

Four Commonly Measured Electrolytes

- The Anion Gap
- Serum Sodium (Na⁺)
- Urine Sodium
- Serum Potassium (K⁺)
- Urine Potassium
- Serum and Urine Chloride (Cl⁻)
- Serum Bicarbonate (HCO₃⁻) or Carbon Dioxide (CO₂)

OBJECTIVES

1. State which of the four commonly measured electrolytes show significant variation in different age groups and in pregnancy.
2. Differentiate between milligrams (mg) and milliequivalents (mEq) in relation to measurements of electrolytes in the serum and in replacement therapy.
3. Give examples of how the serum cations and anions are kept in electrical neutrality by the kidney and by shifts into and out of cells.
4. Explain the effect of water deficit and water overload on serum sodium levels.
5. Describe nursing assessments that might detect clients with increased and decreased serum sodium levels.
6. Identify possible nursing diagnoses for clients with hypernatremia and hyponatremia.
7. Explain why serum potassium levels may not accurately reflect the total body potassium levels.
8. Describe the nursing assessments that might detect clients with increased or decreased serum potassium levels.
9. Identify possible nursing diagnoses for clients with hyperkalemia and hypokalemia.

10. **Explain the clinical significance of the relationship of serum chloride to serum bicarbonate.**
11. **Describe how chlorides are usually replaced in therapy.**

Although many electrolytes are in the blood, when electrolytes (or "lytes") are ordered as a laboratory test, the test is for the four common ones discussed in this chapter. A shorthand method of reporting "lytes" on a client's chart is:

$$\frac{140}{103} \bigg| \frac{4}{27}$$

Sodium and potassium are the two values on top and chloride and bicarbonate are on the bottom. Laboratory evaluations of these four basic electrolytes are critical in the assessment of fluid and electrolyte balance as well as acid–base balance.

This chapter focuses primarily on the serum levels of the first three, as well as on the urine levels of sodium and potassium. Because the reference values for these three electrolytes are essentially the same for all populations after the newborn period, it is expedient for nurses to memorize them. Only bicarbonate is significantly changed according to age and pregnancy.

Bicarbonates will be discussed in the next chapter, in relation to acid–base balance and arterial blood gases. The discussion will explain why some laboratories may report serum bicarbonate levels with a test called the "CO_2 content."

The three less commonly measured electrolytes—calcium (Ca^{++}), magnesium (Mg^{++}), and phosphate (PO_4^-)—are covered in Chapter 7.

INTERPRETING SERUM ELECTROLYTE REPORTS

When interpreting the reports of serum electrolytes, one must always keep in mind that the laboratory report reflects only *serum* levels. It may not be an accurate reflection of the body's total electrolyte level. Generally, the level of electrolytes in the serum is very close to the electrolyte levels in the interstitial fluid with one major exception. Interstitial fluid does not have the plasma proteins found in serum. Because the electrolytes can shift readily from plasma to interstitial fluid, or vice versa, the extracellular fluid remains similar in substances other than the plasma proteins.

But the electrolytic compositions of extracellular (serum and interstitial) fluid and intracellular (cell) fluid are strikingly different. Sodium (Na^+) and chloride (Cl^-) are the two major electrolytes in the extracellular fluid, whereas potassium (K^+), magnesium (Mg^+), and phosphate (PO_4^-) are major intracellular ions (Table 5–1). Shifts of electrolytes do occur between the cells and the extracellular fluid, but not in major amounts. So the measurement of only serum levels cannot always accurately reflect the status of the electrolytes in the individual cells. For example, during a pathological state, such as acidosis, more potassium may shift out of the cells because more hydrogen (H^+) ions are moving into the cell. Thus the serum level may seem normal or even high, yet the cells are becoming deficient in their main electrolyte, potassium.

Serum sodium and chloride levels rarely reflect the total sodium or chloride content in the body because a change in these levels causes a corresponding change in

TABLE 5-1. COMPOSITION OF ELECTROLYTES IN SERUM, INTERSTITIAL FLUIDS, AND CELLS

Fluid	Major Electrolytes	
Extracellular		
Serum	Na^+	Sodium
	Cl^-	Chloride
	HCO_3^-	Bicarbonate
Interstitial	Almost the same as plasma (note no plasma proteins)	
Intracellular		
Cellular	K^+	Potassium
	Mg^{++}	Magnesium
	PO_4^-	Phosphate

the volume of the plasma. Sodium and chloride are responsible for most of the osmotic pressure in extracellular fluids. So if the sodium and chloride ions increase in the plasma, they retain more water in the plasma. Hence the concentration of sodium is still reported as 135–145 mEq and the chloride as 100–106 mEq, both *per liter of fluid*. More sodium and chloride (that is, more salt) in the plasma holds more water in the vascular system and eventually in the interstitial spaces (edema).

MEASUREMENT BY MILLIEQUIVALENTS (mEq)

Electrolytes are reported in measurements of milliequivalents (mEq) rather than in milligrams (mg). The reason is that milligrams measure only the weight of the chemical element, and equal weights do not mean equal chemical activity. For example, it takes 39 mg of potassium (K^+) to equal 23 mg of sodium (Na^+) in a measurement of chemical activity based on a common standard (Table 5-2). The standard of equivalents is based on how many grams of an element or compound liberate or combine with 1 g of hydrogen (Holum, 1983). Because it takes 23 g of sodium to liberate 1 g of hydrogen, the equivalent weight of sodium is 23 g. *A milliequivalent,* the term used in laboratory reports, is one one-thousandth (1/1000) of an equivalent. If it takes 23 *g* to make 1 equivalent, 23 *mg* equals 1 mEq.

TABLE 5-2. CONVERSION OF MILLIGRAMS (mg) TO MILLIEQUIVALENTS (mEq)

Measurement of Weight	Measurement of Chemical Activity[a]
23 mg of sodium (Na^+)	1 mEq
39 mg of potassium (K^+)	1 mEq
35.5 mg of chloride (Cl^-)	1 mEq
30 mg of bicarbonate (HCO_3^-)	1 mEq
Problem 1	
1000 mg of sodium = _____ mEq	
Solution: 1000 ÷ 23 = 43.4 mEq	
Problem 2	
40 mEq of potassium = _____ mg	
Solution: 40 × 39 = 1560 mg	

[a]See text and Holum (1983).

The important point to remember about the standard of equivalents and milli-equivalents is that 1 mEq of one element always has the same chemical activity as 1 mEq of another element. If milligrams or grams are used to measure the amount of electrolytes in diets or medications, a conversion to the amount of electrolyte milli-equivalents must be done to discuss the physiological effect of the drugs or diet. For example, a diet of 1000 mg of sodium (not sodium chloride) would provide about 43 mEq of sodium. This figure is derived from the fact that it takes 23 mg of sodium to make 1 mEq: 1000 mg divided by 23 mg equals 43 mEq. A more detailed discussion about sodium and salt is covered under the section on sodium. Usually sodium is measured in milligrams.

Potassium is the other electrolyte that may sometimes be measured in milligrams in medication or diet prescriptions. A diet that contains 1560 mg of potassium supplies 40 mEq of potassium (as it takes 39 mg of potassium to equal 1 mEq: 1560 mg divided by 39 equals 40 mEq). Medications, such as potassium chloride, may be marked in both milligrams and milliequivalents. It is much easier to understand the physiological effect of electrolytes when the dosage is noted in milliequivalents as well as in milligrams or volume. Although medications list the electrolyte composition clearly, doctors sometimes order—and nurses sometimes record—only that the client took a teaspoon of a potassium supplement and not how many mEq are contained in the teaspoon.

CHEMICAL ELECTRICAL NEUTRALITY

All electrolytes in the serum carry either negative charges (*anions*) or positive charges (*cations*). These negative and positive charges must always be in perfect balance so that the serum remains neutral. The electrical neutrality of the serum is essential in understanding why certain electrolytes may be lost or retained in the serum, even though this upsets acid–base balance.

One way for the body to always maintain an equal number of positive and negative ions in the serum is shifting of electrolytes from the cells or vice versa. For example, when bicarbonate (HCO_3^-) levels are reduced in the serum, other negative ions must replace the missing negative bicarbonate ions. To keep the electrical balance in the serum neutral, chloride can shift out of the erythrocytes (Chan, 1978); this *chloride shift* is discussed in detail later. Another example involves the relationship of the positive ions potassium (K^+) and hydrogen (H^+). When the level of serum potassium (K^+) falls, there is an increased shift of potassium out of the cells to keep the serum potassium (K^+) normal. As potassium comes out of the cell, hydrogen (H^+) diffuses into the cell to replace the loss of positive ions intracellularly. This shifting of electrolytes from plasma to cells and vice versa is actually a more complex situation, because the kidneys are also working to remove any excess ions from the bloodstream.

Because sodium (Na^+), hydrogen (H^+), and potassium (K^+) are all positive ions, a change in one means some change in the others. In the distal tubules of the kidney, sodium (Na^+) is usually reabsorbed in exchange for either potassium (K^+) or hydrogen (H^+) ions. If there is an abundance of hydrogen (H^+) ions to excrete, the kidney does not excrete many potassium ions. On the other hand, if the potassium level in the serum is low, the kidneys have to continue to excrete hydrogen (H^+) ions even when the hydrogen (H) is needed to maintain the acid–base balance of the serum. The relationship of increased potassium levels to acidosis, as well as that of decreased potassium levels to alkalosis, is discussed in the section on potassium.

When the sodium (Na^+) ion is reabsorbed by the kidney, a negative ion of either chloride (Cl^-) or bicarbonate (HCO_3^-) must be reabsorbed also. If one of these two negative ions is low in the serum, more of the other must be absorbed to maintain the proper amount of anions (negative ions). This inverse relationship of chloride (Cl^-) and bicarbonate (HCO_3^-) is an important consideration in some types of metabolic acid–base imbalances.

■ THE ANION GAP

Table 5-3 shows the amount of the positive ions (Na^+ and K^+) compared with the amount of negative ions (Cl^- and HCO_3^-). For the two cations (positive ions) and two anions (negative ions) that are measured in the serum, there seem to be more positive ions than negative ions, because some of the anions are not measured. This difference between the number of cations and the number of measured anions is called the *anion gap* (Smithline & Gardner, 1976). Actually, this gap (of 14 mEq in Table 5-3) is made up of unmeasured anions such as sulfates, phosphates, and organic acids. Usually these unmeasured anions are around 8–16 mEq, depending on the particular references used by a laboratory. Jacobs et al. (1984) note that the anion gap is extensively used for quality control in the laboratory as a check that there is no error in the measurement of electrolytes.

The clinical importance of the anion gap is that it is increased in the types of metabolic acidosis where organic or inorganic acids are increased in the bloodstream. This increase in the anion gap is helpful in identifying the type of acidosis present. If there is no change in the unmeasured anions in metabolic acidosis, the decreased bicarbonate level (a negative ion) is replaced by an increased serum chloride (Cl^-) level (another negative ion). Other much rarer situations may cause some changes in the anion gap, but for general purposes, nurses use only the concept of the anion gap in caring for clients with metabolic acidosis. Wallach (1986) gives examples of how the anion gap is useful in complicated acid–base imbalances.

By this point the reader may be a little bewildered by so many references to acid–base balance when this chapter is supposed to be on electrolytes. Obviously, electrolyte disturbances and acid–base imbalances are so intimately connected that it is hard to learn about one and not the other. Following the summary of acid–base balances in the next chapter, a chart gives general guidelines of how each electrolyte is changed in the four different types of acid–base imbalance. The concept of the anion gap is also explored further in Chapter 6, in the discussion on the three types of metabolic acidosis.

TABLE 5-3. CATIONS AND ANIONS IN SERUM

Positive Ions (Cations)		Negative Ions (Anions)		Unmeasured Anions
Sodium	140 mEq	Chloride	103 mEq	Phosphates
Potassium	4 mEq	Bicarbonate	27 mEq	Sulfates
				Organic acids
Total	144 mEq	Total	130 mEq	(gap of 14 mEq)
		144 − 130 = gap of 14 mEq[a]		

[a]See text for explanation of this anion gap and Smithline & Gardner (1976), Jacobs et al. (1984), and Wallach (1986).

Preparation of Client and Collection of Sample

Most laboratories require about 1 cc of blood to do each of the four electrolyte tests. If electrolytes are done by an automatic analyzer, only 2.5 ml may be needed (see SMA in Chapter 1). Usually, all four are done routinely, but sometimes only one is ordered, particularly the potassium. It is especially important that the blood sample not be traumatized because hemolysis of cells makes the potassium report inaccurate. (Recall that potassium is an intracellular ion.) The serum is obtained by venipuncture and collected in a tube without additives. The client does not need to be fasting.

Reference Values for Common Electrolytes

Sodium (Na$^+$)	135–145 mEq/L
Potassium (K$^+$)	3.5–5.0 mEq/L (slightly more in newborns)
Chloride (Cl$^-$)	100–106 mEq/L
Bicarbonate (HCO$_3$$^-$) (measured as CO$_2$ content)	
Adult	24–30 mEq/L
Pregnancy	19–20 mEq/L (see PCO_2 levels in Chapter 6 for explanation of reason for lower bicarbonate levels in pregnancy)
Infant	20–26 mEq/L
Children	Slightly lower than references for adults

Note that all four electrolytes may be reported in moles per liter (mmol/L) rather than mEq if the Système International (SI) is adopted by a particular laboratory. Because there is no change in basic numbers for these four electrolytes, 24 mEq of HCO$_3$$^-$ is 24 mmol/L (see Chapter 1 on SI).

■ SERUM SODIUM (Na$^+$)

Sodium has the highest concentration of all the electrolytes measured in the serum, and yet changes in its level are not commonly seen, because its concentration is always correlated with fluid balance. As sodium is the primary factor in maintaining osmotic pressure in the extracellular fluid, changes in sodium are hidden because "water goes where salt is." So one must always interpret a change in serum sodium levels in relation to possible fluid overload or dehydration. A rough estimate of the plasma osmolality (discussed in Chapter 4) can be calculated from the sodium level by multiplying the sodium by two. A normal serum sodium of 140 mEq/L times two would equal a normal plasma osmolality of around 280 mOsm/kg water.

The serum level of sodium is not totally dependent on diet because the kidneys can conserve sodium when necessary. The hormone aldosterone causes a conservation of sodium and chloride and an excretion of more potassium. The daily requirement of sodium for an adult is about 100 mEq or 2.3 g. In children, the usual requirement is around 3 mEq/kg daily (Chan, 1978). Many American diets contain much more than these daily minimums. Some authorities estimate that the average diet may contain as much as 6–10 g of sodium. The American Heart Association (1982) suggests a maximum intake of 2 g of Na or 5 g of NaCl per day.

It is necessary to measure sodium, not just sodium chloride, in the diet because sodium is present in forms other than salt. For example, monosodium glutamate is

TABLE 5-4. RELATIVE SODIUM CONTENT OF FOODS

Foods with about 500 mg sodium (21 mEq)	1/4 scant tsp salt (40% of salt is sodium)
	3/4 tsp monosodium glutamate
	1/2 boullion cube
	1 cup tomato juice
	average serving of cooked cereal
	1 hotdog
	1-1/2 oz ham
Foods with about 250 mg sodium (about 11 mEq)	1 oz canned tuna
	2/3 cup buttermilk
	5 salted crackers
Foods with about 200 mg sodium (about 9 mEq)	1 slice bread
	2 slices bacon
	3 oz shrimp
	1/2 oz cheese
	1 tbsp catsup

(Adapted from *Sodium Restricted Diets*, AHA, 1982; and Hill, 1979. Note that processed food, such as a Big Mac from McDonald's Restaurant, has 1510 mg of sodium and a Heinz pickle, 1137 mg of sodium (Hill, 1979).)

added to many foods in the American diet. Most American diets can be substantially reduced in sodium by avoiding very salty foods and not adding extra salt to foods at the table. One gram of NaCl is about 0.6 g chloride and about 0.4 g, or 17 mEq, of sodium (400 mg divided by 23 equals 17.39 mEq). Table 5-4 lists the amount of sodium in different proportions of salt and food substances. Table 5-5 notes the meaning of sodium labels for food.

Reference Values for Sodium

Adult   135–145 mEq/L

The same reference values are used for all age groups. Pregnancy may cause a drop of 2–3 mEq, but the range is still within general values

---

Increased Serum Sodium Level (Hypernatremia)

Clinical Significance. An increase in the serum sodium level becomes apparent only when there is not sufficient water in the body to balance the increasing sodium level. Because sodium has an osmotic action, an increase in serum sodium pulls water

TABLE 5-5. MEANING OF SODIUM LABELS FOR FOOD

"Sodium free"	Less than 5 mg of Na^+ per serving
Very low sodium	35 mg or less of Na^+
Low sodium	140 mg or less of Na^+
Reduced sodium	Process to reduce usual level of Na^+ by 75%
Unsalted	Processed without salt

Note: Also teach clients to note the actual sodium content for specific foods (Table 5-4).

into the vascular system from the interstitial spaces and the cells. When the laboratory test for *serum* sodium level is elevated, the client is depleted in water, not only in the extracellular compartment, but also in the cells (Table 5–6). Thus many cases of an increase in *total body* sodium do not cause an increased *serum* sodium level. For example, clients with congestive heart failure have sodium retention due to the action of the hormone aldosterone. However, the retention of sodium means an equal retention of water, so the serum sodium level remains around 140 mEq per *liter* of fluid.

For the serum sodium level to be increased on a laboratory report, it is necessary that either (1) there is a large increase in sodium *without* a proportional increase in water or (2) there has been a loss of a large amount of water *without* a proportional loss of salt. Under most circumstances, increasing sodium intake without increasing water intake is hard because an increased sodium intake makes a person very thirsty. If the person is receiving intravenous fluid, such as normal saline, that contains a relatively large amount of sodium, it may be possible to overload with sodium. Intravenous solutions of normal saline contain 0.9% NaCl, that is, 0.9 g of salt in 100 cc or 90 g in 1000 cc. This percentage is 154 mEq of sodium and 154 mEq of chloride per liter. Infants who receive exchange transfusions with stored bank blood may become hypernatremic because stored blood has high sodium levels. An intravenous of dextrose 5% in water is given to prevent overload of sodium.

The much more common reason for an increased serum sodium level is a loss of a large amount of water without a proportional loss of sodium. For example, diarrhea or vomiting may cause a severe decrease in total body water, particularly in infants (Chan, 1978). Not all dehydration results in an increased sodium level, however, because just as much sodium may be lost as water; this loss of equal amounts of sodium and water is called *isotonic dehydration* and is the type in 70% of infants hospitalized for a fluid volume deficit due to vomiting or diarrhea (Wink, 1983). In dehydration due to a loss of water or a lack of water intake, the sodium loss is not proportional and hence the dehydration is *hypertonic*. Even in the early stages of hypertonic dehydration, the serum sodium level is not elevated because water is pulled from the interstitial spaces to keep the sodium at a normal dilution in the serum.

When the serum sodium level begins to rise above normal, this is a sign of a very serious deficit of water that has extended to the cellular level. Another term for this type of dehydration is *hyperosmolar dehydration*. The serum is increased in osmolality, not because of a total sodium increase, but because of a total body water deficit.

TABLE 5-6. CLINICAL SITUATIONS COMMONLY ASSOCIATED WITH SERUM SODIUM ABNORMALITIES

Hypernatremia—serum Na increased (↑) 145 mEq/L
  1. Dehydration is the most frequent cause
  2. Overuse of intravenous saline solutions
  3. Exchange transfusion with stored blood
  4. Impaired renal function

Hyponatremia—serum Na decreased (↓) 135 mEq/L
  1. Excessive water—"dilutional" hyponatremia
  2. Loss of sodium by vomiting, diarrhea, GI suctioning, or sweating
  3. Use of diuretics, diabetic acidosis, Addison's disease, or renal disease, which all cause increased loss of sodium via urine

See text for explanation of why fluid volume changes are usually the underlying cause for changes in serum sodium levels. Also see Culpepper (1986) on common causes of hyponatremia.

POSSIBLE NURSING DIAGNOSES RELATED TO HYPERNATREMIA

Fluid Volume Deficit

The initial symptom of hypernatremia is likely to be thirst, which, if the person is unconscious, confused, or very young, is a subjective symptom that is not communicated to the nurse. Other clinical assessments that correlate with a high serum sodium level include elevated temperature, dry, sticky mucous membranes, and little or no urine output. The specific gravity of the urine is high if the kidneys are still able to concentrate urine. The hematocrit is increased when the water deficit is severe. In the infant, a high-pitched cry and depressed fontanels are other signs of severe water deficit. Hyperactive reflexes and irritability may lead to seizures in infants with high sodium levels.

For the adult, each 3 mEq of serum sodium above the usual refrence range represents a deficit of about 1 L of fluid. Thus a serum sodium (Na^+) level of 157 mEq would be about 12 mEq above the reference of 135–145 mEq. This excess indicates a deficit of about 4 L of fluid. Because 1 L of water weighs 1 kg (2.2 lb), a loss of 4 L would mean a weight loss of nearly 9 lb. Obviously this would be very severe dehydration. In a small child, the loss of even a liter of fluid would be severe dehydration because a loss of 2.2 lb may be 10% of the total weight of the child. The most accurate measurement of the amount of water deficit is the client's loss of weight. Daily weights should be part of the nursing assessment for any clients experiencing fluid losses.

Assisting with Treatments. For hypernatremia due to a water deficit, the therapeutic interventions focus on replacing the lost water. If oral intake is not possible, physicians order intravenous fluids to hydrate the client. Dextrose 5% is the best hydrating solution because it contains no sodium. However, the fluid deficit may need to be corrected very gradually, as changing the sodium level too quickly may be dangerous, particularly for infants. The deficit may need to be replaced over 2–4 days if the sodium concentration is above 160 mEq/L. This slow reduction of the sodium level is necessary to prevent cerebral hemorrhage, which may occur with the rapid correction of hypernatremia (Chan, 1978). Fluid orders may need to be changed every few hours depending on the response of the client. Sometimes a fluid challenge will be given and the client monitored with a central venous pressure line (CVP) or, if needed, pulmonary artery diastolic or wedge pressures (Weil & Rackow, 1984). If the dehydration was due to gastrointestinal problems, food is gradually added back to the diet. The BRAT diet (*B*ananas, *R*ice cereal, *A*pplesauce, and *T*ea or *T*oast) is easy on the gastrointestinal tract.

Preventing Sodium Overload. Often the nurse may be able to prevent hypernatremia due to water deficit from developing by careful observation of clients at risk. For instance, clients who are not taking enough oral fluids may become water deficient. Those who are receiving normal saline solutions (0.9% NaCl) should be checked for any signs of hypernatremia. Intravenous solutions for maintenance are usually only one half normal saline (0.45% NaCl) or even one fourth normal saline (0.25% NaCl). Normal saline solutions (0.9% NaCl) are not used for maintenance solutions unless the client has hyponatremia (Keithley & Fraulini, 1982). Infants who receive blood exchange usually have a peripheral line for infusion of dextrose 5% in water, as the stored blood is high in sodium.

Fluid Volume Excess Due to Excess Sodium

When both sodium and water are retained in excessive amounts, the symptoms are very different from when sodium is in excess. The signs and symptoms of increased total body sodium levels are weight gain, elevated blood pressure, dyspnea, and pitting edema (the common signs of fluid retention). In the adult, edema becomes apparent only after about 3 L of water are retained; this amount of water retention would mean 3 kg or 6.6 lb of weight gain before the edema shows. Thus weight gain is the most sensitive detector of early fluid retention (Pflaum, 1979).

Knowledge Deficit Regarding Need for Sodium Restriction

The client with both sodium and water retention is often on diuretics and/or a low-sodium diet. Also, hypertensive clients are usually told to restrict the sodium in their diets (Hill, 1979). A "restricted sodium" diet would mean less than the 2.3 g or 100 mEq as a basic requirement. Thus the most mild restriction of sodium is a 2-g (87-mEq) sodium diet. A moderate restriction of sodium is 1000 mg (43 mEq). A diet of 500 mg is very restrictive as this amount allows only 21 mEq of a sodium a day (500 mg divided by 23 mg equals 21.1 mEq). A teaspoon of salt has 2000 mg of sodium or 87 mEq. (See Table 5–5 on the meanings of sodium labels.)

   The effectiveness of sodium restriction is determined by the absence of fluid retention, *not by the serum sodium level*. Nurses may need to go over this point several times with clients. It may be hard for clients to see a need to restrict sodium and salt intake when the laboratory report is "normal" for sodium. The American Heart Association has excellent teaching material about low-sodium diets. Chloride titrator strips can be used to test the urine to assess a large sodium intake (Luft et al., 1984).

Decreased Serum Sodium Level (Hyponatremia)

Clinical Significance. Like serum sodium increases, serum sodium (Na^+) decreases are not accurate reflections of total body sodium levels because sodium is usually lost with water. The more common reason for a low serum sodium (Na^+) on a laboratory test is an excess of water in the body. The water excess can be caused by giving salt-free intravenous fluids. Also, in stress and severe illness, such as cancer, there may be an increased production of antidiuretic hormone (ADH), which causes an increase in total body water. The syndrome of inappropriate secretion of ADH (SIADH) can also be due to various drugs such as antidepressants and psychotropics (Sandifer, 1983). Most cases of water excess are usually terminated by an increased urine output, which restores the sodium and water balance. (See Chapter 4 on serum and urine osmolality.)

   Although a real water excess is the more common reason for a low serum sodium level, actual sodium depletion can also be a cause of a low serum sodium level. Ordinarily, the hormone aldosterone conserves sodium, but a continual loss of sodium with only water replacement and no sodium replacement eventually leads to a true sodium depletion. For example, a client who is on diuretics and a restricted sodium diet may experience massive sodium depletion from the body. Excessive sodium loss also occurs:

1. In some types of renal failure, in which there is "salt wasting"
2. In diabetic acidosis, in which case polyuria contributes to a great loss of sodium
3. Particularly in young children, in whom vomiting and diarrhea can lead to hyponatremia if gastrointestinal losses are replaced only with water
4. In exercise, in which perspiration can deplete sodium
5. With a lack of adrenal corticosteroids (Addison's disease). The severe hypotension of an Addisonian crisis occurs because the total body sodium is not enough to keep fluid in the vascular system (see Chapter 15 on cortisone tests)

POSSIBLE NURSING DIAGNOSES RELATED TO LOW SERUM SODIUM LEVELS

Fluid Volume Excess Due to Water Intoxication

Although this discussion distinguishes the symptoms of hyponatremia (low sodium level) due to fluid excess from those due to a true sodium deficit, the clinical picture is usually not so clear-cut.

When the low serum sodium level is due to just an excess of body water, one sign is that that client has a weight gain that is equal to the amount of excess liters retained. For example, a client who is maintained on routine intravenous fluids should not be gaining weight because the caloric intake is minimal. (A bottle of 1000 cc of dextrose 5% contains only 50 g of dextrose.) In fact, an adult client who is being maintained on intravenous fluids of dextrose 5% usually loses about half a pound a day. So if the client is gaining weight at all, this weight has to be water. A gain of a pound means the retention of over 500 ml of fluid. (Every nurse should memorize the fact that a liter of water weighs 1 kg or 2.2 lb or a pound for every pint.)

The other symptom of water excess is an increased urine output. If the water excess continues, and if the kidneys cannot get rid of the excess water, the water diffuses into the interstitial spaces and eventually into the cells. The edema that develops is generalized; it is not contained in dependent areas such as the feet. So, for example, the face may look a little puffy. Edema of brain cells causes nausea and vomiting and eventually convulsions when the serum sodium (Na^+) is as low as 120 mEq. This condition is a hyposmolar imbalance.

Careful nursing assessment of the intake and output records, as well as of weight gains, for clients who are susceptible to fluid overload can do much to prevent severe water intoxication. For example, elderly clients may have an increase of antidiuretic hormone that makes them more susceptible to hyponatremia (Goldstein et al., 1983).

Assisting with Treatment. The treatment for water excess is just to restrict fluid intake for a while. To objectively evaluate that the fluid balance is returning to normal, one must keep accurate records of intake, output, and weight loss.

Alteration in Nutritional Requirements Due to Sodium Depletion

Nurses need to be aware of clients who may be developing a true depletion of sodium, because this type of low serum sodium level can often be prevented if early symptoms of sodium depletion are noted. For example, clients on nasogastric suctioning can lose significant amounts of sodium if water rather than normal saline is used to irrigate the nasogastric tube. Repeated tap water enemas in the elderly may also cause hyponatremia as can large doses of diuretics. With mild to moderate depletions of sodium, the serum sodium level remains within the normal reference range. Yet this condition is still an isotonic imbalance, and the urine sodium becomes low. (See the next section on urine sodium levels.) As the total sodium becomes low, the client has anorexia, apathy, and sometimes a sense of impending doom. Confusion may occur, particularly in elderly clients. Muscle cramps, weakness, and diarrhea reflect the lack of sodium for normal muscle contractions. Eventually the low serum sodium leads to hypotension and shock because there is a loss of osmotic pressure in the vascular system. Infants, although they may be lethargic, may also be asymptomatic until the sodium level is low enough to cause edema and seizures.

Assisting with Sodium Replacement. The therapeutic measures for a true sodium depletion are geared toward replacing both sodium and the lost fluid. Usually the intravenous solution used for replacement would be normal saline (0.9% NaCl), although in extreme cases, a hypertonic (3% NaCl) saline solution may be used. Nurses must carefully monitor clients who are receiving hypertonic intravenous fluids, as too rapid an infusion of a hypertonic solution is very dangerous. The hypertonic solution can not only cause hemolysis of red blood cells, but it can also pull a large amount of fluid into the vascular space, leading to circulatory overload. No more than 200 or 300 ml of 3% NaCl should be given in 4 hours (Culpepper et al., 1986). The hypertonic solutions of salt are rarely used now. Either normal saline (0.9% NaCl) or Ringer's lactate (another isotonic solution) can supply enough sodium to make up the deficiency more safely.

Potential Knowledge Deficit Related to Specific Need for Replenishing Sodium

Because the body can conserve sodium, it is not necessary to instruct clients to eat high-sodium content food over a long period. Yet clients who may become sodium-depleted due to vomiting, diarrhea, or vigorous exercise should drink some salty replacement fluids such as broths instead of just water. For infants, special formulas of electrolytes are used to replace gastrointestinal losses. Athletes who do vigorous exercises know to replace lost fluids with special oral electrolyte preparations that are commercially available. In the past, salt tablets were often used by people who engaged in intense physical activity; it is now generally recommended to replace salt more gradually by dietary increases or salty fluids (Darby, 1980). Note that one cup of tomato juice has 486 mg of sodium (see Table 5-8).

As mentioned, the American diet usually contains more than enough sodium. But sometimes clients may follow too restricted a sodium diet. For example, nurses may need to assess the dietary habits of elderly clients to make sure that their sodium restrictions are not too severe, particularly if they are started on diuretics. Children with cystic fibrosis lose extra sodium in their sweat. (See Chapter 18 on the sweat test for CF.) Clients on lithium must also have plenty of sodium in the diet. (See Chapter 17 on lithium toxicity.)

■ URINE SODIUM

Normally the amount of sodium excreted in the urine varies with the sodium intake. Increased amounts of aldosterone in the serum cause a decreased secretion of urine sodium. (See Chapter 15 on serum and urine aldosterone levels, which may also be ordered.) Conversely, a decreased level of aldosterone activity causes an increased loss of sodium in the urine. Diabetic acidosis and diuretics also cause an increased loss of sodium. Various types of renal failure may cause either increased losses or retention of sodium. A urine sodium of more than 40 mEq/L in oliguria suggests acute tubular necrosis (ATN) (Jacobs et al., 1984). The values of the urine sodium must be interpreted in view of the total clinical picture and can be quite complicated to interpret. Wallach (1986) lists 20 conditions which may increase or decrease urine sodium levels.

Preparation of Client and Collection of Sample
See Chapter 3 on 24-hour urine collections. No special preservative is needed. The diet of the client should be noted as to the amount of sodium intake.

Reference Values for Urine Sodium

40–220 mEq/24 hr or 30 mEq/L (diet dependent)
Full-term infants have sodium clearance of about 20% of adult values
  (Tietz, 1983)

■ SERUM POTASSIUM (K⁺)

Potassium is primarily an intracellular ion, but the small amount that is in the serum is essential for normal neuromuscular and cardiac function. Small changes in the serum potassium (K^+) level can have profound effects on the cardiac muscle. In a normal state of health, adequate potassium is easily obtained by eating a variety of foods. The intake of potassium, which is probably around 40–80 mEq/day for an adult, needs to be on a daily basis because potassium, unlike sodium, is not conserved well by the body. The kidneys continue to excrete 40–80 mEq/day even when there is no intake.

Although potassium can also be lost in gastrointestinal drainage, the kidneys excrete almost all of the potassium. The renal mechanism for potassium (K^+) ion excretion is shared with another positive ion hydrogen (H^+). Either a potassium (K^+) or hydrogen (H^+) ion is excreted when a sodium (Na^+) ion is reabsorbed by the kidney. This relationship partially explains why potassium levels are increased in

---

Reference Values for Serum Potassium

3.5–5.0 mEq/L
In pregnancy there may be a fall of about 0.2–0.3 mEq due to increased
  volume. Slightly higher in newborns and infants

---

acidosis and decreased in alkalosis. The shifting of potassium (K^+) and hydrogen (H^+) ions into and out of the cells in acid–base imbalances also contributes to marked changes in potassium levels. (See Chapter 6 on acid–base balances.)

Increased Serum Potassium Level (Hyperkalemia)

Clinical Significance. The major reason for an increased serum potassium level (hyperkalemia) is inadequate renal output (Table 5–7). Thus hyperkalemia is always a problem in the oliguric phase of renal failure unless potassium intake is limited. (See Chapter 4 for the distinction between renal insufficiency and renal failure.)

The intake of too much potassium in medications can also cause an increased serum potassium (K^+) level. An overdose from oral supplements of potassium is unlikely, but the danger is very real with intravenous use of potassium in high concentrations. Other medications, such as penicillin K, which contains potassium ions, can cause hyperkalemia if renal output is not adequate. (See Chapter 4 on BUN and creatinine levels as assessments of renal function.)

Because potassium is primarily an intracellular ion, anything that causes massive cell destruction increases the serum potassium level. Thus massive tissue injury or a burn causes the release of potassium from damaged cells. Although the serum potassium level may increase after cellular damage, the actual total body potassium is decreased. Thus the hyperkalemia that occurs with a burn or injury is followed by hypokalemia.

Because aldosterone and other steroids cause a retention of sodium and an increased secretion of potassium, conditions in which hormones are decreased may cause an increased serum potassium level. For example, in Addison's disease, a malfunctioning of the adrenal cortex reduces the corticosteroid level. The serum sodium (Na^+) levels are decreased and the potassium (K^+) serum levels may be increased. (See Chapter 15 on laboratory tests for cortisone.)

Although almost all diuretics cause an increased loss of potassium, there are three exceptions. Spironolactone (Aldactone) is an aldosterone antagonist and thus causes increased retention of potassium. Triamterene (Dyrenium) does not affect aldosterone, but it too is a diuretic that may cause hyperkalemia. Triamterene acts directly on the distal tubules to cause excretion of Na^+ and retention of K^+ as does amiloride (Midamor). About 10% of clients on amiloride become hyperkalemic (Govoni & Hayes, 1985).

TABLE 5–7. CLINICAL SITUATIONS COMMONLY ASSOCIATED WITH SERUM POTASSIUM ABNORMALITIES

Hyperkalemia—serum K increased (↑) 5 mEq/L (or above 6.5 in newborns)
1. Renal failure
2. Too rapid intravenous infusion of K^+ replacement
3. Initial reaction to massive tissue damage
4. Associated with metabolic acidosis (see Chapter 6)

Hypokalemia—serum K decreased (↓) 3.5 mEq/L
1. Diuretics, particularly thiazides
2. Inadequate intake when n.p.o., vomiting, or on K-free intravenous feedings
3. Large doses of corticosteroids
4. Aftermath of tissue destruction or high stress
5. Associated with metabolic alkalosis (see Chapter 6)

See text and references at end of chapter for further details. Wallach (1986) lists many medical conditions causing changes in potassium. Newborn references from Children's Hospital San Francisco, California.

Hyperkalemia is often associated with metabolic acidotic states. In acidosis, the kidney must excrete more hydrogen ions, which means less secretion of potassium ions by the renal selection mechanism. In addition, an abundance of hydrogen ions in the serum means that some of these ions go into the cells, which drives potassium out of the cells. Thus, in acidotic states, the total body potassium is not increased, but more potassium ions are in the serum. Serum potassium raises about 0.6 mEq/L for every 0.1 decrease in blood pH. If the acidotic state is due to diabetic ketoacidosis, the lack of insulin compounds the problem of hyperkalemia because potassium needs insulin, as does glucose, to be transported into the cell. (See Chapter 8 on ketoacidosis.)

POSSIBLE NURSING DIAGNOSES RELATED TO ELEVATED POTASSIUM LEVELS

Potential for Injury Related to Effect of Hyperkalemia on Heart and Other Muscles

Probably the most important thing to remember about checking for symptoms of increasing serum potassium (K^+) levels is that many of the symptoms are nonspecific. Potassium is important to nerve and muscle function but so are most of the other electrolytes. Early symptoms of hyperkalemia may be irritability, nausea, diarrhea, and abdominal cramping. Later symptoms may include skeletal muscle weakness. The muscle weakness can progress to a flaccid-type paralysis with difficulty in speaking and breathing.

Hyperkalemia is usually an emergency situation because a high serum potassium level can cause cardiac arrhythmias that can lead to cardiac arrest: The heart stops in diastole. Because the clinical signs of hyperkalemia can be confused with other conditions (hypokalemia can also cause paralysis), the level of serum potassium must be assessed by the laboratory report, not just by physical symptoms. Remember that the serum laboratory test may not reflect the total body potassium. The electrocardiograph is a very sensitive indicator of intracellular potassium, even when the serum potassium still seems normal. High-peaked T waves, a prolonged QRS interval, a decreased amplitude of P and R waves, and depressed ST segments are typical electrocardiographic findings that suggest high potassium levels.

Assisting with Medical Interventions. Although there is no *specific* antidote for hyperkalemia, several different medications may be used to treat a high serum potassium level.

1. Sometimes calcium gluconate is given intravenously to lessen cardiac toxicity. Calcium may be particularly useful if the calcium levels were initially low or borderline. It is not used if the client is on digitalis, because digitalis and calcium have a synergistic effect on the heart.
2. Sodium bicarbonate may be given intravenously if acidosis is present. As the pH of the blood returns to normal, potassium shifts back into the cells. Also, when the pH is normal, the kidney can secrete more potassium ions because there is not a demand to excrete so many hydrogen ions.
3. Intravenous solutions with glucose and insulin help promote the reentry of potassium into the cells, even for clients who are not diabetic.

4. In more chronic states of hyperkalemia, sodium polystyrene sulfonate (Kayexalate), given orally or by enemas, is a sodium–potassium exchange resin.
5. For the client with chronically high potassium levels, usually due to renal failure, the treatment may include peritoneal dialysis or hemodialysis.

Knowledge Deficit Regarding Sources of Potassium

The nurse needs to find out whether the hyperkalemia is likely to be a chronic or recurring situation. If so, the client needs to be taught to read the labels on foods and medications, to determine whether they are high in potassium. For example, most salt substitutes are composed of large amounts of potassium. Instant coffee and other prepared foods may have potassium as one of the ingredients.

Dietary teaching about eliminating potassium may also need to be done. To reinforce client behavior, a contract may be written between the nurse and client to keep potassium levels low through diet adherence. Sheckel (1980) has used graphs of potassium levels posted at the foot of the beds of dialysis clients as one way to reinforce diet selections. Thus potassium levels can be one evaluative tool of effective teaching. (Table 5-8 lists foods particularly high in potassium.)

Potential for Injury Related to Subsequent Development of Hypokalemia

If the high serum levels of potassium were due to metabolic shifts in acidosis, the potassium shifts back into the cells when the pH is returned to normal, and clients may have a serum deficit. Also, if the serum potassium level was increased due to cell damage, the potassium lost from injured cells results in a total body deficit. Always consider the possibility that the hyperkalemia of today could result in hypokalemia tomorrow.

Decreased Serum Potassium Levels (Hypokalemia)

Clinical Significance. Because potassium is not conserved well in the body, an inadequate intake results in a low serum level. However, as the daily need of potassium for an adult is only about 80 mEq, insufficient oral intake is usually not the cause for a low potassium unless the person is totally n.p.o. Even in fasting states, the serum potassium level may not drop immediately, because the breakdown of cells for energy causes the release of potassium.

More commonly, hypokalemia results from an excessive loss of potassium. Any loss of fluid from the gastrointestinal tract causes a loss of potassium. Almost all diuretics cause an increased excretion of potassium, except spironolactone (Aldactone), amiloride (Midamor), and triamterene (Dyrenium). Certain hormonal changes also contribute to an excessive excretion of potassium. The corticosteroids cause sodium retention and thus potassium excretion is increased. Certain tumors may produce hormones that act much like the steroids and thus increase potassium excretion. (See Chapter 15 on ectopic hormone production.) Drugs that cause excessive beta-sympathetic stimulation, such as epinephrine, can cause a transient hypokalemia (Struthers et al., 1983). Ritodine (a beta sympathetic drug), used to halt premature labor, has a side effect of hypokalemia (Aumann & Blake, 1982).

TABLE 5-8. FOODS HIGH IN POTASSIUM AND CORRESPONDING SODIUM CONTENT

Potassium at Least 10 mEq or More by Serving	Sodium (mg)
Avocado, $\frac{1}{2}$	5
Banana, 1 medium	1
Cantalope, 1 cup	19
Dates, 10	1
Figs, 5	10
Instant coffee, 3 g	Check label
Molasses, 2 tbsp	3
Orange juice, 1 cup	2
Potato, baked	2
Prunes, 10 (high calories)	9
Salt substitutes (varies, but may be 30–40 mEq in tsp)	Varies. Check label
Soybeans, $\frac{1}{2}$ cup	2
Tomato juice, canned, 1 cup	486! (not good if on low-sodium diet)

Note that the American Heart Association has patient information cards as well as pamphlets about potassium content in foods. Slawson and Slawson (1985) list sodium and potassium content for many over-the-counter drugs including salt substitutes. Narins (1985) discusses renal retention of potassium from fruit.

An alkalotic serum pH (pH above 7.4) is another reason for a lowered serum potassium. In alkalosis, hydrogen ions (H^+) shift out of the cell in an attempt to lower the pH of the serum to normal. When hydrogen (H^+) shifts out of the cell, more potassium shifts into the cell to replace the missing positive ions. Conversely, a low serum potassium level also contributes directly to the development of an alkalotic state because, when serum potassium levels are low, the kidneys must excrete more hydrogen ions in exchange for the reabsorption of sodium by the distal tubule. So either alkalosis may be the cause of hypokalemia, or hypokalemia may contribute to the development of metabolic alkalosis. The role of hypokalemia in the development of metabolic alkalosis is covered in Chapter 6 under the section on bicarbonate changes in acid–base balance.

POSSIBLE NURSING DIAGNOSES RELATED TO HYPOKALEMIA

Potential Injury Related to Development of Muscle Weakness or Arrhythmias

Nurses need to be aware of clients who may be having extra losses of potassium so they can assess for potential hypokalemia. The only objective assessment for a low serum potassium level is the laboratory test, along with the electrocardiograph changes. Although certain clinical symptoms are caused by hypokalemia, these symptoms can also be caused by other clinical abnormalities. Clients with a low serum potassium level may have anorexia, muscle weakness, a decrease in bowel sounds, and abdominal distention due to decreased peristalsis (ileus). Ileus and lethargy are key symptoms of hypokalemia in the newborn too. Flaccid paralysis may develop with more severe hypokalemia, as well as with hyperkalemia, because both potassium imbalances alter the resting potential of muscle cells (Felver, 1980). Low serum potassium levels make respiratory effort difficult, and they can lead to paroxysmal tachycardia, premature contractions, and other arrhythmias. For clients on digitalis, hypokalemia is quite dangerous because the toxic effects of digitalis are more likely to occur when the serum potassium level drops quickly. The typical electrocardiograph in hypokalemia has prominent U waves, and the T waves are flat or even inverted. (In hyperkalemia, the T waves are just the reverse, very peaked.) Sometimes the replacement of severe potassium losses is monitored by electrographic readings because the ECG is a very sensitive indicator of not just serum potassium levels, but also of intracellular potassium levels.

Assisting with Potassium Replacement. Depending on the severity of the hypokalemia, potassium may be replaced in three ways: (1) intravenously, (2) by oral supplements, or (3) by diet.

Potential for Injury Related to Use of Intravenous Potassium
Most preparations of potassium chloride (KCl) for intravenous use are marketed as 2 mEq/ml. Thus, for a dose of 40 mEq, the nurse would add 20 ml to the intravenous fluid. Potassium must *always be diluted*. Potassium chloride is never given directly by intravenous push no matter how severe the deficiency. Usually no more than 40 mEq of potassium is added to 1000 ml of intravenous fluids, although sometimes as much as 80 mEq are added to a liter. Clients should usually not be given more than 10–20 mEq in an hour, although some authorities say 30–40 mEq/hr is safe in severe deficiencies. For example, if the serum potassium is less than 2 mEq, with electrocardiographic changes and paralysis, up to 40 mEq may be given within an hour. The determination of the dosage and the rate of the infusion are the physician's responsibilities, but the nurse must know the limits of safety. As mentioned, ECG monitoring is a useful assessment tool when high levels of potassium are given. Many clients complain of burning at the site of the infusion when more than 40 mEq are added to a liter of intravenous fluid. If the intravenous must be slowed down because of the burning sensation, the solution needs to be made more dilute or a larger vein used for infusion.

Any client who is receiving potassium must have adequate urinary output. In the adult, "adequate" means at least 30 ml/hr. Newborns should produce 1 cc of urine per kilogram per hour. Thus a newborn who weighs 4 kg (8.8 lb) should produce about 4 ml/hr. In older children, 1–2 ml/kg/hr is a minimum output. The urinary output should always be assessed before potassium is added to an intravenous. Once the intravenous is infusing, nurses must continue to make sure that urinary output remains adequate. Otherwise hyperkalemia can develop rapidly.

Knowledge Deficit Regarding Oral Potassium Supplements
Oral preparations of potassium chloride may come marked in various strengths, such as 10 or 20% solutions, or as so many milligrams per teaspoon. On the bottle, however, the dosage in mEq is also given, and this is the dosage form that should be used. One teaspoon of potassium chloride elixir is not as precise as 20 mEq. Every client should be told the dosage exactly in mEq, not just to take a certain amount by volume.

The oral preparations of potassium come in various forms of elixirs, capsules, and tablets, some that fizz when mixed with juice. Most potassium supplements also contain chloride, which may be a needed replacement in metabolic alkalosis (see Chapter 6). The major problem with oral supplements of potassium is the gastrointestinal upsets they can cause, therefore nurses should teach clients not to take potassium supplements on an empty stomach. Liquids should be diluted. Orange juice is a good vehicle, because it has a high potassium level. Overdoses of oral potassium supplements are not common, but it is important that the urinary output always be adequate.

Potassium replacement can also be done with a relatively inexpensive salt substitute that contains potassium chloride. Many salt substitutes contain more than 50 mEq of potassium per teaspoon (Slawson & Slawson, 1985). The client should consult the physician about the use of salt substitutes.

Knowledge Deficit Regarding Dietary Sources of Potassium

The dietary intake of potassium is usually around 40–80 mEq for adults. For clients who are on diuretics or who for other reasons need a higher intake of potassium, it may be wise to assess their dietary habits to see if they can gain extra potassium by dietary intake. Table 5–8 shows the amount of potassium in some common foods. By including some of the potassium-rich foods, clients may be able to reduce or eliminate the need to take potassium supplements. However, Narins and co-workers (1985) note that supplements are usually needed. The serum potassium levels for clients on long-term diuretics should be checked periodically to make sure that dietary intake of potassium is adequate to balance an increased potassium loss. Clients on thiazides who have continued problems with hypokalemia may be put on one of the potassium-sparing diuretics, but this is usually more costly (Licht et al., 1983).

■ URINE POTASSIUM

The amount of potassium in the urine varies with the diet. It also varies with an increased amount of serum aldosterone or cortisol, which causes an increased excretion of potassium. Further, extra potassium is lost in diabetic acidosis and with thiazide diuretics, but a serum potassium is a better measurement of the need for replacement after diuresis. Renal failure causes a decreased excretion of potassium. The primary use of a 24-hour urine potassium is to assess hormonal functioning and to determine if hypokalemia is of renal or nonrenal origin. Excretion of less than 20 mEq/day in the presence of hypokalemia is evidence that the hypokalemia is not from renal loss (Jacobs et al., 1984). (See Chapter 15 on aldosterone and cortisol levels.) Urine potassium levels are also used sometimes in research studies as one indication of the stress level of the body.

Preparation of Client and Collection of Sample

See Chapter 3 for 24-hour urine collections. No preservative is needed.

Reference Values for Urine Potassium

25–125 mEq/24 hr (varies with diet)

■ SERUM AND URINE CHLORIDE (Cl⁻)

Chloride, the major negative ion in the extracellular fluid, is very important, in combination with sodium, for maintaining the osmotic pressure in the serum. A loss or a gain of chloride is often due to the factors that also cause a loss or gain of sodium. Chloride is found in a variety of foods, usually in combination with sodium. A diet restricted in sodium causes a reduction of chloride intake, too, but not to an inadequate level. The kidneys selectively secrete chloride or bicarbonate ions depending on the acid–base balance. In certain types of renal failure, chloride excretion may be impaired. Chloride can be measured in the urine with sodium and potassium as part of a 24-hour specimen (see Chapter 3).

Reference Values for Serum Chloride

All age groups   100–106 mEq
Falls little, if at all, in pregnancy

Reference Values for Urine Chloride

Adult	110–250 mEq/24 hr
Child	15–40 mEq/24 hr
Infant	2–10 mEq/24 hr

Varies greatly with chloride intake (Tietz, 1983). Chloride dip sticks will estimate total sodium intake (Lufts et al., 1984).

Increased Serum Chloride Level (Hyperchloremia)

Clinical Significance. "Hyperchloremia" is a term that is rarely used clinically. An increase in chlorides in the serum is not a primary focus as the increase must always be looked at in relationship to (1) an increase in sodium (Na⁺) levels or (2) a decrease in the serum bicarbonate (HCO₃⁻) level.

Aldosterone, a mineral cordicosteroid, causes retention of both sodium (Na⁺) and chloride (Cl⁻). In most cases, a proportional increase in water retention makes the electrolytes in the serum appear not to be increased. For the sodium and chloride levels to be elevated, there must be a deficit of water or a large intake of sodium chloride. Because in these situations, the chloride level parallels the rise or fall of the sodium level, the sodium level is used to monitor fluid deficits.

In a couple of clinical situations, the rise in chlorides may be even greater than the rise in sodium levels. In certain types of renal failure, the kidneys are unable to excrete chlorides properly; this inability leads to a type of acidosis called *renal hyperchloremic acidosis.* Chlorides may also be greatly increased in the bloodstream if large amounts of normal saline (0.9% NaCl) are infused over several days. "Normal saline" is not really normal in relation to the sodium and chloride content of the serum, even though it is classified as an isotonic solution. Normal saline contains 154 mEq of sodium (Na^+) ions and 154 mEq of chloride (Cl^-) ions per liter. This is a little higher than the serum level of 135–145 mEq for sodium (Na^+) ions and a great deal higher than the 100–106 mEq for serum chloride (Cl^-) (Keithley & Fraulini, 1982).

Chloride levels are increased in some types of acidosis because the chloride is needed to replace the loss of another negative ion, bicarbonate (HCO_3^-), from the serum. If the metabolic acidosis is due to an increase of other negative ions, such as ketoacids, the chlorides are not increased—and may actually decrease—due to diuresis. The changes in the bicarbonate level, in the chloride level, and in the unmeasured negative ions (the anion gap) give useful information about what is causing the acidotic state. The most important thing to remember about the relationship of a high serum chloride level to acidosis is that, if the chlorides are higher than normal, this condition causes a drop in the serum bicarbonate level because there is room for only a set amount of negative ions. If the serum bicarbonate level drops first, then chlorides may be increased to keep the correct number of negative ions in the serum. Increased chloride levels can be either a cause or a result of metabolic acidosis.

POSSIBLE NURSING DIAGNOSES RELATED TO HIGH CHLORIDE LEVELS

Because changes in chloride levels always take place in combination with changes in other electrolytes, assessments depend on nurses' understanding of the basic reason for the increased chloride level. For example, if the chloride level is related to an increased sodium level, then the nursing diagnoses for sodium are to be followed. If the increased chloride level is causing, or was caused by, acidosis, then the symptoms exhibited are those of acidosis. (The care in metabolic acidosis is covered in the section on bicarbonate levels in Chapter 6.)

Decrease in Serum Chloride Level (Hypochloremia)

Clinical Significance. Decreases in the serum chloride level are commonly due to loss from vomiting, gastric suction, diarrhea, and the use of diuretics.

Because sodium, hydrogen, and potassium ions are usually lost with the chlorides, a chloride drain is only part of a larger problem. For example, the loss of chlorides from the serum means that more bicarbonate must be retained to replace the lack of negative ions, thus contributing to the development of metabolic alkalosis. The loss of potassium or of hydrogen ions also contributes to the development of metabolic alkalosis. Conversely, alkalotic states can cause a low chloride level. In any alkalotic state, the bicarbonate level in the serum increases, so the other major negative ion, chloride, must decrease in the bloodstream. (By now the inverse relationship between the negative ions, bicarbonate, and chloride should be clearly apparent.)

As explained in Chapter 6, clients with chronic lung disease often have high serum bicarbonate levels to balance an increased PCO_2 level in the bloodstream. This chronically elevated serum bicarbonate level also causes a decreased serum chloride level. This condition would be considered a normal compensation in clients with chronic lung disease.

POSSIBLE NURSING DIAGNOSIS RELATED TO LOW CHLORIDE LEVELS

Alterations in Nutritional Requirements Related to Chloride Losses

Nurses need always to be aware of clients who may be losing abnormal amounts of chlorides, so that replacement therapy can begin before alkalotic states develop. For example, clients who are on gastrointestinal suctioning are losing not only chlorides, but also potassium and hydrogen ions. All three losses contribute to the development of metabolic alkalosis. Because potassium supplements contain chloride, the use of potassium chloride is one way that lost chlorides are replaced. If necessary, the physician may order some normal saline (0.9% NaCl) to be given intravenously to replace large chloride losses. The use of oral electrolyte solutions for infants or salty broths for adults to replace sodium losses was already mentioned. Nurses must always keep in mind that a loss of electrolytes usually involves several electrolytes and never just chlorides alone.

■ SERUM BICARBONATE (HCO₃⁻) OR CARBON DIOXIDE (CO₂)

Serum bicarbonate levels (HCO_3^-) are routinely part of both "electrolytes" and arterial blood gases. Note that the carbon dioxide combining power (CO_2) is often used as an indirect measure of the serum bicarbonate. The CO_2 is different than the PCO_2 which is a measure of the blood gas. (Both are discussed in Chapter 6.) Because changes in the serum bicarbonate level always signify some changes in the acid–base balance, the relationship of bicarbonate to carbonic acid is important to note. This bicarbonate-to-carbonic acid (as measured by the PCO_2) ratio of 20 to 1 is the most important buffer in the serum. The 20:1 radio is fundamental to understanding the clinical significance of changes in serum bicarbonate levels. The next chapter includes a summary of this ratio before discussing how serum bicarbonate levels decrease and increase in acid–base imbalances.

QUESTIONS

1. Serum electrolytes are measured in milliequivalents (mEq) rather than in milligrams (mg) because milliequivalents are:

   a. More precise for small concentrations of electrolytes in the serum
   b. Easier to compute in an automated laboratory
   c. Not dependent on the metric system
   d. Based on a measurement of chemical activity, not of weight

2. Given the fact that 39 mg of K^+ equals 1 mEq, compute how many mg of K^+ are needed to give a dose of 40 mEq.

   a. 1.56 g or 1560 mg

   b. 0.56 g or 560 mg

   c. 3.9 g or 3900 mg

   d. 1.4 g or 1400 mg

3. Hydrogen ions (H^+) shift into the cell when serum potassium (K^+) levels drop because, as more K^+ diffuses out of the cell:

   a. The fluid balance changes unless electrolytes are shifted into the cell

   b. Another positive ion must enter the cell to keep the electrical charges neutral

   c. The acid–base balance must be maintained by decreasing serum H^+ ions

   d. There is a lack of positive ions to be excreted by the kidney

4. When the total amount of serum Na^+ and K^+ ions (cations) are compared to the total amount of serum Cl^- and HCO_3^- ions (anions), there are fewer anions. This "anion gap" is due to which of the following facts?

   a. There are always more cations (positive ions) than anions (negative ions) in the serum

   b. Some anions, such as organic acids, are not measured

   c. The electrical balance is not always neutral in acid–base imbalances

   d. The loss of electrolytes decreases the total number of anions in the serum

5. When a client has an abnormal serum sodium (Na^+) report, the most useful nursing assessment to help explore the reason for the sodium imbalance would be which of the following?

   a. Dietary intake pattern of salt and sodium-containing foods

   b. Intake and output records and daily weights

   c. Vital signs over last 24 hours

   d. Record of all medications given

6. A laboratory report of an increased serum sodium level would most likely be part of the clinical findings for a client:

   a. With severe congestive heart failure who has pitting edema of the ankles

   b. On corticosteroid therapy for several months for rheumatoid arthritis

   c. Having diarrhea and unable to take fluids by mouth

   d. Maintained on intravenous fluids of dextrose 5% in 0.2% sodium chloride for several days after surgery

7. A laboratory report of a slightly low serum sodium (Na^+) could be due to all of the following conditions *except* which?

   a. Diet containing no more than 2.3 g (100 mEq) of sodium daily

   b. Maintenance intravenous solutions of 5% dextrose in water (D_5W) for several days

   c. Drinking large amounts of water after strenuous exercise

   d. Use of a diuretic that is an aldosterone blocking agent

8. Characteristic assessments expected for a client with a high serum sodium (Na^+) level due to a water deficit would include all but which of the following?

   a. Hypertension   c. Weight loss
   b. Thirst   d. Elevated temperature

9. Characteristic assessments for a client with a low serum sodium (Na^+) level due to total body sodium depletion include all but which of the following?

   a. Confusion   c. Weight gain
   b. Hypotension   d. Muscle cramps

10. An increase in serum sodium (Na^+) levels is usually an indication that the client needs which of the following?

   a. Less sodium in the diet   c. More fluid intake
   b. Less fluid intake   d. Both sodium and water restrictions

11. Which of the following clients is the *least* likely to have an elevated serum K^+ level?

   a. Mary Burden who is in renal failure
   b. Baby Lois who suffered extensive burns today
   c. Candy Phillips who is in metabolic alkalosis
   d. Jack Brown who has Addison's disease

12. A low serum potassium (K^+) may be a potential problem for all these clients *except* which?

   a. Mr. Rhodes who is on long-term diuretic therapy with thiazides
   b. Mary Rogers who has severe morning sickness with vomiting
   c. Jackie, age 8, who is on corticosteroid therapy as part of the treatment for leukemia
   d. Mrs. Cabrillo who has a severe respiratory infection and who is not taking much fluid

13. Which of the following signs or symptoms is the most suggestive of hyperkalemia?

   a. Paralytic ileus (lack of bowel sounds)
   b. Peaked T waves on the cardiac monitor
   c. Skeletal muscle cramps
   d. Depressed T waves on the cardiac monitor

14. Mrs. Forrest, who is scheduled for a cholecystectomy tomorrow, has a serum K^+ of 2.3 mEq. (She has been on thiazide diuretics.) The nurse is to monitor the potassium replacement, which Mrs. Forrest is to receive intravenously. Which of these guidelines about potassium is correct?

   a. Urine output should be at least 100 cc/hr
   b. No more than 10 mEq of KCl should be given in an hour
   c. No more than 80 mEq of KCl should be added to 1000 cc bottle

d. KCl is given IV push only in extreme cases where the serum K^+ is below 2.5 mEq

15. Mrs. Forrest is going home on hydrochlorathiazide (Hydrodiuril) due to hypertension. The doctor has prescribed a potassium chloride (KCl) supplement to be taken in liquid form t.i.d. The nurse should instruct the client to:

a. Dilute the KCl in water, but not in juice
b. Never take the KCl at the same time as any other medicine
c. Not take the KCl on an empty stomach
d. Keep the KCl in the refrigerator

16. Mrs. Forrest asks the nurse about foods that are high in potassium. What item does not contain at least 10 mEq of potassium?

a. Orange juice, 1 cup
b. Cranberry juice, 1 cup
c. Instant coffee, 3 g
d. Potato, 1 baked

17. All of the following clients are likely to have low serum chloride (Cl^-) levels *except* which?

a. Mr. Hagan who has an elevated serum bicarbonate (HCO_3^-) level due to ingestion of baking soda
b. Baby Raggio who has had severe vomiting
c. Mrs. Rhodes who is on loop diuretics and a low-sodium diet
d. Mrs. Nicholls who is in renal failure

18. Methods of replacing serum chloride levels would not include:

a. Potassium chloride (KCl) supplements
b. Intravenous solutions of normal saline (NaCl 0.9%)
c. Ammonium chloride tablets (NH_4Cl)
d. Salty broths or electrolyte solutions containing chlorides

REFERENCES

American Heart Association. (1982). *Salt, sodium and blood pressure.* Dallas, Texas: American Heart Association.

Aumann, G., & Blake, G. (1982). Ritodrine hydrochloride in the control of premature labor. *JOGN, 11*(2), 75–79.

Bullock, B., & Rosendahl, P. (1984). *Pathophysiology.* Boston: Little, Brown.

Chan, J. (1978). Clinical disorders of sodium, potassium, chloride, and sulfur metabolism: Diagnostic approach to children. *Urology, 12*(11), 504–508.

Culpepper, M., et al. (1986). Why is the serum sodium low? *Patient Care, 20*(7), 94–110.

Darby, W. (1980). Why salt? How much? *Contemporary Nutrition, 5*(6), 1–2.

Felver, L. (1980). Understanding the electrolyte maze. *AJN, 80*(9), 1591–1595.

Goldstein, C., Braunstein, S., & Goldfarb, S. (1983). Idiopathic syndrome of inappropriate antidiuretic hormone secretion possibly related to advanced age. *Annals of Internal Medicine, 99,* 185–188.

Govoni, L., & Hayes, J. (1985). *Drugs and nursing implications* (5th ed.). Norwalk, CT: Appleton-Century-Crofts.

Hill, M. (1979). Helping the hypertensive patient control sodium intake. *AJN, 79*(5), 907–909.

Holum, J. (1983). *Elements of general and biological chemistry* (6th ed.). New York: John Wiley & Sons.

Jacobs, D., Kasten, B., DeMott, W., & Wolfson, W. (1984). *Laboratory test handbook with DRG index.* St. Louis: Mosby/Lexi.

Keithley, J., & Fraulini, K. (1982). What's behind that IV line? *Nursing 82, 12*(3), 33–42.

Licht, J., et al. (1983). Diuretic regimens in essential hypertension: A comparison of hypokalemic effects, blood pressure control, and cost. *Archives of Internal Medicine, 143,* 1694–1699.

Luft, F., et al. (1984). Influence of home monitoring on compliance with a reduced sodium intake. Archives of Internal Medicine, *144*(10), 1963–1965.

Metheny, N., & Snively, W. (1978). Perioperative fluids and electrolytes. *AJN, 78*(5), 840–845.

Narins, R., et al. (1985). Renal retention of potassium in fruit. *NEJM, 313*(9), 582–583.

Pflaum, S. (1979). Investigation of intake–output as a means of assessing body fluid balance. *Heart-Lung, 8,* 495–498.

Sandifer, M. (1983). Hyponatremia due to psychotropic drugs. *Journal of Clinical Psychiatry, 44,* 301–303.

Sheckel, S. (1980). Contracting with patient-selecting reinforcers. *AJN, 80*(9), 1596–1599.

Slawson, M., & Slawson, S. (1985). Problem ingredients in OTCs. *RN, 48*(4), 53–61.

Smithline, N., & Gardner, K. (1976). Gaps—Anionic and osmolal. *JAMA, 236,* 1594–1597.

Struthers, A., Whitesmith, R., & Reid, J. (1983). Prior thiazide diuretic treatment increases adrenalin-induced hypokalemia. *Lancet, 1,* 1358–1360.

Tietz, N. (Ed.). (1983). *Clinical guide to laboratory tests.* Philadelphia: W.B. Saunders.

Wallach, J. (1986). *Interpretation of diagnostic tests.* Boston: Little, Brown.

Weil, M., & Rackow, E. (1984). A Guide to volume repletion. *Emergency Medicine, 16*(8), 101–110.

Wink, D. (1983). Fluid-induced hyponatremia in infancy. *AJN, 83*(5), 765–767.

6

Arterial Blood Gases (ABG)

- pH of the Blood
- P_{CO_2} (Partial Pressure of Carbon Dioxide)
- Serum Bicarbonate (HCO_3^-) and CO_2
- P_{O_2} (Partial Pressure of Oxygen)
- Oxygen Saturation
- Lactic Acid or Blood Lactate

OBJECTIVES

1. Demonstrate the four-step sequence in interpreting the meaning of arterial blood gas reports to determine the four primary acid–base imbalances.
2. Explain how the buffering system, the lungs, and the kidneys maintain the serum bicarbonate to carbonic acid ratio of 20:1.
3. Describe the nurse's role when arterial blood gases are drawn.
4. Explain how reference values for blood gases are altered in pregnancy and in the newborn period.
5. Explain the physiological basis for the symptoms of acidosis and alkalosis, both metabolic and respiratory in origin.
6. Identify possible nursing diagnoses for clients with increased and decreased P_{CO_2} levels (respiratory alkalosis and acidosis).
7. Identify the possible nursing diagnoses for clients with increased or decreased serum bicarbonate levels (metabolic alkalosis and acidosis).
8. Explain how electrolytes alter and are altered by changes in the acid–base balance.
9. Explain the concept of the anion gap in relationship to the various kinds of metabolic acidosis.
10. Explain why high concentrations of oxygen may be dangerous for the client with a low P_{O_2} and a high P_{CO_2}.

11. Demonstrate how PO_2 and PCO_2 levels are utilized by the nurse to assist with treatment of respiratory problems.
12. Describe the basic pathological process that produces increased lactic acid in the serum.

This chapter begins with an introductory section about acid–base imbalances. Several charts help to show the fundamental differences in the four primary acid–base imbalances. After this general discussion, pH, PCO_2, and bicarbonate tests are presented first due to their major significance in acid–base imbalances. The last part of the chapter discusses PO_2 and oxygen saturation and measurement of lactic acid as an assessment of dangerous hypoxia at the cellular level.

Each laboratory measurement is discussed as a separate test so that the reader can better understand the clinical significance of both increases and decreases in each value. As in other chapters, possible nursing diagnoses for each change in laboratory test are discussed after the clinical significance.

PURPOSE OF BLOOD GASES

Only the PO_2 and the PCO_2 measurements actually measure blood gases. The "P" before the O_2 and CO_2 stands for the partial pressure of the gases. The respiratory gases include nitrogen, oxygen, carbon dioxide, and water vapor. Dalton's *law of partial pressure* states that the total pressure exerted by a mixture of gases is the sum of the individual partial pressure (Miller & Sherman, 1977). Table 6–1 shows the percentage of gases in the blood and how this determines the partial pressure of each.

Blood gases are used to determine the respiratory status or the acid–base balance of the client. If the primary focus is to evaluate the respiratory status of the client, then the PO_2, PCO_2, and pH levels, as well as sometimes the oxygen saturation, are the most important to evaluate. If the primary focus is to evaluate a metabolic acid–base imbalance, then the PO_2 has little significance. By looking first at the pH, then the PCO_2, and then the HCO_3^-, one can figure out whether the acidosis is either respiratory or metabolic in origin. Signor and Del Bueno (1982) have developed decision trees based on these three components. In some confusing clinical situations,

TABLE 6-1. FOUR GASES IN ARTERIAL BLOOD AT SEA LEVEL

Gas	Percentage of Gas	Partial Pressure (mm Hg)
Nitrogen (not measured)	75.5	574
Oxygen	13.0	99—venous drops to 40 mm Hg
Carbon dioxide	5.3	40—venous rises to 46 mm Hg
Water vapor (not measured)	6.2	47
Totals	100.00	760

Note that the total pressure exerted by a mixture of gases is the sum of the individual partial pressures. See Holum (1983) and Miller and Sherman (1977, 1978a, b) for measurements of gases in atmosphere and in alveolar air.

TABLE 6-2. FOUR STEPS TO DETERMINE THE FOUR PRIMARY ACID-BASE IMBALANCES

Step 1: *Look at pH*	Is the pH above 7.45? If so, the client is alkalotic. Go to Step 2. Is the pH below 7.35? If so, the client is acidotic. Go to Step 3.
Step 2: When the pH is elevated	Is the P_{CO_2} below 40 mm Hg? If so, the alkalosis is respiratory in origin. Is the P_{CO_2} above 40 mm Hg or in the normal range? If so, the alkalosis is not respiratory in origin. Look for metabolic causes. Go to Step 4.
Step 3: When the pH is decreased	Is the P_{CO_2} above 40 mm Hg? If so, the acidosis is respiratory. Is the P_{CO_2} below 40 mm Hg or normal? If so, the acidosis is metabolic in origin. Go to Step 4.
Step 4: Looking at the bicarbon-ate in relation to the pH	Note that in metabolic acidosis, both the pH and the bicarbonate level are decreased. In metabolic alkalosis, both the pH and the bicarbonate are elevated. (See Table 6-4 for compensation.)

Worthington (1979) and Glass and Jenkins (1983) include several case studies as practice for determining acid-base imbalances by looking at laboratory reports in a systematic manner.

clients may have a combination of acid–base disorders, but this chapter focuses on the four basic types. Table 6–2 summarizes the way to interpret blood gas results to determine the primary acid–base imbalance. The last part of the chapter discusses hypoxic states that are not directly related to acid–base imbalances.

SUMMARY OF ACID–BASE BALANCE

The normal pH of arterial blood is between 7.35 and 7.45, with 7.4 taken as the average. Varying a little from this narrow range can be disastrous. Many chemical reactions in the body do not function normally if the pH of the blood is not in the normal range (Holum, 1983). If the pH is below 7.35, this condition is called *acidosis*. If the pH is above 7.45, it is called *alkalosis*. As demonstrated in Table 6–2, if the increased or decreased pH is due to a marked change in the P_{CO_2}, then the acid–base imbalance is respiratory in origin; all other acid–base imbalances are considered metabolic.

Understanding how P_{CO_2} and bicarbonate (HCO_3^-) function in the buffering system of the body is necessary if one is to be able to interpret the meaning of abnormal blood gas values. Buffer systems act as chemical sponges, which can give off or absorb hydrogen ions. There are minor buffers in the bloodstream, such as phosphates and proteins, but these are not measured in evaluating the acid–base balance. The major buffer system is the carbonic acid–bicarbonate buffer system. The carbonic acid level is measured indirectly by the P_{CO_2} level and the bicarbonate level by the bicarbonate level or the total carbon dioxide content (Table 6–3). This carbonic acid–bicarbonate buffer system is often referred to as the *20:1 ratio,* which means one part of carbonic acid for each twenty parts of bicarbonate.

Note that, although the carbonic acid level is not measured directly, it can be figured out because it is always 3% of the P_{CO_2}. Hence a P_{CO_2} of 40 mm Hg indicates 1.2 mEq of carbonic acid in the serum, which must be balanced by 20 parts of bicarbonate or 24 mEq (Shrake, 1979). As long as this ratio is maintained, whether it is 40 to 2 or 10 to 0.5, the pH of the blood stays in the normal range. Thus if the carbonic acid level changes, the kidneys try to compensate by changing the bicar-

TABLE 6–3. THREE LABORATORY TESTS THAT MEASURE THE BICARBONATE-CARBONIC ACID BUFFER SYSTEM

$CO_2 + H_2O$	$\rightleftarrows$	H_2CO_3	$\rightleftarrows$	H	+	HCO_3^-
↓		↓		↓		↓
Carbon dioxide measured by P_{CO_2} (40 mm Hg) Test 2		Carbonic acid not measured directly but is always 3% of P_{CO_2} or 3% × 40 mm Hg = 1.2 mEq		Concentration of hydrogen ions measured by pH (7.35–7.45) Test 1		Bicarbonate level measured by serum bicarbonate (24 mEq) Test 3

P_{CO_2} controlled by lungs   Hydrogen, bicarbonate, and other electrolytes controlled by kidneys

Test 1: pH; Test 2: P_{CO_2}; Test 3: serum bicarbonate

A bicarbonate level of 24 mEq and a P_{CO_2} of 40 mm Hg (carbonic acid of 1.2 mEq) is the desirable 20:1 ratio that maintains the pH of the serum between 7.35 and 7.45.
Modified from diagrams in Shrake (1979), Miller and Sherman (1977), and Holum (1983).

bonate level. For example, because a P_{CO_2} of 34 reflects a carbonic acid level of 1 mEq (34 times 3% equals 1.02), the bicarbonate level must drop to 20 mEq to keep a 20:1 ratio. If the bicarbonate level changes, the lungs change the carbonic acid level, but this type of compensation is more limited because the lungs must continue to function for oxygen exchange.

Only the lungs control the regulation of P_{CO_2}. In the bloodstream, carbon dioxide combines with water to form carbonic acid. If more P_{CO_2} is retained, this condition results in more carbonic acid and hence the person tends toward acidosis. If more carbon dioxide is blown off (hyperventilation), there is less carbonic acid in the bloodstream and the person tends toward alkalosis. By this mechanism, the lungs can shift the pH of the blood in just a few minutes.

The kidneys are also instrumental in the regulation of the pH of the bloodstream. Not only do the kidneys constantly excrete hydrogen ions, but they also control the serum bicarbonate level, as well as retaining or excreting sodium, potassium, and chloride ions. For major corrective shifts, it may take the kidneys several days to restore the pH to normal.

If all these regulatory mechanisms—buffer systems, lungs, and kidneys—are not successful in restoring the pH, clients go with varying speeds either into acidosis, leading to coma and death, or into alkalosis with irritability, tetany, and sometimes death. As a general rule, acidotic states are usually more life threatening than alkalotic states (Miller & Sherman, 1978a).

By looking at three laboratory tests, one can usually determine whether the acid–base imbalance is respiratory or metabolic in origin. Table 6–4 shows the laboratory findings for each of the four basic types of acid–base imbalance *before* compensation occurs, and how compensation changes the laboratory tests. In the actual clinical situation, because the client may have more than one imbalance, a chart does not always pinpoint the origin of the difficulty.

Table 6–4 makes the fundamental difference between respiratory and metabolic acid–base imbalances easy to see. If there is a marked increase or decrease in P_{CO_2}, the acid–base imbalance is respiratory in origin. Otherwise, the imbalance is metabolic, and the change in the bicarbonate level has shifted the pH. Table 6–5 summarizes the common reasons for each type of acid–base imbalance.

TABLE 6-4. CHANGES IN pH, Pco₂, AND HCO₃⁻ AND THE COMPENSATORY MECHANISMS IN ACID-BASE IMBALANCES

	pH	P_{CO_2}	HCO_3^-	Compensation
Respiratory alkalosis	↑	↓	Normal until compensation	Kidneys will eventually reduce HCO_3^- (takes few days to complete)
Metabolic alkalosis	↑	Normal unless lungs compensate	↑	Lungs will try to increase P_{CO_2} slightly. Can do quickly
Respiratory acidosis	↓	↑	Normal until kidneys compensate	Kidneys will eventually retain more HCO_3^-. Takes a few days to complete
Metabolic acidosis	↓	Normal until lungs compensate	↓	Lungs will usually reduce P_{CO_2}. Can do quickly

See text for full explanation. Note that: (1) in respiratory alkalosis and respiratory acidosis, the pH and P_{CO_2} vary inversely; (2) in metabolic alkalosis and metabolic acidosis, the pH and HCO_3^- rise or fall together; (3) the kidneys try to compensate for respiratory imbalances, but the compensation takes several days; and (4) the lungs try to compensate for metabolic imbalances, and their compensation is accomplished in a few minutes, but it is limited.

TABLE 6-5. COMMON REASONS FOR ACID-BASE IMBALANCES

Primary Acid-Base Imbalance	Description of Imbalance	Common Reasons for Imbalance
Respiratory alkalosis	Decrease in P_{CO_2} due to hyperventilation	Anxiety Fever, pain, hypoxia Improperly adjusted respirator
Respiratory acidosis	Increase in P_{CO_2} due to hypoventilation	Chronic lung disease that causes CO_2 retention Respiratory depression from drugs or anesthesia
Metabolic alkalosis	Increase in serum bicarbonate (HCO_3) due to increased intake of bicarbonate or increased loss of chlorides, hydrogen, or potassium ions	Vomiting or gastric suctioning, which causes loss of hydrogen, chloride, and potassium ions Ingestion or infusion of soda bicarbonate
Metabolic acidosis	Decrease in serum bicarbonate due to excess acid production, loss of bicarbonate, or increase in serum chloride levels	Excess acids such as ketone bodies in diabetic acidosis or lactic acid in cardiac arrest Loss of bicarbonate via intestines Increase in serum chloride level—renal failure

See text for explanations and Wallach (1986) for more details.

**TABLE 6-6. POSSIBLE CHANGES IN ELECTROLYTES AND URINE pH
FOR ACID-BASE IMBALANCES**

	Sodium (Na$^+$)	Potassium (K$^+$)	Chloride (Cl$^-$)	Urine pH
Respiratory alkalosis	Usually not changed	May be low if alkalosis persists	Will be increased when HCO$_3^-$ decreases for compensation	High if chronic problem
Metabolic alkalosis	Usually not changed	Low	Low	High or paradoxically pH may continue low
Respiratory acidosis	Usually not changed	May be a little increased	In compensation, the increase in HCO$_3^-$ causes decrease in Cl	Low. Many H$^+$ ions excreted
Metabolic acidosis	Total Na$^+$ is low if diuresis as in diabetic acidosis, serum levels may be normal in some states	May be high although cellular deficit of K$^+$. Serum potassium raises about 0.6 mEq per liter for each 0.1 decrease in pH	May increase to replace lost HCO$_3^-$. If unmeasured anions are high, Cl$^-$ may decrease or be normal	Very low pH as kidneys try to excrete H$^+$ ions

Note: See Chapter 5 for discussion on electrolytes and anion gap and Chapter 3 for urine pH. Also see Chan (1978) for pediatric problems, Jacobs et al. (1984) and Wallach (1986) for details on adult medical conditions.

If the acidosis or alkalosis is metabolic in origin, or if the respiratory problem is chronic enough for the kidneys to be involved, it is also important to look at the laboratory tests for electrolytes. (Refer to Chapter 5 to review (1) the inverse relationship between chloride (Cl$^-$) and the bicarbonate (HCO$_3^-$) ions, (2) the concept about the anion gap, and (3) why hyperkalemia is associated with acidotic states and hypokalemia with alkalotic states. In Chapter 3 there is a discussion about the changes of the urine pH in the different types of acidosis and alkalosis.) Table 6–6 shows the usual electrolyte abnormalities for each of the four primary types of acid–base imbalances.

ARTERIAL BLOOD GASES IN GENERAL

Preparation of Client and Collection of Sample

The physician or other clinician skilled in arterial puncture must collect the blood sample, which can be drawn from the radial, brachial, or femoral arteries. In most hospitals only physicians are allowed to do femoral punctures, whereas nurses with special training may do radial or brachial punctures.

Sumner (1980) gives nurses tips on how to do arterial punctures. The site must be disinfected and allowed to dry. Clients need to be told that the stick will be momentarily painful. If they are very afraid of the procedure or if the attempt to obtain a specimen is prolonged, clients may hyperventilate due to anxiety, and they can thus alter test results. If arterial blood samples are needed frequently, clients usually have an arterial catheter in place. Nurses usually obtain specimens from an arterial line. In neonates, arterial sampling can be done via an umbilical catheter.

After being collected in an airtight, heparinized syringe, the blood must be packed in ice for transport to the laboratory. The airtight container and the ice help to prevent the loss of gases from the sample. Special care units may have facilities for testing the sample immediately in the unit. Biswas et al. (1982) demonstrated that it is necessary to expel all air bubbles within 2 minutes and put the sample on ice if the test is not done within 10 minutes from collection.

The amount of blood needed for arterial blood gases depends on the technique used. Although some of the blood gas analyzers can test less than 0.5 ml of blood, accuracy is more assured with a minimum of 3 ml. Some laboratories may require 5–10 ml of blood. Check with the individual laboratory as to how much heparin should be in the syringe. Too much heparin with a small sample causes inaccurate results.

After the sample is drawn, continuous pressure should be applied to the puncture site for at least 5 minutes if the radial artery is used and 10 minutes for the femoral. If the client has any bleeding problems, the pressure dressing should be taped on and left for several hours.

It is important to note on the laboratory slip whether the client was receiving oxygen at the time the sample was drawn, because there may be quite a difference in PO_2 if the client is having oxygen therapy as opposed to breathing room air. The nurse should note how long the client has been on a specific amount of oxygen, such as "25 minutes on 2 liters by nasal cannula." If the client is on assisted ventilation, the settings for the respirator should be noted in case changes need to be made later. The temperature of the client should also be noted because a fever increases the metabolic rate.

If arterial blood cannot be obtained, capillary blood samples may be used. The area should be warmed for 5 minutes before the sample is taken. The warmed ear site is used in children and adults, whereas the warmed heel is used for infants. (See Chapter 1 for the heel stick technique.)

Continuous Monitoring of Oxygen Levels

A skin surface electrode can continuously monitor the oxygen level in the blood. Dingle et al. (1980) describe this monitoring method for the neonate. The monitor (a Hutch electrode) measures the amount of oxygen diffusing through the skin. The monitor is particularly useful for newborns because the infant's skin is thin with little subcutaneous fat as compared to an adult's. Finger probes and ear probes are used for adults. A more sophisticated instrument is used with a pulmonary catheter and is appropriate for continuous monitoring of mixed venous oxygen saturation (SvO_2 monitoring). Shively and Clark (1986) note that use of this instrument will decrease the need for arterial blood gases in critically ill clients because trends in oxygenation status can be monitored continuously.

■ pH OF THE BLOOD

The pH test measures the alkalinity or acidity of the blood. For chemical solutions, a pH of 7 is the neutral point; above 7 is alkaline and below 7 is acid. For the blood pH, the neutral point is 7.4. It is critical that the blood pH remain within a narrow range because many enzymes and other physiological processes do not function normally when the pH is altered.

TABLE 6-7. RELATIONSHIP OF APGAR SCORES IN NEWBORN TO pH LEVEL

Sign	Score 0	Score 1	Score 2
Heart rate	Absent	Below 100	Over 100
Respiratory rate	Absent	Slow, irregular, hypo-ventilate	Good, crying lustily
Muscle tone	Flaccid	Some flexion of extremities	Active motion/well flexed
Reflexes	No response	Cry, some motion, grimace	Vigorous cry
Color	Blue, pale	Body pink/hands and feet blue	Completely pink

Apgar Score	Estimate of pH
7 or above	7.27
6 or below	7.22

Note: the Apgar score is a simple and practical method to assess the overall physical status of the infant immediately after delivery. It is done at 1 minute and 5 minutes after birth. Wallach (1983) notes fetal blood pH provides best correlation with fetal outcome but in 20% of infants the acid–base status may be misleading.

References Values for pH

Adult	7.35–7.45 (arterial)
	7.30–7.41 (venous)
Newborn	7.3–7.4 (arterial)
	See Table 6–7 for pH in newborns

Increased pH of Arterial Blood (Alkalosis)

Clinical Significance. An increased serum pH indicates that the client is in a state of alkalosis. To determine whether the alkalosis is respiratory or metabolic in origin, it is necessary to look at the Pco_2 and the serum bicarbonate (HCO_3^-) level. If the alkalosis is respiratory in origin, the Pco_2 is markedly decreased. If the alkalosis is metabolic in origin, the serum bicarbonate (HCO_3^-) level is markedly elevated. The common clinical situations that would cause these changes and the reference values are discussed under the Pco_2 and the HCO_3^- tests.

POSSIBLE NURSING DIAGNOSES RELATED TO ALKALOTIC STATES

Potential for Injury due to Neuromuscular Irritability and Possible Tetany

Specific nursing implications depend on whether the alkalosis is respiratory or metabolic in origin. Some general symptoms of both types of alkalosis include tingling in the extremities or nose, facial twitching, light-headedness, muscle tremors, and tetany. The neuromuscular irritability in alkalotic states occurs because calcium is less soluble in an alkaline medium. Many of the symptoms of alkalosis are those of hypocalcemia. (See Chapter 7 on hypocalcemia.) Clients must be protected from falls of convulsive movements.

Alterations in Breathing Patterns
In respiratory alkalosis the respiratory rate is high because hyperventilation is the cause of the alkalosis. Factors causing hyperventilation, an ineffective breathing pattern, are discussed in the section on P_{CO_2} levels. In metabolic alkalosis the respiratory rate is normal to slightly depressed, with slow and shallow breaths. The depressed respirations in metabolic alkalosis is an attempt by the lungs to retain more P_{CO_2} to balance the increased serum bicarbonate level. The effect on the breathing pattern is of minimal importance as discussed under the section on metabolic alkalosis.

Decreased pH of Arterial Blood (Acidosis)

Clinical Significance. A decreased serum pH indicates that the client is in a state of acidosis. To determine whether the acidosis is respiratory or metabolic in origin, it is necessary to look at the P_{CO_2} and the serum bicarbonate (HCO_3^-) level. In respiratory acidosis the P_{CO_2} is increased. In metabolic acidosis the serum bicarbonate level is lower than normal. Each type of acidosis is covered in the discussion about P_{CO_2} and serum bicarbonate levels. Note in Table 6–7 that newborns with low Apgar scores have a proportionately low pH.

POSSIBLE NURSING DIAGNOSES RELATED TO ACIDOTIC STATES

Potential for Alteration in Sensory-Perceptual Awareness Related to Change in Level of Consciousness
Specific nursing implications depend on whether the acidosis is respiratory or metabolic in nature. General symptoms for both types of acidosis include headaches, weakness, lethargy, and confusion. The level of consciousness is depressed as the acidotic state worsens. Unless the acidotic state is corrected, drowsiness leads from a stuporous state, to coma, and eventually to death.

Alterations in Breathing Patterns
As with alkalotic states, the respiratory patterns are exactly the opposite for the two types of acidosis. In respiratory acidosis, the respiratory rate is depressed because hypoventilation is the cause of respiratory acidosis. An ineffective breathing pattern is the major focus of care. In metabolic acidosis, the respiratory rate is faster and deeper than normal (Kussmaul's respirations) because the lungs are trying to compensate for the decreased serum pH by blowing off more carbon dioxide. Because the rate is a compensatory one the breathing pattern is not a focus of care.

■ P_{CO_2} (PARTIAL PRESSURE OF CARBON DIOXIDE)

The P_{CO_2} test measures the partial pressure of carbon dioxide in the arterial blood. As noted earlier, when carbon dioxide is transported in serum, much of it is combined with water to form carbonic acid ($H_2CO_3^-$), which dissociates into bicarbonate (HCO_3^-) and hydrogen (H^+) ions. The actual carbonic acid level in the serum is not measured, but it can always be determined by multiplying the P_{CO_2} by 3%. A P_{CO_2} of 40 mm Hg is 1.2 mEq of carbonic acid ($40 \times 3\%$) (Shrake, 1979). Because the end result is an increase in the amount of free hydrogen ions, an increase in the P_{CO_2} causes the blood pH to drop below 7.35. The special preparation for obtaining blood gases was covered earlier in this chapter.

Reference Values for P_{CO_2}

Adult	35–45 mm Hg (arterial)
	41–51 mm Hg (venous)
	Values are slightly lower in women (Tietz, 1983)
Pregnancy	Values may be as low as 30 mm Hg by the end of the second trimester. 30–37 mm Hg is normal for pregnancy because of hyperventilation. The kidneys compensate by excreting more bicarbonate, so that the pH of around 7.4 is maintained. Research studies have suggested that progesterone may be the cause of the hyperventilation in pregnancy (Milne, 1979)
Altitude	At higher altitudes the atmospheric pressure is less, so the partial pressure of carbon dioxide is proportionally reduced (see discussion for P_{O_2} values)

Increased P_{CO_2} (Hypercarbia or Hypercapnia)

Clinical Significance in Respiratory Acidosis. An increased P_{CO_2} level indicates that the normal amount of carbon dioxide is not being blown off. Any situation that causes hypoventilation, such as a drug overdose that results in respiratory depression, causes an elevated P_{CO_2}. Higher-than-normal P_{CO_2} levels are also present in certain chronic lung conditions where the exchange of carbon dioxide and oxygen is impaired. Clients with chronic obstructive lung disease may have both hypoxia and hypercarbia (elevated P_{CO_2}), although the latter is not always associated with hypoxia. Some acute lung dysfunctions, such as pneumonia, may cause hypoxia but not an elevated P_{CO_2}. Hypoxia does not always lead to a retention of carbon dioxide for two basic reasons: First, carbon dioxide diffuses more readily across alveolar surfaces than does oxygen, so an impairment of respiratory function results in a fall of P_{O_2} before the P_{CO_2} changes. Second, hypoxia is a stimulus for breathing (Pavlin & Hornbein, 1978). If the lungs can respond to the low oxygen level by increasing the respiratory rate, the carbon dioxide level may stay normal or drop to below normal due to the hyperventilation.

The type of hypoventilation that causes an increased P_{CO_2} can be very transitory and self-limiting, such as when the breath is held. The resultant high level of P_{CO_2} cannot be maintained because it becomes an overpowering stimulus for taking a breath—one cannot commit suicide by holding one's breath. Clients with chronic lung disease who have high carbon dioxide levels no longer use carbon dioxide as a stimulus for breathing. Instead, hypoxia becomes the primary stimulus for breathing, and the kidneys compensate for the gradual increase in P_{CO_2} level by increasing the serum bicarbonate level. The normal blood pH is maintained as long as the kidneys can keep the 20:1 ratio of bicarbonate to carbonic acid. It takes the kidneys several days to compensate for increasing P_{CO_2} levels, so a quick increase in P_{CO_2}, or acute respiratory failure, leads to respiratory acidosis.

Clinical Significance in Metabolic Alkalosis. In metabolic alkalosis, the P_{CO_2} is usually more than 40 mm Hg because the lungs are attempting to reestablish the bicarbonate–carbonic acid ratio by increasing the carbonic acid to match the increased serum bicarbonate. This compensatory hypoventilation is not very effective because the respiratory rate cannot be depressed very much without creating hypoxia.

POSSIBLE NURSING DIAGNOSES RELATED TO HYPERCAPNIA

Alteration in Sensory–Perceptual Awareness Related to Change in Level of Consciousness

Nurses must always be aware of the early signs of increasing P_{CO_2} levels. The term CO_2 narcosis, another name for respiratory acidosis, gives a clue that carbon dioxide can be a central nervous system depressant. Early signs of increased P_{CO_2} may be headache, dizziness, and confusion. The confusion may progress to decreasing levels of consciousness until the patient is comatose. The treatment for respiratory depression may include assisted ventilation until the underlying pathophysiology can be medically treated. Nursing interventions are geared toward improving the respiratory status. Frequent arterial blood gases help to monitor the improvement of the client and ensure that increasing carbon dioxide levels are not occurring.

The seriousness of an elevated P_{CO_2} level can be evaluated only in relation to the amount of compensation that has occurred. For example, clients with chronic lung disease may have a higher-than-normal P_{CO_2} with a higher-than-normal bicarbonate level and a resulting normal pH. So they may not be in immediate danger. (In addition to looking at these three laboratory results, also look at the chloride level, which is lower than normal because the negative ion bicarbonate (HCO_3^-) is increased in the serum. See Chapter 5.) A drug that depresses the respiratory center, a respiratory infection, or some treatment that causes a lot of exertion may throw such compensated clients into respiratory acidosis, or CO_2 narcosis.

Potential for Injury in Clients with Chronic Obstructive Disease Related to Use of Oxygen and Sedatives

High doses of oxygen can be lethal for clients who have a chronically high P_{CO_2} because hypoxia has become the respiratory stimulus for the client. The medullary center no longer responds to high levels of P_{CO_2}, which is normally the primary stimulus for respiration, because the chronically elevated P_{CO_2} has made the center insensitive to carbon dioxide as a stimulus for breathing. The only stimulus for breathing is hypoxia. For clients with advanced emphysema, a P_{O_2} of 50–60 mm Hg is "normal." Their color may improve as the hypoxia is eliminated, but their respirations become slower and slower because they no longer have a stimulus to breathe. If these clients are not stimulated to breathe, the P_{CO_2} level rises even higher, and they may die in respiratory acidosis. Goldstein et al. (1984) found that supplemental oxygen could be given at night to clients who have *stable* but severe obstructive lung disease to prevent a fall of P_{O_2} with sleep. This use of O_2 is not for unstable or acutely ill clients.

Note also that very small doses of drugs, such as morphine or diazepam (Valium), can depress respirations to a serious degree, because the response to hypoxia is depressed (Pavlin & Hornbein, 1978). (See the discussion under Po_2 on ways to assess and intervene for hypoxia in both the client with acute and chronic respiratory problems.)

Decreased PCO₂

Clinicial Significance in Respiratory Alkalosis. Just as hypoventilation leads to an increased PCO_2 level, hyperventilation leads to a decreased PCO_2 level. (The terms hypocarbia or hypocapnia are rarely used.) Often hyperventilation is due to severe anxiety. Hysterical or semihysterical people tend to breathe very fast and deeply, with a lot of sighing. Physical conditions, such as fever, pain, or hypoxia, can also cause hyperventilation. No matter what the stimulus, the end result is that, if enough carbon dioxide is blown off to lower the PCO_2, the person will be in respiratory alkalosis.

Some clients may have a slightly low PCO_2 most of the time, but usually this form of chronic hyperventilation is not noticed until the person has an acute anxiety attack (Waites, 1978). It is unusual to see compensation for respiratory alkalosis because severe hyperventilation typically does not last long enough for the kidneys to begin to excrete extra bicarbonate. An exception, however, is the client on a respirator: An improperly adjusted respirator can be responsible for hyperventilation that continues over a long time.

Clinical Significance in Metabolic Acidosis. A lower-than-normal PCO_2 can also be a compensatory mechanism for metabolic acidosis. For example, clients in diabetic acidosis use up much of the bicarbonate buffer in their bloodstream to buffer the ketone bodies. The lungs try to restore the 20:1 ratio by reducing the PCO_2 and hence the carbonic acid part of the ratio (Kussmaul's respirations), but this compensation cannot offset the severe metabolic acidosis.

POSSIBLE NURSING DIAGNOSES RELATED TO HYPOCAPNIA

Alteration in Comfort Related to Neuromuscular Irritability

Most of the symptoms that result from a lowered PCO_2, which can be alarming to the client and to the nurse, can be explained on the basis of the effect of an alkaline pH on serum calcium levels. Because calcium is less soluble in an alkaline medium, less ionized calcium is available when the blood pH rises above normal. Hence the client has symptoms of hypocalcemia. (See Chapter 7 for the symptoms of hypocalcemia.) There may be tingling of the fingers, twitching, muscle tremors, carpopedal spasms, and even tetany. The person may feel light-headed and dizzy. If the hyperventilation is less severe and more of a chronic problem, the person may have only such symptoms as chronic exhaustion or diffuse weakness.

Nurses in emergency rooms or outpatient clinics are the ones most likely to see people who are seeking treatment because of hyperventilation (Sandvik, 1977). Recognizing that the client is hyperventilating is easy, but assessing whether it is due to anxiety or to physical causes may not be so easy. Ruling out fever, pain, or hypoxia as reason for the hyperventilation is important. (If the hyperventilation is due to an underlying metabolic acidosis, there will be no symptoms of alkalosis because the pH remains acid from the metabolic problem.)

Anxiety Related to Unknown Factors
If the hyperventilation is due to functional anxiety, nursing interventions can be instrumental in stopping the hyperventilation. The person needs to be reassured that slower breathing will decrease the symptoms. Breathing into a paper bag helps to increase the P_{CO_2} level. The nurse needs to maintain a calm, soothing environment so the person can gain control and reduce the feeling of anxiety. Hyperventilating may be a recurring problem that warrants a referral for counseling to help the person learn ways to deal with anxiety. If the anxiety level is high, the physician may order drugs to reduce the anxiety. Sometimes the client may need to be taught the proper way to do diaphragmatic breathing. The long-term goal is to help the person deal with the anxiety and to see how the anxiety has caused the breathing problem.

Ineffective Breathing Patterns Related to Hypoxia and Other Causes
The nurse needs to be aware of other situations where hyperventilating may occur. For example, a client in labor may not be doing the breathing exercises correctly and thus go into respiratory alkalosis. Also, clients on respirators need careful monitoring to make sure that the ventilation rate is not too fast. If hyperventilation is due to a stimulus such as fever, then therapeutic measures to reduce the fever will eliminate the hyperventilation. The most likely cause of respiratory alkalosis, other than anxiety, is hypoxia. See the discussion for P_{O_2} levels.

■ SERUM BICARBONATE (HCO_3^-) AND CO_2

Bicarbonate functions as a very important buffer in the bloodstream. To keep the bloodstream's pH between 7.35 and 7.45, the bicarbonate in it is kept at a 20:1 ratio to carbonic acid. The section on P_{CO_2} explained how changes in the P_{CO_2} cause changes in the bicarbonate level. Also, because bicarbonate and chloride are both negative ions in the serum, an increased retention of serum chloride means less retention of bicarbonate (Miller & Sherman, 1978b). Thus serum bicarbonate measurements are useful in both acid–base imbalances and electrolyte imbalances, and they are therefore a routine part of laboratory tests for either "electrolytes" or "arterial blood gases."

Direct and Indirect Methods to Measure Bicarbonate
There are several different laboratory methods to measure the serum bicarbonate level. Some laboratories may do direct measurements of the bicarbonate and report it as such. One indirect method involves measuring the total carbon dioxide content of the serum and calculating the bicarbonate level from this figure. An older method involves measuring the CO_2 combining power of the serum.

Nurses do not need to understand the technicalities of how these various tests are done, but it is important to use the reference values that correspond to the exact method used by a specific laboratory. There is less standardization of bicarbonate measurement than with the other electrolytes. If a laboratory report does not have any item marked "bicarbonate," look for something called "carbon dioxide content" or "carbon dioxide capacity," which reflect the bicarbonate component of the blood. This CO_2 content is different than the P_{CO_2} of blood gases.

Meaning of "Base Excess" or "Base Deficit"

Some laboratories also measure the total buffer base of the body and report this as a "base deficit" or a "base excess." The *buffer base* refers to all the buffer ions in the serum, including not only bicarbonate but also phosphates, hemoglobin, and plasma proteins. The total buffers are usually around 50 mEq/L, but the laboratory just reports so many minus or plus milliequivalents. The normal would be a -2 mEq to a $+2$ mEq. More than a -2 mEq means a *base deficit,* which correlates to a decrease in bicarbonate levels. A result of over 2 mEq signifies a *base excess,* which correlates to an increased bicarbonate level.

Reference Values for Bicarbonate

Adult	24–30 mEq/L
Pregnancy	Falls early in pregnancy by an amount consistent with the fall in the P_{CO_2}. A P_{CO_2} of 34 mm Hg is balanced with a bicarbonate of around 20 mEq to keep the pH around 7.4
Newborn	20–26 mEq/L (Prematures may have even lower reference values)
Children	Slightly lower references than those for adults
Base excess or base deficit	-2 to $+2$ mEq/L

Bicarbonate levels measured by carbon dioxide content.

Increased Serum Bicarbonate Level (Base Excess)

Clinical Significance in Metabolic Alkalosis. The loss of hydrogen, potassium, and chloride ions all contribute to the development of metabolic alkalosis. First of all, any loss of hydrogen ions causes a proportional increase in the bicarbonate side of the bicarbonate–carbonic acid buffering system. Second, as discussed in Chapter 5, when potassium is low in the serum, the kidneys are unable to excrete bicarbonate normally. Third, when chloride, a negative ion, is decreased in the bloodstream, another negative ion is needed to keep the positive and negative ions balanced in the serum (Chan, 1978). Thus the kidneys cause a retention of bicarbonate to replace the missing chloride.

The most common reason for an increase in the bicarbonate level is a loss of gastric contents. Clients who vomit or who have nasogastric suctioning without proper potassium chloride replacement (KCl) are prone to have high bicarbonate levels. Clients on diuretics may also lose abnormal amounts of chloride and potassium and thus develop metabolic alkalosis.

An increase in the serum bicarbonate level can also occur with the ingestion of large amounts of sodium bicarbonate. As a home remedy, clients may take baking soda (soda bicarbonate), which is systemically absorbed. Commercial antacids, such as Maalox, are usually not systemically absorbed, so they do not cause alkalosis, but they may contribute to metabolic alkalosis if there is inadequate renal function. Alkalosis can also occur from overdosage with intravenous soda bicarbonate to treat acidosis. Usually this rebound effect is not a serious problem.

Clinical Significance in Respiratory Acidosis. An increased serum bicarbonate level is a compensatory mechanism for the elevated PCO_2 of the client with chronic lung disease. In this situation, the serum chloride is decreased because the negative ion bicarbonate is increased. The increased bicarbonate level is necessary to keep the pH of the serum normal.

POSSIBLE NURSING DIAGNOSES RELATED TO ELEVATED BICARBONATE LEVELS

Potential for Injury Related to Neuromuscular Irritability
Usually clients in metabolic alkalosis do not have many symptoms directly related to the acid–base imbalance. Their respirations may be a little slow because their lungs are trying to compensate by conserving some carbon dioxide. The change in their respiratory rate is usually too slight to be clinically significant. Other symptoms would be related to the decreased solubility of calcium in an alkaline pH. As with respiratory alkalosis, clients may experience neuromuscular irritability, tingling in the fingers, twitching of the nose or lips, and even tetany or convulsions if the alkalosis is not corrected. Safety measures should be instituted.

Potential for Alterations in Cardiac Output Related to Arrhythmias
Because hypokalemia is associated with metabolic alkalosis the client must be monitored for cardiac arrhythmias and will most likely need both potassium and chloride replacement (Table 6–5). Nursing implications for potassium chloride administration were covered in the last chapter. The client may also be given isotonic solutions to intravenously replenish the loss of chlorides. Fruit juices and broth may be given in less severe depletions of chloride and potassium.

Lack of Knowledge Regarding Potential Danger of Sodium Bicarbonate
If the client has a history of increased intake of soda bicarbonate, then stopping the ingestion is usually enough. Clients need to be taught that baking soda is not a desirable antacid because it is absorbed into the bloodstream. Ammonium chloride, although a systemic acidifier, is rarely used to counteract alkalosis. Determining and correcting the reason for the increased bicarbonate is usually sufficient.

Decreased Serum Bicarbonate Level (Base Deficit)

Clinical Significance in Metabolic Acidosis. Unless the client has a low PCO_2, and thus a low serum bicarbonate level as compensation, a decrease in the serum bicarbonate level is an indication that the client has some type of metabolic acidosis. The severity of the acidotic state depends on how low the blood pH has dropped.

The decrease in serum bicarbonate levels that occurs in metabolic acidotic states can be due to:

1. Utilization of the bicarbonate to buffer acids, such as excessive lactate, ketone bodies, or other toxic metabolics, that contain hydrogen ions (the most common type of metabolic acidosis seen clinically)
2. A primary loss of bicarbonate
3. An increase in serum chloride level

Increased Production of Acids. In a normal state of health, as acids are produced or introduced into the body, they are neutralized by the bicarbonate–carbonic acid buffering system and eventually excreted by the kidneys. With a sudden increase in acids in certain pathological states, the kidneys do not have enough time to excrete the acids or enough bicarbonate to neutralize them.

1. In diabetic acidosis, the acids produced are the ketone bodies
2. In shock, the tissue hypoxia results in an excessive buildup of lactic acid (see test for lactic acid at end of chapter)
3. In renal failure, or in severe dehydration, the kidneys can no longer excrete hydrogen ions or acids such as the phosphates and sulfates
4. In cardiac arrest, there is an immediate buildup of lactic acid (as well as a high PCO_2, so the client has both respiratory and metabolic acidosis)
5. Aspirin overdose floods the system with an acid. (Initially the ASA acts as a respiratory stimulant causing some respiratory alkalosis, but the end result may be acidosis)

CONCEPT OF ANION GAP. The lactates, phosphates, ketone bodies, and other acids that can cause metabolic acidosis are negative ions (anions) in the bloodstream. So an increase in these acids increase the anion gap, which is the amount of unmeasured negative ions or anions in the bloodstream (see Chapter 5). It is determined by comparing the total amount of positive ions in the serum (primarily sodium and potassium) with the total amount of negative ions in the serum (primarily chloride and bicarbonate). When the total positive and the negative ions are compared in the bloodstream, there is a gap because one type of negative ions, namely the acids, are not measured. Usually, the unmeasured acids account for about 8–16 mEq of the total negative ions (Wallach, 1986).

In metabolic acidosis the increase in the negative ions of ketoacids, lactate, phosphate, sulfate, or other acids makes the anion gap larger because more unmeasured negative ions are present in the bloodstream. The anion gap is useful in distinguishing this first type of metabolic acidosis from the other two types because in them there is no increase in the acids that comprise the unmeasured negative ions and therefore no increase in anion gap (Smithline & Gardner, 1976).

Primary Loss of Bicarbonate. A primary loss of bicarbonate can occur with gastrointestinal losses below the pylorus because the intestinal tract and pancreatic secretions are rich in bicarbonate. (As a general rule, gastrointestinal losses above the pylorus, such as vomiting or gastric suctioning, tend to cause alkalosis due to the loss of hydrogen, potassium, and chloride ions. So alkalosis is related to vomiting and acidosis to diarrhea. However, dehydration from either vomiting or diarrhea is likely to result in acidosis due to the kidneys' inability to excrete acid by-products.) The primary loss of bicarbonate (a negative ion) leads to an increased chloride level to keep the positive negative charges balanced in the serum. The anion gap does not increase.

An Increase in the Serum Chloride Level. A primary increase in the serum chloride level means that another negative ion, bicarbonate, must be proportionally decreased. The lowering of the serum bicarbonate level keeps the electrical charges of the serum electrolytes balanced, but it creates acidosis because the buffering ability of the serum is decreased.

This third type of metabolic acidosis (hyperchloremic acidosis) is a much less common clinical occurrence than the first two types. High doses of chlorides in intravenous therapy may raise the serum chloride level. Also, certain types of renal failure result in an inability to properly excrete chloride ions.

POSSIBLE NURSING DIAGNOSES RELATED TO ACIDOTIC STATES

Potential for Injury Related to Alterations in Sensory Perceptions and Level of Consciousness

It is important for nurses to recognize early symptoms of acidosis, because severe acidosis can be life threatening. When a client has a lowered serum bicarbonate level that is creating metabolic acidosis, one of the key symptoms is hyperventilation. This deep and rapid respiration (Kussmaul's breathing) is an attempt to restore the 20:1 bicarbonate–carbonic acid ratio by decreasing the carbonic acid in the blood. (Recall that 3% of the PCO_2 is carried in the bloodstream as carbonic acid.) These fast and deep respirations may look like the client has "air hunger," but they really reflect an attempt to blow off extra PCO_2. This increased respiratory rate may be one of the first clues that the pH is dropping. As the pH drops lower, the client begins to exhibit signs of confusion, lethargy, and eventually coma. (A diabetic coma is a form of severe metabolic acidosis.) Newborn infants can develop severe metabolic acidosis if they are not kept warm and given sufficient calories. Acidosis can develop immediately, such as with a cardiac arrest, or very slowly, as in a client with renal failure. Some diabetics who do not take their insulin may go into a coma within a day or so. A young child who is diabetic may go into acidosis very quickly, whereas an adult diabetic may take several days to develop ketoacidosis. The important thing is to know the type of situation that can lead to metabolic acidosis so any changes can be detected early.

The major goal of treatment is to eliminate the cause of the acidosis. The cold-stressed newborn must be warmed and fed. The diabetic client requires insulin so that glucose, rather than fats, can be used as the primary source of energy. Clients in shock must have increased oxygen perfusion at the cellular level so that there is no longer the anerobic metabolism that has caused a buildup of lactic acid (see lactic acid measurement at end of this chapter).

Potential for Injury Related to Use of Sodium Bicarbonate Intravenously

Although the goal of treatment is to eliminate the cause of the acidosis, the client may need sodium bicarbonate intravenously to bring the serum pH back to normal immediately. For example, in cardiac arrest sodium bicarbonate used to be the first drug administered to counteract the severe metabolic and respiratory acidosis. Some experts do recommend waiting to give the sodium bicarbonate in a witnessed arrest until ABGs are obtained (Gever, 1984). Adrenalin, and many other drugs, are maximally effective only when the pH of the blood is normal. Sodium bicarbonate may be given direct intravenous push or in a continuous intravenous solution. Other drugs should not be mixed with the bicarbonate solution because they may precipitate in an alkaline pH. For example, calcium precipitates in a strongly alkaline pH.

The respiratory rate is one objective assessment of the effectiveness of therapy. When acidotic clients are given sodium bicarbonate, the hyperventilation decreases as the pH of the blood returns to normal. Sometimes the client may be given enough sodium bicarbonate to create a rebound metabolic alkalosis. Symptoms such as tingling can be signs that the pH of the blood is rising too much. However, in most situations where the physician orders low doses of sodium bicarbonate, the acidotic state is a more severe problem than the possibility of a rebound alkalosis. In an acute emergency, such as a cardiac arrest, it is essential that someone, usually the nurse, keep a detailed record of all the medications given the client.

Alteration in Fluid and Electrolyte Balance
Very close monitoring of the intake and output for clients in acidosis is essential to prevent severe dehydration and further electrolyte imbalances. During acidotic states, more hydrogen ions go into the cells, and potassium ions are forced out. The potassium that leaves the cells is eventually excreted by the kidneys so that the aftermath of metabolic acidosis is a depletion of total body potassium. In connection with the anion gap, chloride levels may or may not be increased, depending on whether the metabolic acidosis is due to an increase of acids, which are negative ions. Sodium may also be depleted, particularly in diabetic acidosis where diuresis has been a prominent feature. The nurse caring for a client who is recovering from metabolic acidosis must be aware of all the nursing implications for changes in each of these electrolytes, each of which was discussed separately in Chapter 5.

■ PO_2 (PARTIAL PRESSURE OF OXYGEN)

The PO_2 measures the amount of oxygen dissolved in the blood. The partial pressure is calculated by multiplying the amount of gas in a solution (%) by the total pressure (mm Hg or millimeters of mercury). Hence the laboratory reports the PO_2 as "so

Reference Values for PO_2	
Adult	75–100 mm Hg while breathing room air. May be above 225 mm if breathing 40% oxygen (with normal lungs)
Newborn	60–70 mm Hg are usually given as maximum reference values, or 40–60 mm Hg in some laboratories
Aged[a]	The PO_2 drops about 3–5 mm Hg for each decade after 30. After age 70 a PO_2 of around 85 mm Hg is the maximum reference value
Location	In high altitudes, such as Denver where the atmospheric pressure is 670 mm Hg, the maximum reference value for a person under 30 is around 81 mm Hg

[a] The relationship between age and PO_2 can be approximated by the formula (Tietz, 1983):

$$PO_2 = 104 - (age) \times 0.27$$

many millimeters of mercury (mm Hg).'' In a healthy young person, arterial blood may have about 13% oxygen dissolved in the plasma. At sea level, the partial pressure of oxygen would be 13% times 760 mm Hg or 98.8 mm Hg. As can be seen by the reference values, breathing pure oxygen, moving to a high altitude, or just simply aging makes quite a difference in the partial pressure of oxygen in the bloodstream.

Increased PO_2

Clinical Significance. The only clinical situation that creates a high PO_2 is the administration of high doses of oxygen. 100% oxygen may increase the PO_2 to over 500 mm Hg. Whether high oxygen pressures in the blood can alter certain bodily conditions, such as aging, is a controversial subject that is being explored.

POSSIBLE NURSING DIAGNOSES RELATED TO ELEVATED PO_2 LEVELS

Potential for Injury Related to Prolonged Use of High Levels of Oxygen

It was discovered many years ago that high doses of oxygen can cause irreversible blindness in premature infants. The high oxygen level causes a condition called *retrolental fibroplasia*. Nurses must routinely check the oxygen content of incubators to make sure that the oxygen delivery is correct. More recently it has been discovered that the prolonged use of high concentrations of oxygen can cause airway irritation and eventually damage to the lungs in both children and adults (Nielson, 1980).

Oxygen may also have a toxic effect on the central nervous system when oxygen is delivered under pressures greater than normal. The nurse should question any order for the prolonged use (over 8 hours) of 100% oxygen. In severe and complicated cases of hypoxia, the client may have to be on high concentrations of oxygen for an extended period of time. Frequent monitoring of blood gases is necessary to evaluate whether the oxygen therapy is satisfactory and whether lower concentrations of oxygen can be used. D'Agostino (1983) notes that the general rule is to use the lowest possible amount of inspired air, that is oxygen (FIO_2), to keep the PO_2 no more than 90 mm Hg unless special circumstances, such as carbon monoxide intoxication require higher PO_2 levels. Toxicity to oxygen rarely develops if the FIO_2 is kept below 40%. (See the section on elevated PCO_2 for the special dangers of oxygen therapy with some clients with obstructive disease.)

Decreased Arterial PO_2

Clinical Significance. Many different conditions can cause hypoxia, which is usually defined as a PO_2 of less than 70 mm Hg in the adult. With atelectasis or emphysema there may be ventilation to blood flow abnormalities so that oxygen does not reach the bloodstream. Hypoventilation, such as in the client who has taken a respiratory depressant, causes hypoxia. Anatomical defects, such as when arterial and venous blood intermix, cause hypoxia. In essence, any situation that interferes with the CO_2–O_2 exchange leads to a lowered PO_2.

Because the PCO_2 may be elevated, normal, or decreased with a decreased PO_2, it is important to look at the laboratory reports for both PCO_2 and pH when evaluating the clinical significance of a low PO_2. With many types of hypoxia, the PCO_2 may remain normal because carbon dioxide can diffuse much more readily than oxygen can across alveolar surfaces. If the hypoxia state is causing marked hyperventilation, the PCO_2 may actually drop below normal. For example, with pneumonia, both the PO_2 and PCO_2 may be lower than normal. The infection in the lungs interferes with oxygen exchange more than with carbon dioxide exchange. The hypoxia leads to hyperventilation in an attempt to increase oxygen. The hyperventilation causes more blowing off of carbon dioxide so the PCO_2 becomes lower than normal (respiratory alkalosis). In respiratory depression, such as that caused by general anesthesia, lowered PO_2 levels cannot stimulate increased respirations, so the PCO_2 level rises (respiratory acidosis). In chronic lung disease, there may first be only hypoxia, but eventually an increase in the PCO_2 level as the lung damage becomes worse. The clinical significance of hypoxia, compounded by hypercapnia (high PCO_2), is quite different from hypoxia alone, as noted earlier.

POSSIBLE NURSING DIAGNOSES RELATED TO HYPOXIA OR LOW PO_2 LEVELS

Alteration in Tissue Perfusion Due to Hypoxia

The nurse may be instrumental in preventing serious complications from hypoxia by detecting it before cyanosis occurs, which is a late symptom of hypoxia. Peripheral cyanosis that occurs in the nailbeds reflects poor peripheral perfusion, but not necessarily an extremely low PO_2. Tissue hypoxia is not synonymous with arterial hypoxia (Bullock & Rosendahl, 1984). Central cyanosis is best assessed by looking at the tongue. In the adult the PO_2 is less than 50 mm Hg by the time central cyanosis occurs. The blue color of central cyanosis denotes at least 5 g of unoxygenated hemoglobin in the arterial blood—or over one third of the total hemoglobin in the blood. The nurse needs to look for early symptoms of hypoxia, such as tachycardia and restlessness. By the time this one third or more of the hemoglobin is unsaturated, the client may be in real distress. Lack of oxygen to the myocardium can alter the cardiac output and produce arrhythmias.

Assessing for Cyanosis in Dark-Skinned People. Because cyanosis is difficult to assess in the dark-skinned person, nurses must become familiar with the client's precyanotic color. When cyanosis is suspected, nurses can press on the skin to create pallor. In cyanotic tissue the color returns slowly by spreading from the periphery to the center. Also the lips and tongue become ashen gray in a black person who is cyanotic (Bloch & Hunter, 1981).

Potential for Injury Related to Use of Oxygen

When oxygen is ordered for the client with hypoxia, nurses must make sure that the safety and comfort of the client are maintained. Clients and family need clear instructions about the danger of smoking. Discontinuing oxygen for just a few minutes may cause a significant drop in the PO_2 of some clients, and it may take as much as 20 minutes to restore the previous level (Felton, 1978). Because hypoxia can contribute to the development of severe cardiac arrhythmias, 100% oxygen may be given before and after suctioning a client. The nurse should consult with the physician about whether oxygen therapy can be interrupted for oral temperatures, feedings, or other procedures. The most objective assessment of the need for continual oxygen therapy is the blood gas report. The client on a ventilator may have blood gases drawn frequently to assess if the ventilator is properly adjusted. (See the section on elevated PO_2 levels for the potential danger of prolonged high levels of PO_2.)

Impaired Gas Exchange Related to Factors Other Than Simple Hypoxia

For some clients with hypoxia, oxygen may not be their primary need. For example, if the hypoxia is due to mucus plugs blocking some of the airways, then coughing, deep breathing, and maybe suctioning need to be instituted. If hypoxia is due to an acute condition, such as an asthmatic attack, hydration and bronchodilation would be as important as oxygenation (Rifas, 1983). When a client is allowed to stay in one position, not all areas of the lungs are equally ventilated; so some unoxygenated blood goes back to the left atrium. This is called *physiologic shunting*. By changing the client's position frequently, physiologic shunting does not add to the problem of hypoxia. However, if the hypoxia is due to a poor cardiac output, changing positions often may be tiring to the client and not a top priority. It is very important to understand the basic reason for the hypoxic state so that nursing measures are geared to help the client to utilize oxygen effectively and to conserve energy so that oxygen need is not increased.

The possible nursing implications for clients with a low PO_2 and a high PCO_2 were covered in the section on PCO_2. It is essential for the nurse to understand the potential danger of giving high concentrations of oxygen to clients who have hypoxia coupled with a chronically increased PCO_2. Recall that a client with chronic emphysema who has an elevated PCO_2 and a "normal" PO_2 of 50–60 mm Hg is using the hypoxia as a stimulus for breathing.

Alteration in Comfort Related to Dyspnea

Some clients, such as those with lung cancer or other destructive lung diseases, may have continual problems with dyspnea because their PO_2 is chronically low and oxygen therapy is of limited use. Maxwell (1985) suggests that nurses can help these types of clients recognize their anxiety and how it contributes to their breathlessness. Specific items taught to help restore control and power over the shortness of breath (SOB) include: controlled breathing through pursed lips, relaxation techniques, work simplification measures, and breathing techniques to use in activities of daily living.

■ OXYGEN SATURATION

Because the PO_2 measures the amount of dissolved oxygen in the blood, not the amount of oxygen carried by the hemoglobin, one must determine the oxygen saturation of the blood to evaluate its total carrying capacity. If hemoglobin is carrying the normal amount of oxygen, the oxygen saturation is close to 100%. The oxygen saturation of the hemoglobin is affected by the partial pressure of oxygen, by the temperature, by the pH, and by the chemical and physical structure of the hemoglobin itself. Unless there is a significant change in the last three factors, the oxyhemoglobin dissociation curve can be used to compute the oxygen-carrying capacity of the blood.

References Values for Oxygen Saturation

96–100% (arterial sample)

Comparison with P_{O_2} values (normal pH and temperature):

    98% = P_{O_2} of 100 mm Hg
    95% = P_{O_2} of 80 mm Hg
    89% = P_{O_2} of 60 mm Hg
    84% = P_{O_2} of 50 mm Hg
    35% = P_{O_2} of 20 mm Hg

Note: Venous blood has about 70–75% oxygen saturation.

Decrease in the Oxygen Saturation

Clinical Significance. Shunting of blood from the venous to the arterial system causes decreased oxygen saturation. The oxygen saturation is also very low with carbon monoxide poisoning because CO combines with hemoglobin over 200 times faster than O_2 does. The additional information from the oxygen saturation test is usually part of the assessment of a client who is having cardiac catheterization studies (See Chapter 26). Continuous mixed venous oxygen saturation can be measured by instrumentation (Shiveley & Clark, 1986) and is useful for monitoring critically ill clients and assessing the need for nursing interventions.

■ LACTIC ACID OR BLOOD LACTATE

Lactic acid is produced by anaerobic glycolysis and is a normal by-product of strenuous exercise. Dangerous levels of lactic acid can develop from pathological conditions that cause prolonged hypoxia or severe hypotension such as shock. Liver disease can also cause a buildup. (Lactic acid acidosis is the first type of metabolic acidosis discussed in the section on decreased serum bicarbonate levels.) Lactic acid acidosis can develop in a short time and almost immediately with a cardiac arrest. Lactic acid acidosis can also coexist with other types of acidosis such as those brought on by dehydration or renal failure. Lactic acid acidosis is a probability in any stuporous or comatose client who has a large anion gap (Bullock & Rosendahl, 1984). Jacobs et al. (1984) recommend a measurement of lactic acid when the anion gap is above 20, pH of 7.25, and the P_{CO_2} not elevated. (See Chapter 5 on the anion gap.) Lactic acidosis can also be idiopathic in a seriously ill client and can be fatal within a short time. Treatment involves taking measures to eliminate cellular hypoxia.

Gross hemolysis depresses results. False low values occur with high LDH levels. Elevations of lactate may occur with exercise, epinephrine, alcohol, glucose, and sodium bicarbonate infusions.

Preparation of Client and Collection of Sample

Venous or arterial blood is collected in either a gray top or green top container, depending on the laboratory method. Note on the laboratory slip whether the blood is arterial or venous as values differ. The specimen should be packed in ice and analyzed within 15 minutes after collection.

Reference Values for Lactic Acid

Venous   1.5–2.2 mEq/L   (0.5–19.8 mg/dl)
Arterial   0.6–1.8 mEq/L   (5.4–16.2 mg/dl)

QUESTIONS

1. In the client with no previous metabolic acid–base imbalances, hyperventilation will result in which of the following?

    a. ↓ PCO_2 and ↓ pH of serum
    b. ↓ PCO_2 and ↑ pH of serum

    c. ↑ PCO_2 and ↑ pH of serum
    d. ↑ PCO_2 and ↓ pH of serum

2. In the client with chronic lung disease, the kidneys can compensate for an elevated PCO_2 by which of the following?

    a. Retaining additional HCO_3^- (bicarb)
    b. Excreting more Na^+ and K^+ ions
    c. Excreting carbonic acid
    d. Retaining H^+ ions to balance the PCO_2

3. When a client has blood drawn from the radial artery for arterial blood gases (ABG) the nurse should do all of the following *except* which?

    a. Pack the blood sample in ice for transport to the laboratory
    b. Keep pressure on the puncture site for at least 5 minutes
    c. Transfer the blood sample to a heparinized test tube
    d. Record whether or not the client was breathing room air when the ABGs were drawn

4. Mrs. Candy is admitted in a diabetic coma. The aide reports to the nurse that, on admission, Mrs. Candy's respirations are rapid (38) and seem very deep. The nurse should do which of the following?

    a. Recheck the respirations because it is unusual to have such a high rate as she is retaining CO_2
    b. Check for signs of infection because this is probably causing the increased rate
    c. Notify the doctor that the client is having dyspnea
    d. Know that none of the above actions show an understanding of acid–base balance

5. Which of the following assessments by the nurse does not support the possibility that a client is going into metabolic alkalosis?

   a. Twitching
   b. Irritability

   c. Slow, shallow breaths
   d. Difficult to arouse

6. Michael, a 7-lb newborn, has an Apgar score of 7 (the normal is 10). He lost points for heart rate, respiratory rate, and color. The meperidine (Demerol) given to his mother before delivery has resulted in the newborn having a slight:

   a. Metabolic alkalosis (bicarbonate excess)
   b. Respiratory alkalosis (low P_{CO_2})
   c. Metabolic acidosis (bicarbonate deficit)
   d. Respiratory acidosis (high P_{CO_2})

7. In a normal pregnancy blood gases are which of the following?

   a. The same as in the nonpregnant state
   b. A lower P_{CO_2} and a lower HCO_3^-
   c. A higher P_{CO_2} and a higher HCO_3^-
   d. A lower P_{CO_2} and a higher HCO_3^-

8. High concentrations of oxygen may be dangerous for the client with a chronically elevated P_{CO_2} because the client:

   a. May develop respiratory distress due to oxygen toxicity
   b. Will no longer have hypoxia as a stimulus for breathing
   c. Depends on the P_{CO_2} as a stimulus for breathing
   d. Has a high P_{CO_2}, not a low P_{O_2}

9. Respiratory alkalosis (low P_{CO_2}) could result from all of the following situations *except* which?

   a. Hypoxia   b. Fever   c. Hysteria   d. Narcotic overdose

10. Which *one* of the following clients should be observed for possible signs of tetany if the calcium levels are borderline normal?

    a. Mr. Vick who had a cardiac arrest yesterday
    b. Ms. Rona who tends to hyperventilate when she is anxious
    c. Mrs. Degas who was hypotensive after her delivery today
    d. Baby Fong who is in respiratory distress

11. Deborah, age 18, is in the emergency room. She says she is having an "anxiety" attack. She complains of feeling light-headed and "shaky" all over. Which action by the nurse would *not* be appropriate in this situation?

    a. Have Deborah practice taking rapid deep breaths
    b. Provide a calm, soothing environment
    c. Help her identify what has made her so anxious now
    d. Ask Deborah to breathe into a paper bag

12. Which type of loss from the gastrointestinal tract contributes to the development of metabolic alkalosis (high serum bicarbonate)?

   a. Draining fistula from pancreatic cyst
   b. Gastric suctioning
   c. Diarrhea
   d. Ileostomy drainage

13. Which one of the following conditions does not cause a decrease in the serum bicarbonate HCO_3^- level?

   a. Prolonged decrease in the PCO_2
   b. Increased serum chloride level
   c. Markedly increased serum ketones
   d. Decreased serum potassium level

14. Jimmy, age 6, has lost an abnormal amount of chlorides because of vomiting. The loss of chlorides would contribute to which of the following?

   a. Respiratory alkalosis (low PCO_2)
   b. Respiratory acidosis (high PCO_2)
   c. Metabolic alkalosis (base excess)
   d. Metabolic acidosis (base deficit)

15. Betty Parker was admitted to the hospital with severe hyperemesis gravidarum. She has been unable to retain any meals or liquids. Her dehydrated and near-starvation state make her a candidate for which of the following?

   a. Metabolic acidosis (base deficit)
   b. Metabolic alkalosis (base excess)
   c. Respiratory acidosis (high PCO_2)
   d. Respiratory alkalosis (low PCO_2)

16. Rhonda, a 6-lb, 2-oz newborn, had a normal Apgar score. A half-hour after birth, her temperature is 96.8R. She must burn extra calories because she is cold-stressed. Unless she is warmed and fed, she is likely to develop which of the following?

   a. Metabolic acidosis (base deficit)
   b. Respiratory acidosis (high PCO_2)
   c. Metabolic alkalosis (base excess)
   d. Respiratory alkalosis (low PCO_2)

17. The anion gap is increased (that is, the unmeasured negative ions are increased) in which of these types of metabolic acidosis?

   a. Primary loss of serum bicarbonate
   b. Buildup of organic acids
   c. Increase of chlorides
   d. All of the above

18. Mrs. Landino has been receiving sodium bicarbonate intravenously for an acidotic state. The nursing assessment that would indicate that the sodium bicarbonate has restored the blood pH to normal is which of the following?

   a. Blood pressure is in normal range
   b. Urine output has increased
   c. Irritability and muscle spasms are less
   d. Respirations have returned to normal

19. Blood gases drawn on a client reveal a normal PO_2, a slightly low PCO_2, and

a slightly high pH. Which of the following situations would most likely produce these blood gas results?

a. Mr. Emory who has chronic emphysema

b. Bobby Black who is in diabetic acidosis

c. Mrs. Calhoun who is recovering from anesthesia and has had a lot of muscle relaxants.

d. Mrs. Delgado who has been using breathing exercises during her labor contractions

20. Mr. Cope has been admitted with a diagnosis of respiratory acidosis due to a chronic lung condition. When looking at his laboratory data, which of the following would be indicative of his acid–base difficulty? (Assume some compensation has occurred.)

a. High blood pH, low P_{CO_2}, high HCO_3^-

b. Low blood pH, high P_{CO_2}, high HCO_3^-

c. High blood pH, low P_{CO_2}, low HCO_3^-

d. Low blood pH, high P_{CO_2}, low HCO_3^-

21. Bill Phillips is on a respirator due to a drug overdose. Which of the following set of blood gases would be an indication that the respirator needs to be set at a lower rate?

a. P_{CO_2} 60 mm Hg; P_{O_2} 100 mm Hg, pH 7.32; HCO_3^- 28 mEq

b. P_{CO_2} 40 mm Hg; P_{O_2} 80 mm Hg, pH 7.42; HCO_3^- 25 mEq

c. P_{CO_2} 30 mm Hg; P_{O_2} 98 mm Hg, pH 7.56; HCO_3^- 26 mEq

d. P_{CO_2} 45 mm Hg; P_{O_2} 110 mm Hg, pH 7.42; HCO_3^- 29 mEq

REFERENCES

Bloch, B., & Hunter, M. (1981). Teaching physiological assessment of black persons. *Nurse Educator, 6,* 24–27.

Biswas, C., Ramos, J., Agroyannis, B., & Kerr, D. (1982). Blood gas analysis: Effect of air bubbles in syringe and delay in estimation. *British Medical Journal, 284,* 923–927.

Bullock, B., & Rosendahl, P. (1984). *Pathophysiology.* Boston: Little, Brown.

Chan, J. (1978). Clinical disorders of sodium, potassium, chloride, and sulfur metabolism. Diagnostic approach to children. *Urology, 12,* 504–508.

D'Agostino, J. (1983). Set your mind at ease on oxygen toxicity. *Nursing 83, 13*(7), 55–56.

Dingle, R., Grady, M., Lee, J., & Paul, S. (1980). Continuous transcutaneous O_2 monitoring in the neonate. *AJN, 80*(5), 890–893.

Felton, C. (1978). Hypoxemia and oral temperatures. *AJN, 78*(1), 56–57.

Gever, L. (1984). Administering sodium bicarbonate during a code. *Nursing 84, 14*(1), 100.

Glass, L., & Jenkins, C. (1983). The ups and downs of serum pH. *Nursing 83, 13*(9), 34–41.

Goldstein, R., et al. (1984). Effect of supplemental nocturnal oxygen on gas exchange in patients with severe obstructive lung disease. *NEJM, 310*(7), 425–429.

Holum, J. (1983). *Elements of general and biological chemistry* (6th ed.). New York: John Wiley & Sons.

Jacobs, D., Kasten, B., DeMott, W., & Wolfson, W. (1984). *Laboratory test handbook with DRG index.* St. Louis: Mosby/Lexi.

Maxwell, M. (1985). Dyspnea in advanced cancer. *AJN, 85*(6), 673–677.

Miller, M., & Sherman, R. (1977). Metabolic acid–base disorders, Part I: Chemistry and physiology. *AJN, 77*(10), 1619–1650.

Miller, M., & Sherman, R. (1978a) Metabolic acid–base disorders, Part II: Physiological abnormalities and nursing actions. *AJN, 78*(1), 87–108.

Miller, M., & Sherman, R. (1978b) Metabolic acid–base disorders, Part III: Clinical and laboratory findings. *AJN, 78*(3), 1–16.

Milne, J. A. (1979). The respiratory response to pregnancy. *Postgraduate Medical Journal, 55*(5), 318–324.

Nielson, L. (1980). Pulmonary oxygen toxicity and other hazards of oxygen therapy. *AJN, 80*(12), 2213–2215.

Pavlin, E., & Hornbein, T. (1978). The control of breathing. *Basics of Respiratory Disease, 7*(11), 1–6.

Rifas, E. (1983). Teaching patients to manage asthma. *Nursing 83, 13*(4), 77–82.

Sandvik, J. (1977). The emergency management of hyperventilation. *Journal of Emergency Nursing, 3,* 17–20.

Shrake, K. (1979). The ABC's of ABG's or how to interpret a blood gas value. *Nursing 79, 9*(9), 26–33.

Shively, M., & Clark, A. (1986). Continuous monitoring of mixed venous oxygen saturation: An instrument for research. *Nursing Research, 35*(1), 56–58.

Signor, G., & Del Bueno, D. (1982). A sinfully easy way to interpret ABG's. *RN, 45*(9), 45–49.

Smithline, N., & Gardner, K. (1976). Gaps—Anionic and osmolal. *JAMA, 236,* 1594–1597.

Sumner, S. (1980). Refining your technique for drawing arterial blood gases. *Nursing 80, 10*(4), 65–69.

Tietz, N. (Ed.). (1983). *Clinical guide to laboratory tests.* Philadelphia: Saunders.

Waites, T. (1978). Hyperventilation—Chronic and acute. *Archives International Medicine, 138*(11), 1700–1701.

Wallach, J. (1983). *Interpretation of pediatric tests.* Boston: Little, Brown.

Wallach, J. (1986). *Interpretation of diagnostic tests.* Boston: Little, Brown.

Worthington, L. (1979). What those blood gases can tell you. *RN, 42*(9), 23–27.

7

Three Less Commonly Measured Electrolytes

- Serum Calcium (Ca^{++})
- Urinary Calcium
  Quanititative Method (24-Hour Urine Sample) and Qualitative Method (Sulkowitch Test)
- Serum Phosphorus (P^{++}) or Phosphates
- Urinary Phosphorus
- Serum Magnesium (Mg^{++})

OBJECTIVES

1. Explain the relationship of parathyroid hormone (parathormone) to serum and urine levels of calcium and phosphorus.
2. Identify nursing assessments useful in detecting hypercalcemia or hypocalcemia, including the Sulkowitch test for urine calcium.
3. Plan appropriate nursing interventions to decrease the harmful effects of hypercalcemia.
4. Analyze clinical situations to determine which clients are likely to have changes in serum phosphorus or calcium levels.
5. Describe the nursing diagnoses used for calcium/phosphorus imbalances.
6. Prepare a teaching plan for clients who must decrease or increase calcium and phosphorus intake.
7. Identify nursing assessments useful in detecting serum magnesium excess and deficiency.
8. Identify potential nursing diagnoses for clients with magnesium excess or deficiency.

This chapter covers three electrolytes or minerals that appear in small amounts in the serum: calcium, phosphorus, and magnesium.

Both calcium and phosphorus serum levels are controlled by parathyroid hormone (parathormone or PTH), which also promotes the reabsorption of calcium and the excretion of phosphorus. The end results of an increased secretion of parathormone are an increased serum calcium and a decreased serum phosphorus level. Although the serum calcium level often varies inversely with the phosphorus level due to this hormonal control, both calcium and phosphorus may be increased or decreased together in other clinical situations. Calcium and phosphorus are discussed in separate sections, but the reader needs to be aware that both tests are useful in assessing an imbalance of either electrolyte. In addition, urinary tests for both may give additional information about their overall metabolism. Methods of testing for calcium and phosphorus in the urine are discussed after each section on the electrolytes.

Magnesium is less well understood than the other two electrolytes. It is known that a marked increase in serum magnesium has been shown to decrease the release of parathyroid hormone, and that aldosterone causes a decrease of serum magnesium as it does of potassium. The section on magnesium discusses the interrelationship of magnesium to calcium and potassium in deficiency states.

Unlike the more commonly measured electrolytes discussed in Chapter 5 (Na^+, K^+, Cl^-, HCO_3^-), the three electrolytes in this chapter are not always measured in milliequivalents (see Chapter 5 for a definition of milliequivalent). Because a particular laboratory may use either mg or mEq, reference values using both systems are presented. In addition, some laboratories may use the SI (Systéme International) discussed in Chapter 1. For Na, K, Cl, and HCO_3, the SI and the mEq figures are the same. But with Ca, P, and Mg, the SI figures are different from the mEq. (See Appendix A for the SI equivalents.)

■ SERUM CALCIUM (Ca⁺⁺)

Calcium, a positively charged ion, circulates in the bloodstream both in the free or ionized state and bound to plasma proteins. The bound calcium, carried chiefly by albumin, is about half of the total calcium in the bloodstream. Because most laboratories measure the total calcium level, not just the ionized calcium, a change in the serum albumin level means a change in the total serum reference values. A decrease of 1 g of albumin means that the serum total calcium level is about 0.8 mg less. Because the free, or ionized, calcium affects neuromuscular function, a low calcium level due to a low albumin level does not make the client symptomatic for hypocalcemia. When the serum albumin level is not normal, some laboratories measure the ionized part of the serum calcium to get a clearer picture of any calcium deficiency. Factors that cause decreased serum albumin levels are discussed in Chapter 10.

The amount of calcium in the serum is quite small compared with that present in the teeth and bones. The bones contain a tremendous reservoir of calcium that can be used if needed to keep the serum calcium level normal. Two hormones control serum calcium levels. Calcitonin, a hormone secreted by the thyroid gland, protects against a calcium excess in the serum. Parathormone (PTH), secreted by the parathyroid gland, functions to keep a sufficient level of calcium in the bloodstream; an increase in PTH not only increases the serum calcium level, it also decreases phosphorus levels. Thus, for many types of serum calcium imbalance, it is important to evaluate the serum phosphorus level too. The relationship of phosphorus to calcium is discussed in detail in the next section on serum phosphorus levels.

Calcium is obtained in several food sources, of which milk products are the best: A cup of milk, for example, contains 236 mg of calcium. Other sources that contain a fairly large amount of calcium include vegetables, such as turnip greens, collard greens, white beans, and lentils (Table 7–1). Intestinal cells need vitamin D, a unique vitamin made entirely in the body from cholesterol and a photochemical reaction, to absorb calcium. Thus sunlight and a diet adequate in fat are important to ensure proper levels of vitamin D (Wood, 1977). Protein is also required for the proper utilization of calcium. Chronic nutritional deficiencies of calcium, vitamin D, and protein eventually result in lowered serum calcium levels. Yet, due to the vast reservoir of calcium in the bones, dietary deficiencies do not immediately cause lowered serum calcium levels.

Reference Values for Serum Calcium

Adult	Calcium levels tend to be slightly higher in men 8.5–10.5 mg/dl or 4.3–5.3 mEq/L
Pregnancy	Falls gradually to a level at term about 10% below nonpregnant level. Consistent with the fall in albumin
Newborn	7.4–14 mg/dl or 3.7–7 mEq[a]
Children	Slightly higher in children—may be up to 12 mg

---

[a]Children's Hospital San Francisco considers below 8 abnormal for a 1500 g infant and below 7.5 mg/dl abnormal for an infant below 1500 g.

Infants require 360–540 mg of calcium, depending on age. Children and adults require around 800 mg of calcium. Adolescents, as well as pregnant and lactating women, have the greatest requirement for calcium, which is around 1200 mg (American Academy of Pediatrics, 1978). Calcium supplementation to a total intake of about 1500 mg a day has been shown to inhibit age-related bone loss in postmenopausal

TABLE 7–1. EXAMPLES OF FOODS HIGH IN CALCIUM AND/OR PHOSPHORUS

Food in 100-g Portions	Calcium in mg	Phosphorus in mg
Swiss cheese	925	563
Cheddar cheese	750	478
Brick cheese	730	455
American cheese	697	771
Turnip greens	246	58
Almonds	234	504
Collard greens	203	63
Beans, white	144	425
Milk (100 g = scant ½ cup)	118	93
Frankfurter	32	603
Bologna	32	581
Peanuts	69	401
Whole wheat flour	41	372
Liver	8	352

Modified from Linkswiler and Zemel (1979) with permission.

women (Recker, 1983). Excess calcium is excreted in the urine. The measurement of urinary calcium is covered after the discussion on serum calcium levels.

Preparation of the Client and Collection of the Sample

One ml of serum is needed. Some laboratories require a fasting state, although water is allowed. Remember that if the serum albumin level drops 1 g, the total serum calcium level drops 0.8 mg, even though the ionized calcium remains the same. Always interpret calcium levels in relation to serum albumin levels.

Increased Serum Calcium Level (Hypercalcemia)

Clinical Significance. As with many other tests, dehydration gives a pseudo-high reading for the serum calcium level. An increased level of the parathyroid hormone, PTH, causes a persistently elevated serum calcium level. Because adenomas of the parathyroid gland can cause the gland to produce additional amounts of PTH the physician may order several other tests, including an assay of PTH levels to rule out the possibility that a parathyroid tumor is responsible for hypercalcemia. Often the client may be asymptomatic even though the laboratory report shows a higher-than-normal serum calcium level. In borderline cases, the test may be repeated several times over a period of weeks or months, in addition to other diagnostic studies, such as the parathyroid hormone assay (discussed in Chapter 15). If the high serum calcium level is due to parathyroid dysfunction, the client may need surgery to remove part of the parathyroid gland.

There are several other common reasons for the serum calcium level being higher than normal (Table 7–2). The most common is the release of calcium in metastatic bone disease as bone is destroyed. Also, some of the hormonal changes in malignant states may contribute to raising the serum calcium level. Some tumors produce PTH-

TABLE 7-2. COMMON CAUSES OF HYPERCALCEMIA AND HYPOCALCEMIA

Hypercalcemia (Serum Ca^{++} levels above 10.5 mg/dl or see values for specific laboratory)
  Pseudo-rise due to dehydration
  Hyperparathyroidism (serum P decreased)
  Malignancies
  Immobilization
  Thiazide diuretics
  Vitamin D intoxication (serum P increased)

Hypocalcemia (Serum CA^{++} levels below 8.5 mg/dl or see values for specific laboratory)
Infants have lower values to 8 or 7.5 mg/dl
  Pseudo-decrease due to low albumin levels
  Hypoparathyroidism (serum P increased)
  Early neonatal hypocalcemia
  Chronic renal disease (serum P increased)
  Pancreatitis
  Massive blood transfusions
  Severe malnutrition (serum P decreased)
  Symptoms of hypocalcemia when patient is alkalotic although total serum calcium is normal (see text)

Serum P = Serum phosphorus levels which help with interpretation of serum Ca.
See text for explanation and Chan (1979); Tripp (1976); Canalis et al. (1977); Felver (1980); McFadden et al. (1983); Elliot et al. (1983); Quinlan (1983); and Coward (1985).

like substances. (See Chapter 15 for a discussion on ectopic hormone production.) Long-term immobilization may result in increased serum calcium levels because the lack of normal bone stress causes the release of calcium from bone. Thiazide diuretics are another reason for hypercalcemia. Excessive milk intake (meaning at least 3 quarts of milk a day) is a less frequent cause of hypercalcemia. Vitamin D intoxication can also result in hypercalcemia. Hypercalcemia and elevated serum vitamin D levels may persist for months after the vitamin D supplements are stopped (Butler et al., 1985).

POSSIBLE NURSING DIAGNOSES RELATED TO HYPERCALCEMIA

Alteration in Fluid Requirements Related to Potential for Injury from Formation of Renal Stones

An increased serum calcium level almost always means an increased calcium excretion by the kidneys. Thus, insofar as a high concentration of calcium in the urine may lead to the formation of renal stones (*calculi*), it is very important that a client with hypercalcemia stay well hydrated. Some authorities suggest that the urine volume needs to be above 2500 ml in 24 hours (Smith et al., 1978). Health teaching for the client at home should include information on how to make sure the urine is never concentrated; the person must be aware of the importance of drinking fluids at bedtime and also during the night. A visiting nurse can help make out a schedule for the client or for a member of the family to follow.

Calcium is more likely to precipitate in an alkaline urine. Yet, because the urine pH is normally acid (around 6), precipitation may not be a threat unless the client gets a urinary tract infection, which may make the urine alkaline. Measures, such as the intake of cranberry juice, to change an alkaline urine to acid are discussed in Chapter 3.

For emergency treatment of hypercalcemia forced diuresis with intravenous normal saline is usually used because calcium excretion improves when sodium supplementation is provided (Elliott & McKenzie, 1983). The standard saline solution infusion rate is 1000 ml over 4–6 hours (Elbaum, 1984). The nurse must monitor daily weights and intake and output records to avoid overload. Furosemide (Lasix) may be given concurrently. Thiazide diuretics are never used with hypercalcemia because they exacerbate the condition (Quinlan, 1982).

Potential for Injury Related to Slowing of Reflexes

The client with an increased serum calcium level may demonstrate some slowing of reflexes. Because increased serum calcium levels decrease the permeability of nerve cell membranes to sodium, the depolarization process is affected, and the nerve fibers have a decreased excitability. This condition may result in some lethargy or a general sluggish feeling. Other possible problems may be vague abdominal pains and constipation; confusion may develop and lead to a comatose state.

Potential Alteration in Cardiac Output

An elevated serum calcium level also tends to slow the heart and arrhythmias may develop. If the client is on digoxin, a high serum calcium level may be particularly dangerous because it potentiates the effect of the digoxin.

Potential for Injury and Impaired Mobility Related to Development of Pathological Fractures

If the hypercalcemia is a result of loss of calcium from the bones, the client becomes very susceptible to fractures. These types of fractures are referred to as *pathological fractures* because the bone is made fragile by a pathological process. Clients who are prone to pathological fractures must be handled very gently. The nurse must be alert to any vague symptoms of bone pain. Sometimes just turning in bed can cause a fracture. If ambulation is possible, weight bearing can help to minimize loss of calcium from the weight-bearing bones. A walker or other supportive device is essential for safety. Coward (1985) developed a written information guide for clients with cancer who may develop hypercalcemia. One of the measures to teach clients is to remain as physically active as possible with an emphasis on walking.

Knowledge Deficit Regarding Drug Therapy for Hypercalcemia

Although several drugs may be used to reduce high serum calcium levels, none of them are entirely satisfactory (Elliot & McKenzie, 1983). Sometimes more than one drug is used. With all these drugs the client must remain well hydrated at all times, including during the night.

1. *Calcitonin* (Calcimar), a synthetic preparation of the hormone produced by the thyroid gland, is being investigated as a treatment for certain types of transitory hypercalcemia. Presently calcitonin is used mostly to lower serum calcium levels and to increase bone formation in the client with Paget's disease who has considerable bone destruction. Clients with Paget's disease may take calcitonin injections daily over a long period of time. Often the nurse needs to teach the client how to do the injections at home. Allergic reactions can occur.
2. *Phosphates* decrease serum calcium levels on the principle that an increased serum phosphate level causes a decreased serum calcium level. Presumably, the higher phosphate level promotes the deposition of calcium in the bone and decreases the reabsorption of bone. The disadvantage is that there may be some deposition of calcium in soft tissues as well. The use of phosphates is a slow process, and the client must have good renal function.
3. *Mithramycin,* an antineoplastic drug, is also sometimes used to reduce high serum calcium levels in clients with malignancies. A single dose may reduce elevated serum calcium levels for 3–15 days (Canalis et al., 1977). However, a rebound hypercalcemia, along with many toxic side effects, may result from the use of this drug.
4. Of the *glucocorticosteroids,* prednisone and some others reduce serum calcium levels, but they may take a week to 10 days to do so. The nurse and the client must be aware of the potential side effects from the use of corticosteroids. (See Chapter 15 on hormones.)

Alteration in Nutritional Requirements Related to Possible Dietary Restrictions

Depending on the underlying pathophysiology, the dietary restriction of foods high in calcium may be used to control hypercalcemia. Restricting milk and milk products very dramatically reduces the calcium intake. Other sources of calcium—such as dried legumes, broccoli, and some other dark green leafy vegetables—probably do not need to be restricted if dairy products are reduced or eliminated (Mundy et al., 1977). The nurse needs to consult with the doctor about what degree of diet restriction may help to alleviate the high serum calcium levels. Then any restrictions can be explained to the client. Because hypercalcemia may be due to complex pathological processes, the value of diet restriction must be evaluated in relation to the particular medical problem that exists. For hypercalcemia related to malignancy it is usually *not* necessary to avoid foods high in calcium (Coward, 1985). Table 7-1 gives examples of foods high in calcium.

Decreased Serum Calcium Level (Hypocalcemia)

Clinical Significance. First of all, as much of the serum calcium is bound to albumin it is important to make sure that the lowered serum calcium level is not due to a lowered serum albumin level.

Just as *hyper*parathyroidism causes *hyper*calcemia, *hypo*parathyroidism causes *hypo*calcemia, because the parathyroid hormone, PTH, controls serum calcium levels. Hypoparathyroidism, or a lack of PTH, can be due to accidental damage to the parathyroids during thyroid surgery. The hypocalcemia may be more severe from surgical removal of the parathyroids than from the other various causes of hypoparathyroidism.

Early neonatal hypocalcemia is a clinical condition experienced by many preterm infants in the first 24 to 48 hours of life. The exact reason for this kind of hypocalcemia is not known (Domenech & Maya, 1978).

Hypocalcemia is also commonly seen in clients with renal failure when there is an impaired elimination of acid phosphates. The increase of phosphates in the serum causes a decreased calcium level due to the inverse relationship between these two levels. (See the beginning of the chapter for an explanation of this interrelationship due to PTH control.) Also in chronic renal disease, because the kidney is unable to finish the process of making vitamin D chemically active, calcium absorption is impaired. The tubules of the kidney are responsible for the final active form of vitamin D, which functions as calcitrol, a hormone necessary for calcium absorption. Vitamin D is the only vitamin known to be converted to a hormonal form (DeLuca, 1981). Children who have chronic renal disease may develop rickets because of the lowered serum calcium levels.

Serum calcium levels can also be lowered because calcium is being deposited in tissues. In pancreatitis, the fatty acids that are released can bind up calcium. The pancreas may actually become calcified in areas of necrotic tissue. In massive blood transfusions, the serum calcium level may drop because the calcium ions in the blood are bound by the citrate that the blood bank uses as the anticoagulant. The liver removes the citrate from the circulation, but it may not be able to do so fast enough when a large amount of blood is infused.

Severe malnutrition may eventually lead to hypocalcemia, but, due to the vast reserves of calcium in the bones, a calcium-deficient diet does not immediately cause a drop in serum calcium levels. Hence a pregnant or lactating woman who does not have enough calcium intake continues to have a normal serum calcium level as she loses calcium from the teeth and bones. Children and elderly people who have calcium-deficient diets usually retain normal serum calcium levels too. But the child develops rickets, and the older person develops osteomalacia or a softening of the bones. Osteoporosis, a major health problem for many post-menopausal women, is related to a lack of calcium intake which may have existed for many years (Recker, 1983). A very severe malnutrition that includes a lack of vitamin D and protein eventually causes a lowered serum calcium level when calcium cannot be released from the bones or teeth.

The nurse should bear in mind the effect of pH on calcium solubility. In alkalotic states, even though the total serum calcium does not change, the amount of ionized calcium is less because calcium is less soluble in an alkaline medium. A decrease in the ionized portion of serum calcium causes symptoms of hypocalcemia even though the laboratory test looks normal. (Recall that the serum calcium level measures both bound calcium and ionized calcium.)

When the client is acidotic, the total serum calcium level may be low, but the client has few symptoms as long as he or she is acidotic because more calcium is in the ionized state. When the pH returns to normal, there is less ionized calcium and the symptoms of hypocalcemia become apparent. Thus acidotic states may "mask" a true hypocalcemia state.

POSSIBLE NURSING DIAGNOSES RELATED TO HYPOCALCEMIA

Potential for Injury due to Tetany

The symptoms of hypocalcemia vary depending on how low the level of serum calcium drops and on how abruptly it drops. Hypocalcemia causes muscle twitching and cramps, which may lead to generalized muscle spasms that are called *tetany*. These cramps in the muscles are due to the neuromuscular irritability from the lack of calcium ions. In the client with a low serum calcium level, a tapping of the jaw causes a facial spasm (Chvostek's sign). Some clients, particularly women, may exhibit this sign even though calcium is normal. Another assessment for low serum calcium levels is to look for carpopedal spasms or spasms in the hands. The carpopedal spasms may be elicited when the arm becomes a little ischemic. For example, when the nurse takes the blood pressure, the client's hand may twitch when the cuff is left inflated for a couple of minutes (Trousseau's sign). Very subtle signs of neuromuscular irritability due to hypocalcemia, such as a twitching of the nose, may be overlooked unless the nurse is aware that any neuromuscular irritability should be watched for in a client who is a candidate for hypocalcemia. In the newborn the symptoms may include twitching or convulsions. Treatment for newborns is advocated when levels drop below 7.0 mg/dl (Domenech & Maya, 1978). The symptoms of hypocalcemia often coincide with hypoglycemia in the newborn. (See Chapter 8 for a discussion on hypoglycemia in the newborn.)

Because clients with the potential for hypocalcemia may have a convulsive state, the nurse must be prepared for such a possibility. Calcium gluconate for intravenous administration should be on an emergency cart. After thyroid or parathyroid surgery, an ampule of calcium gluconate is usually kept at the bedside. Clients at risk for hypocalcemia usually have their serum calcium levels measured daily.

Special Emphasis for Symptoms of Hypocalcemia in Alkalosis.
If the client is having symptoms of tetany because less calcium is in an ionized state, the client is not given calcium as the treatment. In alkalosis, the symptoms arise

from a lack of ionized calcium, not from a *true lack* of calcium. When the pH returns to normal, the calcium is once again ionized in the correct amount for neuromuscular functioning. (The possible nursing implications for the client in alkalosis are covered in Chapter 6.)

Potential for Injury Related to Replacement of Calcium
The treatment for hypocalcemia depends on the underlying cause. To prevent tetany and convulsions, the serum calcium level must be raised quickly to normal. If the signs of tetany are severe, the physician orders calcium to be given intravenously. Several different salts of calcium are available, but usually calcium gluconate is given for fast replacement. Unlike potassium, calcium can be given directly by intravenous push. (In most clinical situations, the physician must give medications that are given by intravenous push.) The medication may give the client a feeling of warmth due to the vasodilation that occurs, along with a drop in the blood pressure, for which the client must be monitored.

In less acute situations—when the client is having few symptoms—an ampule of calcium gluconate may be added to a bottle of intravenous fluid. Because calcium precipitates in an alkaline medium, calcium salts can never be added to intravenous fluids with an alkaline pH. Most dextrose and saline solutions are acid in pH, but this point must be carefully checked as an intravenous may also contain sodium bicarbonate.

Before the start of any type of calcium replacement, a blood sample must be drawn to determine the baseline serum calcium level. After or during calcium replacement therapy, other samples may be drawn to make sure that the serum calcium level is not becoming higher than normal. Because calcium has a profound effect on the heart, some physicians may choose to have the client on a cardiac monitor all the while calcium is being replaced. This precaution is all the more likely if the client is also on digoxin, because calcium increases the possibility of digitalis toxicity.

Knowledge Deficit Regarding Use of Oral Calcium Supplements
For mild hypocalcemia, and in chronic states, the client may be given various oral preparations of calcium salts. Newborns may be given oral supplements, once feedings are tolerated. The nurse needs to find out whether the particular preparation being used should be taken on an empty stomach. With some preparations, alkaline foods and milk tend to decrease the absorption of calcium. The calcium of other preparations may have a bitter taste or cause gastrointestinal irritation, so that it is better tolerated with food. Also some preparation may be constipating. Clients on calcium supplements should not take tetracyclines because calcium interferes with the absorption of this type of antibiotic. Metabolites of vitamin D, such as calciferol or calcitrol, are used to increase serum calcium levels. The use of vitamin D supplements requires careful monitoring of serum calcium levels because vitamin D has a cumulative effect. Urine levels may also be monitored (McFadden, et al., 1983). An inexpensive source of calcium carbonate is found in some antacid tablets so clients should discuss with their physician the best type of calcium replacement for them.

Alteration of Nutritional Requirement for Calcium
Calcium requirements are best met by having adequate calcium in the diet. So the nurse must assess the dietary habits of individuals to determine whether their calcium intake is adequate. If the client does not like milk or cheese (which,

as dairy products, are among the best sources for calcium), powdered milk can be added to many dishes without changing their taste. A tablespoon of powdered milk contains nearly 50 mg of calcium (Table 7–3). Foods high in oxalates and phosphates, such as spinach, rhubarb, and asparagus, tend to decrease calcium absorption (Quinlan, 1983). Also, a lack of protein decreases calcium utilization (Tripp, 1976) but a diet with excess protein wastes calcium. Elderly clients may have a decrease in gastric hydrochloric acid which decreases calcium absorption. A form of oral glutamic acid hydrochloride (Acidulin) may be used to improve calcium absorption (Cerrato, 1985).

Knowledge Deficit Regarding Phosphate Binders
Another way to help raise the serum calcium level is to reduce the amount of phosphate intake. (The relationship of high phosphorus levels to low serum calcium levels is discussed next in the section on phosphorus.) Oral antacids that contain magnesium or aluminum (Aludrox) are sometimes ordered with meals to help bind up phosphates so that more calcium can be absorbed. If the low serum calcium level, related to a high serum phosphorus level, is due to renal failure, medications containing aluminum, not magnesium hydroxide, are prescribed to lower the serum phosphorous level because magnesium is not excreted well in renal dysfunction.

■ URINARY CALCIUM

QUANTITATIVE METHOD (24-HOUR URINE SAMPLE)

Preparation of Client and Collection of Sample
All urine for 24 hours is collected in a special bottle that contains 10 ml of hydrochloric acid (HCl). The HCl is to keep the pH of the urine low (pH of 2 to 3) because calcium tends to precipitate in an alkaline medium. The client stays on the usual diet. Any increased intake of protein by the client should be noted because more calcium

TABLE 7–3. COMMON REASONS FOR CHANGES IN SERUM PHOSPHATE LEVELS

Hyperphosphatemia (Serum phosphorus over 4.5 mg/dl in adult)
  Hypoparathyroidism (serum Ca decreased)
  Renal failure (serum Ca decreased)
  Increased growth hormone
  Vitamin D intoxication (serum Ca increased)

Hypophosphatemia (Serum phosphorus below 3 mg/dl in adult)
  Hyperparathyroidism (serum Ca increased)
  Diuresis
  Malabsorption or malnutrition (serum Ca decreased)
  Increased glucose metabolism—carbohydrate loading
  Antacid abuse

Serum calcium Ca^{++} helps in interpretation.
See text and Kreisberg (1977); Chan (1979); Knochel (1977, 1985); and Baker (1985) for more details and for less common medical conditions.

is excreted on a high-protein diet. (See Chapter 3 for general instructions about 24-hour urine collections.)

Reference Values for Urinary Calcium

Adult	50–300 mg/dl depending on dietary intake
Children	Range is around 5 mg-kg of body weight if on normal dietary intake of calcium (Chan, 1979)

Clinical Significance. Normally up to 99% of the calcium filtered by the kidneys is reabsorbed. An increased urinary calcium level is almost always due to an elevated serum calcium level (Chan, 1979). The amount of calcium being excreted in the urine may differ for various types of hypercalcemia, so the 24-hour urine collection may give the physician extra diagnostic clues. For example, a highly elevated urine calcium does not usually accompany primary hyperparathyroidism because the increased amount of PTH promotes additional reabsorption of calcium. In other types of hypercalcemia, such as with malignant tumors, the urine calcium level may be as high as 800 or 900 mg in 24 hours. In conditions where there is a low serum calcium level, the urinary excretion of calcium is very low.

QUALITATIVE METHOD (SULKOWITCH TEST)

This is a test done on one specimen of urine to get a rough indication of the amount of calcium being excreted in the urine. The findings are reported as normal, increased, or decreased. Either the client may be taught to do this test, or a visiting nurse can do it on a visit, as it is easy to perform.

Preparation of Client and Collection of Sample
The client should continue with the usual diet. If hypercalcemia is suspected, the urine should be collected before a meal. If hypocalcemia is suspected, the urine should be collected after a meal. A few drops of calcium oxalate solution are added to the urine specimen to see if precipitation occurs.

Reference Values for Sulkowitch Test

Heavy white precipitate indicates more-than-normal calcium in the urine.
Fine white cloud is considered to be within the normal range.
Clear specimen indicates less-than-normal calcium in the urine specimen.

Clinical Significance of Results. An increased calcium in the urine in an early morning fasting specimen would be a strong indicator of persistent high serum calcium levels. If the specimen remains clear even after meals, there is a strong possibility that the serum calcium level is always abnormally low. Clients may do these tests over a period of weeks to help assess the presence or absence of a problem. If they do, they must record not only the results but also the timing of the specimens in relation to meals.

■ SERUM PHOSPHORUS (P⁺⁺) OR PHOSPHATES

Serum phosphorus levels are actually measured as phosphate ions. Laboratories may report phosphorus levels as phosphorus (P) or phosphate (PO₄) levels. Whereas potassium is the major intracellular *cation,* phosphorus is the major intracellular *anion.* So the majority of phosphorus is in bone tissue and skeletal muscle, and phosphates regulate many enzymatic actions that are critical for energy transformations. Because phosphorus has a very close relationship to calcium, the phosphorous level is usually more useful as a diagnostic tool when looked at in relation to the serum calcium level.

The phosphate electrolyte is the only electrolyte that is markedly different in values for children and adults. (The bicarbonate ion discussed in Chapter 5 does have slight variations with age.) The marked increase in phosphate ions in young children is partially explained by the increased amount of growth hormone that is present until puberty.

The recommended dietary allowances for phosphorus, except in infancy and lactation, is a one-to-one ratio to calcium. Thus an adult requires about 800 mg of phosphorus a day. In the infant and the lactating woman, the need for calcium exceeds the need for phosphorus. In most American diets, however, the intake of phosphorus is probably twice that of calcium: The average calcium intake may be around 700 mg, whereas the average phosphorus intake is about 1500 mg (Linkswiler & Zemel, 1979). This higher phosphorus intake occurs for two reasons. First, phosphorus is abundant not only in dairy products but also in many natural foods. Second, many food additives contain a lot of phosphates. Linkswiler and Zemel (1979), in a detailed discussion of the additional source of phosphorus from food processing, conclude that at the present time there are no data to suggest harm from the extra phosphates in the diet. Processed meat, cheese, and soft drinks are three sources that are quite high in phosphates. Table 7–1 lists other foods that are high in calcium and/or phosphates.

Like calcium, phosphorus is controlled by the parathyroid hormone. Increases in the level of PTH cause a decrease in the serum level of phosphorus and an increased secretion of phosphorus by the kidney.

Additional phosphates are excreted by the kidney. Some phosphate is also excreted in the feces. Drugs, such as aluminum hydroxide (Aludrox) can significantly increase the fecal excretion of phosphates.

Special Preparation of Client and Collection of Sample
One ml of serum is needed. Some laboratories require the fasting state, although water is allowed. Because increased carbohydrate metabolism lowers serum phosphorus levels, the client should not have intravenous solutions of glucose running before the

Reference Values for Serum Phosphorus	
Adult	3.0–4.5 mg/dl or 1.8–2.6 mEq/L Male values are slightly higher than female values
Pregnancy	Slightly lower in pregnancy
Newborn	5.7–9.5 mg/dl. May be higher ranges in prematures and for a few days after birth
Infant and Children	4–6 mg. Levels decline with maturity
Aged	May be slightly lower in the aged

test. If an intravenous of glucose is being administered, note it on the laboratory slip. The serum needs to be sent to the laboratory as soon as possible because the laboratory must quickly separate the serum from the cells.

Increased Phosphate Level (Hyperphosphatemia)

Clinical Significance. The clinical significance of an elevated phosphorus level is always evaluated in relation to the serum calcium levels to get a clearer picture of what may be a very complicated pathological process (Table 7–3):

1. When the phosphorus level is elevated and the serum calcium level is low, hypoparathyroidism may be the reason. The lack of parathyroid hormone (PTH) decreases the renal excretion of phosphates.
2. In some types of renal dysfunction, the kidneys cannot excrete phosphate ions. A high phosphate level in the serum then depresses the serum calcium level through several hormonal actions.
3. Diseases of childhood may sometimes involve an increase in the production of growth hormone. In such a case, the serum calcium level would not be elevated.
4. If the phosphates in the serum are elevated due to vitamin D intoxication or to the excessive intake of milk, then the serum calcium is most likely elevated too.
5. In certain malignant conditions, the serum phosphate level may either remain normal or be somewhat elevated when the serum calcium is elevated.

POSSIBLE NURSING DIAGNOSES RELATED TO ELEVATED PHOSPHATE LEVELS

Potential Alterations in Nutritional Requirements of Calcium and Phosphorus

If the underlying problem is due to hypoparathyroidism, then replacement with calcium and vitamin D corrects the problem. If the phosphorus and calcium levels are both elevated, the client may be put on a moderately reduced calcium and phosphorus diet by limiting dairy products (see the discussion for hypercalcemia diets). If the serum phosphorus level is increased and the serum calcium is normal or decreased, the restriction of dairy products must be countered by calcium supplements. It is hard to significantly reduce the serum phosphorus level by diet alone because phosphorus is abundant in many more foods than is calcium (Mundy et al., 1977). Certain medications may also contain significant amounts of phosphates. For example, sodium phosphate enemas would be contraindicated if hyperphosphatemia is possible (Biberstein & Parker, 1985).

Knowledge Deficit Regarding Use of Phosphate Binders

If the phosphorus level is high and the calcium level is low, as often happens in renal failure, the client may be put on medication to reduce the phosphate level. Aluminum hydroxide gels (AluCaps or Aludrox), given by mouth, unite with the phosphates present in food to form insoluble aluminum phosphate. These insoluble phosphate compounds are then excreted in the feces. Magnesium hydroxide also binds phosphates, but the additional magnesium intake is contraindicated in renal failure. Aluminum hydroxide is continued even after dialysis is started because dialysis cannot efficiently reduce serum phosphate levels.

Decreased Serum Phosphorus Level (Hypophosphatemia)

Clinical Significance. Moderate hypophosphatemia can result from a variety of conditions (Table 7–3):

1. Hyperparathyroidism results in a high serum calcium level and a low phosphorus level.
2. Diuretics may cause a low phosphorus level.
3. Phosphates can be lost in large amounts in some types of renal diseases, although phosphate retention is more common.
4. Drugs that bind up phosphate, such as aluminum or magnesium gels, can cause phosphate deficiency. However, diets are usually high in phosphates so this pharmacological binding of antacids is usually not a major concern.
5. Malabsorption syndromes may eventually lead to low serum phosphorus levels.

Other clinical conditions in which serum phosphorus concentrations may fall are alcoholic withdrawal, diabetes mellitus, the recovery diuretic phase after severe burns, hyperalimentation therapy, and nutritional recovery syndrome. Baker (1985) notes that hypophosphatemia is the most frequent and dangerous electrolyte disorder occurring with hyperalimentation. Exactly why all these clinical conditions cause hypophosphatemia is not completely understood. It is known that, when glucose metabolism is increased (carbohydrate loading), the phosphorus ions become tied up. Also a decrease in serum magnesium ions or a shift in potassium ions tends to create hypophosphatemia. Knochel (1977, 1985) has two extensive reviews of research on hypophosphatemia.

POSSIBLE NURSING DIAGNOSES RELATED TO LOW PHOSPHORUS LEVELS

Potential for Injury Related to Neuromuscular Deficits
It is hypothesized that lowered serum phosphorus levels create central nervous system symptoms such as irritability and confusion. Hence nurses must be aware that clients with any altered electrolyte may not be able to function normally; so safety precautions become very important.

Potential for Injury Related to Replacement Therapies
Therapy for low serum phosphate levels may include administration of phosphate salts in oral or intravenous form. Because clients likely to develop low phosphorus levels may also develop low potassium and low magnesium levels, the nurse must be familiar with all the replacements being used. Potassium phosphate should be given at no more than 10 mEq/hr (Baker, 1985). The greatest hazard of giving large amounts of phosphates is that hypocalcemia may result.

Possible Alteration in Nutritional Requirements
If the client can tolerate oral feedings, milk is a very good source of phosphorus. It is usually not necessary to do long-term health teaching about phosphor-

us intake because in a regular diet phosphates are abundant. The concern with the client who has a low serum phosphorus level is to correct the often complex metabolic problem that has caused the deficiency in the serum. If the lowered serum phosphorus level is due to hyperparathyroidism, surgery is usually done.

■ URINARY PHOSPHORUS

Preparation of Client and Collection of Sample

All urine is collected over a 24-hour period. There is no need for a preservative in the bottle, and the urine does not need to be iced. (Note that for urine calcium a preservative is needed. When both calcium and potassium are to be collected the preservative will not interfere with the test for phosphorus.)

Reference Values for Urinary Phosphorus	
All groups	0.4–1.3 g in 24 hr. Varies with intake. Average is 1 g in 24 hr

Clinical Significance. Urinary phosphorus levels usually reflect the amount of both organic and inorganic phosphates taken in the diet. Because PTH causes a decreased renal reabsorption of phosphorus, hyperparathyroidism causes an increased urinary phosphorus level. This test may help to explain the alterations in serum calcium and phosphorus levels. In renal failure, the excretion of phosphates may be impaired so that the urinary phosphorus level is decreased. However, testing the urine in renal failure usually does not give any additional clinical help. The urinary phosphorus test is most often used when there is a complex metabolic problem, such as an endocrine disturbance or malnutrition problems, and when a very complete investigation of all electrolyte disturbances needs to be done to monitor the progress of the client.

■ SERUM MAGNESIUM (Mg^{++})

Primarily an intracellular ion, magnesium appears in the bloodstream only in very small amounts. The bulk of magnesium is combined with calcium and phosphorus in the bones. Magnesium is essential for neuromuscular function and for activation of certain enzymes in the body. Changes in serum magnesium levels affect other serum ions, too, such as potassium, calcium, and phosphorus. Thus magnesium deficiency is not usually seen alone. Evidently the body can store magnesium, because deficiencies usually develop in chronic conditions not in acute conditions.

Because magnesium is present in a variety of foods, a normal diet supplies the recommended daily allowances. Magnesium requirements for infants and children may range from 60–250 mg, depending on age, but optimum levels for children are not clearly established (Chan, 1979). Adult men need around 350 mg and adult women around 300 mg. Pregnancy and lactation increase the need to around 450 mg. Some studies suggest the present requirement may not be optimal for most people (Seelig, 1982).

Magnesium is excreted primarily by the kidney. The hormone aldosterone causes an increased excretion of magnesium as it does of potassium. Compared to the facts known about potassium, much is still to be learned about how magnesium functions in the body. (See Chapter 5 for a detailed discussion of the effect of aldosterone on potassium levels.)

Preparation of Client and Collection of Sample

The client does not have to be fasting. One ml of serum is needed. Calcium gluconate may interfere with some test methods. Hemolysis of the specimen must be avoided because magnesium is primarily an intracellular ion.

Reference Values for Serum Magnesium

Adult	1.5–2.0 mEq/L or 1.4–2.5 mg
Pregnancy	Gradual fall of about 10–20%
Children	1.54–1.86 mEq/L
Aged	No reported difference

Increased Serum Magnesium Level (Hypermagnesemia)

Clinical Significance. Renal failure is the most common reason for magnesium excess, because the kidneys are unable to excrete magnesium normally. If the renal output is not adequate, an increased magnesium level may result from the administration of medications containing magnesium, such as milk of magnesia (Table 7–4).

Obstetrical clients who receive magnesium sulfate ($MgSO_4$) parenterally for treatment for preeclampsia or toxemia can develop extremely elevated serum magnesium levels if the intravenous rate and the urinary output are not carefully monitored. Therapeutic serum levels for clients receiving $MgSO_4$ are kept in a range of 2.5–7.5 mEq/L (Butts, 1977) or 5–7 mEq/L for premature labor (Elliott, 1983).

POSSIBLE NURSING DIAGNOSES RELATED TO ELEVATED MAGNESIUM LEVELS

Potential for Injury Related to Alterations in Neuromuscular Functioning

Higher-than-normal levels of serum magnesium produce sedation, depression of the neuromuscular system, and some reduction in the blood pressure. If the mother was given $MgSO_4$, the newborn may have lethargy and respiratory depression. Whether the excess magnesium is due to renal failure or intravenous therapy treatment for toxemia, an excess of magnesium can lead from muscle weakness to muscle paralysis, so that deep tendon reflexes are weak or absent. In severe hypermagnesemia (over 10 mEq/L), paralysis of voluntary muscles produces flaccid quadriplegia and respiratory failure (Quinlan, 1983). Severe hypotension occurs. The electrocardiogram (ECG) shows changes similar to those of potassium excess. Thus nursing assessments for the client who is at risk for developing serum magnesium excess should include: (1) frequent blood pressure and pulse monitoring, (2) assessment of the client's level of consciousness, (3) presence of normal reflexes such as the knee jerk, and (4) careful intake and output records.

In addition to muscle weakness the client may be confused and thus less aware of the surrounding environment. The nurse must take whatever measures are necessary to protect the client from injury. If the magnesium excess is causing acute problems, the physician may order calcium gluconate or calcium chloride to be given intravenously because calcium is the antidote for magnesium excess.

Knowledge Deficit Regarding Hidden Sources of Magnesium
Clients with chronic renal failure should not be given any medications that contain magnesium. The nurse needs to do some client teaching because several over-the-counter drugs contain magnesium. For example, antacids used should be those that contain aluminum hydroxide gels, not magnesium hydroxide. A popular cathartic, epsom salts, is a compound of magnesium sulfate. Many other laxatives contain magnesium, and those pose a special threat to the elderly with decreased renal function. The dietary restriction of magnesium intake is not a focus for teaching because most foods contain only a trace of this mineral.

Decreased Serum Magnesium Level (Hypomagnesemia)

Clinical Significance. A decrease in serum magnesium is usually due to some type of chronic problem involving a low intake of dietary magnesium over a long period of time (Table 7-4). For example, people who use alcohol as the primary source of calories may become deficient in magnesium. Deficiencies may also result from impaired absorption, such as that associated with a draining intestinal fistula or with heavy use of diuretics. Cohen and Kitzes (1983) note that a normal serum magnesium level does not rule out the possibility that a digitalis-toxic arrhythmia is being caused by a magnesium deficiency. Because long-term therapy with a diuretic can deplete magnesium, a lymphocyte magnesium content may be better than a serum level to determine true deficiency. One study revealed that clients on digitalis were twice as likely to have a deficit of magnesium as a deficit of potassium (Whang et al., 1985). Various metabolic disorders, such as hypercalcemia, may contribute to magnesium deficiency. Research has suggested that there is a lowering of magnesium levels in long-term insulin-treated diabetics and hypomagnesium appears to be an additional

TABLE 7-4. COMMON REASONS FOR CHANGES IN THE SERUM MAGNESIUM LEVEL

Hypermagnesemia (Serum Mg^{++} level above 2 mEq/L)
   Renal failure

   IV administration of $MgSO_4$ for toxemia

Hypomagnesemia (Serum Mg^{++} level below 1.5 mEq/L)
   Chronic malnutrition (i.e., alcoholism)

   Diarrhea or draining gastrointestinal fistulas

   Diuretics

   Diabetes

   Hypercalcemia or other complex metabolic disorders

See text and Chan (1979); Elbaum (1977); Freeman and Wittine (1977); Felver (1980); Cohen and Kitzes (1983), and Elliott (1983) for more details.

risk factor for the development of retinopathy in diabetics (McNair et al., 1978). Clients with low magnesium levels may also have unexplained hypocalcemia and hypo-kalemia, which causes complex electrolyte imbalances.

POSSIBLE NURSING DIAGNOSES RELATED TO HYPOMAGNESEMIA

Alterations in Nutritional Needs, Less than Body Requirements

An assessment for magnesium deficiency is appropriate for clients who have to be fed by artificial means or who are chronically malnourished. As long as a client is able to take a regular diet, increasing foods that are high in mag-nesium has little practical significance; the trace mineral is sufficient in a regular diet. Recent studies have suggested that magnesium requirements may be in-creased during total parenteral nutrition. The average need for the client on long-term hyperalimentation may be around 400 mg (Freeman & Wittine, 1977). Nurses should be aware of the need for replacement therapy of magnesium for any client who has poor nutrition over an extended period of time. Also the combination of diuretics and digioxin can lead to digioxin toxicity if the magnesium level is low in the cells.

Sleep Pattern Disturbances and Neuromuscular Irritability

Early symptoms of a lack of magnesium are related to neuromuscular irritability: The client may have tremors, muscle cramps, and insomnia. The nurse should assess for any involuntary movements or twitching by the client. See the sec-tion on hypocalcemia on how to check for a positive Chvostek's sign and a positive Trousseau's sign. The client may eventually show symptoms that look very similar to the tetany of hypocalcemia. Often the client may have several deficiencies so that the clinical picture is not so simple. Laboratory tests have to be done to identify exactly which electrolyte imbalances coexist. A low calcium or a low potassium that is unresponsive to treatment may be due to a coex-isting low magnesium (Elbaum, 1977).

Potential for Injury Due to Intravenous Magnesium Replacements

Magnesium deficits are corrected by the intravenous use of magnesium sulfate, which comes in concentrations of 10% and 50%. One gram of $MgSO_4$ is equal to 8.12 mEq or 4.06 millimoles. Usually 2–4 g (17–34 mEq) may be given daily in divided doses. The dosage for children is calculated on the basis of weight. If magnesium is being given intravenously, the nurse must assess carefully for the signs and symptoms of magnesium excess discussed in the section on hyper-magnesium. The intravenous infusion should be stopped if there is a sharp de-crease in blood pressure, extreme sedation, or weak reflexes. The importance of assessing for the patellar reflex (knee jerk) was already stressed.

QUESTIONS

1. A public health nurse is visiting Mrs. Johnson, an elderly woman who lives alone and who does her own cooking. She considers milk to be "for babies." If she

does not wish to drink milk or use it in cooking, which alternative foods would offer the highest calcium intake?

   a. Fresh greens, beans, whole wheat products
   b. Rice, liver, and chicken
   c. Apples, oranges, and other citrus fruits
   d. Potatoes, shellfish, and cornmeal

2. Hypercalcemia (high serum calcium levels) should be assessed as a potential problem for all of the following clients *except* which?

   a. Mr. Robbins, who is in acute renal failure
   b. Mrs. Berry, who has been on bedrest for several weeks with multiple fractures
   c. Mr. Clancy, who has metastatic bone disease
   d. Mr. Berlin, who takes vitamin D capsules and drinks a lot of milk

3. All of the following medications are sometimes used to reduce high serum calcium levels *except* which?

   a. Aluminum hydroxide   c. Mithramycin
   b. Corticosteroids   d. Calcitonin

4. Which nursing action is the most important to prevent complications for clients with a high serum calcium level?

   a. Keeping the pH of the urine alkaline
   b. Checking for signs of tetany
   c. Making sure the client is well hydrated
   d. Checking for tachycardia

5. A lactating mother who drinks only one or two glasses of milk a day will most likely continue to have a normal serum calcium level for which of the following reasons?

   a. Two glasses of milk supply the minimum calcium requirements for lactation
   b. Calcium is also available in most meat products and leafy green vegetables
   c. Lactation causes a decrease in the parathyroid hormone
   d. Calcium is being drawn from the reservoir in the bones and teeth

6. Which of the following is a characteristic symptom of a low serum calcium level?

   a. Flank pain   c. Bradycardia
   b. Carpopedal spasms   d. Constipation

7. Which of the following clients has little possibility of developing symptoms of hypocalcemia?

   a. Baby Lynn, a premature infant born this morning
   b. Mrs. Thomas, who had a subtotal thyroidectomy today
   c. Mrs. Rhoades, who has metastatic cancer of the liver
   d. Jack Benson, who has acute pancreatitis

8. Which of these clients is the most likely to have decreased serum calcium and serum phosphorus levels?

   a. Mr. Lamb, who takes a lot of antacids and milk
   b. Mr. Babiloni, who is in renal failure
   c. Baby Wong, who is on a low-fat diet and who is never taken outdoors
   d. Mrs. Candy, who is in a diabetic coma and who is being treated with glucose and insulin

9. When a qualitative method of testing for calcium in the urine (Sulkowitch test) is being done to assess the possibility of hypocalcemia, the client should be taught to collect the urine specimen when?

   a. Before meals   b. After meals   c. Randomly   d. Upon arising

10. Mr. Jacobs is on therapy to reduce his serum phosphorus level. Which of the following foods is not high in phosphorus content and would thus be allowed on his diet?

    a. Processed luncheon meat   c. Soft drinks
    b. Skim milk   d. Apples

11. In a client with chronic renal failure, aluminum hydroxide may be useful in lowering serum phosphorus levels because the drug:

    a. Causes precipitation of insoluble phosphates in the intestine
    b. Increases secretion of phosphorus in the urine
    c. Counteracts the effect of the parathyroid hormone
    d. Balances the pH of the serum

12. The nurse should be assessing all of the following clients for symptoms of magnesium deficiency *except* which?

    a. Sally, age 5, who has had vomiting and diarrhea for 24 hours
    b. Mrs. Leandro, who is on hyperalimentation therapy
    c. Mr. White, who has a long history of alcohol abuse
    d. Mrs. Warzenkiak, who has a chronic problem with a draining gastrointestinal fistula

13. Mr. Olino is an elderly man who has had poor nutritional habits over an extended period of time. The public health nurse suspects that magnesium deficiency may be one of his problems. Which of the following symptoms would *not* be indicative of a low serum magnesium?

    a. Leg and foot cramps   c. Irritability
    b. Tremors   d. Unusual amount of sleeping

14. Mrs. Long is receiving magnesium sulfate ($MgSO_4$) intravenously as treatment for preeclampsia. Which of the following nursing assessments is an indication that Mrs. Long may be developing a serum magnesium excess?

    a. Rise in pulse and blood pressure

b. Exaggerated patellar reflex (knee jerk)

c. Sedation

d. Seizure activity

15. An antidote for high serum magnesium levels is the administration of which of the following?

a. Potassium chloride

b. Calcium gluconate

c. Aluminum hydroxide

d. Calcitonin

REFERENCES

American Academy of Pediatrics Committee on Nutrition. (1978). Calcium requirements in infancy and childhood. *Pediatrics, 62*(11), 826–833.

Baker, W. (1985). Hypophosphatemia. *AJN, 85*(9), 999–1003.

Biberstein, M., & Parker, B. (1985). Enema-induced hyperphosphatemia. *American Journal of Medicine 79,* 645.

Butler, R., et al. (1985). Calcinosis of joints and periarticular tissues associated with vitamin D intoxication. *Annals of Rheumatic Disease, 44*(7), 494–498.

Butts, P. (1977). Magnesium sulfate in the treatment of toxemia. *AJN, 77*(8), 1294–1298.

Canalis, E., et al. (1977). Hypercalcemia: Diagnosis and therapy. *Connecticut Medicine, 41*(1), 16–21.

Cerrato, P. (1985). Hidden malnutrition in geriatric patients. *RN, 48*(7), 60–62.

Chan, J. (1979). Clinical disorders of calcium, phosphate, magnesium, and hydrogen ion metabolism: Diagnostic approach in children. *Urology, 13*(2), 122–128.

Cohen, L., & Kitzes, R. (1983). Magnesium sulfate and digitalis-toxic arrhythmias. *JAMA, 249*(20), 2808–2810.

Coward, D. (1985). Knowledge of hypercalcemia in patients at risk to develop cancer-induced hypercalcemia. *National Symposium of Nursing Research Abstracts.* San Francisco: Stanford University Hospital.

DeLuca, H. (1981). Modern views of vitamin D. *Contemporary Nutrition, 6*(2), 1–2.

Domenech, E., & Maya, M. (1978). Calcium intake in the first five days of life in the low birthweight infant. *Archives of Disease in Childhood, 53*(10), 784–787.

Elbaum, N. (1977). Detecting and correcting magnesium imbalance. *Nursing 77, 7*(8), 34–35.

Elbaum, N. (1984). With cancer patients, be alert for hypercalcemia. *Nursing 84, 14*(9), 58–59.

Elliott, G., & McKenzie, M. (1983). Treatments of hypercalcemia. *Drug Intelligence and Clinical Pharmacy, 17*(1), 12–21.

Elliott, J. (1983). Magnesium sulfate as a tocolytic agent. *American Journal of Obstetrics and Gynecology, 147*(3), 277–283.

Felver, L. (1980). Understanding the electrolyte maze. *AJN, 80*(9), 1591–1595.

Freeman, J., & Wittine, M. (1977). Magnesium requirements are increased during total parenteral nutrition. *Surgical Forum, 28*(10), 61–62.

Knochel, J. (1977). The pathophysiology and clinical characteristics of severe hypophosphatemia. *Archives of Internal Medicine, 137*(2), 203–225.

Knochel, J. (1985). The clinical status of hypophosphatemia. An update. *NEJM, 313*(7), 447–449.

Kreisberg, R. (1977). Phosphorus deficiency and hypophosphatemia. *Hospital Practice, 12*(3), 121–128.

Linkswiler, H., & Zemel, M. (1979). Calcium to phosphorus ratios. *Contemporary Nutrition, 4,* 1–2.

McFadden, E., Zaloga, G., & Chernow, B. (1983). Hypocalcemia: A medical emergency. *AJN, 83*(2), 227–230.

McNair, P., et al. (1978). Hypomagnesemia: A risk factor in diabetic retinopathy. *Diabetes, 27*(10), 1075–1077.

Mundy, G., et al. (1977). Calcium and the kidney: Renal osteodystrophy and renal calculi. *Connecticut Medicine, 41,* 205–209.

Quinlan, M. (1982). Solving the mysteries of calcium imbalance: An action guide. *RN, 45*(11), 50–52.

Quinlan, M. (1983). Would you recognize this dangerous electrolyte imbalance? *RN, 46*(3), 51–55.

Recker, R. (1983). Osteoporosis. *Contemporary Nutrition, 8*(5), 1–2.

Seelig, M. (1982). Magnesium requirements in human nutrition. *Contemporary Nutrition, 7*(1), 1–2.

Smith, L., et al. (1978). Current concepts in nutrition: Nutrition and urolithiasis. *NEJM, 298,* 87–89.

Tripp, A. (1976). Hyper and hypocalcemia. *AJN, 76*(7), 1142–1145.

Whang, R., et al. (1985). Frequency of hypomagnesemia in hospitalized patients receiving digitalis. *Archives Internal Medicine, 145*(5), 655.

Wood, C. (1977). Calcium metabolism. *Nurse Practitioner, 2*(9), 30–32.

8

Tests to Measure the Metabolism of Glucose and Other Sugars

- Fasting Blood Sugar (FBS)
- Postprandial Blood Sugar (PPBS) or Two-Hour P.C. Blood Sugar
- Random Blood Sugar (RBS)
- Blood Glucose Finger Sticks
- Glucose Tolerance Test (GTT)
- Glycosylated Hemoglobin (GHB) and Hemoglobin A_{1c}
- Serum Acetone or Ketones
- Sugar and Acetone in Urine
- Sugars Other than Glucose in Urine
  Lactose Tolerance Test and Serum Test for Galactosemia

OBJECTIVES

1. Describe the hormonal control of serum glucose levels.
2. Compare the client preparation, usefulness, and limitations of the various tests of glucose to detect diabetes.
3. Describe the expected laboratory findings and related assessments in hyperosmolar hyperglycemic nonketotic coma (HHNK) and in ketoacidosis.
4. Identify appropriate nursing diagnoses for clients with hyperglycemia of varying severity.
5. Compare and contrast the assessment of hypoglycemia in adults, children, newborns, and the elderly.
6. Determine the priority nursing and medical interventions for various types of hypoglycemia, including reactive hypoglycemia.
7. Identify nursing assessments that would indicate the possibility of a rebound effect from insulin (Somogyi effect).
8. Develop a teaching plan to inform clients about urine and blood glucose tests done at home.

9. Analyze the similarities and differences in galactose and lactose intolerances, along with the laboratory tests used to identify each abnormality.

FBS, PPSB, RBS, GTT, and S and A's—these abbreviations should all be familiar
to the nurse because they represent very common measurements of the glucose in
the blood and urine. At the present time there is no general agreement over which
is the best to use for detecting diabetes mellitus. Clinicians may use several of these
tests both to diagnose and to evaluate the therapy for diabetes mellitus, as well as
for other conditions involving an elevated blood sugar level (hyperglycemia) or a low
blood sugar level (hypoglycemia). A newer test (GHB) has made it possible to evaluate
hyperglycemia over a period of about three months.

   Normally, all complex carbohydrates, including sugars and starches, are eventually broken down to glucose. In some metabolic abnormalities, such sugars as lactose and galactose are present in the serum and urine. The tests that may be done
to detect these abnormal sugars are covered in the last part of this chapter.

BRIEF SUMMARY OF GLUCOSE METABOLISM

Although the majority of glucose comes from the dietary intake of carbohydrates,
the liver can convert fats and protein into glucose when not enough glucose is available
for the cells. The liver also stores extra glucose in the form of glycogen. With an
excess of glucose intake, the glucose that is not stored as glycogen is converted into
adipose (fat) tissue. Several hormones influence serum glucose levels:

1. *Insulin,* secreted by the beta cells of the pancreas, is essential for the transport of glucose (and potassium) into the cells. A lack of insulin causes an
   increase in the blood glucose level and a potassium imbalance because the
   glucose and potassium cannot get into the cells.
2. *Glucagon,* secreted by the alpha cells of the pancreas, elevates blood glucose
   levels by promoting the conversion of glycogen to glucose. The role of
   glycogen in the treatment of hypoglycemia is explained in the section on
   hypoglycemia.
3. Other hormones that cause an elevation of blood glucose levels are the *corticosteroids, adrenalin,* and *growth hormone.* The hyperglycemic effects of
   these hormones are discussed under the section on the clinical significance
   of hyperglycemia.
4. In pregnancy, *human placental lactogen* (HPL) promotes increased blood
   glucose levels. Other hormones in pregnancy, *progesterone* and *estrogen,* may
   also either have a "diabetogenic effect" or at least raise the blood glucose level.

The actual presence or absence of diabetes may be difficult to assess, both in pregnant and nonpregnant clients, due to the complex hormonal interactions that control glucose metabolism. Table 8–1 summarizes the effect of hormones on glucose
metabolism.

   For most people, the renal threshold for glucose is around 160–190 mg/dl; that
is, glucose is not spilled into the urine until the blood glucose level is above 160–190
mg/dl. For some people, however, the renal threshold may be higher or lower. For

TABLE 8–1. EFFECTS OF HORMONES ON SERUM GLUCOSE LEVELS

Promote Hyperglycemia	Promote Hypoglycemia
Growth hormone	Insulin
Glucocorticoids	
Epinephrine and norepinephrine	
Glucagon	
Human placental lactogen (HPL)	
Estrogen	
Progesterone	
Thyroxin	

See Chapter 15 for detailed discussion of the tests for hormones.

example, in the elderly with a high renal threshold, glucose may not be excreted by the kidney even though the blood glucose is elevated above normal limits (Hayter, 1981). Urine sugar levels need to be compared to blood glucose levels to determine the specific renal threshold for an individual.

Besides some confusion about which values of urine and blood glucose levels indicate diabetes, there may also be additional confusion over the different testing methods used to determine the amount of glucose in the blood. Laboratories may use either the reducing method or an enzymatic method to measure glucose; the enzymatic methods are more often used because they are specific for glucose only. The differences between these two methods are discussed in Chapter 3 on urine testing for sugar because these two methods give different results in urine too. Usually a laboratory chooses to employ only an enzymatic or only the reducing method for serum or blood glucose levels.

As with other tests, these different methods will not be confusing for nurses as long as they always compare the results of a test to the reference values used by the laboratory. If a laboratory uses whole blood to test for blood glucose, for example, the values are about 10–15% lower than if plasma or serum is used, because the red blood cells are not as rich in glucose as in plasma. In this chapter, reference values for several methods are given so the reader is aware of the possible variations. When values are phrased only in general terms—such as "over 140 mg" or "below 300 mg"—they must be considered practical only as general guidelines to the more precise reference values in a particular setting. In clinical practice, the more general term "blood *sugar* level" is often used interchangeably with the more precise term "blood *glucose* level."

■ FASTING BLOOD SUGAR (FBS)

Special Preparation of Client

For a fasting blood sugar test, the client may not eat for at least four hours, but water intake may continue. If the client has an intravenous infusion that contains dextrose, the test is not valid. If the client is a diabetic being treated with insulin, both food and the insulin are withheld until the specimen is drawn.

The blood is collected in a tube with an EDTA-fluoride mixture as a glycolytic inhibitor. (Gray-topped Vacutainer is usually used, but check with the laboratory for the specific method.)

Reference Values (Serum Values, Not Whole Blood Values) for FBS

Adult	(Average around 70–110 mg/dl, but check with laboratory concerning technique used)
	90–120 mg/dl Folin–Wu method (a reducing method)
	65–95 mg/dl Somogyi–Neison (a reducing method)
	60–105 mg/dl Glucose oxidase (an enzyme method)
Newborn	20–80 mg/dl
	Full-term infants around 30 mg
	Low-weight infants stabilize around 20 mg in 72 hr
	Must consult specific orders in neonatal unit
	May treat premature if less than 40 mg/dl (San Francisco Children's Hospital)
Pregnancy	Slightly higher values may be "normal"
Children	Basically same as adults
Aged	Reference values may be slightly higher with aged, particularly with glucose tests other than FBS. The FBS increases only 1–2 mg per decade (Hayter, 1981)

As a general rule, in an adult, a FBS over 140 mg for 2–3 times indicates probable diabetes.

■ POSTPRANDIAL BLOOD SUGAR (PPBS) OR TWO-HOUR P.C. BLOOD SUGAR

Purpose of Test and Preparation of Client

"Postprandial" means after a meal. Sometimes the patient is given a meal consisting of a standard amount of carbohydrate, but more commonly, the laboratory draws the blood after a regular meal. The purpose of this test is to see how the body responds to the ingestion of carbohydrates in a meal.

The timing of the blood specimen drawing must be accurate. The laboratory technician usually draws the blood sample, but the nurse manages the time of the meal, observes what was eaten, and makes sure the client is available for the blood sample within two hours. All the factors that affect the glucose tolerance test results may also affect the p.c. blood sugar levels. Therefore, general use of this test is not recommended (Tietz, 1983).

Reference Values for PPBS

"Normally" the 2-hr postprandial blood sugar will have returned to the pre-meal levels, but such may not always be the case. A value over 140 mg may suggest diabetes. Because the 2-hr value rises about 5 mg/dl for each decade of life, a person of 60 has a 2-hr p.c. blood sugar about 15 mg higher than a person at age 30 (Hayter, 1981).

■ RANDOM BLOOD SUGAR (RBS)

Purpose of Test and Preparation of Client

Because random blood sugars are not drawn in relation to a meal, there is no specific preparation of the client. Blood sugars may be ordered to be drawn at 4 P.M., at 8

P.M., or at other times to assess the fluctuations of blood glucose levels during a 24-hr period.

Reference Values for RBS

For the nondiabetic person or for a diabetic client in good control, the random blood sugars should be within the normal ranges for fasting blood sugars or elevated only in direct relation to meal times.

■ BLOOD GLUCOSE FINGER STICKS

In the past, most diabetics were monitored by self-testing of urine and occasional blood glucose levels obtained by venipuncture by health professionals. (See Chapter 3 on urine tests for glucose). A "revolution" occurred when self-monitoring of blood glucose became possible with reagent strips, and if necessary, a photometer for a digital readout. Christiansen (1980) noted six types of diabetic clients who benefit the most from frequent self-monitoring of glucose levels. Such clients include those with:

1. Abnormal or unstable renal thresholds
2. Renal failure
3. Unstable-type juvenile diabetes (Type I)
4. Impaired color vision (need meter also)
5. Difficulty recognizing true hypoglycemia
6. Diabetes as a complicating factor of pregnancy

Even before the possibility of client self-monitoring, nurses often used reagent strips (Dextrostix by Ames Products) to test newborns for hypoglycemia. Now adults and parents of young children can do blood glucose monitoring at home with the newer reagent strips such as Visidex II (Ames Products) or Chem-Strip bG (Bio-Dynamics, Inc.). Urine tests are often seen as meaningless tests (Miller, 1986). There are two major drawbacks to the use of blood glucose monitoring for all diabetics; (1) the need to stick oneself, sometimes several times a day, and (2) the cost, which is about $750 a year to self-monitor blood glucose without a meter and $1000 to $2150 with a meter (Bergman & Felig, 1984). Clients can buy a small apparatus to do capillary sticks. Most supply houses sell them. Surr (1983a) gives pictorial instructions for three different types of these mechanical blood obtainers. Usually, the cost is worth the better control.

Preparation of Client and Collection of Sample

A drop of capillary blood is obtained by a finger stick, or in the case of an infant, by a heel stick. The extremity should be warm to encourage vasodilation. (See Chapter 1 on the procedure for heel and finger sticks). For routine monitoring at home, clients may just use soap and water rather than alcohol to clean the site. Several different companies make test strips, so it is crucial to follow the manufacturer's recommendations for a certain product. General guidelines include:

1. Cover the entire reagent pad with a large drop of blood. Do not smear the blood. Squeezing the finger to obtain one large drop of blood is permissible.
2. Begin timing exactly when the drop of blood covers the reagent pad on the

strip. Most strips require contact with the blood for 60 seconds, but 30 seconds is enough for some.

3. Remove the blood drop as recommended by the manufacturer. Some are blotted dry, others require the blood to be rinsed off.

4. Determine how much additional time (60–90 seconds is needed for some strips) is needed before reading.

5. Compare the strip with the color chart on the bottle in which the strip arrived. Each color chart is batch specific. Most strips have a range from 20 to 40 mg to 800 mg or more. The color pads are in 20–40 mg increments. If the sample is between two colors, estimate the result.

6. Most of the strips can be timed and dated so the reading can be double-checked by another person later. Clients may be instructed to bring in a weekly record for review by a health professional. Villeneuve et al. (1985) found that reagent strips do not always hold color for a week—perhaps because of improper storage.

7. Regular insulin may be given to cover the glucose. Guidelines for coverage may be: 180 mg/dl, no insulin; 240 mg/dl, 2–6 units; 400 mg/dl, 5–16 units; 800 mg/dl, 13–26 units. Also clients can learn to fine-tune their own insulin dosages (Robertson, 1985).

Use of Photometers

The strips used to monitor blood glucose can be put into a photometer or reflectance meter that gives a digital readout. The strips and meters are not interchangeable. Dextrostix, for example, is used in the Glucometer made by Ames Products (Ames Product Profiles, 1986), Chem-Strip bG (Bio-Dynamics Product Profile, 1986), in the Accu-Chek bG made by Bio-Dynamics, Inc. (See Chapter 1 for addresses of the major companies that make laboratory test kits.) For the color-blind client, the photometer is essential.

For others, the photometer may be an unneeded extra expense. Insurance companies may reimburse for these nonprescription products if the physician documents that the meter is necessary for clients to do accurate self-monitoring of blood glucose. Surr (1983b) has detailed pictures on how to use four different types of meters. Costs are detailed in a pictorial article by Joyce et al. (1983).

Reflectance meters with built-in timers and digital readouts can also be used with memory chips that record each determination so that when they are connected to a microcomputer, a data base is available for decision making (Villeneuve et al., 1985).

■ GLUCOSE TOLERANCE TEST (GTT)

Purpose of Test

The oral glucose tolerance test used to be considered the best way to diagnose diabetes mellitus (Siperstein, 1975). Yet since so many factors can render the test invalid, the current trend is to rely more on fasting blood sugar levels and, less likely, postprandial blood sugars (Wallach, 1986). Bed rest, infections, and trauma—as well as drugs, such as diuretics, birth control pills, or cortisone—all cause an abnormal glucose tolerance test. Even stress can alter the results. In fact, most clinicians feel that a glucose tolerance test is useless when a client is in the hospital because the person is always under some type of stress that makes the test results questionable.

One objection to the GTT is that normally no one ever sits down and eats pure glucose. Hence the response to the oral glucose load may not reflect the normal response to carbohydrate in food. In puzzling conditions, clinicians may still use the GTT to document the individual's reaction to a measured amount of glucose. Because the glucose tolerance test may be of limited value in any setting, one option is to have the client eat a high-carbohydrate diet for a few days and then draw a 2-hour p.c. blood sugar.

Preparation of Client

The client needs to be on a normal diet for several days before the GTT is done. The test is usually scheduled for early morning after the client has been fasting all night. Water is not withheld so that urine samples can be collected at the proper times.

At the start of the test, blood is drawn for a fasting blood sugar, and urine is obtained for testing for glycosuria. The client is then given 100 g of glucose dissolved in water. The glucose drink may be flavored with lemon juice to make it more palatable. (If the client cannot swallow the glucose, the glucose is sometimes given intravenously; but the intravenous glucose may make the test reflect normal carbohydrate metabolism even less.)

Urine and blood samples of glucose are collected at 1-, 2-, and 3-hour intervals. (Some laboratories may collect in half-hour intervals, and others may continue the test for up to 5 hours.) It is essential that the nurse and the client know the timing for each collection so that the blood and urine samples are all collected at the specified times. Although the client may not eat anything during the test, he or she should continue to drink plenty of water so that all the urine samples can be obtained. Clients are not able to urinate every hour unless they have adequate fluid intake. Even if they cannot void on time, the blood sample should be taken because this is the more important part of the GTT.

The results of all the samples are plotted on a graph to see how long it takes the blood sugar to return to normal. Diabetics may either take longer to return to base line readings or never return at all to fasting levels. Clients with reactive hypoglycemia may drop to subnormal blood sugar levels in response to the glucose load. The meaning of the curve must be carefully interpreted by the physician. The sample reference values that follow are based on information from several sources, and they show some of the differences that may be expected in GTT results.

Reference Values for GTT

	Range of Values Below Age 55	Average After 75	Average in Pregnancy
Fasting blood sugar	80–110 mg/dl	110 mg	90 mg
Blood sugar in 1 hr	120–160 mg/dl	200 mg	165 mg
Blood sugar in 2 hr	80–110 mg/dl	150 mg	145 mg
Blood sugar in 3 hr	80–110 mg/dl	140 mg	125 mg

■ GLYCOSYLATED HEMOGLOBIN (GHB) AND HEMOGLOBIN A$_{1c}$

With prolonged hyperglycemia, some of the hemoglobin remains saturated with glucose for the life of the red cell. So a test of glycosylated hemoglobin is a reflection of serum glucose over a period of weeks. Due to problems with standardization and cost, glycosylated hemoglobin tests were not routine tests in most laboratories in the early 80s (Garofono, 1981).

With improvements in the tests for glycosylated or glycohemoglobin has come a wider use of the test in everyday clinical practice. This test is most useful for assessing overall control in insulin-dependent diabetics (Type I). For non-insulin-dependent diabetics (Type II) there is usually not a need to supplement fasting blood sugars with this more costly test.

Glycosylated hemoglobin refers to the components of hemoglobin that have glucose attached. Beyond 6 months of age, at least 90% of the total hemoglobin is hemoglobin A, and this hemoglobin A contains three components that have the glucose attached. Laboratories may measure one of these components or all three for the glycosylated hemoglobin values. The three minor hemoglobins that have glucose attached are A_{1a}, A_{1b}, and A_{1c}. Hemoglobin A_{1c} is the most abundant of the three so is sometimes used for the test (Metzger, 1983). However, other laboratories will measure all of the hemoglobin A_1 and just call the test glycosylated hemoglobin or glycohemoglobin (GHB). It is important to know which type of testing is being done because hemoglobin A_1 is always 2–4% higher than hemoglobin A_{1c}.

Preparation of Client and Collection of Sample

Usual diet and medications are taken, including insulin or oral hypoglycemic agents. (Diabetics may think they must fast as they do for other routine tests for blood glucose levels.) A 5-ml specimen of venous blood is collected in a lavender-top (EDTA) tube. Put it on ice and send it promptly to the laboratory.

Reference Values for Hb A_{1c} and GHB

Hemoglobin A_{1c} (only measures one component of Hemoglobin A: A_{1c})[a]

2.2–4.8%	Nondiabetic adult
1.8–4.0%	Nondiabetic child
2.5–5.9%	Good diabetic control
6.0–8.0%	Fair diabetic control
> 8.0%	Poor diabetic control

Glycosylated Hemoglobin (measures 3 components of Hemoglobin A: A_{1a}, A_{1b}, A_{1c})[b]

7.5% or lower	Good diabetic control
7.6%–8.9%	Fair diabetic control
9.0% or more	Poor diabetic control

---

[a]From Metzger, 1983.
[b]From White & Miller, 1983.

POSSIBLE NURSING DIAGNOSES RELATED TO ELEVATED GHB

Home Maintenance Management, Impaired

An elevated glycosylated hemoglobin may help motivate the client to relook at the way he or she is managing diabetic control. Metzger (1983) noted that clients took more interest and responsibility for their management of diabetes when they could see that their present regimen was resulting in poor control. White and Miller (1983) have also found the test useful as a motivating factor.

The next section discusses other pertinent information related to helping the client control hyperglycemia.

Possible Noncompliance
White and Miller (1983) found the test useful in identifying clients, including children, who have consciously tried to influence their blood or urine tests to hide noncompliance. Obviously, once noncompliance has been identified, the nurse must help try to discover the reasons for the noncompliance.

Elevated Blood Glucose Level (Hyperglycemia)

Clinical Significance. The most common reason for a persistently elevated blood glucose is diabetes mellitus, in which condition the relative lack of physiologically active insulin results in an increased blood glucose level. With extremely high serum glucose levels, diagnosis is easily confirmed, even though the exact level diagnostic of diabetes mellitus is controversial.

Values that denote diabetic coma are fairly standard:

1. In mild diabetic coma, the blood glucose is usually around 300–450 mg/dl.
2. In moderate diabetic acidosis, the blood glucose is around 450 mg–600 mg/dl.
3. In severe diabetic coma, the blood glucose is usually over 600 mg/dl.

Hyperglycemia from other causes may not be as pronounced as the hyperglycemia in diabetic acidosis. In addition, the test for plasma acetone (covered next) will be positive in diabetic acidosis and not in other types of hyperglycemia. Sometimes acute pancreatitis may cause a diabetic state because the beta cells cannot function properly. More often the exact cause of the diabetic state is not known, because much is still to be learned about the disease labeled "diabetes" and about the other conditions that cause hyperglycemia.

In clinical conditions, when certain hormones are elevated, hyperglycemia may be present.

1. The *glucocorticoids,* for example, tend to raise blood glucose levels due to the breaking down of protein to form new glucose (neoglucogenesis). Clients with Cushing's syndrome or clients on high doses of cortisone may have higher-than-normal blood glucose levels.
2. Because *adrenalin* increases serum glucose levels, any stress such as shock, burns, or trauma may create an elevated blood glucose level.
3. The *growth hormone,* secreted by the pituitary gland, creates an elevated blood glucose by making the cells more resistant to insulin. Tumors or other factors may cause abnormal functioning of the pituitary gland. (See Chapter 15.) Because even a normal amount of growth hormone may make diabetes harder to control, scientists are trying to develop drugs that could selectively inhibit the secretion of growth hormone in diabetics (Press et al., 1984).
4. During pregnancy, several hormones tend to cause some hyperglycemia. The placenta secretes *human placental lactogen* (HPL) or *human chorionic somatomammotropin,* which tends to raise the blood glucose level. In addition, the increased levels of *estrogen* and *progesterone* may cause some increase.

Pregnant clients are classified A through F, according to the severity of the diabetes and of the potential problems that may occur during pregnancy. McAteer

(1979) describes in detail the use of White's classification system, along with the diagnostic testing done in pregnancy and in the newborn. As a general rule, women who become diabetic only during pregnancy (Class A) are not diabetic when the stress of pregnancy is over. Also, diabetics who require additional insulin during the last two trimesters of pregnancy usually return to a lower need or to no need at all for insulin when pregnancy is over (Rancilia, 1979; Schuler, 1979).

Juvenile onset diabetes (before age 15) differs in many ways from adult or maturity onset diabetes. In children, the lack of insulin is usually severe so that diabetic coma or ketoacidosis is much more likely to occur. Diabetics who require insulin are called Type I and those who are non-insulin-dependent are Type II. Adults with Type I have a much greater potential for diabetic coma than do Type II (Stock-Barkman, 1983).

POSSIBLE NURSING DIAGNOSES RELATED TO HYPERGLYCEMIA

Anxiety Related to Potential Diagnosis of Diabetes

Clients with newly elevated blood glucose levels may be very anxious while further testing is being done. The possibility of diabetes may be particularly frightening if they have known someone who had numerous complications from the disease. Assessments may indicate the need for some health teaching while the client is undergoing a diabetic work-up.

1. Excess glucose in the blood can be deposited in the lenses of the eyes, causing blurred vision. It may be several weeks before the sugar deposits are cleared from the lenses (Hayter, 1981). Thus eye examinations for fitting glasses should not be done until the hyperglycemia is controlled.
2. Of course, talking about a specific diabetic diet during testing would be premature. But if the person is overweight, diet counseling may be very appropriate if aimed at motivating the person to shed extra pounds.
3. The importance of exercise in helping the body utilize glucose could also be discussed.
4. Because an elevated blood sugar makes the person more susceptible to infections, cleanliness becomes very important.

Knowledge Deficit Related to Management of a Chronic Disease

If the patient is eventually diagnosed as diabetic, the nurse is instrumental in helping the patient to learn to manage the disease including self-injections of insulin and self-monitoring of glucose levels discussed earlier. Because dietary regimes must be practiced lifelong, every effort should be made to facilitate compliance by a flexible approach (Chait, 1984). One newer approach is the use of a glycemic index, which can be used with the ADA diet. The glycemic index rates carbohydrate-rich foods according to how high they elevate blood glucose levels. For example, glucose (corn sugar) has a rating of 100%, an orange 40%, and soybeans 15% (Cerrato, 1985). By choosing foods with a low glycemic index, the diabetic may require less insulin.

Potential for Fluid Volume Deficits and Electrolyte Imbalances

Two of the most important nursing implications for clients with elevated blood sugars are (1) to keep them from becoming dehydrated and (2) to assess for electrolyte imbalances. Glucose in high concentrations in the bloodstream functions as an osmotic diuretic because it makes the plasma hypertonic (Table 8–2). Extra water is pulled into the vascular system from the interstitial spaces and even from the cells if the hyperglycemia is severe and long-lasting. As excess glucose is excreted by the kidneys, so are enormous amounts of water. Thus the key symptoms of hyperglycemia are thirst (polydipsia) and increased urination (polyuria).

As long as the client can drink large amounts of water, dehydration may not occur, but the continued diuresis causes a loss of potassium and sodium. The loss of these electrolytes leads to some of the specific problems discussed in Chapter 5.

If the hyperglycemia is due to a lack of insulin, then the other two cardinal signs of diabetes, polyphagia and weight loss, eventually occur, because the cells are literally starving for glucose.

When dehydration becomes pronounced, the person has the characteristic signs and symptoms such as the loss of skin turgor, flushed warm skin, and soft eyeballs. The soft eyeballs are due to lack of fluid in the interstitial tissue of the eyeball.

Interventions for Hyperosmolar Hyperglycemic Nonketotic Coma. The progression of the above symptoms is called *hyperosmolar hyperglycemic nonketotic coma* (HHNK). A hyperglycemic coma can occur as a result not only of diabetes but of any pathologic condition entailing a persistently high blood sugar that causes severe dehydration and electrolyte imbalance. The coma is called "nonketotic" because ketones are not part of the pathological problem; the serum ketones (see the test for plasma acetone) do not increase. Therapy is geared to reducing the blood sugar level by replacing fluids and perhaps by giving some insulin to help the body utilize the excess sugar. Since thromboembolic episodes can occur due to the increased viscosity of the blood, nurses should institute measures to decrease the chance of venous thrombi. HHNK can be a complication of hyperalimentation therapy if glucose levels are not closely monitored. (See Chapter 3 on urine sugar levels in hyperalimentation therapy.)

Interventions for Diabetic Coma due to Ketoacidosis. In diabetes, the three levels of glucose intolerance are hyperglycemia, ketosis, and ketoacidosis. Diabetic coma is caused by severe dehydration and by the acidosis resulting from

TABLE 8–2. EFFECT OF ELEVATED GLUCOSE ON SERUM OSMOLALITY

For an estimate of serum osmolality, the formula is:

$$2(Na + K) + BUN/2.8 + blood\ glucose/18 = estimate\ of\ serum\ osmolality$$

Use of formula with normal lab values

$$2(135 + 4.5) + 15/2.8 + 120/18$$
$$279 + 5.36 + 6.66 = 291$$

Change of values with HHNK

$$2(146 + 5.0) + 28/2.8 + 300/18$$
$$302 + 10 + 16.66 = 329$$

Note: Reference values for serum osmolality are 282–295 mOsm Kg H$_2$O, and the values for a calculated one should be within + or − 9 or 10 mOsm (Jacobs et al., 1984; Wallach, 1986). See Chapter 4 for a discussion of the precise measurement of serum osmolality. Also see Hennessy (1983) on HHNK.

the build-up of ketone bodies. When glucose is not available for the cells because of the lack of insulin, fats and sometimes protein are converted to glucose and used as the source for energy. The incomplete oxidation of fats and proteins lead to the buildup of ketones in the bloodstream (ketosis). Eventually the ketones, which are acid, exhaust the buffering capacity of the blood and ketoacidosis occurs. The serum bicarbonate level is decreased. Ketoacidosis, as one type of metabolic acidosis, is discussed in Chapter 6 in the section on decreased serum bicarbonate levels. (Note also that the P_{CO_2} level decreases in an attempt to compensate for an overwhelming acidotic state.) Table 8–3 provides a summary of some of the symptoms of hyperglycemia and of hypoglycemia; Table 8–4 shows the laboratory reports used for diabetic ketoacidosis.

Nursing interventions for ketoacidosis include the careful regulation of intravenous fluid and electrolyte replacements, as for HHNK. Electrolytes must be carefully monitored during the acute stages of diabetic coma. Isotonic saline (0.9% sodium chloride) is usually administered, at a rapid rate, as the first infusion. When the blood glucose falls to 250 or 300 mg/dl, the physician may change the intravenous fluid orders to include dextrose 5% so hypoglycemia will not occur later (McCarthy, 1985). Potassium levels are high in the serum because insulin is needed for optimal transportation of potassium into the cells. Potassium also leaves the cell as more hydrogen ions go into it. (See Chapter 5 on the effect of acidosis on the potassium level.) When the acidosis is corrected, hypokalemia may occur if adequate replacement is not given, and hyponatremia may result from the loss of sodium by diuresis. Because dehydration may cause a pseudo-elevation of serum sodium levels, osmolality tests of serum and urine (Chapter 4) are useful to assess the magnitude of the dehydration.

TABLE 8-3. OUTSTANDING SIGNS AND SYMPTOMS OF HYPERGLYCEMIA AND HYPOGLYCEMIA

Hyperglycemia (Most of symptoms are due to dehydration; occurs gradually)
 1. Frequent urination, (positive for sugar)
 2. Thirst, dry mouth, and skin
 3. Soft eyeballs
 4. Nausea, vomiting, abdominal pain
 5. Weakness, confusion, blurred vision
 6. Severe dehydration and electrolyte imbalance
 7. Possible coma
 8. Urine positive for ketones[a]
 9. Kussmaul's respiration[a]
10. Acetone breath[a]
11. See Table 8–4 for other laboratory tests in diabetic ketoacidosis

Hypoglycemia (Many of symptoms are due to release of epinephrine, also due to lack of sugar for CNS; happens quickly.)
 1. Diaphoresis (see exceptions for newborns and elderly)
 2. Tachycardia, anxiety
 3. Weakness, hunger
 4. Irritability, confusion, behavioral changes
 5. Tremors or convulsions
 6. Coma
 7. Urine negative for sugar
 8. Low blood sugar

Including HHNK as one type of hyperglycemia: see text and Slater (1978); Hennessy (1983); Stock (1985); McCarthy (1985); and McAdams & Birmingham, (1986) for more details.
[a]Present only if ketosis and ketoacidosis develop.

TABLE 8-4. LABORATORY TESTS USED IN DIABETIC KETOACIDOSIS

	Ketoacidosis		
	"Mild"	*"Moderate"*	*"Severe"*
Serum glucose	300–450 mg/dl	450–600 mg/dl	600 mg/dl +
Plasma ketones	4 + in undiluted sample	4 + in 1:1 diluted sample	4 + in 1:2 diluted sample
Serum bicarbonate (see Chapter 6)	More than 15 mEq/L	10–15 mEq/L	Less than 10 mEq/L
pH (see Chapter 6)	More than 7.3	7.2–7.3	Less than 7.2
BUN (see Chapter 4)	Less than 25 mg/dl	25–40 mg/dl	40–100 mg/dl
Urine glucose (see Chapter 3)	2%	2%	2%
Urine acetone (see Chapter 3)	Small	Moderate	Large

See Chapter 4 on osmolality and Walesky (1978); McCarthy (1985); and McAdams & Birmingham (1986) for more details on ketoacidosis.

Administering Insulin. Regular insulin is the only type of insulin used in treating elevated serum glucose levels that may fluctuate every few hours. It is also used to control glucose blood levels during labor and delivery or during surgery, when the unusual stress causes unpredictable levels of hyperglycemia (Wimberley, 1979). The intermediate insulins (NPH and Lente) are begun when the severe hyperglycemia in ketoacidosis has been corrected and the person is in a more stabilized condition. Both urine and blood glucose levels are used to monitor the return of the blood sugar to a lower stable level. The nurse must carefully monitor blood sugar levels because additional units of regular insulin are usually ordered on the sliding scale format, as noted in the earlier section on blood glucose reagent strips.

Urine may also be monitored for S and A. (Chapter 3 contains not only specific instructions on different methods of urine testing for sugar and acetone, but also charts to illustrate the effect of drugs on Clinitest and Tes-Tape.) The disappearance of ketones from the urine is one way to evaluate that ketoacidosis no longer exists. The usefulness of the serum acetone level in comparison with urine testing is discussed in the next section.

■ SERUM ACETONE OR KETONES

When glucose is not available to the cells and the body mobilizes fat and protein as sources of energy, ketone bodies (acetoacetic acid, acetone, and beta-hydroxybutyric acid) are the byproducts. The acidity of these ketone bodies causes the ketoacidosis that results from uncontrolled diabetes mellitus or starvation.

When ketoacidosis is suspected, the laboratory can quickly test a blood sample to determine the relative amount of ketones in the blood. Some laboratories may test acetoacetic acid and acetone rather than just ketones. Normally the levels of ketone bodies should be negative. Various laboratories use slightly different techniques to estimate the presence of ketone bodies, and consequently they report serum ketone or acetone levels in different ways.

Preparation of Client and Collection of Sample

The laboratory usually needs about 2 ml of blood to do any form of these tests, and there is no special preparation of the client. The tablets used for urine testing of ketones can also be used to test ketones in serum or blood (Acetest, Ames Products, 1986). For serum testing, the color of the tablet is compared two minutes after a drop of serum is placed on it. If whole blood is put on the tablet, the clot is removed after 10 minutes and the tablet is compared to the chart. Except when laboratory facilities are not readily available, such as during a home visit or in a camp setting, it is better to let the laboratory do the measurement of serum acetone under more controlled conditions where serum can be separated from whole blood and properly diluted.

Reference Values for Serum Ketones

Acetoacetate plus acetone levels	0.3–2.0 mg/dl
Serum ketone levels:	
Undiluted sample	4+ is considered mild ketoacidosis
1:1 diluted sample	4+ is considered moderate ketoacidosis
1:2 diluted sample	4+ is considered severe ketoacidosis

Some laboratories may just report abnormal results as small, moderate, or large amounts of ketones.

Positive Test for Ketones in Serum

Clinical Significance. The presence of large amounts of ketones in the serum is diagnostic of ketoacidosis. More often, the presence of ketones is assessed by frequent urine testing because ketones are excreted by the kidney. (The specific procedure for testing urine for ketones is covered in Chapter 3.) As ketones enter the bloodstream, the excess is excreted by the kidneys so that the urine test is postive *before* the buildup in the serum is excessive. However, in severe ketoacidosis, the dehydrated state may cause oliguria so that obtaining urine for testing is difficult. Also, when the acidosis is coming under control by therapy, the serum level is more reflective of the current status of the client because the serum levels begin to drop while the urine level remains high. The serum acetone level is thus the more useful as an immediate indicator of the amount of ketones in the bloodstream. When clients have a continuing positive serum acetone level, the nurse may note a fruity odor to their breath similar to the odor of nailpolish remover, which is due to the excretion of some acetone by the lungs.

Low Blood Glucose Level (Hypoglycemia)

Clinical Significance

Hypoglycemia in the Diabetic Client. Hypoglycemia in the diabetic client is caused by: (1) too much insulin, or less frequently, by too high a dose of oral hypoglycemic agents; (2) too little food; or (3) increased exercise without additional food intake. Less insulin is needed for the utilization of glucose when the body's activity is increased by work or exercise. Recall also that, in the case of stressful events, such as infection or trauma, more insulin is needed to control hyperglycemia. Hence, if bouts of hyperglycemia and hypoglycemia are to be prevented, the well-controlled diabetic must have a balance between diet, medication, and exercise, plus a lack of stress.

In the pregnant woman, hypoglycemia is most likely to occur at two times during the pregnancy. During the first three months, because the growing fetus requires additional glucose, the mother may experience some periods of low blood sugar. Again during labor, the extra exertion may also make the woman more prone to hypoglycemia (Schuler, 1979).

Hypoglycemia is always a potential problem in infants whose mothers are diabetic. During uterine life, the infant's pancreas secretes large amounts of insulin due to the high blood glucose levels in the mother. Glucose crosses the placental barrier, but insulin does not. After birth, the infant's pancreas may continue to secrete large amounts of insulin even though the blood glucose levels are much less than in utero. Usually glucose levels drop the lowest an hour or two after birth, reach a plateau in 2–4 hours, and then gradually increase (Vogel, 1979). Infants that are premature or that have a low birth weight are also prone to hypoglycemia caused by a lack of glycogen reserves in the immature liver.

Hypoglycemia in Nondiabetic Clients. Hypoglycemia in nondiabetic clients is not well understood. Two major groups of hypoglycemia are classified as fasting and postprandial. Fasting hypoglycemia is likely to suggest serious organic disease. (Jacobs et al., 1984). In a few clients a low blood sugar level can be traced to a tumor of the pancreas, to a lack of cortisone (Addison's disease), to extensive liver disease, or to pituitary hypofunction. (See Chapter 15 on growth hormone.) Alcohol-induced fasting hypoglycemia can cause death if not identified and corrected (Dipp, 1978).

Most cases of hypoglycemia, however, are termed "functional" because their exact cause cannot be attributed to organic pathology. Sometimes this type of hypoglycemia is termed "reactive" because the hypoglycemic attack may follow a meal of high carbohydrates, particularly one with a lot of sugar. Sometimes this functional hypoglycemia may be related to anxiety and stress.

Glucose tolerance tests may be used to determine the response of the person to a load of sugar. Yet most authorities feel that even a blood sugar as low as 40 mg should not be considered hypoglycemia if the client has no symptoms (Siperstein, 1975). The diagnosis of "hypoglycemia" usually refers to the presence of hypoglycemic symptoms rather than to a certain blood glucose level.

POSSIBLE NURSING DIAGNOSES RELATED TO HYPOGLYCEMIA

Potential for Injury Due to Lack of Glucose for Normal Cellular Function

For clients who are likely to develop hypoglycemia due to too much insulin, the key nursing implication is to assess for early symptoms of hypoglycemia so that treatment is given quickly. Hypoglycemia occurs rapidly and can lead to coma if it is not treated. (In contrast, the coma that may develop from hyperglycemia usually takes much longer to develop as the person gets progressively more dehydrated and as the ketones build up in the bloodstream.)

One of the most outstanding symptoms of hypoglycemia in many adults and children is diaphoresis (excessive sweating). Because infants do not perspire, however, this clinical sign is not useful in the newborn nursery. The diaphoresis, along with weakness, dizziness, and tremors is the result of an increased surge of adrenalin (epinephrine) to raise the blood sugar level. Clients on beta blockers may not exhibit diaphoresis or tachycardia.

If the brain is deprived of glucose for more than a few minutes, the client begins to experience irritability, confusion, and severe behavioral outbursts that may make it impossible to get the person to take some juice. A low blood glucose causes convulsions and coma. Permanent brain damage can result from severe hypoglycemia. The onset of hypoglycemia in the elderly may not show the signs and symptoms of increased epinephrine usually seen in the young. As a result, the episodes of confusion or other cerebral dysfunctions may be wrongly attributed to cerebral arteriosclerosis. Eliopoulos (1978) and Hayter (1981) describe the unique reactions of the elderly person with diabetes.

Interventions to Raise the Blood Sugar Level. Anytime that hypoglycemia is suspected, don't wait for a progression of symptoms; have the person drink a glass of orange juice or eat some candy. If the symptoms are not due to hypoglycemia, the extra sugar does not significantly affect other conditions. But if the symptoms *are* due to hypoglycemia, the concentrated sugar quickly restores the blood sugar level and the symptoms disappear. Four ounces of orange juice contain 10 g of simple carbohydrate. Food with protein and complex carbohydrates, such as milk and crackers, should be given as a follow-up (Stock, 1985). If a client is brought to an emergency room in an unconscious state from an unknown cause, a diagnostic procedure is to draw laboratory blood for a serum glucose level and then immediately give 50 cc of 50% glucose. If the unconscious state is due to hypoglycemia, the client immediately becomes more responsive as the blood sugar returns to normal. Nurses should be aware that alcohol intoxication can cause severe hypoglycemia, for which the mortality rate is 25% in children (Dipp, 1978).

Assessing and Treating Hypoglycemia in the Newborn. In the newborn infant, the symptoms of hypoglycemia are tremors, listlessness, apnea, cyanosis, a shrill cry, changes in muscular tone, and an unstable temperature. When the infant is hypoglycemic, the resultant release of glucagon stimulates the secretion of calcitonin from the thyroid (Vogel, 1979) which may cause a rapid fall of serum calcium, which in turn causes the symptoms of tetany. (see Chapter 7 for a discussion of hypocalcemia.) Usually the newborn of a diabetic mother is fed early with 10–20% glucose by a bottle, by gavage, or by intravenous infusion if necessary. The infant is also frequently tested for blood glucose levels (see the procedure for reagant strips discussed earlier in this chapter). Any infant prone to hypoglycemia is usually kept in a special care nursery for close observation.

Assessing for Hypoglycemia When Clinical Symptoms Are Not Obvious. Clients who have experienced hypoglycemia are usually aware of the beginning of symptoms and take some orange juice or candy to offset the reaction. For some people the early symptoms of hypoglycemia may not be so obvious or the hypoglycemia may occur during sleep. For example, with the intermediate acting insulins (NPH and Lente), the peak action is 8–12 hours after administration and the duration is around 24 hours. Headache and weakness may be the only symptoms.

Two signs of hypoglycemia can be objectively measured by nurses: (1) a fall in temperature and (2) a rise in the systolic blood pressure of about 4–6 mm Hg, with a larger drop in the disastolic blood pressure (Hite and Humphrey, 1979). With objective documentation of these two measurements, nurses can assess drops in blood sugar that might not be otherwise detected. Clients can purchase an alarm to wear on the wrist. The Sleep Sentry (Teledyne Avionics) detects perspiration or a temperature drop on the wrist.

Knowledge Deficit Regarding Use of Glucagon as Treatment for Hypoglycemia

Some physicians may order the hormone glucagon as treatment for an insulin reaction when it is not feasible to give intravenous glucose immediately. The hormone, available in 1 mg ampules, is injected the same way as insulin, and it should be effective in raising the blood sugar in 15–20 minutes (Gever, 1985). Glucagon, secreted by the alpha cells of the pancreas, stimulates the formation of glucose from glycogen stores. So it is not effective for the person who is malnourished and who thus has little stored glycogen. The physician must make the decision as to whether the drug may be useful for a client in a home situation. A member of the family needs to be instructed on how to give glucagon when the client has an insulin reaction that does not respond to oral sugar. If glucagon is used the client needs a feeding of combined simple and complex carbohydrates to replenish the glucose.

Alterations in Nutritional Requirements Related to Changes in Activity

The nurse and the diabetic client receiving insulin need to be aware that unusual exercise increases the chance of hypoglycemia. Because active muscular exercise increases the utilization of carbohydrates, the person requires more food intake or less insulin. When a person is in the hospital, the stress of the hospitalization and the lack of normal muscular activity both contribute to increasing the blood sugar level. When the person is discharged, the stress is less and normal muscular activities are resumed. So the insulin requirement may be decreased. Sometimes in pediatric units, children are taken to a park or playground for a few times before they are actually discharged from the hospital so that insulin maintenance dose matches the food intake and exercise level of the child. This may be very helpful in preventing hypoglycemic attacks after the child is at home.

Knowledge Deficit Regarding Insulin Rebound

With so many variables affecting it, the blood glucose level may fluctuate a lot during a 24-hour period. The Somogyi effect, named after the man who first described the phenomenon (Kaiser 1980), is the occurrence of insulin rebound. After a period of hypoglycemia, several hormones (epinephrine and the glucocorticosteroids) are released to raise serum glucose levels. So repeated episodes of slight hypoglycemia may have the end result of making the person hyperglycemic, which may partially explain why some clients on insulin still have wide fluctuations of blood sugar levels that are not directly related to food intake. Based on this theory, a plan for reducing the insulin dose may bring about a more stable blood sugar because there is no longer the rebound effect from the periods of slight hypoglycemia.

The nurse can be useful in detecting this pattern of slight hypoglycemia reactions followed by hyperglycemia. For example, a client may suddenly have a lot of sugar in the urine after being negative only a few hours before. Perhaps the person feels a little weak or hungry during the time the urine is negative, but eats something and soon feels better. Yet clients may not think that such small symptoms are important enough to report. The nurse may also note that one random blood sugar was unusually low while the next one was unusually high. The client at home may be taught to do blood glucose testing before meals and at bedtime to make sure that slight hypoglycemia is not occurring. The importance of clearly establishing the presence of any slight hypoglycemic attacks is that the client has better control when the insulin is slightly decreased. Having more stable blood sugar levels when the insulin is slightly reduced is considered proof that the Somogyi effect or insulin rebound was creating the problem (Hite and Humphrey, 1979).

Alteration in Nutritional Requirements Related to Functional Hypoglycemia

In contrast to the patient who has hypoglycemia caused by an insulin reaction, the client with functional hypoglycemia does not have symptoms that progress to a coma. The light-headedness, sweating, and palpitations may be relieved by the intake of some carbohydrate. For the long-term management of hypoglycemic attacks, the person is usually advised not to eat concentrated sugars at all because they may cause a surge of insulin in the bloodstream. The diet usually consists of a high-protein, low-carbohydrate diet with frequent feedings. For example, the person should eat cottage cheese and maybe some fruit for a mid-morning snack rather than pastry or a doughnut and coffee. Stimulants such as caffeine should be avoided because the caffeine may cause a sudden rise in blood sugar that stimulates insulin production.

Anxiety Related to Functional Hypoglycemia

The relationship of diet, stress, and anxiety to functional hypoglycemia still is not well understood. The nurse needs to evaluate the potential stress in the environment since this may be a contributing factor for the development of the hypoglycemic symptoms. Emphasis is placed not on the symptoms, but rather on eradicating the stimulus for the symptoms—be it food indiscretions, anxiety, or some yet undetected organic abnormality. Measuring blood glucose during a hypoglycemic attack at home may be helpful in documenting the physiological nature of the symptoms and distinguishing them from anxiety symptoms.

■ SUGAR AND ACETONE IN URINE

Although self-monitoring by blood glucose test strips may be ideal, urine monitoring is the older and less costly method. The techniques for both the enzyme method (Tes-Tape) and the reducing method (Clinitest) are discussed in Chapter 3. Also discussed in that chapter are the differnces between the two methods and the nursing implications for urine testing in general. When a diabetic client is on insulin, the urine is tested before meals and at bedtime. If the client is being controlled on oral hypoglycemic agents, the urine testing is typically done once a day after the largest meal. The client is taught to call the physician or clinic if the sugar is 1–2% for one or two days. In children, one day of spilling 1 or 2% sugar would be reason to notify the physician or clinic (Guthrie, 1980). As noted in the literature (Miller, 1986) urine tests are meaningless when blood glucose levels can be done.

■ SUGARS OTHER THAN GLUCOSE IN URINE

As discussed in Chapter 3, using the copper-reduction technique (Clinitest), rather than the enzyme method (Tes-Tape), is important if an assessment for the presence of sugars other than glucose is to be done. Lactose, fructose, and galactose can be detected only by the reduction method. In the newborn, metabolic abnormalities due to genetic defects can cause various sugars to be present in the urine. The excretion of abnormal sugars begins after the baby is begun on a milk diet. Thus the testing for abnormal sugars must not be done when the baby is still taking just glucose and water. Most of the sugars, such as lactose (discussed next), are fairly benign. The most important other sugar to detect in the urine is galactose, because its presence is a potentially dangerous condition.

LACTOSE TOLERANCE TEST

Lactase, an enzyme found only in the small intestine, is important for digestion of lactose, a sugar found in milk. Due to both genetic and other factors, some people, particularly Black and Oriental, may have a deficiency of lactase.

A lack of this enzyme leads to an intolerance for milk because the lactose in the milk cannot be converted to a simple sugar. (One glass of milk contains 12 g of lactose.) The stools are sour and have a low pH, rather than an alkaline pH, because of the presence of undigested milk. The test for lactose tolerance is to give a measured amount of lactose and then test the blood *glucose* level at various intervals. An increase of less than 20 mg of glucose, associated with gastrointestinal symptoms (bloating or diarrhea) is strongly suggestive of lactase deficiency. The treatment is to use lactose hydrolyzed milk or milk fermented products (Newcomer, 1980).

SERUM TEST FOR GALACTOSEMIA

Galactosemia is an inherited disorder in which galactose cannot be converted to glucose because of a lack of the enzyme galactose-1-phosphate-uridyl transferase or two other enzymes (Tietz, 1983). The galactose is wasted in the urine. Once galactose has been detected in the urine, the test for these enzymes verifies that there is a genetic defect in metabolizing galactose. To prevent mental retardation and other complications, a diet containing no milk products should be instituted within the newborn period. If milk is not eliminated from the diet, cataracts may appear wtihin one month and any neurological defects may be permanent.

All parents, especially those who have home deliveries, need to be aware of the importance of early detection of the presence of any sugar in the urine or any intolerance to milk. Galactosemia is one of the tests sometimes mandated by law for newborns. (See Chapter 18 on genetic screening tests).

QUESTIONS

1. All of the following hormones cause an increase in serum glucose levels *except* which?

   a. Growth hormone
   b. Cortisone

   c. Testosterone
   d. Epinephrine

2. In comparing the tests for fasting blood sugar (FBS), postprandial blood sugar (PPBS), and random blood sugar (RBS), which statement is the most accurate?

   a. The client must be n.p.o. before all three tests are done
   b. An abnormality of any two of the tests indicates diabetes mellitus
   c. RBS gives the most accurate picture of carbohydrate metabolism
   d. The exact timing of the drawing of the specimen is most critical for the PPBS

3. Which of the following would not be considered a reason to postpone a glucose tolerance test? The fact that the person:

   a. Is on bed rest
   b. Has a fever

   c. Is on a reducing diet
   d. Had hypoglycemic symptoms yes-
      terday

4. Which of the following statements is correct about glucose tests in the elderly client (over 65)?

   a. The curve for a glucose tolerance test for the elderly should return to base line as soon as the curve for a person under 50
   b. The renal threshold for glucose is usually decreased in the elderly
   c. The postprandial blood sugar level in the elderly tends to be higher than p.c. blood sugar levels for young adults
   d. Normals for fasting blood sugar tests tend to border on hypoglycemia in the elderly

5. The plasma acetone level is:

   a. Increased in both diabetic coma and hyperosmolar hyperglycemic nonketotic coma (HHNK)
   b. Decreased in both diabetic coma and HHNK
   c. Unchanged in either diabetic coma or HHNK
   d. Increased in diabetic coma and not changed in HHNK

6. Mrs. Forini is a diabetic client in labor. She is on sliding scale insulin coverage for blood glucose above 240 mg/dl. Which type of insulin is used to control hyperglycemia in acute situations such as labor and delivery?

   a. Regular insulin
   b. Lente insulin

   c. NPH insulin
   d. Semi-Lente insulin

7. Which of the following nursing actions would be most appropriate for the client with an elevated blood sugar level of 200 mg/dl?

    a. Testing the urine every 3 hours for sugar and acetone

    b. Restricting all fluid intake to prevent nausea and vomiting

    c. Observing for any signs of infection

    d. Assessing for possible signs of acidosis such as slower-than-normal breathing

8. All of the following clients have the potential for injury related to the development of hypoglycemia *except* which?

    a. Baby Tell, born 4 hours ago to a diabetic mother who is on sliding scale coverage

    b. Ms. Fannin, who is in her first trimester of pregnancy and is insulin-dependent (Lente 20 units)

    c. Mr. Lord, who has been controlled on NPH 40 units, but who now is on bed rest with an infected toe

    d. Mr. Sloan, with a possible diagnosis of functional hypoglycemia, who has just eaten two candy bars to "tide him over" until mealtime

9. A characteristic symptom of hypoglycemia in *both* the adult and newborn is which of the following?

    a. Diaphoresis   **b.** Tremors   **c.** Shrill cry   **d.** Confusion

10. The night nurse discovers Mr. Riley, a newly diagnosed diabetic client, wandering about in his room. He says he has a headache. He appears flushed and warm. The nurse knows that Mr. Riley had 55 units of Lente insulin in the morning and 10 units of regular insulin at bedtime to cover a blood glucose of 240 mg/dl. Which action would be the most appropriate for the nurse to do first?

    a. Get Mr. Riley back to bed and check to see if he has an order for pain relief for the headache

    b. Call the intern to check Mr. Riley for possible diabetic acidosis

    c. Obtain a finger stick for a blood glucose and then give Mr. Riley a glass of orange juice if his blood sugar is low

    d. Assess his vital signs, particularly the temperature and blood pressure, and wait to see if he is becoming diaphoretic

11. Glucagon, a hormone from the alpha cells of the pancreas, is sometimes used to do which of the following?

    a. Treat mild cases of diabetes

    b. Counteract the effect of epinephrine

    c. Help promote conversion of glycogen to glucose

    d. Reduce the blood sugar level in newborns

12. The client who has functional or reactive hypoglycemia needs to be taught to maintain a diet that includes all *but* which of the following?

    a. High carbohydrates   **c.** Low carbohydrates

    b. High protein   **d.** Frequent small feedings

13. Which of the following is *not* characteristic of a client who may be experiencing insulin rebound (Somogyi effect)?

a. Urine and blood sugars that are higher after meals

b. High urine sugars a few hours after negative urine tests

c. Headaches, tremors, and diaphoresis before a meal

d. Wide fluctuations in blood sugars that are not related to meals

14. Mrs. Hobdey, age 54, is being discharged from the hospital. She is on an oral hypoglycemic agent. She does not want to learn to do finger sticks for blood glucose levels. Which of the following should be taught Mrs. Hobdey about testing her urine?

a. She can use either Clinitest tablets or Tes-Tape because the tests are the same and give the same results

b. She should test her urine at least once a day after her largest meal of the day and do so more often only if the test is positive

c. She should test her urine before meals and at the hour of sleep, and report any positive signs immediately

d. She does not need to test her urine because she is not taking insulin

15. Sarah is a 5-year-old with diabetes. Which of these points would *not* be correct to teach Sarah's parents about testing in diabetes?

a. Finger sticks for glucose may be useful to assess for hypoglycemia if Sarah has unexplained behavioral outbursts

b. Regular exercise is important in keeping blood sugar levels more stable

c. If the urine sugar is positive, an acetone should always be done

d. If the sugar and acetone remain positive after more than two days, the clinic or physician should be notified

16. Which of the following conclusions is *incorrect* in comparing galactose and lactose intolerances and the tests done for each?

a. Both galactose and lactose can be detected in the urine by Clinitest tablets

b. Galactose intolerance is a more serious defect than lactose intolerance

c. A nonmilk diet in the infant eliminates the symptoms of both lactose intolerance and galactose intolerance

d. The blood glucose level will be abnormally elevated in both conditions

REFERENCES

Ames Product Profiles. (1986). *Acetest, Dextrostix, Visidex II* and *KetoDiastix*. Elkhart, IN: Ames Division, Miles Laboratories.

Bergman, M., & Felig, P. (1984). Self-monitoring of blood glucose levels in diabetes. *Archives of Internal Medicine. 144,* 2029–2034.

Bio-Dynamics Product Profiles on Chem-Strip bG. (1986). Indianapolis, IN: Bio-Dynamics, Inc.

Cerrato, P. (1985). A new way to help diabetics eat right. *RN, 48*(11), 71–72.

Chait, A. (1984). Dietary management of diabetes mellitus. *Contemporary Nutrition, 9*(2), 1–2.

Christiansen, C., & Sachse, M. (1980). Home blood glucose monitoring. *The Diabetes Educator, 6,* 13–21.

Dipp, S. (1978). Metabolic effects of alcohol. *Arizona Medicine, 35*(10), 651–652.

Eliopoulos, C. (1978). Diagnosis and management of diabetes in the elderly. *AJN, 78*(15), 884–887.

Garofono, C. (1981). A simpler test for diabetes? *RN, 44*(9), 155.

Gever, L. (1985). Administering glucagon in an emergency. *Nursing 85, 15*(1), 66.

Guthrie, D. (1980). Helping the diabetic manage self-care. *Nursing 80, 10*(2), 57–65.

Hayter, J. (1981). Diabetes and the older person. *Geriatric Nursing, 2,* 32–36.

Hennessy, K. (1983). HHNK dehydration. *AJN, 83*(10), 1425–1426.

Hite, A., & Humphrey, J. (1979). How to spot the vicious cycle of insulin rebound. *RN, 42*(7), 44–47.

Jacobs, D., et al. (1984). *Laboratory test handbook with DRG index.* St Louis: Mosby/Lexi.

Joyce, M., et al. (1983). Those new blood glucose tests. *RN, 46*(4), 46–52.

Kaiser, D. (1980). The Somogyi effect. *AJN, 80*(2), 236–238.

McAdams, R., & Birmingham, D. (1986). When diabetes races out of control. *RN, 49*(5), 46–53.

McAteer, J. (1979). Clinical implications of laboratory studies: Diabetic pregnancy and neonatal outcome. *Critical Care Quarterly, 2*(12), 61–72.

McCarthy, J. (1985). The continuum of diabetic coma. *AJN, 85*(8), 878–882.

Metzger, M.J. (1983). A new test for blood sugar. Hemoglobin A. *AJN, 83*(5), 763–764.

Miller, V. (1986). Diabetes, let's stop testing urine. *AJN, 86*(1), 54.

Newcomer, A. (1979). Lactose deficiency? *Contemporary Nutrition, 4*(9), 1–2.

Press, M. et al. (1984). Importance of raised growth hormone levels in mediating the metabolic derangements of diabetes. *NEJM, 310*(13), 810–815.

Rancilia, N. (1979). When a pregnant woman is diabetic: Postpartal care. *AJN, 79*(3), 453–456.

Robertson, C. (1985). How to teach patients to monitor blood glucose. *RN, 48*(12), 24–25.

Schuler, K. (1979). When a pregnant woman is diabetic: Antepartal care. *AJN, 79*(3), 448–450.

Siperstein, M. (1975). The glucose tolerance test. *Advances in Internal Medicine, 20,* 279–323.

Slater, N. (1978). Insulin reactions vs. ketoacidosis: Guidelines for diagnosis and intervention. *AJN, 78*(5), 875–877.

Stock, P. (1985). Insulin shock. *Nursing 85, 15*(4), 53.

Stock-Barkman, P. (1983). Confusing concepts. Is it diabetic shock or diabetic coma? *Nursing 83, 13*(6), 33–41.

Surr, C. (1983a). New blood-glucose monitoring products: Part I. *Nursing 83, 13*(1), 42–43.

Surr, C. (1983b). New blood-glucose monitoring products: Part II. *Nursing 83, 13*(2), 58–62.

Tietz, N. (Ed.). (1983). *Clinical guide to laboratory tests.* Philadelphia: Saunders.

Villeneuve, M., et al. (1985). Evaluating blood glucose monitors. *AJN, 85*(11), 1258–1259.

Vogel, M. (1979). When a pregnant woman is diabetic: Care of the newborn. *AJN, 79*(3), 458–460.

Walesky, M. (1978). Adult diabetes: Diabetic ketoacidosis. *AJN, 78*(5), 872–874.

Wallach, J. (1986). *Interpretation of diagnostic tests.* Boston: Little, Brown.

White, N., & Miller, B. (1983). Glycohemoglobin. *Nursing 83, 13*(8), 55–57.

Wimberly, D. (1979). When a pregnant woman is diabetic: Intrapartal care. *AJN, 79*(3), 451–452.

9

Tests to Measure Lipid Metabolism

- Serum Cholesterol
- Serum Triglycerides
- Lipoprotein Electrophoresis
- High-Density Lipoprotein (HDL) Cholesterol
- Low-Density Lipoprotein (LDL) Cholesterol

OBJECTIVES

1. Define hyperlipidemia and discuss factors that seem to contribute to its development.
2. Describe the client preparation necessary for tests of serum cholesterol and serum triglyceride levels.
3. Discuss the controversial aspects of the relationship of serum cholesterol and serum triglyercide levels to the development of cardiovascular disease.
4. Plan a diet low in cholesterol and saturated fats.
5. Identify nursing diagnoses that may be useful for the client with elevated serum cholesterol levels.
6. Identify assessments that might indicate a lack of essential fatty acids in the diet.
7. Give examples of how serum triglyceride levels are used as an evaluation tool.
8. Describe lipoprotein electrophoresis and explain how the research findings from this test have been applied to clinical situations.

Hyperlipidemia is a broad term that means high plasma concentrations of cholesterol, triglycerides, or the complex lipoproteins. Although cholesterol is the lipid that seems to get the most publicity, it is just one that can be measured in the serum. Other lipids found in the serum include the triglycerides and the phospholipids, such as lecithin and sphingomyelin. Lecithin and sphingomyelin comprise the basis of the L/S ratio, a test done on amniotic fluid to evaluate the maturity of the fetus (see Chapter 28).

Serum cholesterol levels and, less frequently, triglyceride levels are done to evaluate the risk potential for the development of atherosclerosis. According to current knowledge, the serum cholesterol level is the more important laboratory test to assess for hyperlipidemia that may be helped by therapy.

In addition to the use of these two tests to evaluate hyperlipidemia, lipoprotein electrophoresis may be done to evaluate rarer types of lipid abnormalities. Lipoproteins are complex protein molecules that contain several protein and lipid components. Lipoprotein molecules can be separated into four different bands on a strip of paper by using an electric current to cause migration of the molecules. Identification of abnormal patterns for the four bands on the electrophoresis strip has resulted in a classification system of various types of hyperlipidemia. Researchers have discovered that some types of lipoproteins, such as the high-density lipoproteins, may actually be protective against the development of atherosclerosis. HDL-cholesterol and LDL-cholesterol are being used to assess the risk potential for developing coronary vascular disease.

■ SERUM CHOLESTEROL

Cholesterol, a natural constituent of the serum, is essential for the production of bile salts, for the manufacture of many of the steroid hormones, and for the composition of cell membranes. Cholesterol is manufactured from saturated fats in the diet. The liver esterifies cholesterol by combining it with a fatty acid. Most of the cholesterol is present in the bloodstream in the esterified form. Usually only the total cholesterol is measured, unless there is possible liver dysfunction. Because cholesterol has been so closely linked to the development of atherosclerosis there is great concern about how much of this natural constituent should be in the serum (Clark, 1984). At the present time, there is no general agreement about which levels of serum cholesterol are "normal." Only about one third of the adult population in America has cholesterol levels below 200 mg. In other countries, the adult population may have considerably lower values. Cholesterol levels seem to differ greatly depending on such variables as age, diet, geographic location, and genetic influences. Values in the United States used to be considered normal up to around 335 mg, depending on age. Many authorities questioned whether these "normal" values of cholesterol were ideal for optimal health (Kannel, 1976). And a statement by the National Institutes of Health (NIH) Consensus Development Panel (1985a) noted moderate-to-high risk for cardiovascular disease when cholesterol levels are above 200 mg/dl.

Preparation of Client and Collection of Sample

Serum cholesterol requires 2 ml of serum. The client needs to have fasted for a minimum of 4 hours. Because there may be significant variations from day to day in the same individual, the test may be repeated more than once to determine which variations are occurring. The client should be on a regular diet until the fasting period.

Some laboratories may require overnight fasting. Water is allowed. Certain drugs, such as vitamin E, phenytoin, or steroids, may cause false elevations, while other drugs, such as some antibiotics, may cause falsely low readings.

Reference Values for Serum Cholesterol

Adult by age[a]	Less than 30—no higher than 180 mg/dl
	Over age 30—no higher than 200 mg/dl
	These figures are based on NIH Consensus Statement (1985a)
	Women tend to have lower cholesterol levels than men of the same age until after menopause (see Rifkind and Segal (1983) for percentiles for all ages and for both sexes)
Pregnancy	Cholesterol levels increase in pregnancy to around 240–300 mg/dl. Values return to pre-pregnancy values within one month (Hytten & Lind, 1975)
Newborn	90 mg at birth, increases to around 120 mg by third day
Children	From one year, around 130 mg to less than 160 mg/dl by age 19. A cutoff point of 205 mg was used for some studies (Morrison et al., 1979) but NIH (1985a) has lowered all ranges
Aged	Some authorities consider an increase of cholesterol to be proportional to age increases, so that a cholesterol over 220 mg would be acceptable for older adults (see Appendix A). Cholesterol levels may decline in persons over age 70, particularly men

---

[a]Values are for total cholesterol: In liver disease, when liver can not esterify cholesterol, the laboratory may measure "esterified" cholesterol because this value decreases. Normally 65–75% of total cholesterol will be esterified.

Increased Serum Cholesterol Level

Clinical Significance. For the majority of clients, the reason for a high cholesterol level is not known. Much research is being done to try to discover to what extent genetic, dietary, or other environmental factors contribute to high cholesterol levels. Three recognized genetic disorders lead to hyperlipidemia: (1) familial hypercholesterolemia, (2) familial combined hyperlipidemia, and (3) familial hypertriglyceridemia. Although these three disorders affect 0.5–1% of the population and are the most common genetic diseases (Breslow, 1978), they do not cause the vast majority of high cholesterol levels seen in adults.

In some clinical situations, the cause of the increased serum cholesterol level can be identified. For example, liver disease with biliary obstruction, hypothyroidism, and pancreatic dysfunction all cause increased cholesterol levels. Certain drugs, such as corticosteroids, may cause an increased cholesterol level, but the significance of this is not known. Although cholesterol levels are normally high in pregnancy, they rise even higher in preeclampsia (Hytten & Lind, 1975). Also in nephrotic syndromes, the cholesterol level may increase.

POSSIBLE NURSING DIAGNOSES RELATED TO HYPERLIPIDEMIA

Knowledge Deficit Related to Needed Alterations in Diet

Once a client has been definitely identified as having hyperlipidemia, the usual recommendation is to decrease the amount of fat in the diet and to replace saturated fats with polyunsaturated fats. Vegetable oils tend to be high in poly-unsaturated fats, while animal fats are high in saturated fats and cholesterol. Meat, egg yolks, and dairy products are the major source of cholesterol in the American diet (Table 9-1). (See the section on lipoprotein electrophoresis for more details on diet regimens.) Some physicians may recommend a ratio of twice as much polyunsaturated fats as saturated, with a total amount of fat being not more than 30-35% of the total caloric intake. A diet plan may limit cholesterol intake to 200-300 mg per day. Pritikin (1984) advocated a very restricted diet with only 10% fat and less than 100 mg cholesterol a day. A fat-controlled diet may have other health benefits. The National Research Council's study on diet, nutrition, and cancer has supported having total fat intake not more than 30% of the total calories because of the association between high-fat diets and some types of cancer (O'Connor, 1985).

Some dietary recommendations endorsed by the American Heart Association and reported by Rifkind and Segal (1983) are as follows:

1. Caloric intake should be adjusted to achieve and maintain ideal body weight.
2. Reduction in total fat calories should be achieved by a substantial reduction in dietary saturated fatty acids. Saturated fats should be less than 10%, polyunsaturated fats should be at least 10%, and the rest of the fat should come from monounsaturated sources. (Not all dietary plans follow these figures exactly.)
3. Substantial reductions in dietary cholesterol are in order. The average daily intake for adults should be less than 300 mg. If hypercholesterolemia is not controlled, even greater reduction to 250 mg may be warranted.
4. A slight increase in carbohydrate intake can make up the caloric difference resulting from less fats in the diet. Any glucose intolerance must be controlled. If the serum triglyceride level is above the 90th percentile, some carbohydrate reduction may be needed.
5. Avoid excessive dietary sodium. The level of sodium restriction must be determined by the physician based on signs of hypertension and other conditions (see Chapter 5 on low-sodium diets).
6. Other dietary factors, such as alcohol, should be limited if the triglyceride level is above the 90th percentile.

Despite the advertising world's use of "low-cholesterol" labeling to sell food, the need for the strict dietary restriction of cholesterol is controversial. Dietary restrictions do not seem to be the perfect treatment for high serum cholesterol levels because so many factors seem to influence the metabolism of cholesterol (Sodhi & Mason, 1977; Clark, 1984). Some authorities maintain that it is not necessary to restrict cholesterol in the diet, because most studies have failed to demonstrate a consistent relationship between changes in serum cholesterol (Flynn, 1979; Reiser, 1980). However, other studies have shown a reduction in serum cholesterol levels if the change in diet continues for as long as 17 months (Mallison, 1978).

TABLE 9–1. SOURCES OF CHOLESTEROL AND SATURATED FATS IN DIET

	Approximate Amount of Cholesterol (mg)	Approximate Amount of Saturated Fat (g)
Liver	370	2.5
Egg, one	275	1.7
Veal	86	4.0
Pork	80	3.2
Hot dog	75	9.9
Lean beef	73	3.7
Chicken: Light meat	72	1.7
Dark meat	82	2.7
Ice Cream, 1 cup	59	8.9
Fish	59	0.3
Lobster	46	0.07
Whole milk, one glass	33	5.1
Cheese, 1 ounce	30	6.0
Butter, 1 tablespoon	31	7.1
Coconut oil	0	11.8
Palm oil	0	6.7
Olive oil	0	1.8
Corn oil	0	1.7
Safflower oil	0	1.2

Note: All meat is for 3-ounce servings. Oils are for 1 tbsp.
Values collected from several sources published by American Heart Association (1985) and others (Wallis, 1985).

A large study involving 12 lipid research clinics did demonstrate that serum cholesterol levels can be reduced by up to 7% by diet and that the risks of coronary artery disease are definitely less with lower levels of cholesterol (Rifkind & Segal, 1983). Clients should be encouraged to read about this landmark study, which received wide coverage in lay publications such as *Time Magazine*. Wallis (1984) noted this study was the broadest and most expensive research project in medical history.

Potential Noncompliance Related to Need for Long-term Changes in Dietary Patterns

When a client has a high serum cholesterol level, the nurse's role in diet teaching may be crucial. Rather than emphasizing a diet that is based on restrictions (no eggs, no steak, no ice cream, no butter), it may be better to take a more positive approach and stress the foods to choose. Thus the person can be encouraged to choose fish, chicken, and lean beef, polyunsaturated margarine rather than butter, and more fresh fruit for dessert. Clients should also be made aware of the food served in "fast food" places, which specialize in selling food that contains high amounts of fats and calories. Most of the deep-fried chicken parts or doughnuts are cooked in melted lard. On the other hand, the client at home can use corn oil, a polyunsaturated fat, to prepare food.

Harris (1985) reports that some fatty acids in fish oil may actually protect against cardiovascular disease. The client must read current findings on diet changes as such research continues. The American Heart Association has excellent material for teaching patients about low-fat diets. Diet modification for children is especially controversial. Some authorities have suggested that as early as the second year of life, American children should be on the modified low-fat diet described for adults (Breslow, 1978; Glueck, 1986).

Knowledge Deficit Regarding Drug Therapy

If dietary changes are not sufficient to lower cholesterol levels, the physician may order certain medications, such as those listed in Table 9-2. Cholestyramine (Questran) is also used to lower an elevated direct bilirubin because it binds up bile salts. (See Chapter 11 on direct bilirubin.) Other drugs are being investigated as possible aids in reducing serum cholesterol levels.

Nurses must be aware of the information for the specific drug chosen for the client. The client has serum cholesterol, and maybe serum triglyceride levels, checked every few weeks for the first few months. Some drugs, such as clofibrate (Atromid-S) may have more effect on the triglyceride levels than on cholesterol levels. With most of the drugs, the serum level of cholesterol may not drop for 1–2 months. The client needs encouragement to continue whatever diet has been prescribed and to report any side effects of the drug. If there are undesirable side effects, the client is switched to other drugs or is given drugs to minimize the effects (Mathos, 1986). Treatment of hyperlipidemia in children may be treated with intensive dietary therapy for 6 months to a year before drugs are used. Long term studies are being done to see the effect of diet and drugs on pediatric populations (Glueck, 1986).

Alteration in Nutritional Requirements, Less than Body Requirements

Any plan for diet restriction must be looked at in relation to the total nutritional need of the person. The person following a diet very restricted in saturated fats faces the possibility of some vitamin E deficiency. If a client doesn't like skim milk, a calcium deficiency can occur (see Chapter 7). Iron deficiency may occur on low cholesterol diets, too (Cerrato, 1985).

Ineffective Individual Coping Related to the Need to Adopt Healthier Life-style

The nursing implications for the client with a high serum cholesterol level are broader than just teaching about diet and drug therapies because cholesterol seems to be only one of the risk factors for the development of cardiovascular disease. Thus, it is important to identify the other risk factors that may be present, such as lack of exercise, obesity, hypertension, stressful environments, and cigarette smoking (NIH, 1985b). All these risk factors seem to be interrelated, along with other factors such as glucose levels (Ross & Glomset, 1976). For example, hypertension may be a critical factor in the development of atherosclerosis because low pressure areas of the circulation, although bathed in the same lipid-laden blood, do not develop atherotic placques as do the arteries in the body that have the highest pressures (Kannel, 1976). Obesity and stress both contribute to the development of hypertension. For each 5 lb of extra weight, the diastolic pressure rises about 1 mm Hg. It is not enough to tackle just one of the risk factors, because all are part of a still *poorly understood* pathophysiology.

Hence a nurse, skilled in health teaching and counseling, can help the person with a high serum cholesterol level to find ways to achieve a healthier life-style. It is essential that clients know both what is known, and what is still not known, about the role of serum cholesterol and other risk factors in the development of vascular disease. The client can then make choices about what can be changed in his or her style of living to reduce some or all of the risk factors.

Alteration in Health Maintenance Related to Need for Family Follow-ups

Although the influence of genetics cannot be controlled by the person, it is important to consider genetic implications in counseling a client with an elevated serum cholesterol level. Because severe hyperlipidemia may sometimes be partly genetically based, the family members of clients with diagnosed hyperlipidemia need to be screened for the same condition. It is usually considered advisable to screen close relatives when a person has a coronary event before the age of 60. If a familial hyperlipidemia is suspected and a child's lipid levels are normal, rescreening every three to five years is recommended (Breslow, 1978). Most authorities feel the prevention of hyperlipidemia, particularly in young people, begins with basic changes in health practices for the entire family. Williams et al. (1986) offer evidence that men with familial hypercholesterolemia can avoid early coronary death by controlling the known risk factors.

Decreased Serum Cholesterol Level

Clinical Significance. Common conditions that cause low serum cholesterol levels include: (1) *hyperthyroidism,* in which the increased metabolism accounts for an increased utilization of fat; (2) *severe liver damage,* after which the liver can no longer manufacture cholesterol; and (3) *malnutrition,* which eventually leads to a deficiency of cholesterol due to the lack of fats in the diet. Chronic anemia, cortisone therapy,

TABLE 9–2. DRUGS USED TO TREAT VARIOUS TYPES OF HYPERLIPIDEMIA

Drug	Decrease in Cholesterol	Decrease in Triglycerides	Type of Hyperlipidemia[a]
Cholestyramine (Questran)	marked	none	II_A, II_B
Clofibrate (Atromid-S)	mild	marked	II_A, II_B, III
Colestipol (Colestid)	marked	none	II_A, II_B
Dextrothyroxine (Choloxin)	moderate	variable	II_A
Gemfibrozil (Lopid)	mild	marked	II_A, II_B, IV
Niacin (many brand names for nicotinic acid)	marked	marked	II_A
Probucol (Lorelco)	moderate	none	II_A, III

Note: See Antilipemics (1984); Govoni and Hayes (1985); and Mathos (1986) for details about each drug and Yeshurum and Golto (1976) for history of drug use.
[a]See text for definitions of types of hyperlipidemia based on Fredrickson (1967). Also see NIH *Consensus Development Conference Statement* (1985a) for more current trends.

and AIDS also cause lowered cholesterol levels. If the low serum cholesterol level is the result of a disease process, treatment is geared toward the particular pathophysiology. The low serum cholesterol level, by itself, is not of specific concern. Remember that because the "normals" for cholesterol levels are arbitrary, low cholesterol levels are unlikely to cause any symptoms in the client.

If the client is on a diet or on drugs to reduce the cholesterol levels, a gradual lowering of the serum cholesterol levels is an indication of the effectiveness of therapy. Even with drugs, the cholesterol does not usually drop below the lower end of the reference values. After a myocardial infarction, the client may show a low lipid level, but this is a false test result (Silinsky, 1984).

■ SERUM TRIGLYCERIDES

Triglycerides, like cholesterol and the phospholipids, are lipids that are normally present in the serum. The more precise chemical term for this group of lipids is *triacylglycerols,* but the laboratory test is called triglycerides. The triglycerides, the most abundant group of lipids, are neutral fat and oils that come from both animal fat and vegetable oils. A heavy meal or alcohol causes a transient increase in the serum triglyceride level. Excess triglycerides, which are useful for energy, are stored in the body as adipose tissue. The triglyceride test is useful in identifying some types of hyperlipidemia.

Preparation of Client and Collection of Sample
The test should be done in the fasting state, but the client should be on a regular diet before the fasting begins. The laboratory needs 2 ml of serum. Since there is much variation in what is considered "normal," the client usually has the test done more than once if levels are elevated.

Reference Values for Triglycerides	
Adult	90–150 mg/dl. Age- and diet-related. Females slightly lower[a]
Pregnancy	Level rises progressively during pregnancy Note that oral contraceptives also cause an increase (see Appendix D)
Newborn	Lower than 40 mg at birth but rises to 55–60 mg/dl
Children (age 10–14)	Male, 65 mg/dl; female, 75 mg/dl
(age 15–19)	Male, 80 mg/dl; female, 75 mg/dl
Aged (over 65)	130–135 mg/dl

[a]See Rifkind and Segal (1983) for very specific breakdown for all age groups.

Increased Serum Triglyceride Levels

Clinical Significance. Many of the clinical conditions that cause an increase in serum cholesterol levels also cause increases in triglyceride levels. Thus clients with nephrotic syndrome, pancreatic dysfunction, diabetes, toxemia of pregnancy, and hypothyroidism have elevated triglyceride levels. Pancreatitis may cause a very high elevation of triglycerides. Fatty meals and alcohol always raise the triglyceride level for a while. The serum triglyceride level peaks about five hours after a fatty meal. An increase of serum triglycerides is sometimes associated with certain abnormal patterns of lipid metabolism that are probably genetic in origin.

POSSIBLE NURSING DIAGNOSES RELATED TO ELEVATED TRIGLYCERIDE LEVELS

Knowledge Deficit Regarding Diet and Possible Drug Therapy

Clients may need the same instructions on diet as discussed in the section on cholesterol levels. Often weight reduction and a low-fat diet can significantly lower the serum triglyceride level. Some of the drugs used to lower cholesterol also lower triglyceride levels as noted in Table 9–2.

Potential for Ineffective Coping Related to Unhealthy Life-style

The reduction of hyperlipidemia needs to be done in conjunction with other measures to improve the total health of the individual. The American Heart Association considers cigarette smoking, hypertension, and cholesterol as the three major risk factors for cardiovascular disease. The elevated serum triglyceride level is not as firmly established as cholesterol as a risk factor. Because alcohol is a major cause of secondary hyperlipidemia, the possibility of alcohol abuse should be investigated when there are unexplained high levels of triglycerides (Dipp, 1978).

Potential Injury Related to Use of Fat Emulsions

Clients who are deficient in fatty acids can be given fat emulsions intravenously. Because the usual hyperalimentation fluids contain only glucose and amino acids, the fat is given as a separate solution. The fat used for intravenous replacement is composed of soybean oil emulsions and purified egg phosphatides in glycerol and water. This lipid emulsion (Intralipid, Liposyn) can be given via a peripheral vein. Maintaining the emulsion's stability before and during infusion, as well as watching for untoward reactions, are the major responsibilities of the nurse. Specific instructions about how to set up the emulsion are included with the bottle of solution. The client's ability to use lipid emulsions is evaluated by testing the serum triglyceride levels. Within 18 hours after the lipid infusion, the serum triglycerides should return to the baseline (Jacobson, 1979). If the serum triglyceride level remains elevated beyond 18 hours, the client should not be given more fat emulsions.

Decreased Serum Triglyceride Levels

Clinical Significance. A decreased triglyceride level is rarely seen as a clinical problem. Some rare genetic defects may cause low serum triglycerides, and severe malnutrition may lead to low levels. Although hypothyroidism may cause an abnormally high triglyceride level, hyperthyroidism does not contribute to a low level. If the low serum triglyceride level is due to an exhaustion of the body's store of essential fatty acids, the client may have sparse hair growth, scaly and dry skin, poor wound healing, and a decrease in blood platelets, which may lead to some bleeding. The nurse should look for these signs when clients are not getting enough fat in their diet.

■ LIPOPROTEIN ELECTROPHORESIS

Lipoproteins are complex molecules that contain lipids, such as cholesterol and triglycerides, in combination with various proteins. Researchers have been able to make some broad classifications of these lipoproteins based on the varying density of their molecules: HDL, which weigh the most, LDL, and very low-density lipoproteins (VLDL). Electrophoresis can separate these types by using an electric current to cause migration of the molecules. The direction of the different protein molecules

---

Reference Values for Lipoprotein Electrophoresis

A change from the typical pattern in one or more bands on the electrophoretic pattern would be considered abnormal. Several atypical patterns of electrophoresis have been observed and classified as different types of hyperlipidemia. The following brief summary of the six types of patterns are based on several references. The classification system, now a classic, was developed in the late sixties (Fredrickson, 1967).

Type I	Lipoprotein pattern of increased chylomicrons. Serum cholesterol may be normal. Triglycerides are markedly elevated. This is the rarest type of hyperlipidemia. May be treated with just low-fat diet and restriction of all alcohol.
Type II, A	Lipoprotein pattern of increased beta (low-density) lipoproteins. Increased serum cholesterol levels and normal serum triglyceride levels. Therapy would include a restricted cholesterol diet. This is a relatively common pattern of hyperlipidemia and is the most resistant to diet therapy.
Type II, B	Lipoprotein pattern of increased pre-beta and beta lipoproteins. Cholesterol and serum triglyceride are both elevated. This is a relatively common type of hyperlipidemia.
Type III	Lipoprotein pattern shows abnormal type of beta lipoproteins and increased beta lipoproteins. Cholesterol level moderately elevated and triglycerides moderately elevated. Relatively uncommon.
Type IV	This is the most common type of hyperlipidemia. Lipoprotein pattern shows an increase of pre-beta (very low-density) lipoproteins. Serum cholesterol is normal or slightly elevated, with serum triglycerides markedly elevated. Diabetics often show this type of hyperlipidemia. Treatment usually includes control of carbohydrate intake.
Type V	This is an uncommon type of hyperlipidemia. The lipoprotein pattern shows an increase of chylomicrons and of the pre-beta lipoproteins, along with serum cholesterol that is either normal or slightly elevated. Serum triglycerides are elevated.

Types II, III, and IV are particularly associated with the development of coronary artery disease.

is based on size and electrical charge. After the lipoproteins have separated into distinct layers, the layers make a distinct pattern which shows the relative distribution of four bands of lipoproteins: (1) chylomicrons (particles representing dietary fat in transport), (2) pre-beta lipoproteins (VLDL), (3) beta lipoproteins (LDL), and (4) alpha lipoproteins (HDL).

Abnormal Lipoprotein Patterns

Clinical Significance. It has been hypothesized that these six different patterns are due to genetic differences whereas other secondary changes may be induced by high carbohydrate and/or fat intake or by disease states such as diabetes. Some clinicians may feel that identifying the type of hyperlipidemia is important in choosing the correct diet and/or drug therapy. Other clinicians may prefer to designate the hyperlipidemia simply as primary hypercholesterolemia, as primary hypertriglyceridemia, or as a combination of both (Havel, 1977; Rifkind & Segal, 1983).

Since these six categories were developed, much research has been done to establish possible causes for the different types of hyperlipidemia (Ross & Glomset, 1976). Still not known is whether these various types of hyperlipidemia are really separate categories or not. Much of the data from lipoprotein electrophoresis is more appropriate for research purposes than for specific diagnoses. Different authorities have different opinions about the usefulness of this drug or that for different types of hyperlipidemia. However, almost all authorities do agree that the treatment of any primary hyperlipidemia begins with diet changes. The usual diet recommendations for each of the six types of hyperlipidemia are summarized in Table 9-3.

TABLE 9-3. SAMPLES OF DIETARY REGIMEN AS PART OF TREATMENT FOR VARIOUS TYPES OF HYPERLIPOPROTEINEMIAS

Type I	Limit fat intake (25–35 g/day) No alcohol
Type II, A	Increase polyunsaturated fat Reduce cholesterol Limit alcohol
Type II, B	Maintain ideal weight Limit carbohydrate (40% of calories) Normal fat (40% of calories) Increase polyunsaturated fat Reduce cholesterol Limit alcohol
Type III	As in Type II, B
Type IV	Maintain ideal weight Limit carbohydrates (35–40% of calories) Increase polyunsaturated fat Normal cholesterol (up to 500 mg/day) Limit alcohol
Type V	Maintain ideal weight Normal carbohydrate (48–53% of calories) Reduce fat (25–30% of calories) High protein (21–24% of calories) Limit cholesterol (300–500 mg/day) No alcohol

Summary from Kritchevsky and Czarnecki (1980; p. 2), reprinted with permission. See text for discussion on types and Fredrickson (1967) for original description of types of hyperlipoproteinemia. Also see NIH (1985a,b).

The lipid profile, which includes cholesterol, triglycerides, and HDL- and LDL-cholesterols, has essentially replaced the lipoprotein electrophoresis as a clinical assessment of risk for coronary disease (Jacobs et al., 1984).

■ HIGH-DENSITY LIPOPROTEIN (HDL) CHOLESTEROL

The cholesterol component of the HDL (alpha lipoproteins) is measured for this test. Normally about 20% of cholesterol is HDL-cholesterol. Data from the Framingham study, a longitudinal study of the cardiovascular risk for a population in Massachusetts, has supported the theory that low levels of HDL are associated with an increased incidence of coronary vascular disease. Persons with high levels of HDL-cholesterol had less vascular disease. Gordon (1977) presents the statistical evidence for the benefit of higher levels of HDL-cholesterol. Levels above 45 mg/dl are considered to be beneficial in that the client may be less likely to develop atherosclerosis. Levels below 45 mg/dl indicate a higher risk for the development of coronary disease. HDL can be subfractioned, which may have implications for future studies (Kritchevsky & Czarnecki, 1980). Note that the HDL is used to figure out the LDL-cholesterol discussed next.

Preparation of Client
The client should be fasting overnight. Water is allowed. The client should not have had weight changes in the last few weeks. Because many drugs may affect the pattern, drugs should be withheld for 24–48 hours, if possible. Radiological contrast dye interferes with the test.

Reference Values for HDL-Cholesterol

| Adult: | Male | 44–45 mg/dl (average) |
| | Female | 55 mg/dl (average) |

Rifkind and Segal (1983) report percentile reference values for various age groups. Some laboratories report the total cholesterol/HDL cholesterol ratio. The lower the ratio, the lower the risk.

■ LOW-DENSITY LIPOPROTEIN (LDL) CHOLESTEROL

LDLs carry cholesterol in the plasma. Because this type of LDL-cholesterol has been associated with coronary arterial atherosclerosis, it is called the "bad" cholesterol. HDL-cholesterol, discussed above, is the "good" cholesterol. The laboratory can determine the amount of LDL by use of a formula:

LDL-cholesterol = Total cholesterol − (HDL-cholesterol + Triglycerides/5)

For example:

$$\text{LDL-cholesterol} = 200 - \left(55 + \frac{100}{5} \right)$$

$$200 - 75 = 125$$

The formula is not valid for specimens with chylomicrons present or if triglyceride levels are above 400 mg/dl (Jacobs et al., 1984).

Preparation of Client and Collection of Sample

The client should have been on stable diet for at least two weeks before lipid profiles are done. Fasting is required 12 hours before the test. (See notes on total cholesterol levels, as LDL can be calculated from other blood work.)

Reference Values for LDL-Cholesterol

Desirable range for adults is 65–175 mg/dl (Tietz, 1983)[a]
   Pregnancy causes an increase

---

[a]Females have considerably lower ranges than males until menopause. Rifkind & Segal (1983) give percentiles for all age groups.

POSSIBLE NURSING DIAGNOSES RELATED TO HDL- AND LDL-CHOLESTEROL LEVELS

Alteration in Health Maintenance Related to Low Levels of HDL-Cholesterol or High Levels of LDL-Cholesterol

Once clients have been identified as being in a risk group for coronary artery disease they may want information on how to change their cholesterol levels. Some of the recommendations to increase HDL-cholesterol have included eating less meat, consuming fewer calories, drinking 5 to 6 oz of alcohol each week, and eating 1 to 2 tablespoons of lecithin a day. Studies have shown that long distance runners have higher levels of HDL (Smith, 1979). Several studies have also suggested that some alcohol may be protective against coronary heart disease; still, the other negative aspects of alcohol must be considered. Most authorities stress that the best way to increase the amount of HDL-cholesterol is to lose excess weight and then to maintain the proper weight, because HDL-cholesterol concentration decreases with increasing weight (Bradley, et al., 1978), and the total cholesterol increases (NIH, 1985b). The nurse can stress to clients that they should talk to the physician and also read the latest information about HDL. In summary, being at risk for developing atherosclerosic vascular disease can be a strong motivation for clients to evaluate the effect of their total lifestyle on their health and to make changes in other risk factors as discussed throughout this chapter.

QUESTIONS

1. In a female, a rise in the serum cholesterol level is an expected occurrence at all these times *except* when?

   a. About three days after her birth   **c.** During pregnancy

   b. At onset of menses   **d.** After menopause

2. Which one of the following meals contains the least amount of cholesterol?

    a. Steak, baked potato with sour cream, roll and butter, tossed salad with French dressing, and coffee

    b. Lobster, rice, salad with Thousand Island dressing, milk, and apple pie with cheese slice

    c. Chicken, mashed potatoes, green beans, salad with blue cheese dressing, wine, and strawberries with powdered sugar

    d. Liver, rice, peas, cole slaw, tea, and ice cream

3. For clients with hyperlipidemia, the nurse needs to help them assess whether their life-styles contain other high risk factors for the development of a cardiovascular disease. All of the following are considered high risk factors for development of cardiovascular disease except which?

    a. Alcoholic beverages   **c.** Hypertension

    b. Cigarette smoking   **d.** Obesity

4. Mr. Riley, age 44, has been started on drug therapy for a high serum cholesterol level that did not respond to diet and weight control. Which of the following information about hyperlipidemia and drug therapy is appropriate to use to teach Mr. Riley about his disease and drug therapy?

    a. Serum cholesterol levels should show a significant drop in a week or two after drugs are begun

    b. Drug therapy eliminates the need for dietary restrictions

    c. Drug therapy always reduces both cholesterol and triglyceride levels

    d. Family members of Mr. Riley should be screened for abnormal lipid levels because they might need treatment

5. Assessment of a patient who has a decrease in essential fatty acids may include all these findings *except* which?

    a. Sparse hair growth   **c.** increased serum triglyceride levels

    b. Dry and scaly skin   **d.** Decreased serum cholesterol levels

6. Serum triglyceride levels are useful in all the following conditions *except* which?

    a. Evaluating the effect of intravenous fat emulsions

    b. Assessing the presence of hyperthyroidism

    c. Evaluating the effectiveness of some drugs used to control hyperlipidemia

    d. Assessing the type of hyperlipidemia that may be present

7. According to data from the Framingham study, the type of lipoproteins that may offer some protection against the development of cardiovascular disease is which of the following?

    a. Chylomicrons

    b. Pre-beta (very low-density) proteins, VLDL

    c. Beta (low-density) lipoproteins, LDL

    d. Alpha (high-density) lipoproteins, HDL

8. A factor that tends to increase the level of HDL-cholesterol is which of the following?

a. Losing weight if obese   **c.** Eliminating alcohol from the diet

b. Eating meat   **d.** Lack of exercise

REFERENCES

American Heart Association (1985). *Diet and coronary heart disease: Statement for physicians and other health professionals.* New York: American Heart Association.

Antilipemics (1984). *Nursing 84, 14*(3), 57.

Bradley, D., et al. (1978). Serum high density lipoprotein cholesterol in women using oral contraceptives, estrogens and progestins. *NEJM, 299*, 17-21.

Breslow, J. (1978). Pediatric aspects of hyperlipidemia. *Pediatrics, 62*, 510-551.

Cerrato, P. (1985). Making a low cholesterol diet easy to swallow. *RN, 48*(4), 67-68.

Clark, S. (1984). Nutritional control of lipid synthesis. *Contemporary Nutrition, 9*(4), 1-2.

Dipp, S. (1978). Metabolic effects of alcohol. *Arizona Medicine, 35*(10), 651-652.

Flynn, M.A., et al. (1979). Effect of dietary egg on human serum cholesterol and triglycerides. *American Journal of Clinical Nutrition, 32*(5), 1051-1057.

Fredrickson, D.S., et al. (1967). Fat transport in lipoproteins—an integrated approach to mechanisms and disorders. *NEJM, 276*, 215-224.

Glueck, C. (1986). Pediatric primary prevention of atherosclerosis. *NEJM, 314*(3), 175-176.

Gordon, T. (1977). High density lipoprotein as a protective factor against coronary heart disease. *American Journal of Medicine*, (5), 707-714.

Govoni, L., & Hayes, J. (1985). *Drugs and nursing implications.* (5th ed.) Norwalk, CT: Appleton-Century-Crofts.

Harris, W. (1985). Health effects of omega-3-fatty acids. *Contemporary Nutrition, 10*(8), 1-2.

Havel, R. (1977). Classification of the hyperlipidemias. *Annual Review of Medicine, 28*, 195-209.

Hytten, R., & Lind, T. (1975). *Diagnostic indices in pregnancy.* Summit, NJ: Ciba-Geigy Corp.

Jacobs, D., Kasten, B., DeMott, W., & Wolfson, W. (1984). *Laboratory test handbook with DRG index.* St. Louis: Mosby/Lexi.

Jacobson, N. (1979). How to administer those tricky lipid emulsions. *RN, 42*(6), 63-64.

Kannel, W. (1976). Some lessons in cardiovascular epidemiology from Framingham. *American Journal of Cardiology, 37*(2), 269-282.

Kritchevsky, D., & Czarnecki, S. (1980). Lipoproteins. *Contemporary Nutrition, 5*(5), 1-2.

Mallison, M. (1978). Updating the cholesterol controversy verdict—diet does count. *AJN 78*(10), 1681.

Mathos, E. (1986). Quiz on antilipemics. *Nursing 86, 16*(5), 64.

Morrison, J., et al. (1979). Diagnostic ramifications of repeated plasma cholesterol and triglyceride measurements in children: Regression toward the mean in a pediatric population. *Pediatrics, 64*(2), 197-201.

O'Connor, T. (1985). Dietary fat, calories and cancer. *Contemporary Nutrition, 10*(7), 1-2.

National Institutes of Health Consensus Development Panel (1985a). Lowering blood cholesterol to prevent heart disease. *Consensus Development Conference Statement, 5*(7). Bethesda, MD: U.S. Dept. Health and Human Services.

National Institutes of Health Consensus Development Panel (1985b). Health implications of obesity. *Consensus Development Conference Statement, 5*(9). Bethesda, MD: U.S. Dept. Health and Human Services.

Pritikin, N. (1984, August 12). Run, but eat right. *San Francisco Examiner*, pp. 7-8.

Reiser, R. (1980). Diet and blood lipids: An overview. *Food and Nutrition News, 51*, 104.

Rifkind, B., & Segal, P. (1983). Lipid research clinics program reference values for hyperlipidemia and hypolipidemia. *JAMA, 250*(14), 1869–1872.

Ross, R., & Glomset, J.A. (1976). Pathogenesis of atherosclerosis. *NEJM, 295*, 364–377.

Sodhi, H., & Mason, D. (1977). New insights into the homeostasis of plasma cholesterol. *American Journal of Medicine, 63*, 325–327.

Silinsky, J. (1984). Your patient's lipid profile. *RN*, (9), 102–104.

Smith, T. (1979). Medical advice. *Nor-Cal Running Review, 75*, 18.

Tietz, N. (Ed.). (1983). *Clinical guide to laboratory tests*. Philadelphia: Saunders.

Wallis, C. (1984, March 26). Hold the eggs and butter. *Time Magazine*, 56–63.

Williams, R., et al. (1986). Evidence that men with familial hypercholesterolemia can avoid early coronary death. *JAMA, 255*(2), 219–224.

Yeshurum, D., & Golto, A.M. (1976). Drug treatment of hyperlipidemia. *American Journal of Medicine, 60*, 379–392.

10

Tests Related to Serum Protein Levels

- Total Protein (TP) and Albumin/Globulin (A/G) Ratio
- Serum Protein Electrophoresis (SPEP)
- Serum Albumin
- Alpha-1-Antitrypsin (AAT)
- Gamma Globulins
- Immunoelectrophoresis of Serum Proteins (Serum IEP): IgG, IgA, IgM, IgD, IgE
- Urine Protein Electrophoresis and Immunoelectrophoresis (IEP)
- Serum Ammonia (NH_3)
- Alpha-Fetoprotein (AFP)
- Carcinoembryonic Antigen (CEA)

OBJECTIVES

1. Identify the serum proteins measured by electrophoresis and immunoelectrophoresis.
2. Illustrate how cellular and humoral immunity are assessed by specific laboratory tests.
3. Identify nursing diagnoses for clients with low serum albumin levels (hypoalbuminemia).
4. Explain the general clinical significance of various aclonal, monoclonal, and polyclonal patterns of immunoglobulins in serum and urine.
5. Identify basic nursing interventions for any clients who have an abnormal pattern or deficiency of gamma globulins.
6. Describe how the radioallergosorbent (RAST) test is used in the assessment of allergies.
7. Identify the types of medications and food that must be withheld when a patient has an elevated serum ammonia level.
8. Describe the clinical usefulness of AFP and CEA as tumor markers.

This chapter focuses on the most common tests used to measure proteins in the serum. The difference between serum and plasma proteins is that plasma proteins include those involved in the clotting of the plasma. (The plasma proteins, fibrinogen and prothrombin, are discussed in Chapter 13.)

The two serum proteins measured in the test for "total proteins" are albumin and globulin. Albumin is a singular type of protein that is either in the serum in sufficient amounts or not. The tests for globulins are more complex because there are five types of globulins (alpha-1 and -2, beta-1 and -2, and gamma globulins). In addition, there are many singular types of proteins in each of these major classes.

The exact amounts of albumin and of the five major globulin types are determined by a procedure called *electrophoresis*. If certain of the gamma globulins are shown to be abnormal, a further test, *immunoelectrophoresis,* is done to separate out the five major types of gamma globulins. Electrophoresis uses an electrical current to separate the six protein fractions, while *immuno*electrophoresis involves, as an added step, the use of antiserum to cause precipitation of the five gamma globulins (Cawley et al., 1978). The proteins that are identified by these tests are shown in Table 10–1. These tests can be done not only for the serum but also for urine and spinal fluid. One serum protein, alpha fetoprotein, normal in pregnancy and very abnormal otherwise, is discussed at the end of the chapter.

FUNCTIONS OF ALBUMIN IN THE SERUM

Albumin, produced only by the liver, is essential in maintaining the oncotic pressure in the vascular system. A lack of albumin in the serum allows fluid to leak out into the interstitial spaces and into the peritoneal cavity. Albumin is also very important in the transportation of many substances in the bloodstream. For example, when the serum albumin level is less than normal, the total serum calcium level is depressed. (See Chapter 7 on how albumin affects the interpretation of serum calcium levels.)

TABLE 10-1. TESTS OF SERUM PROTEINS

Measured as Total Proteins (T/P)	Measured by Protein Electrophoresis (PEP)	Measured by Immunoelectrophoresis (IEP)	
Serum proteins 6–8.4 g/dl Albumin (3.5–5 g/dl) (52–68%)			
	Alpha-1 globulins (4.2–7.2%)		
	Alpha-2 globulins (6.8–12%)		
Globulins[a] (2.3–3.5 g/dl)	Beta-1 globulins (3–10%)		
	Beta-2 globulins (1–9%)	IgG	75%
		IgA	10–15%
		IgM	7–10%
	Gamma globulins (13–23%)	IgD	Less than 1%
		IgE	Less than 1%

Values are approximate values for adults. See text for variations across life-span.
[a]Note that many of the alpha and beta globulins can be measured by individual tests for alpha-1-antitrypsin, alpha-fetoprotein, and so on. Also, all beta globulins may be reported together as 9.3–15% (Scully, 1986).

Many drugs, lipids, hormones, and toxins are bound to albumin while they are circulating in the bloodstream. Once the drug or other substance reaches the liver, it is detached from the albumin and made less toxic by conversion to a water-soluble form that can be excreted. (See Chapter 11 for further discussion about the role of albumin in the conjugation process of bilirubin.) Albumin is also one of the buffers that function to maintain acid–base balance in the bloodstream, as discussed in Chapter 6.

FUNCTIONS OF GLOBULINS IN THE SERUM

As can be seen in Table 10–1, the globulins are a very complex and diversified group of serum proteins, for which both the alpha and the beta types are synthesized in the liver:

1. *Alpha-1 globulins* contain various lipoproteins, glycoproteins, antitrypsin, and other proteins such as thyroid-binding globulin.
2. *Alpha-2 globulins* contain macroglobulins, haptoglobulin, ceruloplasmin, and hormones such as erythropoietin.
3. *Beta-1 globulins* contain hormones, fat-soluble vitamins, transferrin, and plasminogen, in addition to other lipoproteins.
4. *Beta-2 globulins* contain most of the various components of the complement system and other proteins (Arguembourg, 1975).

Nurses need not necessarily remember what specific proteins go under which type of alpha or beta globulin. The point is that the globulins are composed of many types of proteins. Liver dysfunction is the usual reason for overall changes in alpha and beta globulins. Disease conditions that change an individual alpha or beta globulin, such as the lack of erythropoietin in renal disease, do not cause a major change in the whole broad grouping of serum globulins. (Some of the individual tests for the various components of the complement system, as well as other serological tests involving protein reactions, are covered in Chapter 14.) The lipoprotein electrophoresis, which measures specific alpha and beta globulins involved in fat (lipid) transport, is used to detect certain types of hyperlipidemia. (Lipoprotein electrophoresis is covered in Chapter 9.)

Unlike the alpha and beta globulins, gamma globulins, now called immunoglobulins, are not synthesized by the liver. They are made by B lymphocytes in response to a stimulus from an antigen. Classified as five main types that are designated by the letters IgG, IgA, IgM, IgD, and IgE, these five immunoglobulins are changed considerably in different types of immunological responses. To understand the clinical significance of testing for immunoglobulins, one must recall some basic facts about the concepts of cellular and humoral immunity.

The Immune System
Optimal immunological defense probably depends on interactions between cellular and humoral immunity, but much is still to be learned about the interaction of these two systems.

Cellular Immunity. Cellular immunity, or delayed hypersensitivity, is a function of the T lymphocytes that are controlled by the thymus. The presence of adequate cellular immunity can be demonstrated by a positive response to various skin tests. Cellular immunity is not identified by tests on plasma because T lymphocytes do not produce antibodies, although they may help mediate this function of the B lymphocytes. See Chapter 2 on lymphocytes. Also see Chapter 14 on the test for AIDS.

Humoral Immunity. Because the immunoglobulins secreted by the B lymphocytes are found in the bloodstream and in other secretions such as saliva, tears, and colostrum, this type of immunity is called *humoral*. Humoral immunity is the type directly measured by assessment of the circulating antibodies in serum and in other body fluids, because the antibodies or immunoglobulins are produced by the B lymphocyte system. The *B* stands not for blood but for bursa, because earlier research discovered this type of lymphocyte in the bursa of chickens. In man, the B lymphocytes are thought to be produced in the lymphoid tissue of the gastrointestinal tract. The distinctions between the five types of gamma globulin are discussed under the section on the test of immunoelectrophoresis.

The complement system contains several proteins that are classified by the letter C and a number (such as C_2, C_4, and the like). The complement system enhances the antibody-antigen reaction of the humoral system. The tests involving the complement system are discussed in Chapter 14.

■ TOTAL PROTEIN (TP) AND ALBUMIN/GLOBULIN (A/G) RATIO

The total protein measures albumin and globulin levels in the serum. Albumin divided by globulin equals the A/G ratio. The normal range is 1.0 or above. For example, if albumin is 3.5 and globulin is 2.5 the ratio is 1.4. Because serum protein electrophoresis measures the actual amount of albumin and globulin it is a much more useful test than reporting just a ratio. In addition, the electrophoresis gives much more information about all the types of globulins.

■ SERUM PROTEIN ELECTROPHORESIS (SPEP)

In this test, the laboratory uses an electrical current to separate normal human serum into six distinct protein fractions, through a migration of protein molecules. Various protein molecules, after separating out in a gel mixture or on a coated film, are fixed on a sheet of paper. Albumin, the largest component, has the greatest mobility, so it moves the farthest away from the point of the electrical current. The alpha globulins line up next, then the beta globulins (Cawley et al., 1978). Because the gamma globulins migrate the least from the electrical point, this group makes the last big distinct band on the paper. Once the six protein fractions have been separated out on the strip of paper, the sheet is stained to identify the pattern.

This pictorial representation of the amounts of each protein type is useful as a screening device because significant changes in the patterns can be noted and further testing done if deemed necessary by the clinician. For example, protein electrophoresis is a screening test for multiple myeloma. The pathologist is usually the one to compare the pattern to known abnormal patterns that are seen in various disease states. The strip of paper, or electrophorectogram, can be put into a machine that quantifies the six serum protein fractions and reports the amount in percentages. This report in percentages can be read by the nurse, as the percentages can be compared to reference values for each type of protein fraction.

Preparation of Client and Collection of Sample
The client should be fasting but can have water. One milliliter of whole blood is ample for total protein and electrophoresis. Fresh samples are ideal, but older samples can be used. The dye used for a bromosulfophthalein test makes the results falsely elevated for a couple of days.

Reference Values for SPEP

Essentially, the same for all people. Variations noted for electrophoresis results are as follows:

Total serum protein	6–8.4 g/100 ml
Serum albumin	3.5–5.0 g/100 ml
Serum globulins	2.3–3.5 g/100 ml

Electrophoresis (reported as a percentage of total protein):

Adult	Albumin	52–68%
	Globulins	
	Alpha-1	4.2–7.2%
	Alpha-2	6.8–12%
	Beta-1	3–10% } (some laboratories report
	Beta-2	1–9% } betas together as 9.3–15%)
	Gamma	13–23%
Newborn	Essentially fall in the same distribution with a lowering of beta-1. See details about gamma globulins in text.	
Pregnancy	Albumin falls quickly the first few months and then more slowly during rest of pregnancy. Overall fall is about 1 g/100 ml. The alpha and beta globulins show slight increases whereas the gamma globulins may decrease slightly (Hytten & Lind, 1975).	

Note that oral contraceptives may cause a slight decrease (see Appendix D).

Children	Tend to have slightly greater amounts of alpha-2. Types and amounts of gamma globulins depend on age. See text.	
Age 4–11	Total protein	6.6–7.9 g
Age 12–20	Total protein	6.8–8.4 g
Aged	The gamma globulins, or at least the immunological response, decreases with age (Dharan, 1976). Albumin levels gradually decrease (Jacobs et al., 1984).	

■ SERUM ALBUMIN

Elevated Serum Albumin Level

Clinical Significance. No pathological conditions cause the liver to produce extra amounts of albumin. So an increased value of albumin on a laboratory report is a reflection of dehydration. (Recall that many tests can be falsely elevated by dehydration.) The inclusion of excess amounts of protein in the diet does not raise the serum albumin level because protein is first broken down into amino acids and then used for various purposes, including storage as adipose (fat) tissue.

Decreased Serum Albumin Level

Clinical Significance. (Hypoalbuminemia) Because albumin is totally synthesized by the liver, liver dysfunction is a common reason for a decreased serum albumin level. Reduced albumin levels are not seen in acute liver failure because it takes several weeks of nonproduction before the albumin level drops. The most common reason for a lowered level is chronic liver dysfunction due to cirrhosis. Clients with AIDS have hypoalbuminemia. A loss of albumin in the urine due to renal dysfunction (nephrotic syndrome) can also cause a decrease of albumin in the serum. Although a drop of about 1 g/100 ml is normal in pregnancy, there is even more of a drop in preeclampsia. (Albuminuria, or albumin in the urine, is a key sign of both renal pathology and eclampsia. See Chapter 3.) Severe burns, with the related damage to capillaries and blood vessels, result in a large loss of serum proteins, including albumin. The increased capillary permeability due to the burn damage may cause a continual leak of serum proteins out of the vascular system. Also, the long-term depression of protein synthesis after a burn may last for a couple of months.

If there is inadequate intake of protein, the body begins the breakdown of muscles and of other protein tissue (catabolism) to obtain enough amino acids for the continuing synthesis of serum albumin. Thus albumin levels do not drop in fasting states or in malnutrition until the condition is severe. Protein requirements may be greatly increased during stress, infection, or injury. The patient is in a negative nitrogen balance when the catabolic process is greater than the anabolic process and when the protein deficiency is long-standing. A combination of illness with prolonged protein deprivation is eventually reflected in a reduced serum albumin level. Other test results that indicate malnutrition are a low transferrin level and a low lymphocyte count (See Chapter 2).

In the United States, a true protein deficiency (kwashiorkor) is a rare condition. Certain elderly groups, particularly Black and Spanish-American women, may contain people who have lower than the recommended daily allowance of protein (Palombo & Blackburn, 1980). However, this low-protein diet does not affect serum albumin levels directly unless illness increases the need for more protein. On rare occasions, when children, who require more protein than adults, are placed on an inadequate cult-type vegetarian diet, they may become so depleted in protein that this causes a lowered serum albumin level. Vegetarians who choose a diet with a sufficient variety of grains, nuts, fruits, and vegetables maintain adequate protein synthesis.

TABLE 10-2. FOODS HIGH IN PROTEIN

Food Item	Grams of Protein
Complete proteins	
1 egg	7.0
1 oz meat or fish	7.0–8.0
1 oz cheese	6.0–7.0
8 oz milk	8.5
1 tbsp dried milk	1.6
Incomplete proteins[a]	
1 tbsp peanut butter	4.0
2 slices wheat bread	4.0
1 cup nuts	7.0–8.0
3 oz lentils	7.0
¼ cup garbanzo beans	10.0

Estimates are from various food labels and nutritional pamphlets.
[a]Consult a nutrition text on how incomplete vegetable proteins can be balanced to supply all needed amino acids.

POSSIBLE NURSING DIAGNOSES RELATED TO HYPOALBUMINURIA

Impairment of Skin Integrity Related to Development of Edema

Because albumin is responsible for the oncotic pressure in the vascular system, a reduction in serum albumin causes edema. Edema occurs when the albumin level falls to 2.0–2.5 gm/dl. Without adequate albumin in the bloodstream, fluid leaks out into the interstitial spaces and into the peritoneal cavity. Unlike the edema due to too much volume in the vascular space, this type of edema is not found primarily in dependent areas. For example, clients with an increased volume due to congestive heart failure have edema in the feet if they are sitting up or in the sacral area if in bed. In contrast, clients with edema due to a lack of albumin may also have puffy eyelids or hands and a swollen abdomen due to the leakage of fluid into the peritoneal cavity. (The cirrhotic client who has hypoalbuminemia is also likely to have portal hypertension that intensifies the collection of fluid in the peritoneal cavity.) In addition to weighing these clients and checking their ankles and sacral area for edema, the nurse should also measure the abdominal girth to check the progression of edema. Besides causing edema, the lack of protein also escalates the risk of decubitis ulcers because cellular nutrition is inadequate (Cerrato, 1986). Skin breakdown is always a potential problem. These clients need superb skin care.

Assisting with Interventions to Decrease Edema. A collection of fluid in the peritoneal cavity may make it impossible for the patient to breathe comfortably in a reclining position. Sometimes a paracentesis must be done to take the pressure off the diaphragm (See Chapter 25 on paracentesis). The disadvantage of a paracentesis is that proteins are lost in the peritoneal fluid. Diuretics, along with some restrictions of fluids and sodium, may be ordered because an increased amount of aldosterone may also be contributing to the formation of edema. (See Chapter 5 on hypernatremia.)

Alteration in Nutritional Requirements of Protein

The primary treatment for edema caused by a lack of serum albumin is to increase the albumin level. If the liver can still synthesize albumin, a diet with adequate protein is appropriate for long-term therapy. The recommended daily allowance for protein for healthy adults is around 44–56 g a day depending on age and weight. These general figures are set higher than what may be the minimum needed. Palombo and Blackburn (1980) suggest that many Americans eat as much as 90 g of protein while the minimum needed may be as little as 35–50 g. See Chapter 4 on urinary urea nitrogen as a test for a negative nitrogen balance or protein deficit.

Often the clients who need the protein the most can tolerate it the least because their livers are unable to handle the ammonia that results from protein breakdown. (See the test for serum ammonia at the end of this chapter.) If protein is well tolerated, however, then eggs, cheese, fish, and meat are excellent sources, along with a correct mixture of nuts, grains, and vegetables. If protein needs to be increased in the diet, one egg or an ounce of cheese supplies about 7 g of protein. A glass of milk made from dried milk powder supplies 8 g of protein without increasing the cholesterol intake. (See Chapter 9 for the cholesterol controversy.) Also, dried milk is economical and can be added to many foods and beverages. Commercially made protein supplements can be used, although they tend to be expensive. If the client is also deficient in minerals and vitamins, these liquid diets may ensure a higher level of many necessary nutrients. The client must have plenty of calories from carbohydrates so that protein is not used as an expensive energy source. See Table 10–2 for a comparison for the protein content in various foods.

Potential for Fluid Volume Excess Related to Albumin Replacement Intravenously

For the client who needs albumin replacement immediately, albumin can be given intravenously. Brand names for albumin include Albumisol, Albuspan, Burminate, Albuminar, Albuteen, and Proserum. Some albumin, which is collected from human donors, is obtained from placental blood, which is a significant fact since the infusion of some albumins causes a rise in the alkaline phosphatase level. (See Chapter 12 for this enzyme test.) Albumin does not need to be refrigerated as does whole blood. It does not have any preservatives added so it must be used soon after it is opened.

Albumin comes in a 5% and a 25% concentration. The 25% solution is usually given at a rate no faster than 1 ml a minute. The 5% solution can be given at a rate of around 2 ml to 4 ml a minute (Govoni & Hayes, 1985). The intravenous infusion must be given slowly because of the danger of circulatory overload. Vital signs must be monitored.

As the oncotic pressure returns to normal, edematous fluid is pulled back into the vascular system. The mobilization of edema from the tissues causes an increased urine output. The albumin remains in the bloodstream for several days, but with a severe albumin deficiency, the client may need repeated infusions over time. Serum albumin levels are assessed every few days, or even daily, to determine how much replacement is needed. Giving albumin intravenously is costly and studies suggest that protein by oral feedings helps to raise albumin levels even when protein synthesis seems questionable (Tullis, 1977).

High Risk for Infection

Clients with a lack of protein have a lowered resistance to infection. A decreased absolute lymphocyte count (below 1500 mm^3) is associated with malnutrition. See Chapter 2 for information related to lowered lymphocyte counts and Chapter 16 for nursing diagnoses related to infections.

■ ALPHA-1-ANTITRYPSIN (AAT)

Alpha-1-antitrypsin is an example of a special alpha globulin that can be measured. A decrease or near-absence of ATT can be a factor in chronic obstructive lung disease. The role of antitrypsin is to inhibit the damaging effects from proteolytic enzymes released by bacteria and phagocytes in the lung. The relationship of antitrypsin to the liver is not well understood, but a lack of this protein is found in young children with liver disease (Tietz, 1983). Clients with lung or liver dysfunctions are screened for a lack of this alpha protein. More specific phenotyping is desirable if low levels are found (Jacobs et al., 1984). Alpha-1-antitrypsin deficiency can also be assessed by amniocentesis (See Chapter 28).

Preparation of Client and Collection of Sample

No special preparation of client is necessary. Laboratory needs 10 ml of blood.

Reference Values for AAT

85–213 mg/100 ml

> **POSSIBLE NURSING DIAGNOSIS RELATED TO DECREASED ALPHA-1-ANTITRYPSIN**
>
> **Potential for Ineffective Airway Clearance**
> The key nursing implication for the client with a lack of antitrypsin is to protect the client against respiratory infections. Smoking and polluted environments should be avoided because of high risk for developing emphysema in the third or fourth decade of life.

■ GAMMA GLOBULINS

Clinical Significance. There is usually more diagnostic significance in the patterns of gamma globulins than in the alpha and beta globulins. There may be an increase either of various types (polyclonal) or of only one type (monoclonal), or there may be an absence (aclonal) of gamma globulins. The use of the term "clonal" refers to the origin of the globulins from a particular *clone* of plasma cells (Cawley et al., 1978)

Polyclonal Patterns. This pattern is a reflection of an overproduction of almost all the immunoglobulins in response to antigens. Several different clones of plasma cells are producing increased amounts of various immunoglobulins. The end result is a general hypergammaglobulinemia, a characteristic response to infections (the inflammatory response). Autoimmune diseases and certain liver diseases cause a generalized increase too.

Monoclonal Patterns. In this pattern, only one type of gamma globulin is increased. Patterns of this sort may be more specifically diagnostic because they involve a spike of a single globulin, which can be closely examined by immunoelectrophoresis to detect paraproteins or abnormal varients of an immunoglobulin. Monoclonal patterns are found in a number of situations:

1. A majority of clients with multiple myeloma have a peak of a paraprotein or abnormal globulin. (The discussion on immunoelectrophoresis explores paraproteins.)

2. Sometimes the elderly have a monoclonal pattern that appears to be more the result of the aging process than of a specific disease. However, for clients that show a monoclonal pattern, half may eventually develop multiple myeloma (Dharan, 1976).

3. Macroglobulinemia, an increase in the IgM, is characterized by an increase in just one type of immunoglobulin.

4. Malignant lymphomas and acute infections are other conditions that may cause an increase of only one type of immunoglobulin.

Aclonal Patterns. In aclonal patterns, or hypogammopathies, the gamma globulins are absent or markedly decreased.

1. The lack of gamma globulins may be congenital. Infants with an aclonal pattern may appear normal at birth due to the presence of immunoglobulins from the mother. But then frequent and severe infections begin to occur when the passive immunity from the mother no longer exists.

2. Acquired hypogammaglobulinemia is most often seen with chronic lymphocytic leukemia, malignant lymphomas, or other diseases affecting the bone marrow.

3. Drugs, such as corticosteroids and cytotoxic drugs used for treatment of malignancies, may reduce gamma globulin levels or at least make the gamma globulins ineffective.

4. Radiation therapy and toxins in the environment can also produce an acquired lack of gamma globulins.

POSSIBLE NURSING DIAGNOSES RELATED TO ABNORMAL GAMMA GLOBULINS

High Risk for Infection

The person with either fewer gamma globulins or abnormal gamma globulins is very susceptible to opportunistic pathogens. High levels of abnormal immunoglobulins are always accompanied by lower levels of normal immunoglobulins. So the single most important nursing implication for a client who has an abnormal gamma globulin pattern is to protect the client from infection (Donley, 1976). Bacterial pneumonia is often the cause of death. The client must be protected from others who have upper respiratory infections. Sometimes it may be necessary to initiate reverse isolation to protect the client, particularly with infants who have a severe immuno-deficiency disorder. With the older person, meticulous hand washing is probably the key point, as reverse isolation, with its extra cost, still does not protect persons from the bacteria on their own skin or from the bacteria in food. A concentrated effort should be made to keep the environment relatively free of pathogens. Because the main defense against invading organisms is intact skin and mucous membranes, the nurse must promote good skin care. Proper nutrition with adequate protein is also important for the production of immunoglobulins and lymphocytes. (See the discussion on albumin for ways to ensure adequate protein intake.) The premature infant and the aged person are particularly vulnerable to infections due to their more severe lack of enough antibodies to offer resistance to pathogens.

Potential for Injury Related to Injections of Gamma Globulins

Gamma globulin may be administered to patients to increase immunoglobulin levels temporarily. Immune serum globulin may prevent serious infection if circulatory levels of IgG (discussed next) are kept at about 200 mg/dl. However, immune globulin may not prevent chronic infections of the secretory tissues such as the respiratory tract. The gamma globulin may be needed every three to four weeks. Since now and then serum globulin injections can cause anaphylaxis, the person should be observed for 20–30 minutes after the injection (Govoni & Hayes, 1985). Plasma therapy may also be used if larger doses of passive immunity are needed, as repeated injections are painful and time-consuming.

Knowledge Deficit Related to Technical Aspects of Therapy

In addition to the replacement of normal gamma globulins there may also be an attempt to remove abnormal proteins from the bloodstream by pheresis. *Pheresis* is the process whereby a specific plasma constituent is separated from other blood constituents and removed from the client's plasma. (Pheresis can also be used to obtain platelets for transfusion.) If the client has an excessive amount of abnormal IgM (see the discussion on macroglobulinemia), this protein can be filtered out of the blood by the pheresis machine (Rossmann et al., 1977).

■ IMMUNOELECTROPHORESIS OF SERUM PROTEINS (SERUM IEP): IgG, IgA, IgM, IgD, AND IgE

When a protein electrophoresis demonstrates abnormalities in the gamma globulins, it may be useful to find out exactly which of the gamma globulins are changed. Before 1960, the term "gamma globulins" was used to include those known to give the body immunity against antigens or foreign proteins. According to the World Health Organization, *immunoglobulins* are defined as proteins of animal origin that are endowed with known antibody activity (Arguembourg, 1975). Certain other proteins that do not have antibody activity are also called immunoglobulins. These paraproteins are the type seen elevated in the monoclonal patterns of multiple myeloma and in other abnormal productions of plasma cells. Although there are only five main groups of immunoglobulins (IgG, IgA, IgM, IgD, and IgE), 40 or more fractions can be distinguished by researchers. This discussion is limited to some general knowledge about the five major types of immunoglobulins.

The laboratory uses antiserum preparations to cause a precipitation of each of the five major types of immunoglobulins. The precipitations may be done in a gel or on a glass slide and then transferred to a sheet of paper. The final result is a pattern of bands that have a certain curvature, position, and intensity of color. Abnormalities in any of the immunoglobulins cause the band for that precipitation to be displaced, bowed, lighter in color, thicker than normal, or absent. The laboratory can also quantify each type of immunoglobulin. Some laboratories may report in milligrams and some in grams. Thus the results may be, for example, 0.8–1.5 g/dl or 800–1,500 mg/dl. The reference values used here are in milligrams.

Preparation of Client and Collection of Sample

A fresh sample is the sample of choice, but aged serum or plasma can be used. Depending on the technique, only 2 ml of blood may be needed. Other techniques require more. Any blood transfusions or blood component therapy within the last 6 weeks, as well as any immunizations or vaccines within the last 6 months, should be noted on the laboratory requisition.

Reference Values for Immunoglobulins

Adult	IgG	639–1349 mg/dl (usually about 75% of total)
	IgA	70–312 mg/dl (10–15%)
	IgM	86–352 mg/dl (7–10%)
	IgD	0.5–3 mg/dl (less than 1%)
	IgE	0.01–0.04 mg/dl (less than 1%)
Newborn	IgG	640–1.250 mg/dl
	IgA	0–11 mg/dl
	IgM	5–30 mg/dl
	IgD	—
	IgE	—
Children		Depends on age. By age 6 months to a year, levels begin gradual increase. Adult values may be reached by late teens
Pregnancy		Evidently IgE falls somewhat during pregnancy, while the others show no significant change
Aged		Even healthy older people may show abnormal patterns with increase of paraproteins. (Dharan, 1976). In response to a challenge, such as an infection, immunoglobulin production is likely to be reduced or a less vigorous response

---

Changes In Immunoglobulins

Clinical Significance. The exact significance of changes in immunoglobulins may be determined only in conjunction with other tests such as urine immunoelectrophoresis and perhaps bone marrow studies. Following is a brief summary of the general characteristics of changes in each component of the immunoglobulins. One way to remember which one is the most abundant and which is the least is to use the word *GAMDE ,* because G is the most abundant and E the least abundant in the adult. Kyle and Greipp (1978) contains an extensive review of the studies done on the immunoglobulins.

IgG. This immunoglobulin, which makes up about three-fourths of the total immunoglobulins, is the only one that crosses the placenta. Hence the infant has a high level. which shows some decrease until about 6 months to a year, when the infant begins ample production of IgG.

IgG protects against virus, bacteria, and toxins. It is more for a secondary response. Thus specific IgG antibodies against infections such as hepatitis or rubella indicate past exposure and probable immunity (see Chapter 14). In the newborn IgG levels indicate passive immunity. A lack of IgG causes severe immunodeficiency. IgG increases when the person is desensitized to antigens, and it apparently blocks IgE actions (Voignier & Bridgewater, 1978). Note that injections of immune serum globulin contain primarily IgG.

IgA. The second most common immunoglobulin in the bloodstream, IgA is also present in watery fluids and in surface secretions, such as saliva, tears, and colostrum. These immunoglobulins are thought to be the first line of defense against organisms invading the respiratory, gastrointestinal, or urinary tracts. The infant begins producing IgA after a few months. Deficiencies of IgA may be combined with other deficiencies or be alone.

IgM. In the bloodstream in slightly lower levels than IgA, IgM does not cross the placenta, but the infant may begin synthesizing IgM sooner than IgA. IgM is particularly important for resistance to gram-negative bacteria (Heagarty et al., 1980). IgM is the major component in a primary immune response. IgM antibodies are indicators of an active infection. IgM activates the complement system, its level remaining high as long as the antigen is present. The antibodies to blood group antigens are in the group of IgM immunoglobulins. (See Chapter 14 for discussion of IgM antibodies for hepatitis and rubella.)

Because IgM has a high molecular weight, abnormal increases in it are called *macroglobulinemia.* These immunoglobulins tend to make the blood highly viscous. Normal viscosity of blood is 1.4 to 1.8 as compared with the viscosity of water (Scully, 1986). The increase of macroglobulins also makes the person very sensitive to cold (Dharan, 1976). As discussed earlier, pheresis therapy may be used to remove abnormal immunoglobulins (Rossmann et al., 1977).

IgD. This immunoglobulin is in the bloodstream in very small amounts. The exact functions of IgD are unclear at the present time.

IgE and the RAST (Radioallergosorbent Test for IgE Antibodies). IgE, which is in the bloodstream in very small amounts, increases in allergic states and in the event of parasitic infestation. Evidently IgE is responsible for severe hypersensitive reactions. A measurement of specific IgE antibodies in the serum helps to establish the diagnosis of allergic disease by identifying which allergens are causing clinical symptoms such as hay fever, asthma, or skin rashes (Hamburger, 1978).

The RAST measures the quantity and the increase of antigen-specific IgE present in the serum. Hence the exact quantities of antibodies to a variety of pollens, such as animal dander or food, can be tested. Although more expensive than conventional skin testing, the RAST gives precise information without causing any hypersensitivity reactions. The test has become the most reliable for the diagnosis of food allergy of the immediate type. No satisfactory laboratory test is available to aid in the diagnosis of delayed (up to 5 days) food allergy (Breneman, 1979).

■ URINE PROTEIN ELECTROPHORESIS AND IMMUNOELECTROPHORESIS (IEP)

The techniques for doing electrophoresis and immunoelectrophoresis of urine are similar to those for serum testing. If an abnormal amount of protein is discovered in the urine, these tests can identify exactly which kinds of proteins are being excreted. (See Chapter 3 for the screening technique for proteinuria.) Normally, a 24-hr urine has a protein content of around 40–150 mg, with no more than 10 mg in a random specimen. The dipstick used for screening registers 1 + when there are about 30 mg in the specimen; less than 30 mg causes a trace showing.

The dipstick method of screening for proteinuria tests primarily for albumin so a dipstick for protein is not reliable as a screening test for proteins other than albumin. The laboratory uses other methods to screen for abnormal proteins, such as Bence Jones protein which may occur with multiple myeloma. The electrophoresis and, if necessary, an immunoelectorphoresis are used to follow up a quantitative or qualitative report of abnormal protein in the urine.

Protein in the urine may not always be pathological. Glomerular permeability increases in some people when they are in the upright position (orthostatic proteinuria). Another nonpathological reason for protein in the urine is vigorous exercise.

Reference Values for Urine Protein Electrophoresis

Three main types of pathological patterns may be identified by separating out the protein fractions in urine (Cawley et al., 1978 p. 74).

1. There may be a marked increase in the albumin fraction and some increase in alpha and beta globulins. This signifies increased glomerular permeability such as that seen in some renal disease and in eclampsia.

2. There may be a marked elevation in alpha and beta globulins with a decrease in albumin. This most likely signifies tubular damage.

3. There may be various abnormal proteins or paraproteins, such as those found in multiple myeloma or in other disorders of the gamma globulins. This is considered a prerenal pattern. Just as in the serum, immunoelectrophoresis can then be used to identify exactly which globulins are present.

■ SERUM AMMONIA (NH₃)

The liver normally converts ammonia, a byproduct of protein metabolism, into urea, which is excreted by the kidneys. When the liver is unable to convert ammonia to urea, toxic levels of ammonia accumulate in the bloodstream. In severe liver failure, the blood urea nitrogen (BUN) drops as the ammonia level rises. (See Chapter 4 on the use of the BUN as a test for renal function.)

Preparation of Client and Collection of Sample

Some laboratories may require a fasting state; water is allowed. Either 2 ml of venous or arterial blood can be used. The blood is put into a heparinized tube (green-top Vacutainer) and packed in ice for transport to the laboratory. If the client is on antibiotics (such as neomycin) for treatment of hepatic coma, write this fact on the laboratory slip.

Reference Values for Serum NH_3

Adult	35–65 mcg/dl
Newborn	90–150 mcg/dl
Children	45–80 mcg/dl (tested by enzymatic method, Children's Hospital, San Francisco, California)

Values may vary considerably from laboratory to laboratory. See Appendix A for another set of values.

Increased Ammonia Level

Clinical Significance. Increased ammonia levels, which occur in liver dysfunction, may be due either to blood not circulating through the liver well or to actual hepatic failure. For example, in Reye's syndrome, an increasing ammonia level signifies major liver damage. In terminal cirrhosis, the client has an elevated ammonia level. Cirrhotic clients who have portal-caval shunts done to relieve portal hypertension may have increased ammonia levels after surgery because blood is shunted away from the liver.

POSSIBLE NURSING DIAGNOSES RELATED TO INCREASED AMMONIA LEVELS

Potential for Injury Related to Sensory-Perceptual Alterations

Although high levels of ammonia occur in hepatic coma (hepatic encephalopathy), the ammonia may not be what actually causes the neurological symptoms. Most likely, many toxins in hepatic failure cause the symptoms of disorientation and tremors seen in hepatic encephalopathy. The client should be checked for a certain kind of tremor of the hand called liver flap or *asterixis* (which can also be caused by high levels of uremia or other central nervous system toxins). Ask the client to extend his or her arms out in front of the body, spread the fingers, and hold the hands in a dorsiflexed position. Clients who have a high level of ammonia in their blood and who are developing hepatic encephalopathy cannot hold their palms up in a steady manner. The hands will flap. Asking the client to write his or her name or to draw a star are other ways to assess the neurological dysfunction. The nurse may often be the first one to notice subtle changes in the client's ability to perform simple tasks that require coordination and mental alertness. The lack of mental alertness and coordination may progress to a coma unless treatment is begun. Budd & Rothwell (1983) note that in children with Reye's syndrome there are five stages of neurological involvement. Early detection of changes in level of consciousness is crucial.

Alterations in Nutritional Requirements Related to Need to Reduce All Sources of Ammonia from Protein Breakdown

Because a rising serum ammonia level indicates an inability of the liver to handle the breakdown of protein, the client should have limited protein intake until the ammonia level returns to normal. Hepatic-Aid, an enteral amino acid formula, may be used but the overall improvement in neurological function is questionable (Lieber, 1983). If the patient in hepatic failure has a gastrointestinal bleed, this makes the progression to hepatic coma faster because ammonia is produced when the blood proteins in the intestine are broken down. Enemas and gastric lavage may be needed to get as much of the blood out of the gastrointestinal tract as possible. Because intestinal bacteria produce ammonia by breaking down protein, the amount of bacteria may also be reduced by giving neomycin, a nonsystemic antibiotic, which may be given orally or by enemas.

Resuming Protein Intake. When the ammonia level returns to normal, protein is cautiously put back into the diet in increasing amounts. The diet may be limited to only 20 g of protein/day for awhile. (See Table 10–2 for a list of the protein content of foods.) As the protein level in the diet is increased, the nurse must watch carefully for any signs of hepatic encephalopathy. Serum ammonia levels are useful in evaluating the ability of the liver to once again handle protein. Lactulose, an ammonia detoxicant, may be given orally or rectally to help reduce ammonia levels. Oral lactulose may be continued for a long time (Govoni & Hayes, 1985).

Potential for Injury Related to Use of Sedatives and Diuretics

In addition to the amount of protein in the diet, other factors that contribute to the development of hepatic coma include hypokalemia and the use of sedatives and narcotics. The body is less able to handle ammonia when the potassium level is low or when alkalosis is present. Thus diuretic therapy (which often causes potassium loss) may be contraindicated when the client has an increased ammonia level. In addition, the failing liver is unable to detoxify many drugs, including sedatives and narcotics. When a client has a rising ammonia level, all previous drug orders need to be reevaluated to see if they are still appropriate in respect to the change in the client's condition.

■ ALPHA-FETOPROTEIN (AFP)

Normally this globulin, formed only in the yolk sac and liver of the fetus, disappears from the bloodstream after birth, except for trace amounts, which may be detected by radioimmunoassay (RIA). (See Chapter 15 for a description of RIA.) The test for alpha-fetoprotein is done on amniotic fluid to detect certain congenital defects (see Chapter 28) as well as in the serum of pregnant women and other adults to detect a specific pathology.

The serum alpha-fetoprotein has the distinction of being the first maternal serum test to screen for a genetic defect in the fetus. In the fetus, if the neural tube fails to close properly, enormous amounts of fetal protein leak out into the amniotic fluid all during the pregnancy. In the pregnant woman, levels above the usual reference values for a particular gestational age may indicate a neural tube defect in the fetus. (See Chapter 18 for a detailed discussion of this test.) The alpha-fetoprotein level is also usually increased in the serum of the mother when the infant has died in utero (Hytten & Lind, 1975).

In the nonpregnant adult, a markedly increased alpha-fetoprotein level is associated with primary carcinoma (hepatoma) of the liver and certain types of testicular cancer (Ostchega & Culnane, 1985). Metastatic cancer to the liver does not cause such a rise. Very small amounts are present in some nonmalignant liver diseases in children and adults. The appearance of a fetal protein in an adult malignancy gives support to the theory that cancer somehow arises from very primitive cells. Other fetal proteins may also be present in some types of malignancies. As a group, these antigens are called oncofetal antigens (OFA). See the CEA test discussed next.

Preparation of Client and Collection of Sample

There is no special preparation of the client for a serum sample. The laboratory needs 2 ml of clotted blood.

Reference Values for AFP

Fetal	200–400 mg/dl
After infancy (1 year)	Less than 30 ng/ml (Tietz, 1983)
Pregnancy	Serum levels increase during pregnancy to levels of 2.1–16.5 μg/dl (See Chapter 18)

■ CARCINOEMBRYONIC ANTIGEN (CEA)

CEA, a glycoprotein that circulates at high level during fetal life, is detectable in only tiny amounts in the blood of healthy adults. CEA is elevated in certain types of malignancies, such as colon cancer and metastatic breast disease, and thus is useful as a tumor marker. About 70% of clients with colon cancer have elevated CEA levels (Tietz, 1983). (See the above discussion on alpha-fetoprotein as another example of a fetal protein used as a tumor marker.) Although CEA may be used as part of a diagnostic work-up for cancer of the colon, the CEA is most useful as a marker to determine the effectiveness of treatment. For example, CEA levels usually return to normal about 6 weeks after a colon malignancy is surgically removed (Ostchega & Culnane, 1985). If the CEA begins to rise after treatment, this is an indication of a return of the malignancy. CEA is helpful but not conclusive, and thus of little value, in a diagnostic work-up for cancer of the colon because: (1) not all people with cancer of the colon show elevated CEA levels and (2) several conditions other than colon cancer may cause elevated CEA levels (Fletcher, 1986). Some other conditions causing elevated CEA levels are heavy cigarette smoking, cirrhosis, ulcerative colitis, diverticulitis, rectal polyps, peptic ulcer disease, pancreatitis, and many malignancies (National Institutes of Health, 1981).

Preparation of Client and Collection of Sample
Venous blood is collected without an additive. A large amount is needed (20 ml). The specimen must be sent on ice (See Appendix A, Table 5).

Reference Values for CEA

0–2.5 ng/ml

Note: Smokers may have values as high as 5.0 ng/ml or even higher (Tietz, 1983).

POSSIBLE NURSING DIAGNOSES RELATED TO ELEVATION OF CEA OR AFP

Potential for Ineffective Coping Related to Severity of Malignancy and Possible Need for More Treatments
As noted above, both the CEA and AFP are tumor markers, so persistent or rising levels indicate that the tumor is still active and prognosis is thus less favorable. Additional treatments may be needed and the client and family may need

help in coping with the less than favorable news from the physician. Fletcher (1986) notes that the value of the test depends on whether information about a bad prognosis is used humanely.

QUESTIONS

1. Protein electrophoresis is a more useful test than the albumin/globulin ratio for the measurement of serum proteins because electrophoresis does what?

   a. Identifies specific proteins other than albumin and globulin
   b. Reports the percentages of both albumin and the five globulins
   c. Measures two types of albumin as well as the various types of globulins
   d. Requires less sophisticated technical equipment

2. The only clinical condition that creates an elevated serum albumin level is which of the following?

   a. Early liver dysfunction   **c.** Dehydration
   b. Increased protein intake over a   **d.** Kwashiorkor
        long period

3. A lowered serum albumin level (hypoalbuminemia) is likely to be a clinical problem for all these clients *except* which?

   a. Mrs. Lehman, who is in her last trimester of pregnancy and has been admitted for preeclampsia
   b. Tommy, age 6, who has severe nephrosis
   c. Mr. Buber, who has advanced cirrhosis
   d. Shirley, age 17, who has been on a very restricted diet (only juices) for the past 8 days

4. The major clinical manifestation of the client with a lowered serum albumin level is which of the following?

   a. Decreased susceptibility to   **c.** Loss of weight
        infection
   b. Edema   **d.** Tendency to bleed

5. Mr. Buber is receiving a 25% solution of albumin intravenously because his serum albumin level was 2 g/100ml. Which of the following nursing actions is *inappropriate?*

   a. Run the solution no faster than 1 ml a minute
   b. Observe the client frequently for possible circulatory overload
   c. Tell Mr. Buber he will probably have increased urination over the next several hours
   d. Keep the albumin refrigerated until 30 minutes before it is hung

6. For the client who can tolerate oral feedings, the most efficient and economical way to increase protein intake is to do which of the following?

   a. Use commercially prepared protein mixtures or powders
   b. Add extra tablespoons of powdered milk to foods and beverages
   c. Increase meat consumption
   d. Reduce carbohydrate intake so the person can eat more protein

7. The major nursing diagnosis for the client who is deficient in alpha-1-antitrypsin is which of the following?

   a. Potential for ineffective airway clearance related to repeated upper respiratory infections
   b. Knowledge deficit related to needed dietary changes
   c. Alteration in cardiac output related to fluid volume excess
   d. Impairment of skin integrity related to edema

8. Which of these clients is the *least* likely to have low levels of immunoglobulins?

   a. Baby Federini, a premature infant born yesterday
   b. Mrs. Patch, who is a month pregnant and diabetic
   c. Mr. Regoni, who is on corticosteroid therapy and is malnourished
   d. Mrs. Adams, who is 85 years old and has been admitted for a malignancy

9. The single most important nursing diagnosis in caring for any client with an abnormal gamma globulin pattern is which of the following?

   a. Fluid volume deficit
   b. Fluid volume excess
   c. High risk for infection
   d. Impairment of skin integrity

10. Which immunoglobulin crosses the placenta and provides immunity for the newborn for several months?

    a. IgG   b. IgA   c. IgM   d. IgD

11. The radioallergosorbent test (RAST) is useful to do which of the following?

    a. Measure all the various types of immunoglobulins in the serum
    b. Distinguish between cellular and humoral immunity
    c. Measure the quantity of antigen specific IgE antibodies in the serum that increase in immediate allergic reactions
    d. Discriminate the globulins of high molecular weight (macroglobulin) from other globulins

12. Mr. Buber is a client with cirrhosis who has an ammonia level of over 100 mcg/100 ml. He states he wants "something to eat." Which diet would be appropriate for Mr. Buber this morning?

    a. Eggs, toast, jelly, and coffee
    b. Grapefruit juice, cereal, and a glass of milk
    c. Orange juice and sliced banana
    d. Pancakes, syrup, butter, and coffee

13. In a nonpregnant state, what might the continuing presence of large amounts of alpha-fetoprotein in the serum indicate?

a. Infertility   **c.** Congenital enzymatic defect

b. Lack of adult proteins   **d.** Active malignancy

REFERENCES

Arguembourg, P. (1975). *Immunoelectrophoresis* (2nd ed.). Basel, Switzerland: S. Karger.

Breneman, J. (1979). Food allergy. *Contemporary Nutrition, 4*(3), 1–2.

Budd, R., & Rothwell, R. (1983). Spotting Reye's syndrome while there's still time. *RN, 46*(12), 39–42.

Cawley, L., et al. (1978). *Electrophoresis and immunochemical reactions in gels* (2nd ed.). American Society of Clinical Pathologists, Chicago: Educational Products Division.

Cerrato, P. (1986). How diet helps the skin fight pressure sores. *RN, 49*(1), 67–68.

Dharan, M. (1976). Immunoglobulin abnormalities. *AJN, 76*(10), 1626–1628.

Donley D. (1976). Nursing the patient who is immunosuppressed. *AJN, 76*(10), 1619–1625.

Fletcher, R. (1986). Diagnostic decision: Carcinoembryonic antigen. *Annals of Internal Medicine, 104*(1), 66–73.

Govoni, L., & Hayes, J. (1985). *Drugs and nursing implications* (5th ed.). Norwalk, CT: Appleton-Century-Crofts.

Hamburger, H. (1978). Diagnostic usefulness of specific IgE antibody measurements. *Mayo Clinic Proceedings, 53,* 459–462.

Heagarty, M., et al. (1980). *Child health: Basics for primary care.* Norwalk, CT: Appleton-Century-Crofts.

Hytten, F., & Lind, T. (1975). *Diagnostic indices in pregnancy.* Summit, NJ: Ciba-Geigy Corp.

Jacobs, D., Kaston, B., DeMott, W., & Wolfson, W. (1984). *Laboratory test handbook with DRG index.* St. Louis: Mosby/Lexi.

Kyle, R., & Greipp, P. (1978). Laboratory investigation of monocloncal gammopathics. *Mayo Clinic Proceedings, 53*(10), 719–739.

Lieber, C. (1983). Alcohol–nutrition interaction. *Contemporary Nutrition, 8*(12), 1–2.

National Institute of Health Consensus Statement (1981). CEA as a cancer marker. *Consensus Development Conference Summary, 3*(7).

Ostchega, Y., & Culnane, M. (1985). Tumor markers. *Nursing 85, 15*(9), 49–51.

Palombo, J., & Blackburn, G. (1980). Human protein requirements. *Contemporary Nutrition, 5*(1), 1–2.

Rossmann, M., et al. (1977). Pheresis therapy: Patient care. *AJN, 77*(7), 1135–1141.

Scully, R. (Ed.). (1986). Normal reference laboratory values. *NEJM, 314*(1), 41, 49.

Tietz, N. (Ed.). (1983). *Clinical guide to laboratory tests.* Philadelphia: Saunders.

Tullis, J. (1977). Albumin. *JAMA, 237*(1), 355–360.

Voignier, R., & Bridgewater, S. (1978). Allergies in children: Testing, treating and teaching. *AJN 78*(4), 617–621.

11

Tests to Measure the Metabolism of Bilirubin

- Total Bilirubin (van den Bergh Reaction)
- Indirect Bilirubin
- Direct Bilirubin
- Urine Bilirubin
- Urine Urobilinogen
- Fecal Urobilinogen
- Bilirubin in Amniotic Fluid

OBJECTIVES

1. Diagram the normal pathway for bilirubin excretion and explain the five laboratory tests used as assessment tools.
2. Distinguish between prehepatic, intrahepatic, and post-hepatic jaundice in regards to etiologies, symptoms, and changes in laboratory values.
3. Compare and contrast the nursing diagnoses appropriate for increased indirect and/or direct serum bilirubin levels in the infant and the adult.
4. Describe the role of the nurse in assisting with medical interventions for newborns with markedly elevated serum indirect bilirubins.
5. Describe the nurse's role in assisting with medical interventions for clients with elevated serum direct bilirubin.
6. Discuss the psychological impact of jaundice on the client and on significant others.
7. Explain the clinical significance of measuring the bilirubin content in amniotic fluid.

This chapter begins with a discussion about the normal pathway of bilirubin excretion and differences between the two types of bilirubin, conjugated and unconjugated. The clinical symptom of any elevated bilirubin is jaundice, but the nursing implications are somewhat different depending on whether the jaundice is prehepatic, posthepatic, or hepatic in origin. The chapter ends with a discussion about general nursing diagnoses for any patient with an elevated bilirubin (jaundice), along with some more specific implications depending on the origin of the jaundice. Understanding the various laboratory tests is the first step in understanding which pathophysiological process is creating the jaundice.

PATHWAY OF NORMAL BILIRUBIN EXCRETION

Bilirubin is a normal component of red blood cells (erythrocytes). When the reticuloendothelial system breaks down old or nonuseful red blood cells, bilirubin is one of the waste products. This "free" bilirubin, which is not water-soluble, is a lipid-soluble waste product that needs to be made water-soluble to be excreted. So it is carried by albumin to the liver, where it is conjugated by the liver and made water-soluble. Only water-soluble conjugated bilirubin can be excreted in the urine.

The liver handles bilirubin in a similar way to other poorly water-soluble compounds such as steroids, drugs, and toxins (Schmid, 1972). In general, such substances are carried by the plasma proteins (see Chapter 10) to the liver, where they are detached from the protein and made less toxic by conversion to a form that can be excreted.

An enzyme, glucuronyl transferase, is necessary for the transformation, or conjugation, of bilirubin. Either a lack of glucuronyl transferase or the presence of drugs that interfere with this enzyme renders the liver unable to conjugate bilirubin.

Urine, however, is not the major pathway of excretion for conjugated bilirubin, almost all of which is excreted as one of the components of bile salts. In fact, bilirubin, a vivid pigment, gives bile the characteristic bright greenish-yellow color. When the bile salts reach the intestine via the common bile duct, the bilirubin is acted upon by bacteria to form chemical compounds called *urobilinogens*. Technically, the breakdown of conjugated bilirubin in the intestine creates several other compounds, but the end product that is measured in both urine and feces is labeled as urobilinogen. These breakdown products give feces their dark color; hence an absence of bilirubin in the intestine causes clay-colored stools. Most of the urobilinogen is excreted in the feces, while some is reabsorbed and goes through the liver again and still another small amount is excreted in the urine. Thus tests for fecal and urine urobilinogens can detect abnormalities in bilirubin excretion.

Because the bilirubin is chemically different after it goes through the conjugation process in the liver, laboratory tests of the serum can differentiate between the bilirubin that is free (prehepatic) and the bilirubin that is conjugated (posthepatic). The laboratory therefore reports the test results either as total bilirubin or as "direct" or "indirect" bilirubin, terms that refer to the way the two types react to certain dyes (sometimes referred to as the Van den Bergh reaction):

1. The conjugated water-soluble (posthepatic) bilirubin reacts *directly* when dyes are added to the blood specimen.
2. The non-water-soluble, free (prehepatic) bilirubin does not react to the reagents used for the test until alcohol is added to the solution; hence their measurement is *indirect*.

The exact technical procedure for the test is not of major concern for nurses. They should know, however, enough about how the tests are done so that the words "direct" and "indirect" make some sense when laboratory reports are being interpreted. A newer method of bilirubin measurement can also measure fractions of the conjugated bilirubin and the results are listed as *BU* for unconjugated bilirubin and *BC* for conjugated bilirubin. To understand the clinical significance of changes in one or both types, nurses must clearly understand the origin and route for each type of bilirubin. Table 11–1 can be used as a quick summary of how each of the bilirubin tests is related to the normal pathway of bilirubin excretion. Table 11–2 summarizes how each of the five tests of bilirubin is changed in the three types of jaundice (prehepatic, intrahepatic, and posthepatic).

■ TOTAL BILIRUBIN (VAN DEN BERGH REACTION)

Preparation of Client and Collection of Sample

Most laboratories require the client to fast for 8 hours before the test because a large intake of fat interferes with the chemical testing. The test requires 1 ml of serum. The specimen should be protected from bright light because bilirubin is broken down by exposure to sunlight or to high-intensity artificial light. The test should not be done for 24 hours after a dye has been used for x-ray studies. For neonatal use, blood is drawn from a heel stick using a capillary pipette (see Chapter 1). This "micro" bilirubin only measures totals and is appropriate for the first 10 days of life (Jacobs et al., 1984).

TABLE 11–1. RELATIONSHIP OF NORMAL BILIRUBIN EXCRETION TO THE FIVE TESTS USED TO MEASURE BILIRUBIN METABOLISM

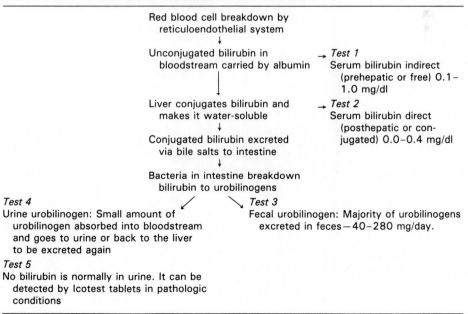

Red blood cell breakdown by
reticuloendothelial system
↓
Unconjugated bilirubin in → *Test 1*
bloodstream carried by albumin   Serum bilirubin indirect
(prehepatic or free) 0.1–
1.0 mg/dl
↓
Liver conjugates bilirubin and → *Test 2*
makes it water-soluble   Serum bilirubin direct
(posthepatic or con-
jugated) 0.0–0.4 mg/dl
↓
Conjugated bilirubin excreted
via bile salts to intestine
↓
Bacteria in intestine breakdown
bilirubin to urobilinogens

Test 4   *Test 3*
Urine urobilinogen: Small amount of   Fecal urobilinogen: Majority of urobilinogens
  urobilinogen absorbed into bloodstream   excreted in feces—40–280 mg/day.
  and goes to urine or back to the liver
  to be excreted again

Test 5
No bilirubin is normally in urine. It can be
  detected by Icotest tablets in pathologic
  conditions

TABLE 11-2. CHANGES IN SERUM, URINE, AND FECES IN THREE TYPES OF JAUNDICE

	Indirect Serum Bilirubin	Direct Serum Bilirubin	Urine Bilirubin	Urine Urobilinogen	Fecal Urobilinogen
Reference values	Average 0.5 mg/dl	Average 0.1 mg/dl	None	0.4–1 mg/day	40–280 mg/day
Prehepatic jaundice (hemolytic)	Elevated usually not more than 5 mg in adults. May be above 20 mg in newborns	Normal	None	Up to 10 mg	Up to 1,400 mg
Hepatic jaundice	Elevated—may be 15 to 20 mg in severe liver failure	Elevations depend on amount of stasis of bile	Elevated if obstruction present	Normal or increased (see text)	Normal or little decreased (see text)
Posthepatic jaundice (obstruction)	Normal in beginning	Elevated—may be 30 to 40 mg if obstruction complete	Elevated—urine dark orange and foams	Slight decrease or normal	Absent—clay-colored stools

Wallach (1986) gives more details on differential diagnosis of various liver diseases.

Reference Values for Serum Bilirubin

Most laboratories report only the figures for the total and the direct. The indirect is calculated by subtracting the direct from the total.

Adult and children past
  newborn stage

Indirect bilirubin	0.1–1.0 mg/dl Mean 0.5 mg	This is the prehepatic, free, or unconjugated bilirubin
Direct bilirubin	0.0–0.4 mg/dl Mean 0.1 mg	Posthepatic, conjugated bilirubin (water-soluble)
Total bilirubin	0.1–1.0 mg/dl	Includes both types of bilirubin
Newborn		See text for explanation of physiological jaundice in newborns. Examples used here, from Tietz (1983), reflect *total* bilirubins. Check with individual laboratory for newer methods using a layered technology for neonatal bilirubin
Term infant	First 24 hr Up to 48 hr 3–5 days	2–6 mg 6–7 mg 4–12 mg
Premature infant	First 24 hr Up to 48 hr 3–5 days	1–6 mg 6–8 mg 10–15 mg
Pregnancy		Bilirubin levels usually remain in normal ranges, but several studies have shown that about 15% of normal pregnancies may have total bilirubins as high as 10 mg (Hytten & Lind, 1975; p. 16)

■ INDIRECT BILIRUBIN

Increased Level (Unconjugated Bilirubinemia)

Clinical Significance. An increase in the indirect portion of bilirubin can be caused in two different ways:

First, the breakdown of red blood cells can increase, thus causing an excess of free bilirubin in the bloodstream. Many conditions cause an increased destruction (hemolysis) of red blood cells:

1. Sickle cell disease
2. Autoimmune diseases
3. Hemorrhage into a body cavity when the red blood cells are broken down
4. Drug toxicity
5. Any physical or physiologic stress (a slight increase)
6. A transfusion reaction caused by incompatible blood (see Chapter 14 on transfusion reactions)
7. RH or ABO incompatibility in an infant

The indirect bilirubin of a newborn with Rh incompatibility (erythroblastosis fetalis) is often above 20 mg. Usually the indirect bilirubin, in an adult, does not go much above 5 mg due to hemolysis. The indirect bilirubin is around 6 mg with sickle cell disease (Wallach, 1986).

Second, the indirect portion of bilirubin can be elevated when the liver's ability to conjugate the free bilirubin that circulates in the bloodstream is decreased. Liver dysfunction causes high elevations of the indirect bilirubin in both adult and newborns. In severe liver disease, the indirect bilirubin may be over 20 mg. Although the most common reason for severe liver dysfunction in the adult is cirrhosis, hepatitis may also make the liver less capable of conjugating bilirubin. As a rare example, some people have a lack of the enzyme glucuronyl transferase (Gilbert's syndrome), which is necessary for the conjugation of bilirubin in the liver. The lack of this specific enzyme results in an increased amount of indirect bilirubin. Drugs, viral diseases, and other toxins may also injure the liver or interfere with enzymatic actions, so that the liver cannot conjugate bilirubin efficiently. About 20% of the hospitalized cases of jaundice in the elderly are related to drug reactions (Mar, 1982).

Jaundice in the Newborn. An increase in the indirect bilirubin is a physiological occurrence in the newborn that is due both to an increased hemolysis and to a slower conjugation by the liver. The infant is born with a large number of fetal red blood cells that have a short life-span. So the hemolysis that occurs after birth is a normal adaptation to the new environment. Yet, since the newborn's liver has inadequate glucuronyl transferase, the liver takes longer to conjugate and to remove bilirubin from the bloodstream. Then the synthesis of the enzyme occurs a few days after birth in a full-term infant and a little longer in a premature. Due to these events, about 50% of newborns have some physiological jaundice that disappears in a few days.

Distinguishing this physiological jaundice from any other kind is important. If the indirect bilirubin rise is elevated the first day, or if it does not begin to drop after three to five days, the jaundice may be pathological rather than physiological. For example, the infant with Rh incompatibility has a high indirect bilirubin immediately after birth. (See Chapter 14 for other tests done for Rh babies.) Lowered serum albumin levels, hypoxia, cold, stress, drugs, and other metabolic factors may also cause abnormal rises in the indirect bilirubin by interfering with the transportation or conjugation of bilirubin. Thaler (1977) explains all the causes for elevations of both indirect (unconjugated) bilirubin and direct (conjugated) bilirubin, as well as how to distinguish these from the physiological jaundice of the newborn.

In a few instances, breast feeding may intensify the physiological jaundice because an enzyme present in some women's milk inhibits the action of glucuronyl transferase. Gartner, one of the original researchers into neonatal jaundice and breastfeeding, does not consider an elevated bilirubin to be significant if the bilirubin is below 20 mg for the first week and if the infant is otherwise healthy (White, 1979). The potential danger of a high level of indirect bilirubin in the newborn is covered in the section on nursing implications of patients with elevated bilirubin levels.

The newborn is particularly susceptible to environmental contaminants because the epidermis is thinner and percutaneous absorption is thus greater. The faster respiratory rate also increases the intake of any environmental contaminant. For example, two epidemics of neonatal hyperbilirubinemia were linked to the use of a phenol disinfectant detergent (Wysowski, 1978). Several infants had very high indirect bilirubins after a new detergent was used to clean bassinets.

■ DIRECT BILIRUBIN

Increased Level (Conjugated Bilirubinemia)

Clinical Significance. Normally the amount of conjugated bilirubin circulating in the bloodstream is very small because the larger portion of this type of bilirubin is excreted via the bile salts into the intestine. Thus a marked increase in the direct bilirubin is an indication of an obstruction in the normal flow of bile. Jaundice due to an elevation in direct bilirubin is called *obstructive jaundice.* The obstruction may be in the collecting channels in the liver, in the hepatic ducts, or in the common bile duct. For example, a gallstone lodged in the common bile duct prevents the normal excretion of bile salts (which contain the conjugated bilirubin) into the intestine. The conjugated bilirubin is thus absorbed into the bloodstream in much larger amounts than normal. In complete biliary obstruction, the direct bilirubin may be as high as 30–40 mg. Another example of an obstruction would be cancer of the head of the pancreas, for which jaundice is often the first symptom. Newborns with a congenital malformation in the biliary tree (biliary atresia) also have high direct bilirubins.

Sometimes the direct bilirubin may be elevated even though biliary obstruction is not apparent. Certain drugs, notably contraceptive steroids and some of the phenothiazines such as chlorpromazine (Thorazine), may cause a stasis of bile in the liver (intrahepatic cholestasis). The bile tends to be viscous, and the small bile ducts in the liver become dilated. The direct bilirubin is elevated due to this partial obstruction to the normal outflow of bile. A similar condition of stasis occurs in what is called the "benign jaundice" of pregnancy. The rise in bilirubin is an occasional occurrence in pregnancy, and the bilirubin returns to normal after delivery (Seymour & Chadwick, 1979). Inflammation of the liver, as in hepatitis, or scarring, as in cirrhosis, may also cause partial obstruction to the flow of bile out of the liver and thereby cause an elevation of the direct bilirubin.

Combination of Direct and Indirect Elevations

Although the previous discussion has attempted to make a clear distinction between elevations of direct and of indirect bilirubin, clinical situations often entail elevations of both (Wallach, 1986). Any clinical condition, any drug, or any toxic condition that causes obstruction to the flow of bile may eventually cause some increase in the indirect bilirubin too, because the stasis of bile in the collecting ducts eventually impairs the normal functioning of the liver. Intrahepatic disease, such as cirrhosis or hepatitis, and drug toxicity may cause elevations in both the direct and indirect bilirubins. Urine bilirubin, urine urobilinogen, and, less frequently, fecal urobilinogen tests may give additional information about the nature of the jaundice. Table 11-2 summarizes the usual findings in jaundice that is prehepatic (hemolytic), intrahepatic (liver dysfunction), or posthepatic (obstruction).

For clinical jaundice, tests other than those for bilirubin and urobilinogen may also be needed. For example, alkaline phosphatase, GTT, 5'N, and LAP are enzymes normally excreted in the bile and are elevated in biliary obstruction. The transaminases are also elevated in most types of liver disease. (See Chapter 12 on using these enzymes in detecting liver and biliary disease.) For cholestatic jaundice, ultrasound (Chapter 23) or oral cholecystograms (Chapter 20) may detect gallstones. Transhepatic cholangiograms (Chapter 20) and endoscopic cholangiography (Chapter 27) are two other diagnostic approaches to obstructive jaundice (Scharschmidt et al., 1983).

■ URINE BILIRUBIN

Because only the water-soluble conjugated (direct) bilirubin can cross the glomerular filter, it is the only type of bilirubin even found in the urine. Normally even this type of bilirubin is not in the urine in detectable amounts because it has been converted to urobilinogen in the intestine. Bilirubin becomes apparent in the urine when there is an obstruction to the normal pathway of conjugated bilirubin. This test is therefore used to detect obstructive jaundice, and it is sometimes said incorrectly to be a test for "bile" in the urine. Because the test is likely to be positive for bilirubin before the person has signs of clinical hepatitis, it may be a screening procedure done on populations that were known to be exposed to hepatitis. It may also be useful to screen out potential blood donors, food handlers, and the like when controlling the spread of subclinical cases of hepatitis is imperative.

Preparation of Client and Collection of Sample

A few millileters of freshly voided urine are needed. The urine must be fresh because oxidation affects the results, and exposure to strong lights also changes the chemical composition of the bilirubin.

Sometimes the nurse or client may test urine for bilirubin by using either a tablet or a dipstick. For the Icotest (Ames Products), 5 drops of urine are placed on a special test mat. A tablet is then placed on the mat and 2 drops of water are added. If the mat turns blue or purple within 30 seconds, the test is positive for bilirubin. With the dipstick method, the positive reaction is a tan-to-purple color. The dipstick method is 2–4 times less sensitive than the tablet method (Ames Product Information, 1986). Drugs that change the color of the urine may mask the color change on the tablet or strip of paper. (See Chapter 3 for a list of drugs that cause color changes in urine, as well as for a dipstick method to check for ascorbic acid, as this may interfere with the bilirubin tests.)

Reference Values for Urine Bilirubin

| All groups | Normally bilirubin is present in such small quantities in the urine that it is not detected by routine screening procedures |

POSSIBLE NURSING DIAGNOSIS RELATED TO BILIRUBIN IN THE URINE (BILIRUBINEMIA)

Alteration in Elimination Patterns Related to Beginning of Obstructive Jaundice

Bilirubin makes urine a dark-orange color, and it also makes urine foam when it is shaken (shake test). Urine does not foam or become dark if it contains only urobilinogen. Because the nurse or client may be the first to notice that the urine color is abnormal, the color of urine and stools should always be a priority assessment when an obstruction of the common bile duct is suspected. (The stools will become clay-colored when complete obstruction occurs.)

■ URINE UROBILINOGEN

Urobilinogen is formed in the intestine from the conjugated bilirubin normally present in bile salts. Most of the urobilinogen is excreted in the feces, but a small amount that finds its way into the bloodstream either goes through the liver again or is excreted in the urine. This test may be used to detect hemolytic jaundice or early liver dysfunction.

An increase in urine urobilinogen follows an increased breakdown of red blood cells, with the increase in fecal urobilinogen even more pronounced than that in urinary urobilinogen. Because some of the urobilinogen that is in the feces is picked up by the portal circulation and carried to the liver again, and because urinary urobilinogen excretion is increased when the liver cannot excrete the recycled urobilinogen, urinary urobilinogen can also be used to detect early liver dysfunction. The inability of the liver to handle urobilinogen occurs before bilirubin excretion is affected (Lewis, 1985).

In obstructive jaundice, the lack of bilirubin excreted into the intestine causes a decrease in the amount of urobilinogen in the urine, which is not important to measure as it is very small even in normal health. The amount of urinary urobilinogen also decreases when there is a lack of intestinal flora to convert bilirubin to urobilinogen; this effect, however, is more of academic interest than of clinical usefulness.

Preparation of Client and Collection of Sample

If a 24-hour specimen is needed, a preservative must be used. (See Chapter 3 for tips on 24-hour urine collection.) The more common procedure is to collect a 2-hour urine sample in the afternoon, because the excretion of urobilinogen is at a maximum from mid-afternoon to evening when food is being digested. The urine should be taken to the laboratory immediately after collection. Strongly acid urine may make the results inaccurate; so if a client is on drugs, such as high doses of salicylates, note this fact on the laboratory slip. Drugs that color the urine also interfere with the test. Laboratories may report in milligrams or in units.

The nurse can also check for urobilinogen by using a dipstick, which shows 0.1–1 Ehrlich units as normal. For amounts from 2 to over 12 Ehrlich units, the color goes from dark yellow to orange when read after 45 seconds (Ames Product Information, 1986).

Reference Values for Urine Urobilinogen

All groups　0.3–1.0 Ehrlich units in a 2-hr sample (1–3 P.M.)

　　　　　　0.5–4.0 Ehrlich units in a 24-hr sample (ask laboratory about preservative)

　　　　　　0.4–1 mg a day. Note specific color chart if doing by dipstick method

---

■ FECAL UROBILINOGEN

The amount of urobilinogen in the feces depends on the amount of conjugated bilirubin that is excreted via the bile salts into the intestine. Since urobilinogen is the end product of conjugated bilirubin, a lack of bacteria to break down the bilirubin may reduce the urobilinogen in the intestine, and thus the feces become lighter in color. The test for fecal urobilinogen is not often done because urine and serum tests may give enough information about the cause of the impaired bilirubin excretion.

The fecal urobilinogen is significantly increased when there is an increased breakdown of red blood cells (hemolytic jaundice) because much more bilirubin is conjugated by the liver and excreted into the intestine. A lack of fecal urobilinogen occurs in obstructive jaundice because the conjugated bilirubin cannot be excreted into the intestine. A lack of conjugated bilirubin in the intestine is apparent to the eye because the feces are clay-colored. In the infant, this condition may not be apparent because the stools are normally light-colored.

Preparation of Client and Collection of Sample
The laboratory gives specific instructions if a specimen of feces is to be saved for 24 hours or for several days. Usually clients can collect the specimen if they are given the correct container. Having clients do so is desirable both to avoid their embarrassment and to protect the nurse from possible contamination in transferring feces (see Chapter 14 on hepatitis precautions). Special waxed containers are used for stool collections.

Reference Values for Fecal Urobilinogen

75–350 mg/100 g of stool
40–280 mg in a 24-hr period

POSSIBLE NURSING DIAGNOSES RELATED TO HYPERBILIRUBINEMIA

Knowledge Deficit Related to Clinical Signs of Jaundice
Although the serum tests are used to monitor the exact level of the bilirubin from day to day, the nurse should also record color changes on a daily basis. Because clients may be the best judges of day-to-day changes in their own skin color, this source of data should never be overlooked and clients should be instructed on what changes are important to note. An excess of serum bilirubin, either the direct or indirect type, gives a yellowish coloration to the sclera of the eyes, skin, and mucous membranes. The symptoms of jaundice begin to appear when the total bilirubin is around 2–4 mg in the adult or older child. In the infant, jaundice may not be apparent until the total bilirubin is around 5–7 mg (Heagerty, 1980). Often the yellow color is noted first in the sclera of fair-skinned people. In dark-skinned people, the inner canthus of the eye may show more change. In dark-skinned or Oriental people, the yellowish tinge also becomes apparent in the mucous membranes of the hard palate (Roach, 1977). Blanching the skin of newborns by pressing on the sternum makes the jaundice of the skin more apparent. With proper lighting, one can see jaundice in the abdomen nearly as easily as in the sclera. Observations for jaundice should be done in natural daylight, if possible.

In a community health setting or clinic, the nurse may be the first one to notice the beginning of jaundice. In high-risk populations composed of abusers of alcohol or other drugs, inspections of the eyes and skins would be especially important to detect liver damage.

Differences in Indirect and Direct Bilirubin. Nurses must also know whether the direct or indirect bulirubin is elevated because the nursing implications vary for each type of elevation. Some of the implications, such as changes in body image or ways to assess for jaundice, are the same for both types. However, the potential danger to the central nervous system, itching, discomfort, and bleeding are problems associated more with one type than the other.

Anxiety of Parents Related to Potential for Central Nervous System Damage in the Newborn

In older children and adults, an increase in the indirect (unconjugated) bilirubin is not in itself dangerous or uncomfortable for the client. After infancy, a blood-brain barrier prevents the indirect bilirubin from affecting the central nervous system. (Very rarely, an extremely high indirect bilirubin in an adult may affect the brain.) High indirect bilirubins in newborns, however, are of grave concern. In infants, indirect bilirubin does leak through the vascular walls and can damage the central nervous system. *Kernicterus* (kern = kernel + icterus = yellow) is the term used to describe the central nervous system damage that results from high indirect bilirubins (usually over 20 mg) in newborns.

No one figure—such as ''over 20 mg''—defines the upper limits of indirect bilirubin that necessitate interventions in the newborn. The physician must consider many factors, such as whether the bilirubin level is rising rapidly or not falling after the first few days. In an individual case, the physician may determine that the bilirubin should not be more than 15 or 18 mg.

New parents, on the other hand, usually need a figure to hold on to so that they can make sense of the laboratory report that is given. A mother may be anxiously awaiting the laboratory report of the bilirubin each day because the bilirubin that exceeds the limit for the newborn may mean that the baby will have to stay in the hospital a few days longer. This news can be devastating to the new parents. Nurses may be able to alleviate some anxiety by a brief explanation about how elevated bilirubins are usually treated in their hospital. The mother and father may prefer not to see the heel sticks done to obtain blood.

Potential for Injury Related to Treatments to Decrease the Indirect Bilirubin in Newborns

Three different methods are used in the newborn to reduce indirect bilirubin:

Exchange Transfusions. These are used primarily for severe cases of blood type incompatibility. (See Chapter 14 for safety needs with transfusions.)

Phototherapy. High-intensity light is used to help break down the indirect bilirubin to a nontoxic substance. Phototheraphy converts bilirubin to derivatives that apparently can be excreted in the bile and urine without being conjugated by the liver. It is important that the baby's eyes be protected under the lights, because the lights can damage the eyes. It is also crucial to monitor the temperature to prevent hypo- or hyperthermia. Extra fluids need to be given to prevent dehydration. The skin becomes lighter in the areas under the light. Evidently, turning the baby so that no areas are shaded is not important because the rapidity of the bilirubin level drop is due to the dose of light, not to the amount of skin illuminated (Tan, 1975).

Because the indirect bilirubin itself is not of danger to the older child or adult, little effort is made to decrease the level itself. Theoretically, sitting in the sun would be beneficial to the child or adult who has a high indirect bilirubin, but it is more important to correct the pathophysiologic process causing the elevation.

Drugs. Another method of treating high levels of indirect bilirubin is the use of drugs. Phenobarbital is given to help promote the hepatic clearance of bilirubin, and it may be given to the woman during pregnancy as well as to the newborn. If the mother received barbiturate therapy, the newborn may have withdrawal symptoms 1 to 14 days after birth (Govoni & Hayes, 1985, p. 987).

Alteration in Comfort Related to Pruritus

It is presumed that the severe itching (pruritus) that often accompanies an elevated direct (conjugated) bilirubin is due to something toxic in the "bile salts" deposited in the skin. Keeping the environment cool is useful because perspiring may accentuate the pruritus. Soothing baths and lotions may also give some relief. Aveeno, a colloidal oatmeal bath for irritated skin, contains no soaps or synthetics that can harm the skin. The bath soothes and cleanses naturally because of its unique adsorption action. Oatmeal baths can be used for infants as well as adults who have pruritus. Children may need to be restrained from scratching. Excess bilirubin levels may also irritate connective tissue in the sclera (Taylor, 1983). Clients may have photophobia and thus a need to avoid bright lights.

Although there is no direct evidence that the pruritus is directly attributed to bile salts, the use of medication that binds the bile salts may relieve the itching. Cholestyramine, (Questran) is a resin that is taken orally to bind bile salts in the intenstine so that there is a larger increase in the feces (Govoni & Hayes, 1985). This treatment may be helpful when the obstruction is not complete. To prevent constipation, the person taking cholestyramine needs a large intake of fluids and a diet high in roughage. Because the drug may bind up other drugs, it should be given at least one hour before or four hours after other drugs. Supplements of fat-soluble vitamins may be needed if the client is on long-term therapy with the drug. (Cholestyramine is also used as a drug to lower cholesterol levels. See Chapter 9.)

Potential for Injury Related to Bleeding Due to Hypoprothrombinemia

For fats and fat-soluble vitamins to be emulsified and absorbed from the intestine, there must be adequate bile salts. For this reason, a client with an elevated direct bilirubin may develop a tendency to bleed. Without bile salts, fat-soluble vitamins, including vitamin K, are not absorbed from the small intestine. If vitamin K is not absorbed into the bloodstream, the liver cannot make enough prothrombin and other factors needed for normal blood clotting. Clients with obstructive jaundice thus often have increased prothrombin times. Clients with elevated prothrombin times due to obstructive jaundice are given parenteral injections of vitamin K. Parenteral vitamin K can reach the liver because the bile salts were not needed to get the vitamin from the intestine into the bloodstream. Specific actions on how to prevent bleeding when the client has an increased prothrombin time are covered in Chapter 13 on clotting tests.

Potential for Pain Related to Certain Types of Obstructive Jaundice

Although jaundice due to an elevation of indirect bilirubin is painless, pain, other than that associated with pruritus, may or may not be associated with jaundice due to an elevation of the direct bilirubin. Because obstruction of the biliary tree by a pancreatic tumor may be painless for quite awhile, the first indications of biliary obstruction would be jaundice and a tendency to bleed. On the other hand, jaundice due to a gallstone in the common bile duct tends to cause severe abdominal pain in the right upper outer quadrant. In such a case, the client may need narcotics to relieve the pain. Characteristically, the pain tends to radiate to the right shoulder, and it may be intensified by an attempt to eat fatty foods.

Alteration in Nutritional Needs Related to Inability to Tolerate Fats and Other Nutrients

Clients with an elevated direct bilirubin usually have marked intolerance to fatty foods. Their nutritional status must be carefully assessed so that their caloric needs are met. If indicated, surgery is done to relieve the obstruction. Before surgery, the client may need intravenous feedings to maintain hydration and caloric intake. Fat-soluble vitamins can be added to intravenous fluids. Even with just a partial or clearing obstruction, the client may have little appetite for food, so the nurse must plan meals carefully. (As a general rule, an increase in the indirect bilirubin does not seriously interfere with appetite unless the liver is involved and then anorexia can be profound.)

Hepatitis, which causes cholestasis, is accompanied by anorexia. Even if foods are not desired, the client should be encouraged to drink fruit juices. These provide some calories and help flush out the water-soluble direct bilirubin into the urine. As the client's appetite returns, food is needed to supply adequate calories and protein for liver regeneration. Protein in the diet would be encouraged only if serum ammonia levels are normal (see Chapter 10). Otherwise, hepatic coma can result from too much protein. Fats can be allowed as tolerated.

Alteration in Self-Concept Related to Body Image Changes

A concentration on the physical aspects of care for clients with an elevated bilirubin must not overshadow their psychological needs. Nurses need to be aware that jaundice is a definite change in the body image of the person. Jaundice may be very upsetting not only to clients but to their families as well. Some clients are afraid to look in a mirror, and others may prefer not to have any visitors. If these clients must come to a clinic, they may not want others to stare at them. (In addition, other clients may be afraid that the jaundice is catching.) Soft, subdued lights make the jaundice less apparent while treatments are begun to reduce the bilirubin level.

Clients' reactions, of course, can also be unexpected. A young man was once admitted to the hospital with severe jaundice due to cirrhosis. Blue dye for a lymphogram (Chapter 20) turned the man's sclera and skin from yellow to green. One might jump to the conclusion that the client would not want anyone to see him and that he would be upset by the parade of nursing students, residents, and interns who came to examine the "green man." On the contrary, the client enjoyed all the extra attention from being unique and seemed a little disappointed when his color began to return to normal. So, as with all generalizations about nursing implications, nurses must choose which ones are applicable for a certain client in a certain setting. Nurses should also recognize that a change in body image due to a specific *external* source (such as the dye) may be quite a different experience from the longer-term and less specific *internal source* such as jaundice due to an inoperable tumor.

■ BILIRUBIN IN AMNIOTIC FLUID

It is not known for sure how bilirubin reaches the amniotic fluid; some of it may diffuse across the skin. The bilirubin in the amniotic fluid is the indirect, non-water-soluble type, and cannot be excreted in the urine of the fetus. The bilirubin content of amniotic fluid is often high during early pregnancy, but it should fall progressively after mid-pregnancy. (See Chapter 28 for a discussion on the procedure of amniocentesis.) The importance of measuring the bilirubin content of amniotic fluid is to determine whether the normal downward progession of bilirubin concentration in the last half of pregnancy is continuing. If the bilirubin content is not dropping, or if it begins to rise for the fetus of a Rh negative mother, medical interventions may be necessary to save the fetus. Laboratories may use either light or chemical methods to determine the amount of bilirubin in the amniotic fluid. (See Chapter 14 for Rh antibody titers and the Coombs' test, which are used to determine the need for amniocentesis.)

QUESTIONS

1. When the body is utilizing the normal pathway of bilirubin excretion, which laboratory test will be negative?

   a. Serum bilirubin level (indirect portion)
   b. Fecal urobilinogen
   c. Urine urobilinogen
   d. Urine bilirubin

2. Which of the following terms is *not* a synonym for direct bilirubin?

   a. Conjugated bilirubin   **c.** Posthepatic bilirubin
   b. Water-soluble bilirubin   **d.** Free bilirubin

3. The laboratory slip on Mrs. Fong's chart shows a total bilirubin of 3.0 mg and a direct bilirubin of 0.3 mg. Her indirect bilirubin is which of the following?

   a. Unknown at the present time   **c.** 2.7 mg/dl
   b. 3.3 mg/dl   **d.** 3.9 mg/dl

4. Which of the following assessments is *not* found in a client with an elevated direct bilirubin?

   a. Urine dark and foams when shaken

    b. Clay-colored stools

    c. Urine bilirubin negative

    d. Urine urobilinogen slightly decreased or normal

5. In an infant, clinical jaundice becomes apparent when the total bilirubin level is around which of the following levels?

    a. 2–4 mg/dl   **b.** 5–7 mg/dl   **c.** 7–9 mg/dl   **d.** Over 9 mg/dl

6. In an adult, clinical jaundice becomes apparent when the serum bilirubin (total) is about which of the following levels?

    a. 2–4 mg   **b.** 5–7 mg   **c.** 7–9 mg   **d.** Over 9 mg

7. The indirect part of the serum bilirubin is increased in all these clinical situations *except* which?

    a. Mrs. Rhoades, age 31, who has anemia due to a lack of iron in her diet

    b. Baby Holmes, 2 days old, on breastfeeding and slightly jaundiced

    c. Shirley, age 7, who has been admitted to the pediatric unit in a sickle cell crisis

    d. Mr. Smith, age 42, who has terminal cirrhosis

8. An increase in the direct part of the serum bilirubin would be an expected assessment finding in all these client care situations except which of the following?

    a. Mrs. Fonolini, who has gallstones in the common bile duct

    b. Mr. Petersen, who is undergoing surgery (Whipple procedure) for cancer of the head of the pancreas

    c. Baby Jones, who has a malformation in the biliary tree (biliary atresia)

    d. Reggie, age 7, who had a transfusion reaction due to incompatible blood

9. Key nursing actions for the client with an elevated bilirubin (indirect or direct) would include all *except* which of the following?

    a. Evaluating the effect of jaundice on the body image of the person

    b. Assessing in natural daylight, the color of the sclera, mucous membrane, and skin

    c. Charting the color of both urine and stools

    d. Encouraging foods that are high in fat-soluble vitamins

10. When jaundice is due to a high elevation of the direct bilirubin, rather than of the indirect bilirubin, nursing diagnoses may include all of the following *except* which?

    a. Alteration in comfort due to pruritus

    b. Potential for bleeding related to hypoprothrombinemia

    c. Alteration in nutritional needs related to intolerance for fats

    d. Potential for injury due to central nervous system damage

11. The most common method used to treat high levels of indirect bilirubin in the newborn is:

a. Complete elimination of breast milk to reduce the factors that interfere with glucuronyl transferase in the liver

b. Exchange transfusions to remove toxic products from the bloodstream

c. Phototherapy with high-intensity lights to help break down the bilirubin

d. Drug therapy with phenobarbital to promote the hepatic clearance of bilirubin

12. All of the following therapeutic interventions may be used for the person who has jaundice due to an elevated direct bilirubin *except* which?

a. Vitamin K by injection to return the prothrombin time to normal

b. Cholestyramine (Questran) to bind up bile salts in the intestine

c. Surgical interventions to remove the obstruction

d. Use of phototherapy to break down the bilirubin

REFERENCES

Ames Product Profiles on Icotest. (1986). Elkhart, IN: Ames Division, Miles Laboratories.

Govoni, L., & Hayes, J. (1985). *Drugs and nursing implications* (5th ed.). Norwalk, CT: Appleton-Century-Crofts

Heagarty, M., et al. (1980). *Child health: Basics for primary care.* Norwalk, CT: Appleton-Century-Crofts.

Hytten, F., & Lind, T. (1975). *Diagnostic indices in pregnancy.* Summit, NJ: Ciba-Geigy Corp.

Jacobs, D., Kasten, B., DeMott, W., & Wolfson, W. (1984). *Laboratory test handbook with DRG index.* St. Louis: Mosby/Lexi.

Lewis, S. (1985). What bilirubin tests can tell you. *RN, 48*(3), 85–86.

Mar, D. (1982). Drug-induced hepatotoxicity. *AJN, 82*(1), 123–124.

Roach, L. (1977). Color changes in dark skin. *Nursing 77, 7*(1), 48–51.

Schmid, R. (1972). Bilirubin metabolism in man. *NEJM, 287,* 703–709.

Scharschmidt, R., et al. (1983). Current concepts in diagnostic approach to the patient with cholestatic jaundice. *NEJM, 308,* 1515–1519.

Seymour, C., & Chadwick, V. S. (1979). Liver and gastrointestinal function in pregnancy. *Postgraduate Medical Journal, 55*(5), 343–351.

Tan, K. L. (1975). Comparison of the effectiveness of single direction and double direction phototherapy for neo-natal jaundice. *Pediatrics, 56*(4), 550–553.

Taylor, D. (1983). Jaundice, physiology, signs and symptoms. *Nursing 83, 13*(8), 52–54.

Thaler, M. M. (1977). Jaundice in the newborn: Algorithmic diagnosis of conjugated and unconjugated hyperbilirubinemia. *JAMA, 237,* 58–62.

Tietz, N. (Ed.). (1983). *Clinical guide to laboratory tests.* Philadelphia: Saunders.

Wallach, J. (1986). *Interpretation of diagnostic tests.* Boston: Little, Brown.

White, M. (1979). Information please on jaundice. *LaLeche League News, 21,* 71–72.

Wysowski, D., et al. (1978). Epidemic neo-natal hyperbilirubinemia and use of a phenolic disinfectant detergent. *Pediatrics, 61*(2), 165–170.

12

Tests to Measure Enzyme And Isoenzyme Levels

- Alkaline Phosphatase (ALP)
- Gamma-Glutamyl Transferase (GGT) or Gamma-Glutamyl Transpeptidase (GGTP)
- 5′ Nucleotidase (5′N)
- Leucine Aminopeptidase (LAP)
- Acid Phosphatase or Prostatic Acid Phosphatase (PAP)
- Alanine Aminotransferase (ALT) or Serum Glutamic-Pyruvic Transaminase (SGPT)
- Aspartate Aminotransferase (AST) or Serum Glutamic-Oxaloacetic Transaminase (SGOT)
- Creatine Kinase (CK) or Creatine Phosphokinase (CPK)
- Lactic Dehydrogenase (LDH)
- Serum Aldolase
- Serum Amylase
- Urinary Amylase
- Serum Lipase

OBJECTIVES

1. Identify factors, other than pathological processes, that tend to cause elevations in the majority of the serum enzyme tests.
2. Explain the usual clinical significance of an elevated serum ALP level and compare to the GTT.
3. Explain the primary purpose of the serum acid phosphatase level as an assessment for a malignancy.
4. Describe possible nursing diagnoses when a client has marked elevations of the transaminases, ALT (formerly SGPT), and AST (formerly SGOT).
5. Descriminate between the cardiac enzymes—CK, AST (SGOT), and LDH—

in relation to the onset, peak, and duration of elevation after a myocardial infarction.

6. Explain why isoenzymes of CK and LDH are often more valuable than the measurement of the total amounts of the enzymes.
7. Identify the most important nursing diagnosis for the cardiac client who has unexpected normal levels of cardiac enzymes.
8. Plan an appropriate activity schedule for a client who has an elevated CK level due to a muscular disorder.
9. Explain how serum amylase and lipase and urinary anylase are used as assessment tools for pancreatitis.
10. Identify the nursing diagnoses for clients who have marked elevations of serum amylase and lipase levels.

This chapter covers the most common enzymes measured in the serum. As an additional assesment, only two of the enzymes, amylase and (less likely) LAP are measured in the urine. Almost all cells contain the major enzymes, although some types of tissue contain larger concentrations of particular enzymes. So when tissue cells are damaged, the enzymes leak out into the serum.

Although the enzymes are not tissue-specific, various types of tissue have isoenzymes with different chemical and physical properties. Isoenzymes of a particular enzyme all control the same specific metabolic function even though their molecular forms vary slightly from one to another. The enzyme LDH, for example, which is abundant in most tissues, can be separated into five distinct types of isoenzymes. LDH_1 is abundant in heart tissues, while LDH_5 is abundant in liver tissue. Each of the five LDH isoenzymes is still not organ-specific, however, because the heart or liver may have more than one type of isoenzyme and isoenzymes may come from several different tissues. Nonetheless, the use of isoenzymes narrows the possibilities of the origin of the elevated enzyme in the serum. (The various isoenzymes are separated by the electrophoresis method, explained in Chapter 10 for protein electrophoresis.)

Enzyme names are generally easy to understand and recognize. Particular enzymes are often named for the reaction that they catalyze. For example, lipase is an enzyme used for the reaction of a lipid or fat, and transaminases transfer amino groups in energy production. Enzymes are easy to recognize because their names almost always end in -ase (Holum, 1983). However, since many of the serum enzyme tests are known by initials rather than by names, there is no way to know that CPK is an enzyme test unless one sees it written out as creatine phosphokinase, and more recently CPK has become just CK for creatine kinase.

To make matters more confusing, the transaminases, which until recently were called SGPT and SGOT, are now called ALT and AST because the new names are more correct in a chemical sense. The enzyme that used to be called serum glutamic-pyruvic transaminase (SGPT) is now called alanine aminotransferase (ALT). The transaminase serum glutamic-oxaloacetic transaminase (SGOT) is now called aspartate aminotransferase (AST). Laboratory reports may use both the old and new names, or only the new names. Older reference books will, of course, use the terms SGPT and SGOT. To lessen the confuson during this transition time, both abbreviations for the transaminases are used in this chapter.

There is a movement to have all enzyme tests reported in a standard way by the use of international units. By convention, the IU is expressed as so many "International Units per liter.'' However, various laboratories may still use different methods to measure enzymes. Results are reported as Bodansky units, Somogyi units, or other units, which usually bear the names of the originators of the method. In this chapter, the IU system for reference values is emphasized, but examples of other values are given too. *Caution:* The only reliable reference values are those determined by the laboratory doing the testing. For example, even two laboratories using Bodansky units may have slightly modified the testing method for their respective laboratories.

Table 12–1 summarizes the most important enzyme elevations for several common pathologic conditions. With a quick glance at the table, the reader sees that none of the enzyme tests is totally specific and that many are changed by several pathological conditions. Also, various nonpathological factors, such as vigorous exercise, cause elevated serum enzymes. Apple and McGue (1983) found marked increases in the CK, LDH, and ALT of men training for marathons. Certain treatments, such as intramuscular injections and the administration of opiates, cause serum elevations of some enzymes. Improper handling of the specimens also brings about elevations due to hemolysis.

In this chapter, each of the factors that affects a particular enzyme is discussed with the specific test. The enzymes are usually not affected by food. The exact timing of each specimen must be documented because several of these enzymes peak quickly and are of short duration, while others do not show up in the bloodstream until a couple of days after tissue injury. For most of the enzyme tests, only elevations of the enzymes or isoenzymes are clinically significant. However, decreased ALP levels and, very rarely, decreased transaminase levels may be clinically significant.

■ ALKALINE PHOSPHATASE (ALP)

Two types of phosphatases are measured in the bloodstream: alkaline and acid. These two types of phosphatases are so termed because their activity is best measured in a pH around either 10 (alkaline) or 5 (acid).

The ALP is a more common clinical test because the enzyme is abundant in several organs. ALP is found in the tissues of the liver, bone, intestine, kidney, and placenta. Its three isoenzymes can be identified by electrophoresis:

1. Band I: Liver, vascular endothelium, and lung
2. Band II: Bone, kidney, and placenta
3. Band III: Intestinal mucosa

However, unlike the other isoenzymes, the isoenzymes of ALP are not commonly used in clinical evaluations of pathology.

Except in pregnancy, most of the serum ALP is made up of liver and bone isoenzymes. Because ALP is increased with new bone formation (osteoblastic activity), children have much higher levels than adults, and because the placenta is a rich source of ALP, a high level of this enzyme is also normal in pregnancy. The ALP from liver tissue is normally excreted into the bile, so biliary obstruction causes an increase of ALP. The ingestion of a fatty meal also causes a temporary increase of serum ALP.

Preparation of Client and Collection of Sample
If the client is on oral contraceptives, phenothiazines, or morphine, note the use of the drug on the laboratory slip, because elevations in the enzyme level may be related to the drug. The laboratory needs 1 ml of serum. Some methods require immediate refrigeration of the sample.

TABLE 12-1. ENZYME ELEVATIONS IN COMMON PATHOLOGICAL CONDITIONS

Serum Enzymes	Eclampsia	Cancer of Prostate	Biliary Obstruction	Bone Metastasis	Liver Malignancy	Hepatitis	Cirrhosis	Myocardial Infarction	Infectious Mononucleosis	Hemolytic Disease	Pulmonary Infarction	Muscular Necrosis or Inflammation	Pancreatitis	Brain Tissue Injury
1. Alkaline phosphatase	↑	↑	(↑)	(↑)	(↑)	↑	↑		↑				↑	
2. Acid phosphatase	↑	(↑)			↑					(↑)				
3. GGT			(↑)		(↑)	↑	↑							
4. 5'N			(↑)		(↑)		↑							
5. Leucine aminopeptidase	↑		(↑)		(↑)		↑						↑	
6. ALT or SGPT	↑		↑	↑	↑	(↑)	↑	(↑)	(↑)		↑	↑	↑	
7. AST or SGOT	↑	↑	↑	↑	↑	(↑)		(↑)	(↑)	↑	↑	↑	↑	
8. CPK or CK (total)								(↑)			↑	(↑)		↑
CK I (BB)														↑
CK II (MB)								(↑)						
CK III (MM)												(↑)		

254

9. LDH Total

   LDH$_1$

   LDH$_2$

   LDH$_3$

   LDH$_4$

   LDH$_5$

10. Aldolase

11. Amylase

12. Lipase

↑ = Significant Elevation. Note that any tissue injury causes *slight* increase in many of these enzymes.

(↑) = Used as Major Diagnostic Tool. See text for elaborations.

Reference Values for ALP	
Adult	13–39 IU 1.4–4.4 Bodansky units 4.5–13 King–Armstrong units
Pregnancy	Levels increase because of production by placenta. Levels may be as high as 107 IU by late pregnancy. Levels return to normal about three weeks after delivery (Hytten & Lind, 1975)
Prematures	50–100% above normal (Tietz, 1983)
Infants and Children	Up to 104 IU 5–14 Bodansky units 15–30 King–Armstrong units Levels remain elevated until puberty when the epiphyses close
Aged	Values tend to be slightly higher than in younger adults

Increased ALP Level

Clinical Significance. A markedly increased ALP level in a nonpregnant adult is a general warning of a bone or liver abnormality. An elevation several times normal is usually the case with liver or bone pathology (Burke, 1978). If there is question of whether bone or liver is the origin, other enzyme tests more specific for hepatobiliary disease may be done. (See discussion on GTT, 5'N, and LAP.)

In Paget's disease, with considerable bone destruction and bone rebuilding, the ALP level is higher than normal. Metastatic cancer to the bone also often causes an elevated ALP if the body attempts to continue to form new bone. If bone is only being broken down (osteolytic process), ALP is not elevated. However, most types of osteolytic processes are accompanied by some osteoblastic activity. A healing fracture causes a modest rise in the ALP level. Conditions such as hyperparathyroidism and vitamin D or calcium deficiencies cause an increased amount of ALP, even though bone growth may be abnormal.

Liver dysfunction is the other main reason for increased ALP levels. The elevation may be due either to actual liver tissue damage or, because ALP is excreted in the bile, to an obstruction of bile flow. Morphine sulfate may cause some spasm of the sphincter of Oddi, and thus it may elevate the ALP level. Conditions that cause obstructive jaundice, such as a stone in the common bile duct or cancer of the head of the pancreas, cause a markedly elevated ALP.

Certain drugs, such as the estrogens and phenothiazines, may cause a stasis of bile (cholestatic effect), thus elevating the ALP in the serum. It has also been postulated that some drugs may induce a synthesis of increased amounts of ALP and other liver enzymes (Rock, 1980). The elevation of the ALP may be the first indication of an adverse reaction to a drug and indicates that the drug should be stopped.

In eclampsia, the ALP levels are increased above the normally high levels of pregnancy, probably because of a liver dysfunction.

Often patients with liver problems, such as cirrhosis, receive albumin intravenously. (See Chapter 10 for a discussion on albumin deficiency.) In such cases, the fact that the placenta is normally a rich source of ALP is important to remember. Administration of albumin derived from placentas causes an elevation of the serum ALP level.

POSSIBLE NURSING DIAGNOSES RELATED TO INCREASED ALP LEVEL

Potential Injury Related to Pathological Fractures

One of the most common uses of the ALP test is to screen for the possibility of bone metastasis in patients with malignancies. The possibility of bone metastasis is an indication that the patient may be prone to pathologic fractures and thus should be handled very carefully and protected from injury. Remember that the metastatic destruction of bone causes an increase of ALP only if osteoblastic activity is occurring along with bone destruction. So not all bone metastasis causes elevated ALP levels. In metastatic disease, any elevated ALP is usually followed with a bone scan (See Chapter 22) to determine the exact points of bone destruction.

Alteration in Comfort Related to Development of Obstructive Jaundice

If the elevated ALP is due to any type of obstruction in the common bile duct, specific nursing implications are related to the presence of obstructive jaundice. (The problems associated with obstructive jaundice are discussed in Chapter 11 in the section on direct bilirubin levels.)

Knowledge Deficit Related to Need to Change Therapeutic Regime

If the client is on drugs that can cause cholestasis, such as estrogens or phenothiazines, even a small increase in the ALP level may be an indication that the patient should not continue on the drug (Burke, 1978). The client who is on oral contraceptives that contain estrogen needs information about other forms of birth control. The physician must be consulted about any needed changes in medication regimens such as a change in tranquilizers.

Decreased ALP Level

Clinical Significance. In the child before the onset of puberty, a decrease of ALP to adult levels indicates a lack of normal bone formation. This condition may be due to pathologic conditions, such as hypothyroidism, celiac disease, cystic fibrosis, or chronic nephritis. Very low levels of ALP are seen in scurvy. Adults with a lack of bone formation due to malnutrition or excessive vitamin D intake may have lowered ALP levels.

POSSIBLE NURSING DIAGNOSIS RELATED TO DECREASED ALP LEVEL

Alteration in Nutritional Needs Related to Malnutrition

The exact nursing implications depend on the reason for a lack of normal bone formation. Usually a dietary plan is needed to ensure an adequate intake of protein, vitamins, and minerals for optimal bone growth.

■ GAMMA-GLUTAMYL TRANSFERASE (GGT) OR GAMMA-GLUTAMYL TRANSPEPTIDASE (GGTP)

GTT, an enzyme that is useful in amino acid transport, is found chiefly in the liver, kidney, prostate, and spleen. When ALP is elevated, the GTT may be used to assess whether or not the increase is due to liver and biliary involvement, because the GTT is more specific for the hepatobiliary system whereas the ALP can be elevated in bone or liver disease. Also, the GTT is said to be a more sensitive indicator of liver disease in childhood than is ALP (Tietz, 1983). (ALP isoenzymes can be tested as discussed in the ALP section, but the GTT, 5'N, or LAP tests have pretty much replaced them.) The GTT is affected by drugs such as phenytoin (Dilantin) and phenobarbital, so the 5'N or LAP tests may be the ones used for clients maintained on these drugs. (These two tests are discussed later in the chapter.) The GTT is also markedly raised by alcohol and hepatotoxic drugs and thus is useful to monitor drug toxicity and alcohol abuse.

Preparation of Client and Collection of Sample:
Some laboratories may require fasting for 8 hours with water allowed. Serum is collected in a red-top tube.

Reference Values for GGT	
Adult: Male	5–38 U/L
Female	5–29 U/L
Children	
1 to 2 years	3–30 U/L
5–15 years	5–27 U/L
Newborn	Levels 5 times childhood values (prematures have 10 times childhood values) (Tietz, 1983)

Clinical Significance. Markedly elevated levels of GTT are seen in liver disease and posthepatic obstruction. Liver damage from alcohol and many drugs, including cancer chemotherapy, causes moderate elevations. Because liver damage from alcohol causes immediate increases, the GTT may be used to monitor a decrease in alcohol intake as part of a withdrawal program. However, some heavy drinkers do not show increased GTT levels (Jacobs et al., 1984).

■ 5' NUCLEOTIDASE (5'N)

5'N, an enzyme used in controlling nucleic acid production, is found in high concentrations in the plasma membranes of liver cells and biliary canaliculi. Significant elevations are associated with hepatobiliary disease. When the ALP is elevated (see ALP discussed above) the 5'N will help determine if the ALP elevation is due to cholestasis. Thus the 5'N is very similar in use to the tests for GGT and to LAP.

Preparation of Client and Collection of Sample
Fasting not required. Serum collected in red-top tube.

Reference Values for 5'N

Adult	2–17 U/L
Pregnancy	Increased in third trimester

Increased 5'N Level

Clinical Significance. 5'N is elevated in common bile duct obstructions such as from a gallstone or a tumor. Drug-induced cholestasis, such as with chlorpromazine (Thorazine), also causes an elevation, as does cirrhosis. Hepatobiliary diseases cause elevations, but malignancies of the bone do not, so the test is helpful in further work-ups for an elevated ALP. Also, the 5'N is less sensitive but more specific than the GTT for liver malignancy (Rock, 1980).

■ LEUCINE AMINOPEPTIDASE (LAP)

Like GTT and 5'N, LAP is a test for another enzyme elevated in biliary obstruction or cholestasis. LAP, a proteolytic enzyme, occurs chiefly in the mucosa of the small intestine and in pancreatic extracts. Of the three tests, LAP is the one used least. LAP can be measured in urine, also, but is not commonly done.

Preparation of Client and Collection of Sample
No fasting needed. Collect 1 ml serum in red-top tube.

Reference Values for LAP

Adults	12–33 IU/L
Pregnancy	Increased in last trimester, returns to normal in 6–8 weeks postpartum (Tietz, 1983)
	Also increases with use of oral contraceptives

Increased LAP Level

Clinical Significance. Elevations are seen with cirrhosis, obstructive jaundice, tumors in the liver, primary cancer of the pancreas, and in some instances, pancreatitis. Severe preeclampsia also causes rises above the normal rise expected in pregnancy.

POSSIBLE NURSING DIAGNOSES FOR ELEVATED GTT, 5'N, AND LAP

Note that all three of these enzymes are related to liver damage and/or biliary stasis. For diagnoses related to liver damage, see the discussion on AST/SGPT in this chapter. For diagnoses related to biliary stasis, see the discussion on obstructive jaundice in Chapter 11.

■ ACID PHOSPHATASE OR PROSTATIC ACID PHOSPHATASE (PAP)

Acid phosphatase is found in high concentrations in the prostate gland, erythrocytes, and platelets. Because this enzyme is excreted in the seminal fluid, a test for acid phosphatase is sometimes done on vaginal secretions as supportive evidence for alleged rape. Because the prostatic portion of the enzyme is in such small amounts in the serum, the laboratory may use radioimmunoassay to measure the prostatic isoenzyme. The test is a tumor marker for prostatic cancer (Ostcheya & Culnane, 1985).

Preparation of Client and Collection of Sample

There is no special preparation of the client. It is important, however, that the specimen not be hemolyzed since the erythrocytes are rich in acid phosphatase. The specimen should be examined within 1 hour or stored as frozen serum. The laboratory needs 1 ml of serum. The enzyme is subject to circadian rhythm, so it should be drawn at the same time each day (Jacobs et al., 1984).

Reference Values for Acid Phosphatase

Adult	Total: 0–3 IU/L
Female	Total: 0.01–0.56 Sigma units/ml
Male	Total: 0.13–0.63 Sigma units/ml
	Prostatic isoenzyme: 0.0–0.5 Fisherman–Lerner units/100 ml
Newborn	Increased levels due to hemolysis
Pregnancy	Very little change, if any

Increased Serum Acid Phosphatase Level

Clinical Significance. Operative trauma or instrumentation of the prostate gland, such as a cystoscopy, can cause a transient increase in the acid phosphatase level. However, the major reason for a marked elevation of the prostatic portion of this

---

POSSIBLE NURSING DIAGNOSIS RELATED TO INCREASED SERUM ACID PHOSPHATASE LEVEL

Anxiety Related to Coping with a Life-threatening Illness

The major use of the serum acid phosphatase level is to evaluate carcinoma of the prostate gland. Usually the man is elderly and may have other physical problems besides the malignancy. The client needs help in coping with what may be a terminal illness. If the tumor is successfully treated by surgery, the acid phosphatase levels decrease in a few days. If etrogen therapy is used as the treatment for the prostatic cancer, the levels of acid phosphatase may not return to normal for several weeks. (See Chapter 15 for nursing diagnoses related to hormone therapy.) An increasing acid phosphatase level may signal a much worse prognosis for the client.

enzyme is cancer of the prostate that has invaded the capsule surrounding the gland. Conditions that cause an increased destruction of red blood cells, such as the various hemolytic anemias, also cause an increase of the nonprostatic portion of acid phosphatase. Acute renal impairment, liver dysfunction, and some diseases of the bone may also cause an increase in the total acid phosphatase level, but this test is not used to evaluate these conditions.

■ ALANINE AMINOTRANSFERASE (ALT) OR SERUM GLUTAMIC-PYRUVIC TRANSAMINASE (SGPT)

Formerly known as SGPT, this transaminase is found in the largest concentration in liver tissue, but it is also present in kidney, heart, and skeletal muscle tissue. Like the other transaminase (AST or SGOT), ALT is increased in various types of tissue damage and so it is not very specific. ALT (or SGPT) may be used if there is a specific need to evaluate the possibility of liver tissue necrosis or liver damage from drugs. ALT has been seen as potentially useful in screening blood donors to reduce the incidence of non-A non-B hepatitis (Apple & McGue, 1983). The ratio of the two enzymes, AST (SGOT) to ALT (SGPT), can also help to evaluate liver diseases.

Preparation of Client and Collection of Specimen
The client does not need to fast. The specimen can be refrigerated after it is clotted, but it is important that the blood not be hemolyzed. The exact time that the specimen was drawn should be noted because serial measurements give useful information about the progression or lessening of liver damage. The laboratory needs 1 ml of blood. Various antibiotics, narcotics, and salicylates may cause false elevations of liver enzymes.

Reference Values for ALT or SGPT

Adult	1–21 U/L
	5–35 Sigma–Frankel units
Aged	Very slight increase

Labor and delivery or other active exercise may cause slight elevations. Newborns have higher levels.

Increased ALT or SGPT

Clinical Significance. In severe hepatitis, the ALT is often over 1000 IU and may rise to 4000 IU. In chronic hepatitis and cirrhosis, the levels are not so markedly elevated. Infectious mononucleosis, which often involves the liver, causes a significant rise in the ALT. (See Chapter 14 for tests for infectious mononucleosis.) Shock, Reye's syndrome, congestive heart failure, and eclampsia all cause an increased ALT due to some liver tissue damage. Hydatidiform moles also cause elevations of the ALT. (Chapter 15 discusses the diagnosis of hydatidiform moles by hormone assay.) A comparison of the ratio of AST (SGOT) to ALT (SGPT) can help to evaluate liver disease. AST (SGOT) levels are greater than ALT (SGPT) in cirrhosis and metastatic carcinoma of the liver. In acute hepatitis and nonmalignant hepatic obstruction, the AST (SGOT) is usually lower than the ALT (SGPT) (Rock, 1980).

POSSIBLE NURSING DIAGNOSES RELATED TO INCREASED ALT LEVELS

Potential for Injury Related to Hepatic Failure
Because a markedly elevated ALT or SGPT may be indicative of severe liver tissue damage, nurses must carefully assess for any signs of liver insufficiency, which could progress to a hepatic coma. (See Chapter 10 for the test of ammonia levels as a sign of liver dysfunction and for details of the symptoms that may be present. Chapter 11 discusses the special needs of the jaundiced patient.)

Alteration in Nutritional Needs
The basic ingredients for the encouragement of liver tissue regeneration are the promotion of rest, the avoidance of drugs toxic to the liver, and the provision of a nutritious diet that is high in calories, protein, and vitamins.

Activity Intolerance Related to Fatigue
Nurses may need to do some teaching to help patients learn how to conserve energy. For clients at home, someone should be available to see that they do indeed rest. Rest is not a luxury here; it is often *the* basic therapy. Enzyme levels, tested over a period of weeks, may be used to gauge the amount of activity allowed. Boredom and depression can occur due to a long convalescent period with prolonged restrictions on usual activities.

■ ASPARTATE AMINOTRANSFERASE (AST) OR SERUM GLUTAMIC-OXALOACETIC TRANSAMINASE (SGOT)

Formerly called SGOT, AST is found predominantly in heart, liver, and muscle tissue, although all tissues contain some of the enzyme. Because the transaminases are very important to energy transformation, the highest amounts of them are found in high-energy cells such as the heart, liver, and skeletal muscles. As discussed in the previous section, the highest concentration of ALT or SGPT is in the liver, and it is used primarily to detect liver necrosis. AST or SGOT can also be used to detect liver necrosis, since both transaminases rise before there are any signs of jaundice. Neither the ALT or AST is used to evaluate skeletal muscle necrosis because two other enzymes (CPK and aldolase) are more specific for muscle tissue necrosis. The AST or SGOT is most often used as one of the cardiac enzymes to detect the occurrence of a myocardial infarction. (ALT or SGPT is not elevated significantly in cardiac damage.) However, if isoenzymes of the other two cardiac enzymes (LDH and CPK) are available, the AST or SGOT may not give any additional information. A summary of the use of all the cardiac enzymes follows the dicussion about each separate cardiac enzyme.

Special Preparation of Client and Collection of Specimen
The client is prepared and the specimen collected in the same way and under the same conditions as for the other transaminase, ALT or SGPT. Note that various drugs may interfere with the test.

Reference Values for AST or SGOT	
Adult	7–27 U/L
	5–40 Sigma–Frankel units
	Female values tend to be slightly lower than male but only marked increases are significant
Pregnancy	Labor and delivery cause slight increases
	Vigorous exercise also tends to increase transaminase levels
Newborn	Values are 2–3 times higher (Jacobs, et al., 1984)
Aged	Slight increase

Increased AST or SGOT Level

Clinical Significance. With the necrosis of tissue that accompanies myocardial infarction, AST is released from the damaged cardiac cells. If the client experiences chest pain for other reasons, such as angina or pericarditis, the AST level is not markedly elevated because there is no actual cell death. The amount of enzyme released depends on the severity of the inflammation. After an acute infarction, the serum level of AST begins to rise in about 6–12 hours. A peak of 100–150 IU is reached in a couple of days, and the enzyme returns to normal in another 2 or 3 days. Comparison of the onset, peak, and duration of AST with the time frames for CPK and LDH is shown in Table 12-2.

In hepatitis, the AST or SGOT may reach levels greater than 500 IU (Wallach 1986), and it is elevated in the bloodstream even before jaundice appears. The return to normal may take weeks to months after hepatitis. Other types of liver involvement, such as that with shock, trauma, or cirrhosis, may cause lesser elevations of the AST. Reye's syndrome and pulmonary infarction are other causes of an elevated AST. The ratio of AST (SGOT) to ALT (SGPT) is useful in distinguishing various types of liver pathology as discussed in the section on ALT. Also the GTT will help distinguish liver involvement.

TABLE 12-2. TIME FRAME FOR CHANGES IN SERUM ENZYME LEVELS AFTER AN ACUTE MYOCARDIAL INFARCTION

	Appears in Serum (Hours)	Peaks (Days)	Duration (Days)
CPK or CK (Isoenzyme II-B)	4–8	0.5–1.5	About 3
AST (Formerly known as SGOT)	6–12	1.5–2.0	4–6
LDH (Isoenzyme LDH_1 and LDH_2 as a "flipped" LDH)	12–24	2–6	8–14

Note: These time frames are general approximations based on several references. Not all clients fall exactly into these patterns. See text for elaboration of relative efficiency of different tests. Also see Gann (1978), Tietz (1983), and Ryan (1984) for discussion of combination of tests.

**POSSIBLE NURSING DIAGNOSES RELATED TO ELEVATED
AST OR SGOT**

Because the AST or SGOT can be elevated from many different causes, nursing care must be based on the underlying pathophysiology. If the AST level is due to hepatic damage, the nursing diagnoses for ALT or SGPT elevations would be useful as general guidelines. If the AST or SGOT is being used to rule out the possibility of a myocardial infarction, the enzymes must be carefully interpreted in relation to other clinical assessments of the patient. Nursing diagnoses related to elevated cardiac enzymes follow the discussion on the CPK and LDH tests.

Decrease in Transaminases ALT (SGPT) and AST (SGOT)

Clinical Significance. Because the levels of transaminases are normally very low, a decrease is unlikely. In *rare* instances, both transaminases ALT (SGPT) and AST (SGOT) are decreased or nonexistent due to severe liver dysfunction because the liver can no longer make the enzymes. Uremia sometimes causes a pseudo-decrease (Jacobs et al., 1984), as can chronic dialysis and ketoacidosis (Wallach, 1986).

■ CREATINE KINASE (CK) OR CREATINE PHOSPHOKINASE (CPK)

CPK, or CK as it is now called, is very important in energy utilization, and is involved in the reaction that changes creatine to creatinine. Because almost all of the circulating CK comes normally from muscular tissue, muscular activity and intramuscular injections are two common ways that CK values are elevated. CK can be measured as one total enzyme in the serum, or it can be separated into three different isoenzymes. The three types of CK isoenzymes are:

1. CK-I (BB): Produced primarily by brain tissue and smooth muscle
2. CK-II (MB): Produced primarily by heart tissue
3. CK-III (MM): Produced primarily by muscle tissue

The isoenzymes of CK are particularly useful in detecting myocardial infarction and progressive muscular diseases that cause muscle necrosis.

Preparation of Client and Collection of Specimen
Because physical activity causes a transient increase in CK, clients should not engage in vigorous activity before the blood sample is drawn. Since intramuscular injections may triple the amount of CK in the serum, such injections should be delayed until the test is drawn if doing so is feasible. Otherwise, the fact that the client has received intramuscular injections should be noted on the laboratory slip. The timing of the drawing for the CK is crucial because the enzyme may disappear from the bloodstream in less than 24 hours after a myocardial infarction. The laboratory needs 1 ml of serum of blood, which should be refrigerated if it cannot be sent to the laboratory immediately.

Reference Values for CK

All groups			
Female	Total: 10–79 U/L		
Male	Total: 17–148 U/L		
Isoenzymes	CK-I	(BB)	Brain 0%
	CK-II	(MB)	Heart 0–5%
	CK-III	(MM)	Muscle 95–100%
Pregnancy	Levels are reduced in first half of pregnancy but rise in second half of pregnancy. Slight increase during labor and delivery. Surgical procedures, such as an episiotomy, cause more increase. Also, intramuscular injections and vigorous exercise elevate the CK		
Newborns	Newborns have higher values and may be very high due to birth trauma		

Increased Serum CK (CPK)

Clinical Significance

Elevation of CK-II. CK, the first enzyme to be elevated after a myocardial infarction, begins to rise in 3–6 hours and may peak in the first 24 hours (Table 12–2). In some clients the CK returns to normal within 16 hours after the chest pain. Gann (1978) gives evidence that one test of CK-II (MB) on admission and another after 12 hours are usually enough to diagnose or to exclude myocardial infarction occurring within 24 hours of admission. Some physicians may order a third one in 24 hours (Jacobs et al., 1984). It is generally agreed that the CK-II (MB) is very useful in the initial detection of an infarction, but it is not useful if the client has had chest pain for a day or two before coming to seek medical help. For some clients, the duration of CK may continue for about 3 days but the peak is missed; in such cases, LDH isoenzymes are more helpful.

Elevation of CK-III. CPK-III (MM) elevations are never diagnostic of a specific muscular disease, but high levels are an indication for further specific testing of muscular function. In the early stages of muscular dystrophy, CK is as high as 3000

POSSIBLE NURSING DIAGNOSES RELATED TO CHANGED LEVELS OF CK

Potential Alteration in Cardiac Output Related to Extension of Myocardial Infarction
Because this CK is the first cardiac enzyme to be increased and has a short duration in the serum, it should not be elevated after the first few days of an infarction. A sudden increase in the CK after a day or two should be reported to the physician immediately and the patient assessed for the possibility of an extension of the infarction. A general summary of key points in planning nursing care for the client with elevated cardiac enzymes follows the discussion on the LDH test.

Knowledge Deficit Regarding Diagnostic Procedures for Muscle Necrosis
If the elevated CK is related to muscle necrosis, the client may need to undergo a battery of tests to discover the exact problem. Women who are found to be carriers of the sex-linked gene for muscular dystrophy may need to be referred to genetic counseling if they desire pregnancy (see Chapter 18). The enzyme aldolase is another test for muscular inflammatory diseases. Some general nursing implications for patients with myositis are covered in the section on aldolase later in this chapter.

IU/L. As the disease progresses, the CK levels drop, and, by the time the person is bedridden, they may be normal. Healthy female carriers of X-linked Duchenne muscular dystrophy have raised levels of CK. Once these women are pregnant, however, the lowering of the CK in the first half of pregnancy may mask the elevation (Hytten & Lind, 1975).

Elevation of CK-I. The third type of isoenzyme, CK-I (BB) may be elevated in the case of extreme shock, of brain tumors, or of severe cerebral accidents. CK-I is being investigated as a tumor marker for certain types of adenocarcinomas (Jacobs et al., 1984).

■ LACTIC DEHYDROGENASE (LDH)

LDH is an enzyme that helps remove a water molecule from lactic acid. LDH is found in large amounts in the heart, liver, muscles, and erythrocytes. It is also present in other organs such as the kidney, pancreas, spleen, brain, and lungs. Like the enzyme CK, LDH can be separated into various isoenzymes:

1. LDH_1 is primarily from the heart and erythrocytes
2. LDH_2 comes mostly from the reticuloendothelial system
3. LDH_3 is from the lungs and other tissue
4. LDH_4 comes from the placenta, kidney, and pancreas
5. LDH_5 is largely from the liver and striated muscle

Total LDH and LDH_1 and LDH_2 are most often used in detecting a myocardial infarction. LDH is not typically used to assess liver function or muscle function, because other enzymes are more specific. (See Table 12–1 for elevations of LDH isoenzymes in various pathologic states.)

Preparation of Client and Collection of Specimen
The sample must be handled carefully because any hemolysis of the red blood cells falsely elevates the results. Even if the hemolysis is not enough to turn the serum pink, there is still an increased LDH. The client does not need to be fasting. The laboratory needs 1 ml of serum.

Increased Serum LDH

Clinical Significance. In myocardial infarction, the LDH begins to rise about 12–24 hours after the cardiac damage. The peak, usually around 300–800 IU/L is in 2–6 days, and the enzyme remains in the bloodstream for up to two weeks. (See Table 12-2 for a comparison of this time frame with the other cardiac enzymes.) The measurement of the isoenzymes 1 and 2 gives an even more specific indication that damaged cardiac tissue is causing the elevation. As noted in the reference values, LDH_2 is usually higher in concentration than LDH_1. In a myocardial infarction the greatest rise is in the LDH_1 isoenzyme and thus it becomes higher than LDH_2. This

---

Reference Values for LDH

Adult	45–90 U/L (Reference ranges highly method dependent)	
Pregnancy	Normal in pregnancy but increases slightly during labor and delivery, as with other vigorous exercise.	
Newborn	First week of life: 160–450 U/L	
Children	60–170 U/L	
Aged	55–102 U/L (Tietz, 1983)	
Isoenzymes[a]	LDH_1 (erythrocytes, heart tissue)	25%
	LDH_2 (reticuloendothelial tissue, kidney)	40%
	LDH_3 (lungs, lymph nodes, spleen, and various other tissues)	25%
	LDH_4 (kidney, placenta, liver tissue)	5%
	LDH_5 (liver tissue, skeletal tissue, kidney)	5%

[a]See specific laboratory reports for ranges for isoenzymes.

---

change in the percentage ratio between LDH_1 and LDH_2, called a *flipped LDH,* is considered to be highly suggestive of a myocardial infarction. A flipped LDH, or the reversal of the ratio of LDH_1 to LDH_2, is apparent sooner than the rise in the total LDH. It also remains evident for 3–4 days after the total LDH returns to normal after a myocardial infarction.

Other possible causes of LDH elevations are as follows:

1. Hemolytic and macrocytic anemias tend to cause elevations in LDH_1 and LDH_2.
2. In pulmonary infarction and infectious mononucleosis, LDH_2 and LDH_3 are elevated.
3. Leukemia and malignancies, in general, cause large increases in LDH_3.
4. Liver damage increases the last two isoenzymes, LDH_4 and LDH_5. Because the last two isoenzymes make up but a small portion (10%) of the total LDH, such an increase may not change the total drastically.
5. Shock and trauma may cause an elevation of all the isoenzymes, as does heart surgery. If the heart-lung machine is used, the LDH will be 4–6 times the normal reference values.
6. In pregnancy, placental disturbances, such as abruptio placenta, effect an elevation in the isoenzymes.
7. Hepatitis causes a more modest increase in the total than that accompanying myocardial infarction.
8. A LDH of 2000 IU or more is almost always due to either megaloblastic anemia or cancer (Burke, 1978: p. 78). LDH is a tumor marker for non-Hodgkin's lymphoma (Ostcheya & Culnane, 1985).

POSSIBLE NURSING DIAGNOSIS RELATED TO INCREASED LDH

Alteration in Cardiac Output Related to Extension of Infarction or Other Complications

Although almost any type of tissue damage can change the LDH, the major use of this test is to determine the presence of a myocardial infarction. (The use of isoenzymes is even more definitive, of course.) Because LDH may remain elevated for a couple of weeks after a myocardial infarction, it is useful in monitoring the client who is convalescing from an infarction. If the LDH begins to rise again after the first week, the physician should be notified immediately because this rise may signal an extension of the infarction. Sometimes a second infarction is "silent," because the client experiences no symptoms of chest pain, or it may be unnoticeable because the client has been heavily medicated with morphine sulfate.

The sudden increase in LDH does not always mean a worsening of the infarction because other things may cause a rise. For example, pulmonary infarctions can occur as a complication of the bed rest. To pinpoint the exact reason for an increasing LDH in a client recovering from a myocardial infarction, a thorough medical assessment and other tests, such as repeat electrocardiograms (Chapter 24) and lung scans (Chapter 22) may be needed. Some general nursing implications for the client with a change in the cardiac enzymes are summarized in the following section.

When the presence of an infarction is open to question, it is prudent to continue to treat the client as a possible myocardial infarction until the condition is definitely ruled out. The key nursing actions are to promote physical and mental relaxation and to watch the vital signs carefully. Ideally, such clients should be in a coronary care unit so that they can be monitored very closely. The use of the cardiac monitor does not take the place of the nurse. The nurse must be able to recognize that the client is having a potentially dangerous arrhythmia so that early treatment can be initiated. The nurse can also detect distended neck veins or slight dyspnea as signals of a potential fluid overload. Even a slight change in vital signs may indicate impending cardiogenic shock (Wenger et al., 1980). This very careful watching of the client is essential any time there is a question of myocardial infarction. (See Chapter 24 for more information on monitoring.)

POSSIBLE NURSING DIAGNOSES RELATED TO CHANGES IN THE CARDIAC ENZYMES (AST OR SGOT, CK, AND LDH)

Potential for Impaired Tissue Perfusion Related to Extent of Myocardial Damage

Understanding the Limitations of Enzymes as Assessment Tools. The real client in the clinical area is never quite as predictable as the one indicated by the textbook tables. So, although the diagnostic interpretation of cardiac enzymes is the responsibility of the attending physician, the nurse caring for cardiac clients needs some general knowledge about standard practices when enzyme levels are puzzling. Usually, in a client with a myocardial infarction, the changes in the cardiac enzymes roughly follow the time frames given in Table

12–2. If all the enzymes, including the isoenzymes, are normal for a couple of days, then the client most likely has not had a myocardial infarction. If the cardiac isoenzyme of CK-II (MB) is elevated and the LDH remains normal, the diagnosis is in question. The client may have had myocardial ischemia rather than an actual infarction. However, angina does not usually cause elevations, and the LDH may not always be positive (Gann, 1978). As a general rule, the flipped LDH is considered highly suggestive of a myocardial infarction. A flipped LDH is present in 80% of myocardial infarctions (Ryan, 1984). The routine use of AST (SGOT) may not be necessary when the CK isoenzymes and LDH isoenzymes are available. Galen (1975) has suggested that the four most important criteria for the diagnosis of a myocardial infarction are: (1) a positive new Q-wave in the electrocardiogram, (2) a classical acute clinical history, (3) the presence of CK-II (MB) over 3%, and (4) a flipped LDH (LDH_1 greater than LDH_2). The important point for nurses to remember is that they must always interpret the enzyme levels in the context of the client's overall clinical picture.

Recognizing Clinical Situations That Cause Pseudo-Elevations of Myocardial Enzymes. When isoenzymes are not available, the enzyme tests may be even more likely to give a pseudomyocardial pattern. For example, if the client has any disease of the biliary tract, then the use of opiates, such as morphine or codeine, can cause a spasm of the sphincter of Oddi. This temporary narrowing or obstruction of the common bile duct can cause an increase in the LDH, and it may make the AST or SGOT markedly increase. Nurses must also remember that intramuscular injections significantly increase the total CK level.

Strenuous exercise can significantly elevate the CK, the AST or SGOT, and the LDH. Evidently the amount of increase of these enzymes is related directly to the vigor of the exercise and inversely to the level of training before the exercise (Statland, 1979). So a man in poor physical condition from a lack of training may have chest pain after a vigorous run or a handball game and the cardiac enzymes may be elevated even though he has not had an infarction. Even men in good shape may have an elevation of LDH and CK when training for a marathon (Apple & McGue, 1983). Again the point is that the enzymes are never diagnostic when used alone.

Recognizing the Importance of Timing of Enzymes. Just as an elevation of serum enzymes is not always proof positive of an infarction, a lack of enzyme elevations does not always mean that an infarction can be ruled out. Table 12–2, in showing the importance of timing in relation to the serum levels of the enzymes, also demonstrates that missing the peak of the enzyme in the serum is possible. According to Wenger et al. (1980), it takes at least a gram of necrotic myocardial tissue to release enough enzymes to cause elevated serum levels. Fatal arrhythmias can result from a very small infarct or from ischemic heart tissue. Thus normal cardiac enzymes must not give nurses a false sense of security.

■ SERUM ALDOLASE

Like most of the other enzymes in this chapter, aldolase is present in all cells. Its highest concentrations are found in skeletal muscles, heart, and liver tissue. Because damage to muscular tissue causes marked elevations of aldolase, it is a diagnostic test for certain types of muscle damage. (CK, discussed earlier, is a more common test for muscular damage.)

Preparation of Client and Collection of Sample

Fasting is not necessary. Aldolase is in erythrocytes, so the specimen must not be hemolyzed. The laboratory needs 2 ml of fresh serum.

Reference Values for Aldolase

Adult	1.3–8.2 U/L
Newborn	Up to 4 times adult level (Tietz, 1983)

Increased Serum Aldolase Level

Clinical Significance. Muscular disorders that cause inflammation of the muscles (myositis) cause an elevation of aldolase. In the event of muscular wasting due to a muscular disease of the central nervous system, such as myasthenia gravis or multiple sclerosis, the aldolase level is not elevated. In progressive muscular dystrophy, the level may be 10–15 times normal in the early stages of the disease, but the level subsides as muscle wasting continues. In some types of acute myositis the levels of aldolase return to normal when corticosteroid treatment is effective. Aldolase testing may be used in conjunction with more specific diagnostic measures to identify the exact reason for muscle necrosis.

POSSIBLE NURSING DIAGNOSES RELATED TO INCREASED ALDOLASE SERUM LEVEL

Self-Care Deficit Related to Muscle Fatigue

The key nursing implication for the client with a skeletal muscular problem is to help the person to be as independent as possible while conserving muscle strength. If the muscular disorder is due to an acute condition, the person is comforted to know that the lack of muscle strength is temporary. Return of muscle strength occurs after the enzymes return to normal. Nursing care during the acute phase may center most on preventing any complications from the disuse of muscles. (The other enzymes that become elevated in acute muscular myositis are the transaminases and CK and these may also be used to monitor recovery.)

Potential for Ineffective Coping Related to Problems of a Chronic Muscular Disease

If the muscular disorder is a chronic problem, such as muscular dystrophy, the client is faced with learning how to cope with a progressively debilitating disease. Because each case of muscle disease differs from all others, the nursing care plan must be individualized to the severity of the disease and to its effects on the person. The community health nurse may be very involved in helping clients adapt to a crippling disease. Janul (1977) gives such clients many helpful hints on ways to be independent in doing personal care and housekeeping, while using their limited energy wisely. The nurse needs to emphasize to clients that a schedule that allows frequent and short rest periods is much better than one with a long rest period. Clients may be able to do much more if they are not hurrying to accomplish several activities in a limited time. In addition to emphasizing a planned exercise and rest schedule, the nurse may also need to do some health teaching about the expected effects of the prescribed medications and the necessity for follow-up diagnostic tests.

■ SERUM AMYLASE

Amylase, an enzyme that helps with the digestion of starch, is found in high concentrations in the salivary glands and in the pancreas, each of which contains a different isoenzyme. These two isoenzymes can be separated, but doing so is not clinically useful because any disease of the parotid gland (mumps) is evident from the swelling of the gland.

Amylase is the only enzyme that is measured in both serum and urine as a routine test. The serum amylase is often done as a stat procedure in clients with acute abdominal pain to distinguish pancreatitis from other acute abdominal problems that would require surgery.

Preparation of Client and Collection of Sample

About 60% of the total amylase is from the salivary gland. If health workers talk over an uncovered urine or blood sample, this can falsely elevate amylase levels (Sobel & Ferguerson, 1985). Drugs that cause spasm of the sphincter of Oddi, such as the opiates, may cause an elevation of the serum amylase. The increase is at a maximum five hours after drug administration. So, if possible, the stat amylase should be drawn prior to the use of opiate drugs. Thiazide diuretics and diagnostic dyes may cause false elevations.

The client does not need to be fasting. Hemolysis does not affect the results of this test. The laboratory needs 1 ml of serum.

Reference Values for Amylase	
Adult	4–25 U/ml
	60–150 Somogyi units
Pregnancy	Pregnancy causes moderate increases. Females taking oral contraceptives will have slightly increased amylase levels
Newborn	Usually absent. Presence may indicate disease process (Tietz, 1983)
Aged	May have higher values (Lawson, et al., 1986)

Increased Serum Amylase Level

Clinical Significance. Pancreatitis is the most common reason for marked elevations of serum amylase, which begins to increase about three to six hours after an attack of this disease. (See Table 12–3 for a comparison with serum lipase, the other

TABLE 12-3. PANCREATIC ENZYMES USED TO DIAGNOSE ACUTE PANCREATITIS

	Begins Elevation[a]	Peaks[a]	Duration[a]
Serum amylase	3–6 hours	20–30 hours	2–3 days
Urine amylase	6–10 hours after serum levels	Varies	1–2 weeks
Serum lipase	Increases after amylase	Varies	Up to 14 days longer than amylase

[a]Time frames are *general* approximations based on several references. See Lawson (1986).

pancreatic enzyme.) The severity of the disease is not always directly related to the levels of the enzyme. In fact, about 10% of patients with fatal pancreatitis have normal serum amylase levels. High levels in alcoholism, pregnancy, and in diabetic ketoacidosis are of salivary rather than pancreatic origin (Jacobs et al., 1984). Renal failure may also cause abnormal elevations not related to pancreatic disease.

In the adult, the two most common reasons for pancreatitis are alcohol abuse and gallstones. Evidently, the obstruction of the pancreatic ducts or pancreatic ischemia triggers an acute inflammatory response, and autodigestion of the pancreas begins. Oral contraceptives, hyperlipidemia, and hyperthyroidism are less common reasons for such response. Ruptured ectopic pregnancies, perforated ulcers, and other acute abdominal conditions may cause some elevation of the serum amylase level due to trauma to the pancreas. In children, pancreatitis is rare and often of an unknown cause. Sometimes it appears to have a hereditary base. In a study done by Sibert (1979), obesity and the beginning of puberty were related to the incidence of pancreatitis in female children.

POSSIBLE NURSING DIAGNOSES RELATED TO INCREASED SERUM AMYLASE LEVEL

Potential for Fluid Volume Deficit
If the client has massive hemorrhagic necrosis, the mortality rate may be as high as 50–80%. If the pancreatitis is not hemorrhagic, the prognosis is much better, but fluid loss can still lead to shock. Thus one key nursing implication for the client with an elevated serum amylase level is to observe for any change in vital signs that may indicate hypovolemia from the loss of pancreatic fluids or blood.

Alteration in Comfort due to Pain
Clients with pancreatitis usually have severe abdominal pain. Comfort measures and pain relief are important. Often meperidine (Demerol) is used to relieve pain rather than morphine because opiates may cause spasms of the sphincter of Oddi (Lawson et al., 1986). (Recall that the potential effect of opiates on the sphincter of Oddi can cause the elevation of the pancreatic enzymes, as well as of liver enzymes such as the transaminases and ALP.)

Alteration in Nutritional Needs Related to Measures to Decrease Pancreatic Stimulation
Stimulation of the pancreas needs to be minimized as much as possible. So the client must be n.p.o. and maintained on intravenous fluids. Atropine, an

anticholinergic drug, may be ordered to decrease gastrointestinal activity. A nasogastric (NG) tube may be used to decompress the bowel until the acute inflammation has subsided although Loiudice et al., (1984) found a NG tube was needed only if ileus or emesis was present and atropine and cimetidine were of little help in resolving the disease process. Bowel sounds may be hypoactive or absent if the inflammation is severe.

Potential for Infection
Antibiotics are used to prevent a secondary infection of the necrotic tissue in the pancreas. (See Chapter 2 on WBC differentials to assess infections.)

Potential for Injury Related to Possible Hypocalcemia, Hypokalemia, Hyperglycemia, and Jaundice
When the client has pancreatitis, often laboratory tests and diagnostic procedures influence nursing care:

1. Calcium levels: Serum calcium may be lowered because calcium is deposited in the pancreas due to fat necrosis. The hypocalcemia may be severe enough to cause tetany. (See Chapter 7 for possible nursing diagnoses for clients with a deceased serum calcium level.)
2. Potassium levels: Hypokalemia may result from a lack of intake and a loss of body fluids. (See Chapter 5 for the implications of a lowered potassium level.)
3. Glucose levels: Hyperglycemia may be brought about because the damaged pancreatic cells may not be able to produce sufficient insulin. (See Chapter 8 for serum glucose levels.)
4. Bilirubin levels: Direct bilirubin may increase if the pancreatic inflammation is due to obstruction of the common bile duct. (See Chapter 11 for the implications when the client has obstructive jaundice.)
5. Triglyceride levels: Triglyceride levels may be high, particularly if alcohol was a triggering event. (See Chapter 9.)
6. Assessing for chronic complications: Once the client is over the acute stage of pancreatitis, the most common complications are abcess formation in the pancreas or pseudocysts, which are collections of fluids in sacs outside the pancreas. Gallium scans (Chapter 22) may be used to detect abcesses, whereas sonograms (Chapter 23) may show the presence of the pseudocysts.

Knowledge Deficit Regarding Measures to Prevent Recurrent Attacks
Clients who have had an elevated serum amylase level may benefit from discharge planning that focuses on the ways that recurrent attacks can be reduced. Alcohol in all forms should be avoided for several months. If alcohol abuse was the precipitating factor, the client may need to seek professional help to deal with a chronic problem. If gallstones are present and a cholecystectomy is to be done later, dietary modifications may be needed.

■ URINARY AMYLASE

Amylase, the enzyme elevated in the serum in acute pancreatitis, can also be measured in the urine. The amylase may be elevated in the urine for as long as two weeks after an acute episode of pancreatitis. Monitoring the amylase levels in urine may be useful after the acute peak in the serum has diminished. (See Table 12–3 for a comparison of the time frames for serum and urine amylases.)

Preparation of Client and Collection of Sample

Usually the test is done on a collection of urine for a 2-hour time period, but sometimes a 24-hour specimen is used. The 24-hour specimen needs to be iced. See Chapter 3 for tips on collecting 24-hour urine specimens.

Reference Values for Urinary Amylase

24–76 U/ml
260–950 Somogyi units in 24 hours

■ SERUM LIPASE

Lipase is a pancreatic enzyme that breaks down fat into glycerol and fatty acids. In acute pancreatitis (see Table 12–3) lipase rises later in the serum than amylase. So lipase may be used as a secondary test for pancreatitis when the diagnosis is questionable. Other types of pancreatic pathology, such as carcinoma or trauma, cause some release of the enzyme into the serum. See the discussion of amylase for nursing diagnoses related to acute pancreatitis.

Preparation of Client and Collection of Sample

The precautions are the same as those for amylase. The laboratory needs 1 ml of serum.

Reference Values for Lipase

All groups	2 U/ml or less Cherry and Crandall method: 1–1.5 U Maclay method: less than 0.3 U
Pregnancy	Increase in late pregnancy to around 15 IU (may be related to high levels of circulating lipids)

QUESTIONS

1. Which one of the following factors is the *least* likely to cause elevations in most of the common serum enzymes?

   a. Eating food four hours before the test
   b. Vigorous physical activity
   c. Administration of intramuscular injections of morphine sulfate
   d. Hemolysis of the serum sample

2. A markedly elevated alkaline phosphatase level is a general warning of either:

   a. increased bone formation *or* obstruction to bile flow

   b. mycardial infarction *or* angina

   c. cancer of the prostate *or* of the liver

   d. increased bone destruction or liver dysfunction

3. Administration of intravenous albumin solutions may cause an elevated serum alkaline phosphatase level for which of the following reasons?

   a. Albumin obtained from placentas is rich in this enzyme

   b. Alkaline phosphatase is transported by albumin

   c. The oncotic pressure is increased in the serum

   d. The method used to purify albumin causes the release of the enzyme

4. The main use of serum acid phosphatase levels is to diagnose and to evaluate malignancies of which of the following?

a. Liver	**c.** Prostate gland
b. Ovaries	**d.** Kidney

5. When a client has a marked elevation of the transaminases ALT (formerly SGPT) and AST (formerly SGOT), the key nursing implication is observation for signs and symptoms of which of the following?

   a. Liver dysfunction

   b. Muscle weakness

   c. Dehydration

   d. Hemorrhage or other cardiovascular problems

6. In myocardial damage, which of these enzymes is most useful for detecting myocardial damage in the first 24 hours after an episode of chest pain?

   a. CK   **b.** AST or SGOT   **c.** LDH   **d.** ALT or SGPT

7. A flipped LDH is one of the characteristic signs of an acute myocardial infarction. A flipped LDH means that LDH_1 is which of the following?

   a. Greater than LDH_2

   b. Less than LDH_2

   c. In an abnormal form

   d. Greater than LDH_4 and LDH_5

8. Mr. Marx is a 50-year-old businessman who was admitted to the coronary care unit with severe chest pain yesterday. His enzyme levels (CPK, LDH, and AST or SGOT) done on admission were normal. Because he wants to make several business calls, he has asked where he can find a phone. Which nursing action is appropriate?

   a. Allow him to go to a phone via a wheelchair, as his enzyme levels are normal

   b. Tell him he has had a heart attack so he must stay on complete bedrest

    c. Make sure that Mr. Marx understands the need for further assessment of ECG readings, serial enzyme levels, and a medical exam to rule out a possible myocardial infarction

    d. Tell him that phone calls are not allowed and continue to observe him for arrhythmias, hypotension, or distended neck veins

9. Mrs. Jackson is a 44-year-old mother with two teen-aged girls. She has increased CK and aldolase levels due to a still-undiagnosed muscular disease. Which advice by a community health nurse would be the most appropriate?

    a. "Schedule most of your activities for the morning when you have the most strength."

    b. "Ask your teen-agers to take care of your personal needs such as baths and shampoos."

    c. "Why not hire someone to do all your housework?"

    d. "Try to alternate each small activity with a short period of rest."

10. Mr. Bigelow is a 35-year-old artist who has been admitted with recurring pancreatitis. Both his serum and urine levels of amylase are markedly increased. The nurse should assess for any signs of which of the following?

    a. Hypocalcemia   **c.** Circulatory overload

    b. Hypoglycemia   **d.** Hyperkalemia

11. Mr. Bigelow's amylase levels have returned to normal, and he is being discharged. When he returns to the clinic next week, it would be *most important* to reemphasize a diet plan that includes which of the following?

    a. Decreased intake of starches and other carbohydrates

    b. Total restriction of alcoholic beverages

    c. Foods high in fat-soluble vitamins

    d. Frequent small feedings with an emphasis on high-caloric foods

REFERENCES

Apple, F., & McGue, M. (1983). Serum enzyme changes during marathon training. *American Journal of Clinical Pathology, 79*(6), 716–718.

Burke, D., et al. (1978). Laboratory studies: When to act on unexpected test results. *Patient Care, 12,* 14–87.

Galen, R.S., et al. (1975). Diagnosis of acute myocardial infarction: Relative efficiency of serum enzyme and isoenzyme measurements. *JAMA, 232,* 145–147.

Gann, D., et al. (1978). Optimal enzyme test combination for diagnosis of acute myocardial infarction. *Southern Medical Journal, 71*(12), 1459–1462.

Holum, J. (1983). *Elements of general and biological chemistry* (6th ed.). New York: Wiley.

Hytten, F., & Lind, T. (1975). *Diagnostic indices in pregnancy.* Summit, NJ: Ciba-Geigy Corp.

Jacobs, D., Kasten, B., DeMott, W., & Wolfson, W. (1984). *Laboratory test handbook with DRG index.* St. Louis: Mosby/Lexi.

Janul, L. (1977). Polymyositis—dermatomyositis: A perplexing disorder. *AJN, 77*(7), 1184–1186.

Lawson, T. et al. (1986). Tracking and treating acute pancreatitis. *Patient Care, 20*(1), 76–109.

Loiudice, T., Lang, J., Mehta, H., & Banta, L. (1984). Treatment of acute alcoholic pancreatitis: The roles of cimetidine and nasogastric suction. *American Journal of Gastroenterology, 79*(7), 553–558.

Ostcheya, Y., & Culnane, M. (1985). Tumor markers. *Nursing 85, 15*(9), 49–51.

Rock, R. (1980). Recent advances in the diagnostic enzymology of liver disease. *Continuing Education for Physicians, 13*(7), 64–70.

Ryan, A. (1984). What cardiac enzymes tell you about acute MI. *RN, 47*(3), 46–49.

Sibert, J.R. (1979). Pancreatitis in childhood. *Postgraduate Medical Journal, 55*(3), 171–175.

Sobel, D., & Ferguerson, T. (1985). *The people's book of medical tests.* New York: Summit Books.

Statland, B. (1979). Strenuous activity and serum enzyme values. *JAMA, 241,* 404.

Tietz, N. (Ed.). (1983). *Clinical guide to laboratory tests.* Philadelphia: Saunders.

Wallach, J. (1986). *Interpretation of diagnostic tests.* Boston: Little, Brown.

Wenger, N., et al. (1980). *Cardiology for nurses.* New York: McGraw-Hill.

13

Coagulation Tests And Tests to Detect Occult Blood

- Prothrombin Time (PT or Pro Time)
- Partial Thromboplastin Time (PTT)
- Activated Coagulation Time (ACT)
- Hemophilia Tests: Factors VIII and IX
- Platelet Count and Mean Platelet Volume (MPV)
- Bleeding Time: Modified Ivy, Simplate, Duke Method, Aspirin Tolerance Test
- Clot Retraction Test
- Fibrinogen
- Fibrinogen Degradation Products (FDP) or Fibrin Split Products (FSP)
- Thrombin Time: Fibrinogen Screen, Thrombin Clotting Time with Reptilase
- Plasminogen/Plasmin Assay
- Occult Blood: Hematest, Hemoccult, and Other Guaiac Tests

OBJECTIVES

1. Describe the four major stages of the coagulation process, as well as the difference between the intrinsic and extrinsic systems of clotting as a basis for laboratory tests.
2. Describe clinical situations where vitamin K is useful for returning the PT to normal.
3. Identify important nursing diagnoses for the client who has a bleeding tendency due to a lack of clotting factors.
4. Devise a teaching plan for a client who is discharged on long-term coumarin therapy.
5. Compare and contrast the two most common coagulation tests, PT and PTT.
6. Describe possible nursing interventions when a client has an abnormally decreased PT or PTT or other signs of hypercoagulability.

7. Explain the screening tests and confirmatory test for classical hemophilia (hemophilia A).
8. Identify possible nursing diagnoses for clients with increased and decreased platelet counts.
9. Identify the changes in fibrinogen levels, along with the changes in other laboratory tests, that are clues that disseminated intravascular clotting (DIC) or consumption coagulopathy may be occurring.
10. Describe the important facts a nurse should know about tests used to detect occult blood in the feces or other specimens.

The delicate balance of the coagulation process makes it possible for a healthy person to experience neither hemorrhage nor thrombus formation. Tests such as the PT, PTT, and platelet counts are routine tests for the clotting ability of the blood. Tests of individual factors are needed to detect specific diseases, such as hemophilia A (test for Factor VIII). Other tests, such as fibrinogen assays, help to assess severe coagulation problems, such as DIC.

Besides the common tests for clotting ability, this chapter also includes information on guaiac and other tests that are used to detect hidden or occult blood. Occult blood tests are used not only to detect bleeding tendencies, but also to screen for rectal cancer.

Laboratory tests both for clotting functions and for bleeding tendencies are of use to the nurse in three primary ways. First, these tests may alert the nurse to the possibility that the client is vulnerable due to an increased bleeding tendency. Second, some of these tests may indicate that the client is vulnerable due to an increased risk of thrombus formation. Third, three of these tests are specifically used to monitor the effects of anticoagulant dugs. The role of the nurse in anticoagulant therapy is stressed. No "magic number" determines when a client will bleed or become subject to thrombus formation. At the very best, these laboratory tests are only guidelines for helping the nurse assess the potential problems.

THE COAGULATION PROCESS

Twelve factors are involved in the clotting process. Remembering all the factors is not necessary, but knowing which test measures which factors is useful. A list of the 12 factors, along with the tests that show the deficiencies and the relation of vitamin K, is included in Table 13–1. Vitamin K was named K because it is the "Koagulation" factor. If the liver cannot obtain vitamin K, four coagulation factors cannot be manufactured: Factors II, VII, IX, and X. Note that the table contains 13 numbers, because one factor (VI) was found to really be part of another factor. The factors were numbered, instead of named, in the order of their discovery, so there could be a universal understanding of which factor was being discussed.

Table 13–1 illustrates that both the PT and PTT test several factors, but not always the same ones. Although the PTT is a broader screening test, certain deficiencies can be assessed by using both the PT and PTT. Also the laboratory can add one factor at a time to see which factor is missing.

The coagulation process can be initiated two ways. With the *extrinsic system,* the clotting is triggered by the release of tissue thromboplastin. With the *intrinsic system,* the coagulation process requires only the factors that are present in the plasma.

TABLE 13-1. COAGULATION FACTORS TESTED BY SPECIFIC TESTS AND RELATIONSHIP TO VITAMIN K

Name of Factor	Test of Deficiency	Vitamin K Needed for Production by Liver
I (fibrinogen)	Fibrinogen level[a] PT, PTT	
II (prothrombin)	PT, PTT	Yes
III (thromboplastin)		
IV (calcium)		
V (labile or proaccelerin)	PT, PTT	
VI (unassigned at present time)		
VII (stable factor or proconvertin)	PT	Yes
VIII (antihemophilic globulin)	PTT	
IX (partial thromboplastin component, Christmas factor, PTC)	PTT	Yes
X (Stuart-Prower factor)	PT, PTT	Yes
XI (plasma thromboplastin antecedent)	PTT	
XII (Hageman factor)	PTT	
XIII (fibrin stabilizing factor)		

[a]Specific assays can be done to test for each factor (see the reference values in Appendix A, Table 4).

Regardless of how the process is initiated, the coagulation process occurs in four stages. Stage I involves the release of platelet factors that begin the clotting process. Stage II is the generation of thromboplastin, as calcium and other factors interact. Stage III is the conversion of prothrombin to thrombin, and Stage IV is the formation of fibrin from fibrinogen. Some sources list three stages of coagulation because Stages I and II are combined as parts of Stage 1. Table 13-2 outlines the stages of clotting.

TABLE 13-2. STAGES OF CLOTTING AND COMMON LABORATORY TESTS

Time of Stage	Stage	Factors Involved	Major Tests for Stage
	I	Platelets initiate clotting	Platelets, clot retraction
Takes 3-5 minutes	II	Thromboplastin (Factor III) is generated by reaction of Factors VIII, IX, X, XI, and XII. Factor IV, Ca^{++}, also needed	PTT very sensitive
Takes 8-16 minutes	III	Factor II (prothrombin) is converted to thrombin. Accelerator Factors V, VII, and X are involved	PT very sensitive
Almost instantly	IV	Factor II (fibrinogen) is converted to fibrin. Factor XIII, the fibrin stabilizing factor, is needed	Fibrinogen levels

Note that some references combine Stages I and II so that:
    Stage I: Formation of thromboplastin or activation of Factor X
    Stage II: Prothrombin to thrombin
    Stage III: Fibrinogen to fibrin
See Tietz (1983); Jacobs et al. (1984); or Wallach (1986) for more details on the stages of clotting and tests used for differential diagnosing.

The importance of calcium in the clotting process should be noted. Usually a defect in calcium is not a problem due to the tremendous reservoir of calcium in the bones and teeth (see Chapter 7 on calcium). About 90% of all clotting defects occur in Stage II, the thromboplastin generation stage. Thus the PTT is a useful screening tool for many bleeding disorders.

■ PROTHROMBIN TIME (PT OR PRO TIME)

Prothrombin, or Factor II, is a plasma protein that is produced by the liver. The confusing thing about the test is that, although it is called prothrombin time, it does not measure just prothrombin, but also several other factors (see Table 13-1.) Remembering the specific names of these other factors is not necessary. The point to remember is that a major change in any, or all, of these factors causes an abnormal PT. Just like prothrombin, these other factors are manufactured in the liver and most of the factors require vitamin K for their manufacture.

The PT is used to test for a pathological lack of clotting factors due either to liver dysfunction or to an absence of vitamin K. While the absence of vitamin K may be due to an absolute lack in the body, more often it occurs because the body is unable to absorb the vitamin due to an obstruction in the common bile duct. The PT is also the specific, and the only, laboratory test used to measure the effectiveness of the coumarin type of anticoagulant drugs, such as warfarin sodium (Coumadin). Although heparin, a different type of anticoagulant, in large doses may change the PT level, two other tests are used to monitor heparin therapy. These are the PTT and the ACT, both of which are discussed later in this chapter. Although the abbreviations, PT and PTT, are very similar and thus often confusing to the novice, the tests are very different and used for two very different anticoagulants (Table 13-3).

Measurement in Seconds and Percentages
Prothrombin results may be reported (1) as time in seconds and (2) as a percentage of normal activity. The seconds reflect how long the blood sample takes to clot when certain chemicals are added. To obtain a control value, the laboratory also tests a known "normal" sample of blood by the same technique. It is important for each laboratory to establish control values because many environmental variables may change the PT results by several seconds. If the client's blood sample is deficient either in prothrombin or in one of the other clotting factors that affect the test, the client's PT in seconds will be higher than the control PT in seconds.

While many laboratories report the PT only in seconds, others report the percentage too. The percentage figure is a little harder to understand than the one in seconds. The percentage is a way of expressing the client's clotting ability as compared to the normal or control activity. In other words, the activity of the factors being tested is considered to be 100% in a control or normal blood sample. With no straight-line relationship between time and percentage, a graph has to be plotted to convert seconds to a percentage. The laboratory dilutes the normal sample to various concentrations. These various dilutions, or percentages of concentrations, are then measured to see how long each takes to clot. A graph is made that plots how percentage equals time. If a client's blood sample clots in, say, 19 seconds, then the laboratory can look at the curve and see where 19 seconds intersects wtih a certain percentage. The time of 19 seconds may reflect 50% of normal clotting ability.

TABLE 13-3. COMPARISONS OF PT AND PTT

	PT	PTT (Activated)
Drugs monitored	Coumarin-type drugs, i.e., bishydroxycoumarin (Dicumarol), warfarin sodium (Coumadin), phenprocoumon (Liquamar).	Heparin
Reference values (control)	60–140% activity 12–15 seconds	No report in percentage 25–37 seconds
Desirable therapeutic levels	1.3–2.5 times control[a]	1.5–2.5 times control
Time of drug to affect laboratory test	Oral coumarin takes several *days* to achieve therapeutic level.	Intravenous heparin acts immediately. (Subcutaneous not usually used except for prophylaxis.)
Usual timing of laboratory test	On daily basis until stabilized. Then 2–3 times per week, and eventually once every 3–4 weeks for long-term control.	Once daily if continuous intravenous or ½–1 hour before the next intermittent dose. (PTT not changed if mini doses of heparin used as prophylaxis.)
Measures used to return laboratory test to normal	1. Reduction of dosage 2. Whole blood 3. Vitamin K$_1$ parenterally (Aqua Mephyton)	1. Reduction of dosage 2. Whole blood 3. Protamine sulfate parenterally
Time of reversability	1. Varies with dosage reduction 2. Immediate with transfusion 3. Several hours for vitamin K	1. Varies with dosage reduction 2. Immediate with transfusion 3. Immediate with protamine

Examples of common[b] drugs affecting results of test	Increase PT time:
	  Alcohol
	  Anabolic steroids
	  Antibiotics
	  Cimetidine (Tagamet)
	  Salicylates
	  Sulfonamides
	  Thyroxine
	  Quinidine (plus many others)
	
	Decrease PT time:
	  Barbiturates
	  Ethchlorvynol (Placidyl)
	  Glutethimide (Doriden)
	  Griseofulvin
	  Oral contraceptives
	  Vitamin K in nutritional supplements, such as Ensure
		Increase PTT time:
		  Salicylates
		  Dipyridamole (Persantine)
		
		May decrease PTT time:
		  Digitalis
		  Tetracyclines
		  Antihistamines
		  Nicotine

[a]Some authorities consider 2 times the control as ample anticoagulation (Errichetti et al., 1984).
[b]See text for explanation and Kirschenbaum and Rosenberg (1982); Gever (1983); Govoni and Hayes (1985); and McConnell (1986) for more details.

Percentages may vary somewhat because each laboratory must make its own graph for correlating times and percentages. Because the percentages must be based on dilution curves, their use may lead to inaccuracy. It is important to realize that 19 seconds may be translated into two different percentages by two different laboratories. In a general sense, the percentage is useful in illustrating how the client's clotting ability compares to the control. For example, a client with a PT of only 20% has only about one-fifth of the clotting ability of the "normal" person used as the control. One might suppose that the greatest clotting factor ability that a client could have would be 100%. Yet remember that for a percentage of normal activity there is a range in "normal." So a figure over 100% can result for the client who has a clotting time that is faster than the control picked by the laboratory. Thus percentages of 60–140% are considered normal individual variations. See Appendix A for percentage values for all the other factors that may be measured. Note that some have as wide a variation as 50–200%.

Relationship of Time to Percentage

An increase in time always means a decrease in percentage of activity, and vice versa, because as the clotting activity of the blood decreases, the blood takes longer to clot. If the percentage of activity is below 60%, the client's PT in seconds is increased to more than the control time. On the other hand, if the client's PT in seconds decreases from, say, 20–12 seconds, then the percentage of clotting activity has increased or risen to somewhere near the 100% normal activity. PT results in textbooks or on charts are sometimes reported just as an "increased PT." This notation means an increase in *time,* not in activity. An increase in the PT time means the percentage of activity is less than normal.

Special Preparation of Client

Note that many drugs can affect the PT (see Table 13–3). Make a note on the laboratory slip of any heparin dosage, because the PT may be affected at the peak of heparin activity. Venous blood (4.5 ml) is collected in plastic tubes with 3.8% sodium citrate (blue top).

Increased PT (Increase in Time and Consequent Decrease in Percentage) or Hypoprothrombinemia

Clinical Significance. A variety of pathologic conditions cause an increased PT. (Remember that an "increased" PT means an *increase* in the seconds and a *decrease* in the percentage. It is easier to speak of an increased PT, rather than spelling it out.)

A client may have an increased PT because the liver is unable to make prothrombin and the other factors measured by the PT test. An increased PT is very characteristic of advanced cirrhosis of the liver. In cirrhosis, a lot of scar tissue takes the place of functioning liver cells, and these nonfunctioning liver cells can no longer make prothrombin. PT is a valuable tool in assessing the amount of liver damage in the client with liver disease. Unlike other situations where the PT is increased, vitamin K injections usually do not help much with advanced liver disease. The inability of the liver to respond to vitamin K, as evidenced by little change in the PT after the vitamin K injection, demonstrates that the liver is so damaged that it cannot produce more prothrombin and other factors, even with abundant vitamin K.

Another clinical reason for an increased PT is the body's inability to absorb vitamin K from the gastrointestinal tract. Because vitamin K is a fat-soluble vitamin, absorption depends on the presence of bile salts. With an obstruction of the com-

---

Reference Values for PT

Adult	Control 11–16 seconds (+ or − 2 seconds). Percentage of normal activity should be close to 100%, but most sources consider a range of 60–140% to be normal variations in percentages.
Newborn	Certain clotting factors are lower than adults', so reference values may be around 12–21 seconds. Prematures may have even higher reference values in seconds.
Pregnancy	In late pregnancy, certain clotting factors are increased, so reference values may be slightly decreased for time in seconds (Howie, 1979). Oral contraceptives also cause increase in clotting factors (see Appendix D).

---

mon bile duct, bile salts cannot be released into the duodenum. So a client who has obstructive jaundice, which is caused by an obstruction in the common bile duct, has an increased PT because the liver cannot get vitamin K.

Much rarer is a true deficiency of vitamin K in the body, because humans do not depend much on dietary sources for vitamin K. This vitamin is manufactured by the bacteria that normally reside in the intestinal tract. So if a client is on long-term antibiotic therapy that wipes out the normal bacteria in the gastrointestinal tract, the client may have an increased PT caused by an absolute deficiency of vitamin K. For example, clients receiving a beta-lactum antibiotic, may also receive 10 mg of vitamin K weekly to prevent hypoprothrombinemia (Govoni & Hayes, 1985). Unlike the client with a failing liver, the client with a vitamin K deficiency or malabsorption problem has an increased PT that can be returned to normal by the administration of vitamin K. When the vitamin is given parenterally, it is absorbed into the bloodstream and bypasses the digestive step that requires bile salts. (See Chapter 11 for more discussion on obstructive jaundice and hypoprothrombinemia in relation to the test of direct bilirubin.)

The newborn's prothrombin time is slightly prolonged because infants do not have the same quantity of some of the clotting factors as adults. Newborns also do not have a store of vitamin K, and they have not yet acquired the normal intestinal bacteria to produce the vitamin. Newborn infants of mothers who are deficient in vitamin K are thus susceptible to a disease called *hemorrhagic disease of the newborn*. A dose of vitamin K, given prophylactically to all newborns, guards against the possibility of hemorrhage in the first few days.

Another hemorrhagic situation with an increased PT is in the complex bleeding disorder called DIC. This clinical situation is discussed in detail at the end of this chapter, along with fibrinogen levels.

Effect of Coumarin on PT. In all the situations discussed above, an increased PT time of 24 seconds, with a corresponding percentage of normal activity of around 20–25%, would be indicative of a severe pathological state. For a patient who is anticoagulated with one of the coumarin-type drugs, such as warfarin sodium (Coumadin), the therapeutic goal is usually to have the PT time about 1.5–2.5 times the control. Some clinics may have the upper limit at 2 times the control (Errichetti et al., 1984). Coumarin-type drugs cause a decrease in the production of prothrombin and of other factors because these drugs interfere with the liver's use of vitamin K. Because the coumarin-type drugs work in this indirect way, by depressing liver function, the change in the PT does not occur for a day or longer. It usually takes several days to get the PT time 1.5–2 times the control. Vitamin K, taken orally or parenterally, reverses the effects of these drugs, returning the PT to normal within several hours. Obviously, a PT in the normal range may be dangerous for the client who needs to be anticoagulated in the first place. Refer to Table 13–3 for a summary of information about coumarin drugs and PT monitoring.

POSSIBLE NURSING DIAGNOSES RELATED TO INCREASED PT

Potential for Bleeding Related to Hypoprothrombinemia

The nurse caring for a client with an increased PT needs a clear understanding of whether this person is likely to be vulnerable to bleeding for a long time or if this abnormal PT is of short duration. For example, if the client has an increased PT as a result of obstructive jaundice, vitamin K brings the PT back to normal within a few hours or at most within a day or so. In this case, one should not need to burden the client and family with a long list of all the possible ways to protect the person from bleeding. On the other hand, the client who is being discharged on a coumarin-type drug needs to know that a PT of 24 seconds and a 20–25% normal clotting activity makes a person vulnerable to bleeding. These clients and their families need detailed instructions on how to treat bleeding episodes. Vitamin K is one antidote for coumarin overdosage (whole blood is the other), but many physicians do not want clients to carry this drug if they are close to a medical facility. Clients with severe liver disease may also be functioning with an increased PT that is of a chronic nature. They need to be taught how to protect themselves from bleeding episodes. As mentioned earlier, probably vitamin K will not help this PT very much. Clients with liver disease are very likely to eventually have severe bleeding episodes.

Assessing and Preventing Bleeding Episodes. Nurses must always be looking for symptoms that could indicate that a client might be bleeding, because a bleeding episode is the possible consequence in any client with an increased PT. Nurses must also be aware of the ways to prevent bleeding. They must use their own judgment about which parts of the following assessment and interventions are needed for an individual client. The degree of client involvement in protecting him- or herself from bleeding depends on the level of illness and the setting of home or hospital. Nurses must assess the client's level of understanding, readiness for information about the condition or treatment, and willingness and ability to participate in health care.

When caring for a client who has a bleeding tendency due to an abnormal PT and other factors, nurses need to be aware of all the subtle clues that can be a symptom of bleeding. As the persons who probably spend the most time with the client, nurses have the opportunity and responsibility to detect these subtle changes before a bleeding episode becomes a major catastrophe. So a complete assessment and prevention of bleeding would include the following:

1. Headaches or changes in the neurological status could indicate bleeding into the cranium. A headache would be of particular concern if the client has had a head injury.
2. Clients with increased PT must be protected from falls. Sports or other activities that could lead to head blows are risky.

3. Shaving should be done with an electric razor to prevent bleeding from accidental cuts.

4. Epistaxis (nose bleeding) and gum bleeding may occur too. So too vigorous tooth brushing, hard coughing, or blowing the nose may trigger a bleeding episode. Nose bleeding in these clients can be a serious matter.

5. Nurses must be particularly careful when suctioning a client who has a bleeding tendency.

6. Vomiting or coughing up blood can be quite serious. The physician should be notified immediately, even if the vomitus contains only a small amount of blood. Often the small amount of blood that is vomited first is just the first indication. Fresh blood looks like blood. Older blood, which has been acted upon by the gastric juices, has a characteristic dark brown color that is called "coffee-ground."

7. In a client with a nasogastric tube, the drainage may be coffee-ground color rather than the yellowish to pale green color of normal stomach contents. Not all coffee-ground drainage from nasogastric tubes means the client is having a lot of bleeding. Sometimes just the presence of the nasogastric tube causes enough irritation to have minimial and nonsignificant bleeding. Yet for a client with an increased PT, any bleeding may be serious.

   Tests can be done to detect occult bleeding in gastric secretions. Yet, obviously, if there is frank blood, doing a guaiac test is a waste. The nurse must also be very careful about the irrigations of a nasogastric tube for a client with bleeding tendencies. Iced saline lavage may be used to control gastric bleeding. Antacids and cimetidine (Tagamet) may be ordered to decrease gastric hyperacidity. (See the section on guaiac and other tests at the end of this chapter.)

8. The client with severe liver disease may also have esophageal varices (varicosities) that can be the source of a massive bleed. The client with suspected varices may have diet restrictions so that only soft foods are served.

9. Abdominal or flank pain may indicate slow internal bleeding. Internal bleeding can be very subtle in the beginning, with few symptoms, because the bleeding usually takes place at a slow rate. A client may complain of a backache that cannot be relieved with back rubs, a change of position, or the administration of a mild analgesic. No one may think about a possible connection to the anticoagulant the client is receiving until the client faints when he or she tries to get out of bed. Then it is discovered that the client has been slowly bleeding into the retroperitoneal area.

   Internal bleeding can cause pain because of the increasing pressure as blood collects. If the bleeding is into the gastrointestinal tract, however, there will probably not be any associated pain because the blood does not cause undue pressure, and if the client has an ulcer, the blood acts as a buffer (Decker, 1985). The blood eventually passes into the stool, but it may be occult, or hidden.

   So clients with a bleeding tendency should periodically test the stools for occult blood. Hematocrits will be useful to assess the exact amount of blood loss (see Chapter 2). The tests for occult blood, described at the end of this chapter, are simple enough that clients can be taught to do a test at home if the situation warrants doing so. If the bleeding is fairly copious and high enough in the gastrointestinal tract to be in contact with the digestive juices, the stools take on a dark black color that is described as "tarry." Straining at stool may cause bleeding, especially if the client has hemorrhoids, so the nurse needs to help the client find ways to avoid constipation.

10. Dark or smokey-looking urine may indicate blood in the urine. Hematuria is often the first indication of overdosage with anticoagulants. Sometimes the blood is bright red if it is fresh. Some physicians may order daily urine tests to check for the presence of red blood cells in the urine. While the laboratory can check for red cells by a microscopic examination, which is more sensitive for intact erythrocytes, nurses may do dipstick tests for blood in the urine too. (See Chapter 3 on hematuria.) Clients who have catheters may bleed from the irritation of the catheter. Nurses should make sure the catheter is securely anchored with tape so it does not slide up and down the meatus. Female patients with bleeding tendencies due to an abnormal PT will probably have heavy menses, and they should be aware of this possibility.

11. Pain in or immobility of a joint can indicate bleeding into the joint. Nurses must think of all the things necessary to protect the client from falls and trauma. When active children are clients, doing so may be a real challenge to the parents and to the nurse. Specific points about bleeding due to classic hemophilia (hemophilia A) are discussed under the test for Factor VIII.

12. Taking blood pressure and the pulse are two other ways to detect bleeding. A slight but steady increase in the pulse rate may be a subtle sign of bleeding, long before the blood pressure drops.

13. Some hospitals have a policy of avoiding intramuscular injections, if at all possible, for clients with bleeding tendencies. If an intramuscular injection must be given, choose the smallest gauge needle possible and apply pressure for ten minutes after the injection.

Also alert laboratory personnel to the client's bleeding tendency. Place a note on the kardex so everyone is aware of the client's bleeding tendency. When laboratory personnel come to draw blood, a nurse needs to remind them of the potential bleeding problem. The fingerstick method to obtain blood should be used whenever possible if the bleeding tendency is severe. (See Chapter 1 for the fingerstick procedure.) Laboratory personnel do not usually look at the kardex, so another good idea is to make a notation about bleeding on the laboratory requisition. Some hospitals put a sign on the client's door to alert all personnel to the bleeding tendency. The nurse can be inventive in particular settings to make sure everyone who will be doing things with the client knows about the bleeding tendency.

Special Needs for the Surgery Client. If a client with an increased PT must go to surgery, it is imperative that the PT be medically corrected before the operation. To get the PT back to a safe level for surgery, vitamin K injections may be ordered. For example, clients who have had valve replacements are usually on long-term anticoagulation therapy to prevent thrombus formation around the valve. If the client needs an emergency appendectomy, the conversion to a normal PT is done in conjunction with heparin replacement as an anticoagulant. When anticoagulant therapy is necessary during a surgical procedure, the client will be switched to heparin because this short-term anticoagulant can be more easily controlled (see PTT) and quickly reversed with protamine. Whole blood should always be available for the client with an abnormal PT who must have surgery because whole blood supplies the missing clotting factors. A type and cross match are done as part of the preoperative preparation. (See Chapter 14 on type and cross match.)

Knowledge Deficit Related to Long-term Anticoagulation

Clients on coumarin therapy are usually on this anticoagulant for a long time. No matter how long they are taking the drug, they must continue to have prothrombin tests (PT) done periodically. It is critical that clients understand the importance of continuing the PTs because the balance between maintaining the needed anticoagulation and preventing bleeding episodes is always precarious. The PT should remain within the predetermined range considered therapeutic for that client. It can be very dangerous for clients to take anticoagulants if they are not followed well with frequent assessments of the PT. Once a client is on a maintenance dose of the drug, the PT may be drawn monthly.

Clients also need explicit *written* instructions about the anticoagulation medicine and the date to return to the clinic office. Some clients may also need to be referred to a public health nurse for a follow-up visit, to more fully assess their health needs if they do not return to have their PT drawn at the clinic. Laboratories all over the world can check PTs. For example, if a person travels to Europe, arrangements can be made to get PTs done at various labs.

When the client is on coumarin-type drugs, a wide variety of other drugs may interact with them so as to cause changes in the PT, either to increase or to decrease the PT. Aspirin and other salicylates potentiate the effect of coumarin, thus increasing the PT time. Often the client is not aware that many pain medications, such as cold remedies, contain aspirin. Brand drugs, such as Percodan, Empirin, or Darvon Compound, all contain aspirin. In fact, more than five hundred aspirin-containing compounds are available commercially. Certainly the client needs to be instructed not to take any medication without consulting the physician who is prescribing the anticoagulant. The coumarin-type drugs are responsible for more adverse drug reactions than any other group. Govoni and Hayes (1985) describe in detail the interactive effect of over 100 drugs with coumarin anticoagulants. (See Table 13–3 for some common interactions.)

Decreased Prothrombin Time

Clinical Significance. Sometimes clients may have a PT time of 8 or 9 seconds, compared to a control of 11 or 12 seconds, or their percentage of activity may be greater than 100%. The reduced prothrombin time may be associated with medications such as oral contraceptives, barbiturates, digitalis, diuretics, or vitamin K. It may also reflect pathology, such as thrombophlebitis or certain malignancies. The reduced prothrombin time, however, is not of clinical significance as a diagnostic tool.

POSSIBLE NURSING DIAGNOSIS RELATED TO REDUCED PT

Potential for Injury Related to Formation of Venous Thrombi
A reduced prothrombin time may indicate hypercoagulability of the blood. Hypercoagulability of the blood, venous stasis, and injury to the venous wall are the three conditions that contribute to the formation of *venous* thrombi. Prolonged bedrest and surgery also increase the possibility of thrombus formation. (Note that the condition associated with *arterial* thrombosis is atherosclerosis. See Chapter 9 on lipid metabolism.) It is thought that at least two of the three conditions (Virchow's triad) must be present to have thrombosis formation in the veins. Venous thrombi are found most often in the deep veins of the legs or in pelvic veins.

When a client has known hypercoagulability of the blood, the primary goal of the nurse is to decrease the possibility of venous thrombi formation by such measures as leg exercises, adequate hydration, and no venous constrictions, such as crossing the legs. (See the discussion under PTT on the effectiveness of low doses of heparin to prevent deep-vein thrombosis.)

■ PARTIAL THROMBOPLASTIN TIME (PTT)

The PTT, a nonspecific test, can demonstrate a lack of any of the various clotting factors, except Factor VII (stable factor), that function in the intrinsic clotting system (see Table 13–1). Because some clotting tests, such as the PT, bypass the intrinsic clotting system, they are not useful to screen for general plasma deficiencies. The PTT, on the contrary, is very useful in detecting the presence of many types of bleeding disorders caused by defective or deficient circulating factors that compose the intrinsic system. If the PTT is abnormal, further tests are needed to pinpoint exactly which factor is defective or deficient.

The other purpose for the PTT is to monitor heparin therapy because heparin, a short-acting anticoagulant that circulates in the plasma, increases the PTT. Table 13–3 summarizes the use of the PTT for monitoring heparin.

Essentially, the laboratory technique for measuring the PTT involves adding certain chemicals to the client's blood sample and timing, in seconds, the formation of a clot. If chemicals are also added to accelerate the clotting time, the result is reported as an "activated" PTT. The client's results in seconds are compared to a control that was tested using the same method. Like the PT, a control is done on

---

Reference Values for PTT

Adult	25–38 seconds for activated PTT or 60–90 seconds if not activated
Pregnancy	May be normally decreased by a few seconds Also may be decreased with oral contraceptives (see Appendix D)
Newborn	Range is increased above adult level

"normal" blood because so many environmental variables can affect each individual situation. Unlike the PT, there is no percentage report.

The specific techniques may vary from laboratory to laboratory.

Special Preparation of Client and Collection of the Sample
Venous blood is collected (4.5 ml) in a tube containing 3.8% sodium citrate (blue Vacutainer). If the patient is being anticoagulated, note the time, dosages and route of the heparin dosage.

Increased PTT

Clinical Significance. An increased PTT, when the client is not on heparin, signifies a bleeding disorder. Further tests must be done to determine which factor is deficient. The abnormality, or the lack of a factor, may be either acquired or hereditary.

The most common hereditary disorder is lack of Factor VIII (antihemophilic globulin), which results in the classical hemophilia, or hemophilia A. An inherited deficiency in Factor IX (plasma thromboplastin component or Christmas factor) results in the condition known as Christmas disease, or hemophilia B. Often the client's history gives clues that the increased PTT is due to a familial condition. (See the tests for Factors VIII and IX). Specific assays for different factors in the plasma definitively establish the diagnosis.

Acquired deficiencies may be more subtle and difficult to connect to any specific cause. The PTT becomes elevated in a complex bleeding disorder where the clotting factors are used up at an abnormal rate. This disorder, DIC, is discussed in detail at the end of this chapter, along with fibrinogen levels. Autologous blood transfusions may cause an elevated PTT (Gillott & Thomas, 1984).

If the client is on heparin, an increase in the PTT is the result of the effects of the circulating anticoagulant in the plasma. Usually the PTT is kept about 1.5–2.5 times the control value. So if the control is 36 seconds, a range of 54–90 seconds would be desirable for the client. A report of 110 seconds would indicate more-than-adequate anticoagulation for that moment when the blood was drawn. A report of 45 seconds would indicate inadequate anticoagulation for the moment the blood was drawn. (At the very best, the PTT reflects only heparin activity at the moment the sample was taken, because heparin activity in the blood varies from moment to moment.)

POSSIBLE NURSING DIAGNOSES RELATED TO ELEVATED PTT

Potential for Injury Related to Increased Risk for Bleeding
An abnormal PTT necessitates postponement of surgery unless it is an emergency. If the PTT is being used as routine check before surgery, such as a tonsillectomy, the test must be done early enough so that the reports are on the chart before the client goes to surgery. Easy bruisability does not always mean a bleeding disorder, but any evidence of past bleeding difficulties needs to be assessed medically before operative or other invasive procedures, such as an arteriogram, are done. See Chapter 25 for the risk of bleeding with invasive procedures.

Anxiety Related to Bleeding Disorder
If the PTT is elevated, several tests may be needed to evaluate the client's clot-

ting ability. Nurses may also be helpful in allowing the client and the family to express their concerns and anxieties about an unknown medical diagnosis. Any client with an elevated PTT has an increased tendency to bleed and thus client teaching for preventing bleeding, discussed earlier, would be appropriate. Griffin (1986) notes that stress may activate the bleeding process so biofeedback and imagery may be useful tools to decrease the client's stress.

Potential for Injury Related to Heparin Therapy

Heparin may be given subcutaneously, intravenously every 4 hours or every 6 hours, or continuously by intravenous drip. The various techniques for giving heparin vary widely from hospital to hospital and from location to location (Sohn, 1981). Before assuming responsibility for heparin administration, the nurse should check to see the results of the latest PTT. To maximize the usefulness of the PTT, nurses must know the time that the PTT was drawn in relation to the last heparin dose. The medical decision to give or not to give the antidote for heparin, protamine sulfate, depends partially on being able to establish how long the PTT was abnormally high. An abnormally high PTT should always be reported immediately before the next dose of heparin is administered. Failure to report an increased PTT has led to a law suit (Northrop, 1986). The nurse must also note if the PTT is *below* the therapeutic range. The PTT report should be called to the attention of the doctor at once, so he or she can reevaluate the situation and readjust the dosage accordingly. It can be as dangerous for the client to remain *under*-anticoagulated as *over*-anticoagulated.

Because heparin activity may vary from moment to moment, it would be a mistake to think that all one needs to adjust the dosage is one PTT. Seeing the range of the PTT gives guidelines to the physician in adjusting the dosage for each individual. Some hospitals use flow sheets so that the PTT can be charted with the dosage of heparin and compared over an extended period. This chart makes it easier to get a clearer picture of the ongoing status of the anticoagulant therapy. Note that a heparin-associated thrombocytopenia can develop, so platelet counts should be ordered (King & Kelton, 1984). See the discussion later in this chapter.

Checking for Drug Interferences. Drugs that interfere with the action of heparin are not as numerous as those that interfere with the coumarin-type drugs, but certain drugs do affect the PTT. The use of digitalis, tetracyclines, nicotine, and histamines may partially counteract the effect of heparin. The potential interaction of these drugs may be significant if they are added or deleted during the time the client is on heparin therapy. Because drugs containing aspirin increase the bleeding time, they should be avoided when the client is on heparin. The reason is that when a client is anticoagulated, platelet aggregation is the main defense against bleeding, and aspirin decreases the adhesiveness of platelets, thus potentiating the bleeding tendency from any type of anticoagulation.

Use of Heparin in Mini-Doses. There is one type of clinical situation in which the PTT need not be checked, even though the client is on heparin. This is when heparin is given in low doses of usually about 5000 units subcutaneously every 8–12 hours. The purpose of the mini-dose is to prevent the possible occurrence of thromboembolic episodes in clients who are high risk due to certain surgical procedures or prolonged bedrest. Studies have shown that the prophylactic use of heparin in small doses can significantly decrease the risk of pulmonary embolus in high risk clients (Sherry, 1976). Heparin may also be combined with dihydroergotamine, which decreases venous stasis (Multicenter Trial Committee, 1984). These doses of heparin are small enough so that they do not significantly affect the PTT. A base-line PTT may be ordered, but nurses do not need to check PTT results before giving each small prophylactic dose of heparin.

Knowledge Deficit Related to Possible Need for Long-term Anticoagulation

Because heparin must be given parenterally and requires close medical supervision, clients do not usually go home on heparin therapy. Client teaching—about drugs to avoid, when to return for tests, and the like—is not a necessity as it is with long-term anticoagulants. If long-term anticoagulants are necessary to prevent other thromboembolic episodes, the usual pattern is to begin with a coumarin-type drug after 5–6 days of heparin therapy and continue both types of anticoagulants until the PT is within the desired range. For example, long-term anticoagulation might be needed for a client who has had a pulmonary embolus (DeMeester et al., 1978). During this switch from heparin to long-term oral anticoagulants, both the PT and PTT need to be monitored and clients need the instructions about coumarin discussed above.

Decreased PTT

Clinical Significance. A PTT lower than the control sample is not diagnostically significant, but it may be a clue reflecting hypercoagulability. (See the discussion under PT for the conditions that may cause increased clotting and how nursing care can help to prevent venous thrombus formation.) Some degree of hypercoagulability is normal in pregnancy, but it can lead to problems (Redman, 1979).

■ ACTIVATED COAGULATION TIME (ACT)

Although the PTT is usually used to monitor heparin therapy, the activated coagulation, or clotting, time can also be used. The ACT, done at the bedside, is commonly used during cardiovascular surgery and in intensive care units. The ACT may also be used to screen for some coagulation deficiencies. This test has replaced the older Lee-White coagulation test (Jacobs et al., 1984).

As with the PTT, the results are not significant unless the timing is correlated with heparin administration. For a clearer picture of the true anticoagulated state of the client, clinicians need to use a flow sheet that lists all the test results with the time and route of dosage given. If the coagulation time is not in the desired therapeutic range, the nurse has the responsibility to notify the physician. The nursing implications for a client with bleeding tendencies are covered under the discussion on PT and PTT. The nurse must always keep in mind that a client on any anticoagulation therapy can bleed, even if laboratory results indicate a satisfactory condition.

Preparation of Client and Collection of Sample

The test is done at bedside by a technologist or other clinician. Whole blood is drawn into special tubes that contain an activator such as siliceous earth (tubes and syringes should be warmed to 37°C). Time to clot is monitored immediately. If the client is on continuous heparin drip, use the other arm to obtain venous sample.

Reference Values for ACT

70-120 seconds (depends on type of activator used)
Desirable range for anticoagulation may be 150-190 seconds

■ HEMOPHILIA TESTS: FACTORS VIII AND IX

The two main types of hemophilia are called A (classical hemophilia) and B (Christmas disease). Classical hemophilia has been the curse of several royal families in Europe. Christmas disease was named for the family who was studied with the genetic defect of Factor IX. The specific diagnosis of classical hemophilia is made by assay of Factor VIII and for Christmas disease by assay of Factor IX. The cause of over 80% of all hemophilias is a deficiency of Factor VIII (Dressler, 1980). Because the PTT is prolonged in hemophilia, it is a screening test for bleeding disorders. The client has normal prothrombin time (PT) and platelet counts.

Preparation of Client and Collection of Sample
Venous blood (4.5 ml) is collected in plastic tubes with 3.8% sodium citrate (blue Vacutainer).

Reference Values for Factor VIII and IX

Factor VIII (antihemophilic globulin)	50–200%
Factor IX (plasma thromboplastic cofactor)	60–140%
See Appendix A, Table 4, for reference values for other factors.	

POSSIBLE NURSING DIAGNOSES RELATED TO DEFICIENCY IN FACTORS

Impaired Home Maintenance Management
The general nursing implications for a client with bleeding tendencies were discussed in the section on PT. Because factor replacement therapy is available, many bleeding episodes can be prevented or treated before damage occurs to joints or to other vital areas. Older children and their parents are also taught to mix the factor concentrate and to do the intravenous infusion (Dressler, 1980). Home therapy for children with hemophilia has been successful, and research (McGuire, 1985) has shown children treated at home displayed improved social adaptive skills as well as improved physical capabilities. Govoni and Hayes (1985) describe the nursing implications of factor therapy.

Anxiety Related to Transmitting a Genetic Disease
See Chapter 18 for a discussion on genetic counseling. Both A and B are in-herited as X-linked recessive traits. In other words, female carriers transmit the gene to half their daughters and to half their sons. The females who receive the defective gene do not have the disease because they also have another "healthy" X. On the contrary, any male who receives the defective X shows symptoms because he does not have a healthy X to balance the effect. Hemo-philia may be mild, moderate, or severe, depending on how much of the factor is produced. Hemophilia can also result from spontaneous mutations.

■ PLATELET COUNT AND MEAN PLATELET VOLUME (MPV)

Sometimes platelets are considered as a third type of blood cell in the plasma. (See Chapter 2 for RBC and WBC). Actually, platelets are not intact cells but only frag-ments of cytoplasm whose only role seems to be in the blood coagulation process. As platelets adhere to the wall of an injured vessel, they clump together (or aggre-gate) and release a substance that begins the coagulation process. Platelets are formed by the bone marrow and removed by the reticuloendothelial system when they are old. The spleen is a major component of the reticuloendothelial system.

Special Preparation of Client and Collection of Sample
The laboratory uses 0.5 cc of blood. EDTA is used as the anticoagulant (lavender top). The count is usually done by a machine, but, if the count is low, it is confirmed by a hand count. Smears can also be done to estimate the number of platelets.

Reference Values for Platelets

Adult   150,000–350,000/mm³
Females have a significantly decreased platelet count for the first few days of
   menses (Wallach, 1986).
Platelets are increased after labor and delivery
Newborns have lower values

Note that the mean platelet volume (MPV) can be measured. Reference values are 7.4 to 10.4 μm³. Larger platelets apparently have better hemostatic function.

Increased Platelet Count (Thrombocytosis)

Clinical Significance. Malignancies, especially advanced or metastatic cases, may cause an elevated platelet count or thrombocytosis. Many clients with an "unexpected" high platelet count are found to have a malignancy. Clients with polycythemia very often have high platelet counts too. (Polycythemia is discussed in Chapter 2 under the section on red blood cells.) Another reason for an increased platelet count is the removal of the spleen, or splenectomy, which causes a temporary increase in the plate-let count. Clients with sickle cell disease have increased platelets (Wallach, 1986).

POSSIBLE NURSING DIAGNOSES RELATED TO ELEVATED PLATELET COUNTS

Potential for Injury Related to Thromboembolic Episodes

A logical assumption is that an increased amount of platelets tends to make the blood more coagulable. As discussed in the section on decreased PT and hypercoagulability, dehydration could be dangerous for a client with a high platelet count. Venous stasis may be of particular concern. Depending on the reason for the thrombocytosis, thrombus formation may or may not be a possibility. For example, the increased platelet count after a splenectomy does not seem to cause any problems.

If thrombus formation is considered a possibility, aspirin, which is used as a mild anticoagulant in certain situations, is sometimes ordered to decrease the adhesiveness of platelets. To prevent gastric irritation, the client needs to be taught either to take aspirin with milk or to dilute it with water.

Potential for Injury Related to Bleeding

Surprisingly, an increased number of platelets does not always mean an increased tendency to clot. In fact, it may mean an increased tendency to bleed. This paradox can be partially explained by the fact that sometimes the increased number of platelets are abnormal ones that cannot function properly in the coagulation process. Thus a client with thrombocytosis may need to be watched for bleeding tendencies. See the detailed assessment guide in the section on PT.

Low Platelet Count (Thrombocytopenia)

Clinical Significance. If the cause of the low platelet count, or thrombocytopenia, is unknown, the condition is called "idiopathic" (unknown cause) thrombocytopenia purpura. "Purpura" refers to bruising. Children who have idiopathic thrombocytopenia purpura often have spontaneous remissions. A low platelet count may occur after a viral infection (Koch, 1984) and is common with AIDS (Wallach, 1986). A low count can be associated with some types of anemias or other hemolytic disorders. Substances that depress bone marrow function, such as chemotherapeutic drugs or radiation, also depress the platelet count. King (1984) lists over 50 drugs that can cause thrombocytopenia. An overactive spleen (hypersplenism) or an enlarged spleen (splenomegaly) destroys platelets at too fast a rate. Severe thrombocytopenia often follows any type of extracorporeal bypass or autotransfusion (Gillott & Thomas, 1984). Because heparin can cause thrombocytopenia, a platelet count may be done every third day while the client is on heparin. (Ramirez-Lassepas et al., 1984).

POSSIBLE NURSING DIAGNOSES RELATED TO THROMBOCYTOPENIA

Potential for Injury Related to Bleeding

When a client has a low platelet count, the major nursing concern is protecting the person from bruising and bleeding. Petechiae are the most common manifestations of thrombocytopenia because the many microscopic injuries that occur continuously in the capillaries are not immediately sealed off due to the lack of platelets. A decrease in the platelet count to 20,000 or less/mm^3 usually puts clients at risk for spontaneous hemorrhage (Silinsky, 1985). Yet some clients may bleed with higher counts. Certain activities may need to be curtailed until the platelet count is returned to normal. In the case of an active child, protection from trauma requires a lot of ingenuity on the part of the nurse and the parents. Symptoms that indicate bleeding are described in detail in the section on nursing implications for an increased PT. Clients may be embarrassed by the bruises on their arms and legs, and so they appreciate clothing to conceal the bruises from curious onlookers.

Potential for Infection Related to Leukopenia, Anemia or Drug Therapy

If the thrombocytopenia is a result of general bone marrow depression, the implications about leukopenia (low white cell count) and anemia (low red cell count) must also be considered. (Related nursing diagnoses are covered in Chapter 2.) Adult clients, and sometimes children, with a low platelet count may be put on corticosteroid therapy, which is given to raise the platelet count to normal (Froberg, 1986). The potential for infection is created by the use of the cortisone-type drugs. (See Chapter 15 on cortisone therapy for other nursing diagnoses.)

In idiopathic thrombocytopenia purpura, sometimes the removal of the spleen is necessary to get the platelet count back to normal. If such surgery is scheduled, the nurse can help to prepare the client for the surgical experience. Adult clients usually have few problems after the spleen is removed because the role of the spleen can be taken over by other parts of the reticuloendothelial system. For children, a splenectomy is usually not done because the spleen is important for antibody production.

Potential for Injury Related to Platelet Transfusions

If thrombocytopenia results from a malignancy or from treatment with chemotherapy drugs, platelet transfusions may be given. Clients with counts of less than 10,000/mm^3 usually require platelet transfusions, while those with more may receive transfusions only if hemorrhage begins (Wroblewski & Wroblewski, 1981). Because patients may become sensitized to the platelet concentrates, transfusions are reserved for those who are at great risk. Three of the major problems in platelet transfusions are allergic reactions, hypervolemia, and bacterial sepsis (Hernandez, 1980).

■ BLEEDING TIME: MODIFIED IVY, SIMPLATE, DUKE METHOD, ASPIRIN TOLERANCE TEST

Bleeding time is a screening test for disorders of platelets or for certain vascular defects in the clotting process. The laboratory technologist does the test at the bedside. For the modified Ivy method a commercial device (Simplate Bleeding Time Device by General Diagnostics) is used to make two small puncture wounds in the forearm. (The Ivy method was done freehand.) If the arm cannot be used, the ear lobe is used (Duke method).

Preparation of Client and Collection of Sample

The technologist places a blood pressure cuff on the client's arm. The pressure is kept at 40 mm Hg. After two small puncture wounds are made on the forearm, the bleeding time is measured by a stopwatch. The bleeding area is blotted with filter paper every 30 seconds. There is a small possibility of scar formation from the wound punctures so some laboratories have the client or guardian sign a consent form (Jacobs et al., 1984). A small dressing is placed over the site. The client should not have had any aspirin or anticoagulants for at least a week before the test. Sometimes the test is done before and after aspirin dosage to assess the effect of the aspirin on the bleeding time (aspirin tolerance test).

Reference Values for Bleeding Times

Duke Method (earlobe)	1–4 minutes
Modified Ivy	2–9 minutes
Simplate	3–9.5 minutes
Borchgrevink	3–12 minutes

■ CLOT RETRACTION TEST

Platelets have a major role in clot formation and in making it become very firm by causing retraction. If the platelets are lacking or defective, the clot does not shrink or retract but stays soft and watery. Also, if fibrinolysins are present in the serum, no clot retraction takes place. Fibrinolysis is discussed next under the section on decreased levels of fibrinogen.

Reference Values for Clot Retraction

50–100% in 2 hours

■ FIBRINOGEN

Fibrinogen (Factor I) is a plasma protein that is manufactured by the liver. Vitamin K is *not* necessary for the formation of this factor, as it is for many of the others manufactured by the liver (see Table 13–1). The sole purpose of fibrinogen seems to be the formation of fibrin as the end-product (Stage IV) of blood coagulation (See Table 13–2).

Preparation of the Client and Collection of Sample

Venous blood (4.5 ml of plasma) is collected in a tube with sodium citrate (blue-top tube).

Decreased Levels of Fibrinogen

Clinical Significance. Low fibrinogen levels can result from rare genetic disorders or from severe liver disease, either of which might first be detected with the PTT.

Reference Values for Fibrinogen

Adult	0.15–0.35 g/dl
	Women tend to have slightly higher levels
Pregnancy	Values may be as high as 0.60 g/dl
	Note that oral contraceptives may cause an increase in fibrinogen levels (see Appendix D)

More commonly, however, the decrease of fibrinogen is due to DIC. DIC is a pathologic overstimulation of the coagulation process. It is also called consumption coagulopathy or the defibrination syndrome.

Not a primary disorder, DIC is secondary to other severe illnesses (O'Brien, 1978; McGillick, 1982). The theory is that widespread tissue injury somehow triggers the clotting mechanism so that a pathological formation of small thrombi occurs in the microcirculation. Paradoxically, the client begins to bleed because the clotting factors are eventually depleted. Besides the low fibrinogen level, the PT is increased, the PTT is increased, and the platelet count is lowered. Thrombocytopenia is a cardinal diagnostic finding (Griffin, 1986). Because the placenta is a rich source of tissue thromboplastin, such abnormalities as abruptio placenta and fetal death can trigger massive clotting problems. Pregnant women have a reduced activity of the fibrolytic system. The increase of clotting factors and the decrease in fibrolysis protect against major hemorrhage, but these changes can also contribute to coagulation problems in pregnancy (Howie, 1979). Other clients that are the most likely to develop this abnormal clotting process are clients with toxemia of pregnancy, metastatic cancer, shock, sepsis, or burns. Respiratory distress syndrome, malaria, snake bite, and extracorporeal bypass may also contribute to DIC.

If some of the PT, PTT, or platelet count tests are positive for DIC, additional tests to check for fibrinolysis and fibrin degradation products may be ordered. (See the following section for values for these tests.)

POSSIBLE NURSING DIAGNOSES RELATED TO DECREASED FIBRINOGEN LEVELS

Potential for Injury Related to Bleeding and Clotting in the Microcirculation

Because a low fibrinogen level is often part of a complex pathological situation, the clients who are the most likely to develop DIC are usually those who are already in an intensive unit with a primary illness. Shock is often present. In the obstetrical area, women with toxemia or with any pathology of the placenta should be observed for DIC. The nurse giving direct care may be first to notice signs of bleeding, such as bruise marks or the appearance of blood in drainage tubes or on dressings. (Refer to the section on PT to review all the ways a nurse can make objective assessments for occult or hidden bleeding.) If thrombi have developed in the microcirculation, the client may have unexplained pain or symptoms of poor circulation to specific areas, such as cyanosis of the fingers or toes.

Assisting with Medical Interventions. Whole blood or blood components may be given intravenously to replace the clotting factors. Nurses must understand the correct rate of flow for the particular blood component used, as well as the complications that may occur. Because blood components are obtained from a pool of donors, hepatitis is something that may happen later. (See Chapter 14 for tests used to screen blood products.) Not only is bleeding occurring, but thrombus formation may be taking place too. So heparin may be part of the therapy for this complex situation (Griffin, 1986). Either the ACT or the PTT is used to monitor heparin therapy to prevent injuries from over-anti-coagulation.

■ FIBRINOGEN DEGRADATION PRODUCTS (FDP) OR FIBRIN SPLIT PRODUCTS (FSP)

The FDP test measures the products that result from the breakdown of fibrin clots by the action of the enzyme plasmin. Fibrin degradation products are found in the clotting disorder, DIC, discussed above. In addition to being useful in diagnosing the presence of DIC, the FDP may also be used to monitor fibrinolytic therapy with streptokinase (Streptase) or urokinase (Abbokinase). Tests of fibrin metabolism may also be used to evaluate the clot formation that occurs after pulmonary embolism (Bynum et al., 1979). Hypofibrinogenemia and fibrin split products occur after autologous transfusions (Gillott & Thomas, 1984).

Preparation of Client and Collection of Sample
Venous blood (4.5 ml) is collected in a special tube that contains thrombin and an antifibrinolytic agent. Blood should be drawn before heparin therapy is begun.

Reference Values for FSP

For screening tests no agglutinations at 1:4 dilution
Quantitative tests $<10\mu g$

■ THROMBIN TIME: FIBRINOGEN SCREEN, THROMBIN CLOTTING TIME WITH REPTILASE

The thrombin time measures the time it takes blood to clot when thrombin is added to the sample. If a clot does not form immediately, a fibrinogen deficiency is present. Heparin therapy will also keep the blood sample from clotting. A reagent called reptilase (derived from snake venom) has an action similar to thrombin as it clots fibrinogen. However, reptilase is not inhibited by heparin so it can be substituted for the conventional thrombin time test when the client is heparinized. In addition to assessing for certain bleeding disorders, the thrombin time is also used to monitor the client receiving fibrinolytic therapy. During treatment with streptokinase (Streptase) or urokinase (Abbokinase) the thrombin time is generally kept about two times the baseline and checked every 3–4 hours (Govoni & Hayes, 1985).

Preparation of Client and Collection of Sample
Use whole blood, 4.5 ml, collected in a plastic tube with NA citrate (blue top). For reptilase test, obtain special tube from hematology laboratory.

Reference Values for Thrombin Time and Reptilase Time	
Thrombin time	14–16 seconds or within 5 seconds of control
Reptilase time	18–22 seconds

■ PLASMINOGEN/PLASMIN ASSAY

Plasminogen is the inactive precursor of plasmin, an enzyme that has the ability to dissolve clots. The amount of these two substances is useful information when the client is on thrombolytic agents such as streptokinase (Streptase) or urokinase (Abbokinase). These tests may also be used to evaluate the client who has DIC. A decrease in plasminogen activity may be associated with the tendency for thrombosis.

Preparation of Client and Collection of Sample
Venous blood is collected in a special tube with a plasmin inhibitor.

Reference Values for Plasminogen
3.8–8.4 CTA units

CTA is the council of thrombolytic agents (Jacobs et al., 1984). If laboratories are using the newer (chromogenic) method, the values will be reported in percentage of activity or mg/dl. Check with the laboratory.

■ OCCULT BLOOD: HEMATEST, HEMOCCULT, AND OTHER GUAIAC TESTS

Occult (hidden) blood can be detected by simple tests that cause color changes in the presence of blood. Although all tests for blood in stool, urine, or other secretions are sometimes called "guaiac tests," not all of them use the chemical guaiac. Some tests, Hematest being the common one, use another chemical, orthotolidine. Although tests such as Hematest and Hemostix (Ames) can be used to detect occult blood in urine, a microscopic examination is needed to detect intact erythrocytes. (See Chapter 3 on tests for hematuria). The various tests for occult blood can also be done on emesis, but note that cimetidine may make the test falsely positive (Mar, 1981) and a low pH falsely negative. Gastroccult (Smith Kline Diagnostics, 1982) is specifically designed to test for occult blood and the pH of gastric secretions. Nurses may use Gastrooccult for on-the-spot assessment of occult blood in emesis or nasogastric drainage. Only a drop of gastric juices is needed.

Nurses can also do on-the-spot assessments for blood in the stool by obtaining a small amount of feces by digital examination if necessary. Hemoccult, which uses a guaiac-impregnated paper, seems to be the best screening test for stools (Glouberman & Szokol, 1978; Tietz, 1983). However some studies (Ahlquist et al., 1985) have found Hemo-Quant (University of Minnesota) a more reliable test. The most important use of such tests as Hemoccult is to screen patients for cancer of the bowel, because bleeding is one of the very early symptoms (Miller & Knight, 1977). A screening for blood in the stool is much easier and less expensive than a sigmoidoscopy.

Preparation of Client and Collection of Sample

The client may be instructed to avoid meat and to eat a high roughage diet for 1–3 days before a screening test of the feces. Meat, especially red meat, may make a false positive and a high-fiber diet increases the chances of finding occult blood if a lesion is present in the gastrointestinal tract. Some places may restrict the client's diet only after an initial screening test is positive. More than one stool specimen may be needed to detect intermittent bleeding. At least three are recommended. Stool specimens do not need to be tested immediately but must be protected from sunlight.

Nurses should be aware of potential influences on these tests. Vitamin C (more than 250 mg) may produce false negative results, whereas iron pills may give false positive results. Turnips and horseradish, which contain peroxidase, may also make a false positive; aspirin and antiinflammatory drugs, which tend to cause slight gastrointestinal bleeding, should be avoided a couple of days before the test. Long-distance runners may have occult blood in the feces after a vigorous run.

The collection of stool can be done at home by the client, who is given a commercially prepared filter paper in a protective cover (Hemoccult by Smith Kline Diagnostics). The written instructions tell the client to collect a small specimen of stool on an applicator and smear the stool on Part A of the paper. A second specimen from a different part of the stool is put on Part B of the paper. After three samples are collected and brought to the clinic or laboratory, two drops of a commercially prepared developing solution are placed on each smear, and the color change is noted after 30 seconds.

Another technique involves the use of a filter paper as toilet paper. The stool is then tested for blood by spraying the paper (Early Detector by Warner-Lambert). The use of these newer techniques may become more widespread in the future, because clients do not have to handle their feces and thus may be more willing to do the test. Another test (EZ-Detect, Self-Care Systems, Inc.) uses a pad which is thrown into the toilet after a bowel movement. The pad turns blue if there is blood. Screening tests done at home will need validation by the laboratory. Refer to current research literature for the sensitivity of the newer tests.

Reference Values for Occult Blood in Stool

Appearance of a blue color indicates the presence of blood. A second test may be done to confirm a positive report.

POSSIBLE NURSING DIAGNOSIS RELATED TO OCCULT BLOOD

Knowledge Deficit Regarding Health Maintenance by Checking for Occult Blood

Nurses may be involved in instructing clients on how to do stool testing for blood as a screening measure at home. For example, the San Francisco Public Health Department offers a program of colorectal screening to all people. The screening, which includes the Hemoccult test done at home, is provided free to any senior citizen. Nurses can educate the public about the importance of the resources available in their communities. As discussed in Chapter 1, screening for occult blood in the feces is one of only a few tests that are generally recommended routinely for even apparently healthy people over age 40. The community health nurse or the family nurse practitioner can offer this screening test to clients. See Chapter 27 for information on sigmoidoscopies, which may be needed as a follow-up to the screening test for occult blood in the feces.

QUESTIONS

1. Mrs. Rodriguez has just been started on hyperalimentation therapy because she is severely malnourished. The hyperalimentation therapy consists of amino acids, a concentrated glucose solution, minerals, and water-soluble vitamins. How could this situation affect the PT drawn today? It is likely the:

   a. Percentage and seconds will both be increased
   b. Percentage will be increased and seconds decreased
   c. Percentage and seconds will both be decreased
   d. Percentage will be decreased and seconds increased

2. The charge nurse is scanning the laboratory reports that were just sent to the unit. A PT of 25% and 28 seconds (with a control of 14 seconds) would be evidence of an adequate therapeutic intervention for:

   a. Mr. Ramos, who is on coumarin therapy
   b. Mr. Wong, who is on heparin therapy
   c. Mrs. Saxon, who is scheduled for a liver biopsy
   d. Mrs. Java, who had an injection of vitamin K_1 yesterday

3. A prophylactic injection of vitamin K_1 is given to newborns because the:

   a. PT of newborns is increased in seconds
   b. Fibrinogen level of newborns is decreased
   c. Platelet count may be lowered in some cases
   d. Intestinal bacteria may destroy the vitamin K

4. Vitamin K injections are less likely to return the PT to normal for which client?

   a. Mr. Richards, who is suffering from malnutrition
   b. Mr. Ringer, who has liver dysfunction
   c. Mrs. Saxon, who is on long-term coumarin therapy
   d. Mrs. Java, who has obstructive jaundice caused by a pancreatic tumor

5. Mr. Ringer, a patient with cirrhosis, has had two episodes of gastrointestinal bleeding but seems stabilized now. His PT is 20 seconds (control 13 seconds) and his platelet count is 100,000 mm³ (reference value 150,000–350,000 mm³). He is on a regular diet but has little appetite. The *most important* instruction for the nurse to give Mr. Ringer when he goes home is for him to:

   a. Maintain a balanced diet with emphasis on foods containing vitamin K

b. Check his pulse regularly and report a rate above 100

c. Always drink a glass of milk when he takes aspirin

d. Report any dark colored or black stools to his physician immediately

6. Mrs. Bender is being discharged on long-term coumarin therapy. When the nurse formulates a discharge teaching plan the *least important* topic to include is the necessity of:

a. Carrying identification that she is on long-term anticoagulant therapy

b. Having periodic PT drawn

c. Not taking nonprescription drugs which contain aspirin

d. Assessing the amount of vitamin K and fat in her diet

7. Mrs. Jones has a PTT of 130 seconds. (Control is 35 seconds.) She is on an intravenous heparin drip at a rate of 700 U/hr. Which action by the nurse is most appropriate after the physician is notified of the laboratory result?

a. Prepare an injection of vitamin K for emergency use by the physician

b. Increase the heparin rate, as ordered, since this will decrease the PTT time

c. Encourage ambulation to increase circulation

d. Keep the patient on bedrest and assess the patient often for any symptoms of bleeding

8. Mr. Jacobs, age 66, is a postoperative client who had a deep-vein thrombosis (DVT) after a previous surgery. His PTT is slightly lower than the normal control value. He is on a "mini-dose" of heparin as a preventive measure. Thus, the nursing action that has the highest priority is to:

a. Assess frequently for bleeding

b. Encourage as much ambulation as possible

c. Ascertain if protamine, the antidote for heparin, is readily available

d. Monitor fluids to prevent circulatory overload

9. If a client has a low platelet count, the initial physical assessment is most likely to reveal:

a. Large hematomas on abdomen and back

b. Delayed capillary filling when the skin is blanched

c. Evidence of gastrointestinal bleeding such as a positive test for blood in the feces

d. Petechiae from small injuries at the capillary level

10. Which of the following nursing actions is the *most appropriate* for Sally, who is complaining of a headache and asking if she may take an over-the-counter medication for pain. Her platelet count today is 20,000 mm³. (Reference value is 150,000–350,000 mm³.)

a. Allow her to take her usual over-the-counter medication for headache because it is usually very effective

b. Offer her fluids to decrease the viscosity of her blood

    c. Obtain an order for aspirin for her headache

    d. Assess her for any changes in level of consciousness (LOC)

11. Sally has a platelet count of 10,000 mm³ due to idiopathic thrombocytopenia; John has a platelet count of 780,000 mm³ due to a malignancy (reference values 150,000–350,000 mm³). Because of these laboratory reports *both* of these clients should be assessed for the potential of:

    a. Bone marrow depression and polycythemia

    b. Thrombus formation in lower extremities

    c. Bleeding episodes from minor trauma

    d. Infection of mucus membranes

12. Which of the following changes in laboratory tests are most indicative of the complex bleeding disorder that is called disseminated intravascular clotting (DIC) or consumption coagulopathy?

    a. Increased PT, increased PTT, and increased platelet count

    b. Decreased PT, decreased PTT, and decreased fibrinogen levels

    c. Increased PT, decreased platelet count, and increased fribrinogen levels

    d. Increased PT, decreased platelet count, and decreased fibrinogen levels

13. Johnny, age 8, is scheduled for a tonsillectomy and adenoidectomy (T and A) tomorrow. The test that will most clearly demonstrate that he has an intact intrinsic clotting system is the

    a. Fibrinogen level

    b. PTT

    c. Platelet count

    d. PT

14. Mr. Ringer is scheduled for a liver biopsy tomorrow. He has a tentative diagnosis of cirrhosis caused by alcohol abuse. Which two of these laboratory tests are used in assessing adequate liver function prior to the invasive procedure of a liver biopsy?

    a. PTT and fibrinogen levels

    b. PT and platelet counts

    c. Fibrinogen levels and platelet counts

    d. PT and anti-hemophilic factor (Factor VIII)

15. Linda Everett, age 32, delivered a premature infant yesterday. Because of massive blood loss she received three units of blood. Today she is having only slight vaginal bleeding. The laboratory data to best substantiate the need for continued close observation of vital signs would be:

    a. PT 120% (control 100%)

    b. Fibrinogen 0.10 g/dl (reference value 0.15–0.60 g/dl)

    c. PTT 37 seconds (control 35 seconds)

    d. Platelet count 400,000 mm³ (reference value 150,000–350,000 mm³)

16. Two days ago, Mr. Frank, age 58, had major abdominal surgery for cancer of the colon. He has a nasogastric tube, which is draining greenish drainage. He is ambulatory with help. Today's laboratory reports show a PT of nine seconds (control 12 seconds), a PTT of 30 seconds (control 34 seconds), and a platelet count of 350,000 mm³ (reference value 150,000–350,000 mm³). *Based on this laboratory data,* a priority nursing action is to:

a. Encourage ambulation of the client

b. Check the nasogastric drainage for occult (hidden) bleeding

c. Check stools for occult (hidden) bleeding

d. Monitor the client for infection or other signs of bone marrow depression

17. Important facts about the guaiac test (Hemoccult) for stool are all the following *except* which?

a. Red meat may cause false positive results in the feces

b. The test is very useful as a screening test for cancer of the colon

c. The stool specimen must be tested within 2–4 hours after collection

d. A blue color indicates a positive reaction for the presence of blood.

REFERENCES

Ahlquist, D. et al. (1985). Fecal blood levels in health and disease. A study using HemoQuant. *NEJM, 312,* 1422–1428.

Bynum, L., et al. (1979). Diagnostic value of tests for fibrin metabolism in patients predisposed to pulmonary embolism. *Archives of Internal Medicine, 139,* 283–285.

Decker, S. (1985). The life threatening consequences of a GI bleed. *RN, 48*(10), 18–27.

DeMeester, T., et al. (1978). Pulmonary embolism therapy. *Patient Care, 12,* 14–71.

Dressler, D. (1980). Understanding and treating hemophilia. *Nursing 80, 10*(9), 72–73.

Errichetti, A. (1984). Management of oral anticoagulation therapy. *Archives of Internal Medicine, 144*(10), 1966–1968.

Froberg, J. (1986). Would you have recognized this deadly disease? *RN, 49*(3), 22–25.

Gever, L. (1983). Warfarin sodium. *Nursing 83, 13*(9), 17.

Gillott, A., & Thomas, J. (1984). Clinical investigation involving the use of the haemonetic cell saver in elective and emergency vascular operations. *American Surgeon, 50*(11), 609–612.

Glouberman, S., & Szokol, A. (1978). Melena and occult blood in the stool. *Arizona Medicine, 35*(6), 399–400.

Govoni, L., & Hayes, J. (1985). *Drugs and nursing implications* (5th ed.). Norwalk, CT: Appleton-Century-Crofts.

Griffin, J. (1986). The bleeding patient. *Nursing 86, 16*(6), 34–40.

Hernandez, B. (1980). Platelets: A short course. *RN, 43*(6), 35–41.

Howie, P. W. (1979). Blood clotting and fibrinolysis in pregnancy. *Postgraduate Medical Journal, 55*(5), 362–366.

Jacobs, D., Kasten, B., DeMott, W., & Wolfson, W. (1984). *Laboratory test handbook with DRG index.* St. Louis: Mosby/Lexi

King, D., & Kelton, J. (1984). Heparin associated thrombocytopenia. *Annals Internal Medicine, 100*(4), 535–540.

King, N. (1984). Controlling bleeding when the platelet count drops. *RN, 47*(9), 25–27.

Kirschenbaum, H., & Rosenberg, J. (1982). Coumadin. *RN, 45*(10), 54–56.

Koch, P. (1984). Thrombocytopenia. *Nursing 84, 14*(10), 55–57.

McGillick, K. (1982). DIC: The deadly paradox. *RN, 45*(9), 41–43.

McGuire, P. (1985). Home therapy for children with hemophilia: Development, implementation and evaluation. *Syllabus of Abstracts for National Symposium on Nursing Research.* Stanford, CA: Stanford Hospital, Department of Nursing.

Mar, D. (1981). Cimetidine update. *AJN, 81*(5), 1026–1027.

Miller, S. F., & Knight, R. (1977). Early detection of colon-rectal cancer. *Ca, 40,* 945–949.

Multicenter Trial Committee (1984). Dihydroergotamine-heparin prophylaxis of postoperative deep vein thrombosis. *JAMA, 251*(22), 2960–2966.

Northrop, C. (1986). Look and look again. *Nursing 86, 16*(1), 43.

O'Brien, B., & Woods, S. (1978). The paradox of DIC. *AJN, 78*(11), 1878–1880.

Ramirez-Lassepas M., et al. (1984). Heparin induced thrombocytopenia in patients with cerebrovascular ischemic disease. *Neurology, 34,* 736–740.

Redman, C. W. (1979). Coagulation problems in pregnancy. *Post Graduate Medical Journal, 55*(5), 367–371.

Sherry, S. (1976). *Low dose heparin therapy: A retrospective review.* Princeton, NJ: Excerpta Medica Offices.

Silinsky, J. (1985). What you can learn from the platelet count. *RN, 48*(1), 87–88.

Smith Kline Diagnostics (1982). *Product instructions: Hemoccult slides and tapes.* Sunnyvale, CA: Smith Kline Diagnostics.

Sohn, C. (1981). Rescind the risks in administering anticoagulants. *Nursing 81, 11*(10), 34–41.

Tietz, N. (Ed.). (1983). *Clinical guide to laboratory tests.* Philadelphia: Saunders.

Wallach, J. (1986). *Interpretation of diagnostic tests.* Boston: Little, Brown.

Wroblewski, S., & Wroblewski, S. (1981). Caring for the patient with chemotherapy-induced thrombocytopenia. *AJN, 81*(4), 746–749.

14

Serological Tests

- ABO Grouping
- Rh Factor
- Rh Antibody Titer Test
- Direct Antiglobulin (Coombs) Test
- Antibody Screening Test (Indirect Coombs)
- Hepatitis B Surface and e Antigens (HB_sAg and HB_eAg) and Antibodies Against Hepatitis B Antigens
- Hepatitis A Tests: anti-HAV, IgM, IgG
- Acquired Immune Deficiency Syndrome (AIDS) Test: Antibodies for HTLV-III or HIV
- Serological Tests for Syphilis (STS)
  VDRL and RPR, FTA-ABS and MHA-TP
- Cold Agglutinins or Cold Hemagglutinins
- Febrile Agglutinins for Typhoid Fever, Paratyphoid, Brucellosis, and Tularemia
- Infectious Mononucleosis
- Streptococci Infections
- Rubella
- Toxoplasmosis (TPM, Toxo)
- Amebiasis
- Cytomegalovirus (CMV) Titers
- Herpes Simplex Virus (HSV) Antibodies
- Torch Screen
- Fungal Antibodies: Histoplasmosis, Coccidioidomycosis, and Blastomycosis
- Fungal Antigens
- Rickettsial Disease: *Proteus* OX-19, *Proteus* OX-2, and *Proteus* OX-K (Weil–Felix Reaction)
- C-Reactive Protein (CRP)

- Complement Activity: C_3, C_4, and C_1 Esterase Inhibitor
- LE Prep
- Antinuclear Antibodies (ANA)
- Antibodies to Native DNA (Anti-DNA)
- Rheumatoid Factor (RF)
- Thyroid Antibodies

OBJECTIVES

1. Explain the basic procedures used for serological tests for blood bank procedures, microbiology, and immunology.
2. Describe the role of the nurse in the prevention and assessment of transfusion reactions from ABO incompatibility.
3. Explain the rationale for the administration of Rh immunoglobulins after certain deliveries.
4. Identify the most important nursing diagnoses when a client has a positive report for HB_sAg (hepatitis B surface antigen) or for hepatitis A.
5. Describe the usefulness of the test for antibodies against HTLV-III or HIV in prevention of the spread of AIDS.
6. Describe what a client should be taught about the various serological tests for syphilis (STS).
7. Describe the clinical usefulness of serological tests for common bacterial, viral, fungal, and rickettsial diseases.
8. Describe the information that should be given to a woman of childbearing age who has a negative titer of rubella antibodies.
9. Explain why positive serology tests or skin tests may not be indicative of an active infection.
10. Describe how C_3 and C_4, two components of the complement system, are altered by antigen-antibody reactions.
11. Describe how humoral antibodies, such as RF, ANA, and others, are useful in assessing possible autoimmune pathology.

The category of serology tests is very broad, including blood bank procedures (immunohematology), identification of antibodies against infectious diseases (microbiology), and studies of immune diseases (immunology). The basic principle underlying serology tests is that a reaction between an antibody and antigen results in a recordable event. In some tests, the client's blood sample is mixed with an antigen to see if there are antibodies in the serum. In other tests, antibodies may be added to the blood sample to see if the antigen exists.

Serological tests alone, however, are usually not specific enough to establish a diagnosis. For example, clients may have antibodies against an infectious agent, such as a fungus, but they may not have the disease when the test is administered. As another example, two clients may both have a high level of RF, which is a type of immunoglobulin. Yet one client has all the symptoms of rheumatoid arthritis, while the other has no symptoms. Likewise, some clients with syphilis may be what is termed "seronegative," while some who do not have the disease are "seropositive." This lack of total specificity is a common problem of all serological tests. Drugs, infections, and such diseases as carcinomas often cause unpredictable changes in immunological response.

The first part of this chapter covers the techniques used in blood banking procedures. The blood types of ABO demonstrate in a dramatic way the antigen–antibody basis for tests. Blood cross matching also uses several antibody titer tests.

The second part of the chapter discusses the common serology tests used in microbiology. (Specific microbiological tests, such as cultures and microscopic examinations, are covered in Chapter 16.) Serology tests are only indirect tests for the presence of an organism, such as a virus, which may have many different antigens. Laboratory tests can detect specific antibodies to a bacterial, viral, fungal, protozoan, or rickettsial antigen or antigens.

The last part of the chapter contains a discussion on the common serology tests used to assess immunological diseases, such as systemic lupus erythematosus (SLE). Serological testing in autoimmune diseases is rapidly growing more common, as research discovers more about the antigen–antibody reactions that occur in these baffling diseases. This chapter may be viewed as a continuum in that tests of antigen–antibody reactions in ABO typing are very predictable, whereas tests such as the new ones for ANA are much less predictable in clinical use.

COMMON TECHNIQUES IN SEROLOGICAL TESTING

As noted above, serological testing is based on the fact that antigen–antibody reaction causes an observable event. From a nursing point of view, the exact testing technique is not of prime interest. Nonetheless, to understand the description of the test, nurses do need to be familiar with the general meaning of the techniques. Six different techniques are commonly used in serological tests:

1. Agglutinations and titer levels
2. Complement fixation (CF)
3. Immunofluorescence antibody tests (IFA)
4. Radioimmunoassay (RIA)
5. Enzyme-linked immunoabsorbent assay (EIA or ELISA)
6. Immunoglobulin electrophoresis

Agglutination and Titer Levels. Agglutination, or clumping, which often occurs when antibodies attach to an antigen, is the most basic type of serology testing. Febrile agglutins, cold agglutins, and the Coombs test are three examples of an observable clumping of cells in the blood sample when there is a certain ratio of antibodies to antigens.

The serum is diluted with normal saline in graduated amounts. For many serological tests, rather than reporting just agglutination (positive) or no agglutination (negative), the laboratory represents the results as a certain *titer,* which is the last dilution at which a reaction occurred. For example, the laboratory would use the standard dilutions in Table 14–1 to test for antibodies against an antigen streptolysin-O that is produced by group A-beta hemolytic streptococci. In the example in the table, the last dilution to cause a reaction was 1:170, which would be the titer reported. In essence, this finding means that the client's serum contained enough antibodies still to cause a reaction with the antigenic material when the serum was diluted 1:170.

TABLE 14-1. TITER DILUTION CHART FOR ASO

1:60	Positive
1:85	Positive
1:120	Positive
1:170	Positive
1:240	Negative
1:340	
1:480	
1:680	
1:960	
1:1360	
1:2720	

ASO = Anti-Streptolysin O Antibodies.
Note that an antibody titer is reported as the last dilution that causes an antigen-antibody reaction or agglutinization. Thus, in this example, the laboratory report would read "ASO titer 1:170." See text for further explanation.

One titer does not give as much information as do two titers separated by a time interval, because a *rise* in titer is more significant than any one high number. So, to catch a rise or fall, the timing of titers is very important. A fourfold increase in titer between an acute and a convalescent sample is usually necessary to confirm the presence of an infection (Weinstein & Farkas, 1979). The time interval between acute and convalescent phase depends on the organism causing the disease.

Complement Fixation. Complement factors are a group of proteins in the blood-stream that enter into certain antigen–antibody reactions. One or more of the constituents of complement (see the test for C_3 and C_4) can be consumed during an antibody–antigen reaction. Since the complement used in the reaction is fixed, it cannot be used again. The tests using complement fixation are hard to standardize, so the newer techniques of IFA, RIA, and ELISA are being used if the laboratory is equipped to do these newer tests. The now-outdated Wasserman test for syphilis is an example of a test using CF.

Immunofluorescence Antibody (IFA) Tests. The IFA test can be direct or indirect. In the direct method, an antibody labeled with a fluorescent dye (fluorescein) is mixed with a sample of blood from the client. If an antigen is present, the antigen–antibody complex can be seen under a microscope with an ultraviolet light source. With the indirect method, the known antigen is mixed with the serum and any antigen–antibody complex is then mixed with fluorescein-labeled anti-immunoglobulin antibodies.

An example of a fluorescent type of test is the FTA-ABS for syphilis. The "FTA" stands for fluorescent treponemal antibody, and the "ABS" stands for a special absorption technique that helps to get rid of some of the nonspecific antibodies that may also get stained with the fluorescent dye. Another example of an IFA discussed in this chapter is the IFA for toxoplasmosis. The IFA test can be falsely positive if the serum contains ANA. (See the ANA test at end of the chapter.)

Radioimmunoassay (RIA). The use of radioactive-tagged antigens is discussed in Chapter 15 in relation to hormone assay.

Enzyme-Linked Immunoabsorbent Assay. The use of enzymes to tag antigens is also briefly discussed in Chapter 15. A test developed to test antibodies against HTLV-III or HIV uses ELIA.

Immunoglobulin Electrophoresis. See Chapter 10 for a discussion of how gamma globulins can be separated into patterns on a graph. The specific identification of immunoglobulins supplements the information gained from serologic testing. IgM antibodies are indicative of an acute infection and IgG antibodies are indicative of past exposure and probable immunity. For examples, see the discussion on tests for rubella and hepatitis.

IMMUNOHEMATOLOGY TESTS

The tests done on blood used for transfusions are often given the name "immuno-hematology," raher than the broader term of "serology."

Screening Blood for Transfusions

Several routine laboratory tests are done on a unit of donor blood (see Table 14–2). Each of these tests is discussed in detail in this chapter. Because transmission of syphilis is possible only in fresh blood that is less than 3 days old, the need for routine STS has been questioned (Kazak, 1979), but it is still a routine test. Hepatitis is a much greater danger from transfusions, as was AIDS before the screening tests were developed. An alternative to transfusions with blood-bank blood is the use of an autologous blood recovery unit that recycles the client's blood lost in the surgical field. The cost is considered greater than blood-bank units if less than two units are salvaged and used (Cozad, 1985). Complications are usually minor if strict protocols are followed. Some diminished coagulability may be observed posttransfusion (Gillott & Thomas, 1984).

Blood banks take several precautions to ensure not only that donor blood is safe to give to a client, but also that it is safe for the person to donate blood. For example, the donor must weigh at least 110 lb (50 k) and have a hemoglobin level of 13.5 g for men and 12.5 g for women. (See Chapter 2 on the measurement of hemoglobin levels.) The donor must have a temperature no higher than 98.6°F (37°C), a heart rate of 50–100 with no irregularities, and a blood pressure between 200/100 and 100/50. The blood bank physician may modify these guidelines depending on the individual situation. Overall, the donor must be in generally good health with no upper respiratory infections or allergies. Blood donations are not taken from people

TABLE 14–2. ROUTINE TESTS ON DONOR BLOOD AND FOR TYPE AND CROSS MATCHING

Donor Blood
1. ABO typing
2. Rh factor and other variations
3. STS
4. HB$_s$Ag and other tests for hepatitis
5. HTLV-III or HIV antibody screen for AIDS
6. Other antibody screens

Type and Cross Matching
1. ABO typing (compatibility)
2. Rh typing (compatibility)
3. Direct Coombs
4. Antibody screening
5. Antibody titer
6. Identification of unusual antibodies and antigens

who have ever had hepatitis, malaria, jaundice, or a venereal disease. Pregnancy or a blood transfusion excludes donors for 6 months. Travel to other countries also excludes donors for 6 months. (Note that the incubation period for hepatitis B is 6 months.) Dental surgery or teeth extraction in the 72 hours prior to the donation excludes a donor. [See Chapter 16 on how even minor dental work can cause transient bacteria in the bloodstream (bacteremia).]

Typing and Cross Matching of Blood (T&C). To do a T&C, the laboratory needs at least 45 minutes to make sure that the donor unit of blood is compatible with the blood of the recipient. The client's blood type and Rh factor are determined so that a matching unit of blood can be taken from the blood bank. Yet it is never safe to assume that any unit of A positive blood can be given to any client with A positive blood. So the cross match mixes a small sample of the two bloods to see if any clumping occurs. When the two serums and cells are combined and incubated, compatibility is demonstrated by the absence of clumping. The full range of tests for a type and cross matching are noted in Table 14–2. In an emergency, the laboratory may do a less-than-full cross match by eliminating items 5 and 6. The physician, however, must notify the blood bank that the shortened version of the cross match is permissible for an emergency case.

Typing and Screeening (T&S). If there is only a faint possibility of the blood being needed, the physican may order a typing and screening (T&S) rather than a cross match. In a screening, the client's blood is tested, so that, if blood is needed, the actual cross matching can be done in less than 30 minutes. The advantage of the screening is that it does not tie up a unit of blood when the potential need is slight. For example, if two units of blood are typed and cross matched for a surgical client, those two units of blood cannot be used for another client until the surgery is done and the blood is released for re-cross matching with another client. In one study, 4762 units of blood were cross matched for elective surgical procedures, and only 200 were actually needed (Lang & Drozda, 1979).

Typing for Packed Cells. If the client needs red blood cells but not serum, the physician orders a unit of packed cells. A unit of packed red blood cells contains only about a half of the amount of plasma as a unit of blood. Typing and cross matching are just as necessary for packed cells as for whole blood. Packed cells are now more commonly used for blood transfusions than whole blood. The major advantage of packed cells is the prevention of volume overload. In this discussion a "blood transfusion" refers to either whole blood or packed cells.

Preparation of Client
There is no special preparation of the client for type and cross matching or for type and screening. For either procedure, the laboratory needs 10 ml of whole blood. Dextran, a plasma expander, should not be started before a type and cross match because it will interfere with the cross matching.

■ ABO GROUPING

All humans can be grouped into four major blood types—A, B, AB, and O—which are genetically determined. Even though Type A has subgroups, one can generally speak of only four types, the frequency of which is shown in Table 14–3 along with

TABLE 14–3. ABO BLOOD TYPING

Estimated Percentage of Population	Type	Description
46	O	No A or B antigens on RBCs. Antibodies against A and B antigens[a]
41	A	Antigen A on RBCs. Antibodies against B antigens
9	B	Antigen B on RBCs. Antibodies against A antigen
4	AB	Antigens A and B on RBCs. No antibodies against A or B antigens

[a]From birth, the person has the antibodies, even with no exposure to the antigens. In contrast, the Rh negative person does not have antibodies against the RH factor until exposed to the factor.

a description of the antigens and antibodies in each type. Besides the ABO grouping, which is the most important variable, the matching of donor and recipient must take into account many other factors.

Understanding the concept of the universal donor and recipient may help the nurse visualize, in a simple way, the significance of antibody-antigen response in immunological testing. Type O blood is theoretically the "universal donor" because there are none of the major antigens on the red blood cells of people with type O blood. Type O blood does have antibodies against A and B, but, in one unit of donor blood, the donor antibodies become so diluted in the plasma of the recipient that the antibodies are of minor importance. The person with AB has both A and B antigens on the red blood cells, so the plasma contains no antibodies against A or B antigens. Thus Type AB people are sometimes called "universal recipients." It is interesting to note that a person born with one type of ABO antigens has the antibodies against the other antigens, even though the person has never had contact with the other types of blood. In contrast, an Rh negative person does not have antibodies against the Rh factor until there is sensitization. (The Rh factor, which, like ABO types, is genetically determined, is discussed later in this chapter.)

Clients must *never* be given a type of blood that contains foreign A or B antigens. For example, a client with Type A blood who is given a unit of Type B blood would undergo a severe hemolytic reaction. The antibodies against the B antigen, which are present in the A client, attack the red blood cells of the Type B donor blood. The hemolysis of the red blood cells causes the release, directly into the bloodstream, of free hemoglobin, which can be very damaging to the renal tubules. The end result of a transfusion of incompatible blood may be renal failure and death.

POSSIBLE NURSING DIAGNOSIS RELATED TO BLOOD TRANSFUSION

Potential for Injury Related to Complications of Blood Transfusion

In most institutions, at least two people must check the client's nameband against the unit of blood to be administered. Obviously, typing and cross matching are of no value if the blood is inadvertently given to the wrong client. Not only the client's name, but the medical record number, too, must match the identification number of the unit of blood. After the unit of blood is hung, the nurse's responsibility is to see that the blood is given correctly. Birdsall (1985) notes that most transfusion-related problems are due to human error. (See also Chapter 13 for a discussion on platelet transfusion and Chapter 2 for leukocyte replacement.)

Assessing for Complications. The nurse must also be aware of the signs and symptoms of an adverse reaction to a blood transfusion. The most severe hemolytic reaction is due to donor–recipient ABO incompatibilities. Rh and other factors may also cause some hemolysis, but usually not as pronounced. (See the next section on laboratory tests done after a hemolytic transfusion reaction.) Checking of vital signs before and during the blood transfusion is the basic nursing action. Also, running the blood slowly for the first 20 minutes minimizes the severity of a reaction, should it occur. Cullins (1979) and Querin and Stahl (1983) describe the nurse's role in the detection and treatment of hemolytic transfusion reactions, as well as of other transfusion reactions, such as allergic reactions, febrile reactions, circulatory overload, and air embolism.

Laboratory Tests for Hemolytic Transfusion Reactions. If a client begins to exhibit symptoms such as fever, chills, and low back pain, it is essential that the nurse not let the transfusion continue. Normal saline can be infused to keep the intravenous line patent when the unit of blood is discontinued.

The unfinished unit of blood must be sent back to the laboratory, along with another specimen of the client's blood, for the laboratory to try to determine what caused the reaction. The client's blood and the donor's blood are re-cross matched to see if they are truely incompatible.

Since one of the dreaded complications of an incompatible blood transfusion is renal failure, the laboratory also needs a urine specimen to check for the presence of hemoglobin in the urine. The client should be on strict intake and output, and all urine should be saved for laboratory examination for at least 24 hours.

The laboratory also checks for free hemoglobin in the plasma, as well as for other substances, such as indirect bilirubin and haptoglobin, that would indicate hemolysis. (See Chapter 11 for an explanation of why the indirect bilirubin is elevated with hemolysis.) Haptoglobin is a serum glycoprotein whose role is to bind free hemoglobin released from destroyed red blood cells. Evidently, haptoglobin is diminished in severe hemolysis because it cannot be replaced quickly enough. Reference values for haptoglobin vary considerably depending on the methods of evaluation used.

Assessing for and Preventing Bacterial Contamination. In addition to the tests for hemolysis, the laboratory may also do a blood culture from the donor bag. (See Chapter 16 on culture reports from blood specimens.) Blood at room temperature becomes a very attractive culture medium for bacteria. Nursing actions to prevent sepsis from blood transfusions include the aseptic technique for starting the transfusion, hanging the blood within 30 minutes after it is taken from the blood bank, and ensuring that the entire unit is transfused within two to four hours.

■ Rh FACTOR

The Rh factor is named after the rhesus monkey used in the original research on this factor. Actually, several different Rh factors have been identified, but usually only the main factor is significant. The Rh factor, like the ABO types, is genetically determined.

There are two different nomenclatures for the Rh factors. In the Weiner system the main Rh factor is Rh_0. In the Fisher-Rose system, the main Rh factor is called D. In the literature, "Rh_0" or "D" is often called the "Rh factor." In this discussion, the term "Rh factor" specifies the main factor involved when one speaks of Rh positive or Rh negative blood. Table 14–4 provides a description of Rh positive and Rh negative.

Normally, the person with Rh negative blood does not have any antibodies against the Rh factor. The Rh negative male can become sensitized (that is, develop antibodies against the Rh factor) by transfusion with Rh positive blood. The Rh negative female can develop antibodies against the Rh factor not only through blood transfusions with Rh positive factors, but also through a pregnancy where the fetus is Rh positive. Once the Rh negative person has developed antibodies against the Rh factor, another transfusion with Rh positive blood, or another pregnancy with a Rh positive fetus, can have serious consequences. The specific nursing implications for blood transfusions and for the Rh factor in pregnancy are discussed next.

Rh Factor in Blood Transfusions

To keep the Rh negative person from developing antibodies against the Rh factor, the Rh negative person is given only Rh negative blood. Hence Rh typing is one of the components of cross matching. The administration of Rh positive blood to an Rh negative person who has developed antibodies against the Rh factor (that is, who is sensitized) causes a hemolytic reaction because the person's antibodies attack the red blood cells that contain the Rh factor. The severity of this hemolytic reaction is usually not as great as it is in ABO incompatibility, but it is nevertheless to be avoided. (See the nursing implications above when a client has any kind of transfusion reaction.)

Rh Factor in Pregnancy

An Rh negative mother and an Rh positive father can produce either an Rh negative or Rh positive baby, depending on the gene passed from the father. Laboratory tests can be done to determine if the Rh positive father has either two positive genes for

TABLE 14–4. Rh FACTOR

Estimated Percentage of Population	Type	Description
85–90	Rh +	Rh antigen on RBCs. No antibodies against Rh factor
10–15	Rh −	No Rh antigen on RBCs. Develops antibodies against Rh factor if sensitized by transfusion of Rh positive blood. Also, the pregnant woman can be sensitized by an Rh positive infant

---

POSSIBLE NURSING DIAGNOSIS RELATED TO THE Rh FACTOR

Knowledge Deficit Related to the Use of Rh Immunoglobulins

About 13% of all Rh negative mothers become sensitized (that is, they develop antibodies against the Rh factor) by their first pregnancy with a Rh positive fetus. If the woman is not immunized by the administration of Rh immuno-globulins, each subsequent pregnancy with an Rh positive fetus incurs a fur-ther 13% risk of starting antibody production. RhoGAM, Gamulin Rh, and Win Rho are some of the brand names of Rh immunoglobulins (Govoni & Hayes, 1985). The use of Rh immunoglobulins is based on the principle of passive immunity. Because the mother has been given a dose of antibodies against the Rh factor, her body is not stimulated to begin an active production of an-tibodies against the Rh factor. The injection of immunoglobulins provides the needed temporary serum level of antibodies to block the effect of the antigen from the fetus, so the mother is not stimulated to begin producing her own antibodies. With each subsequent pregnancy with an Rh positive fetus, the Rh negative mother must receive RhoGAM (or other brand names) after delivery or a smaller dosage (MICRhoGAM or Mini-Gamulin Rh) after an abortion. To be effective, these passive antibodies or immunoglobulins must be given with-in 72 hours after a birth or an abortion. Some physicians also give the immune globulins at 28–32 weeks as an added precaution. These passive antibodies are not useful if the mother has already developed Rh antibodies, which can be measured in the serum. (The Rh antibody test is discussed later in this chap-ter.)

Nurses who work with women in the childbearing years should have a good understanding of the Rh factor so that they can help these women understand the possible implications in relation to pregnancy. The laws of some states make it mandatory that any woman who is bloodtyped must be told the results of the Rh factor. For the Rh negative pregnant women, Ortho Diagnostics (1981) has a pamphlet that explains, in lay terms, what Rh negative women should know about immune globulin therapy.

Rh or one positive and one negative. (Note that an Rh positive mother can carry an Rh negative fetus without any Rh-related problem.)

A potential problem occurs when an Rh negative mother is carrying an Rh positive child. Hemolytic disease of the newborn, formerly called erythroblastosis fetalis, oc-curs when an Rh negative mother produces antibodies against the Rh positive red blood cells of her fetus. With the first pregnancy, the fetus is usually not affected because the mother has not had time to build antibodies against the Rh factor. However, at the time of the infant's separation from the placenta (a full-term birth or an abortion), some of the red blood cells from the fetus enter the mother's general circulation and trigger the production of antibodies against the Rh factor. Subse-quent pregnancies with another Rh positive fetus may present problems because the woman's serum is now sensitized against Rh positive antigens.

■ Rh ANTIBODY TITER TEST

The Rh antibody titer test is used to monitor the course of the Rh negative woman who is carrying an Rh positive fetus. If the mother is in a second pregnancy and did not receive RhoGAM after a first pregnancy or abortion, the rise of the titer helps to determine the need for medical interventions, such as exchange transfusions or an early delivery.

Preparation of Client and Collection of Sample
The laboratory needs 10 ml of blood. Note that this test may also be done on a sample of cord blood.

Reference Values for Rh Titer

The normal Rh antibody titer is negative. A rising titer may indicate the need for immediate medical intervention to prevent serious damage to the fetus or newborn. (See Chapter 28 on amniocentesis for titers of 1:16 or above.)

■ DIRECT ANTIGLOBULIN (COOMBS) TEST

In certain types of sensitization, such as to the Rh factor, the erythrocytes become coated with antibodies or immunoglobulins. The Coombs test is used as a screening test to detect whether immunoglobulins have become attached to the red blood cells.

The test is referred to as a "direct" antiglobulin test (as opposed to the indirect or antibody screening test discussed next), because the red blood cells are tested without any intervening manipulations. A sample of the client's blood is mixed with Coombs serum, which is a rabbit serum that has antibodies against human globulins. If the client's red blood cells are coated with immunoglobulins, agglutination occurs. The Coombs test is done:

1. To screen blood for cross matching: If a client's erythrocytes have been exposed to incompatible blood, the erythrocytes are coated with an antibody or globulin complex.
2. To check for hemolytic transfusion reactions.
3. To assess hemolytic disease in the newborn: In hemolytic disease of the newborn, the antibodies from a sensitized Rh negative mother cross the placenta and coat the fetal red cells. (See Chapter 28 on amniocentesis.)

Other factors may also cause the client's red blood cells to be coated with immunoglobulins. For example, many drugs, as well as autoimmune diseases that cause hemolytic anemia, may cause a positive Coombs reaction. If necessary, further testing can be done to identify the specific immunoglobulins present. (See Chapter 10 on immunoglobulin testing.)

Preparation of Client and Collection of Sample
In the newborn, the blood sample is taken directly from the umbilical cord. In children and adults, a venous sample is used. Note that this test is routine for one aspect of typing and cross matching, which requires 10 ml.

Reference Values for Coombs Test

The Coombs test should be negative. A positive test indicates that some type of globulin is coating the red blood cells.

TABLE 14–5. COMMON SEROLOGICAL TESTS USED IN MICROBIOLOGY

Test	Organism	Remarks
VDRL RPR FTA-ABS MHA-TP	*Treponema pallidum,* which causes syphilis	Confirming tests are done if screening tests are positive
HB$_s$Ag	Hepatitis B virus (formerly called serum hepatitis)	Can also measure antibodies against HB$_s$Ag and other antigens
Anti-HAV	Hepatitis A virus (formerly called infectious hepatitis)	See Table 14–6 for all tests for Hepatitis A and B
HTLV-III or HIV	Virus associated with AIDS	Only tests antibodies for the virus. See current literature for update
Cold agglutinins	Eaton agent of pleuropneumonia-like organism (PPLO) may cause atypical pneumonia	Positive in some cases, not all
HSV	Herpes simplex virus	Not used routinely. See Chapter 16 for other tests
CMV	Cytomegalovirus	Problematic in pregnancy and for immunosuppressed clients
HAT Monospot Monoscreen Monotest	Epstein–Barr virus of infectious mononucleosis	Also see WBC with differential in Chapter 2
ASO Anti-DNase-B Streptozyme test	Group A-beta hemolytic streptococci	Measures antibodies *after* an acute infection with streptococci. Not useful during initial infectious stage
Rubella titer	Rubella virus (3-day measles)	Even a low-antibody titer probably indicates immunity
TPM or Toxo	*Toxoplasma gondii,* a protozoan that causes toxoplasmosis	Most tests are indirect measurements of the protozoan
Hemagglutination for amebiasis	*Entamoeba histolytica* (causes amebic dysentery and hepatic abcess)	Stool cultures also done (see Chapter 16)
Fungus antibody tests	Histoplasmosis Coccidioidomycosis Blastomycosis	Cultures also done (see Chapter 16)
Proteus OX-19 OX-2 OX-K	Rickettsiae, such as *Rickettsia akari,* which causes Rocky Mountain spotted fever, and *Rickettsia prowazekii,* which causes epidemic typhus	Rickettsiae can be cultured, but the reaction to *Proteus* is an easier method to get presumptive evidence

Note: A TORCH screen includes *T*oxoplasmosis, *O*thers such as syphilis or hepatitis, *R*ubella, *C*ytomegalovirus, and *H*erpes.

TABLE 14-6. TESTS USED TO DIAGNOSE HEPATITIS A AND HEPATITIS B

Name of Test	Explanation
Anti-hepatitis A virus (anti-HAV) IgM IgG	Measures antibodies to the hepatitis A virus. Antibodies of IgM type indicate *current* infection, whereas IgG represent past infection and probable immunity. Used to diagnose or rule out hepatitis A in a suspected case of hepatitis.
Hepatitis B surface antigen (HB_s Ag)	Measures surface antigen of hepatitis B virus. Indicates infection with hepatitis B and carrier state if persists. Used to screen potential blood donors and to diagnose or rule out hepatitis B in suspected cases of hepatitis.
Hepatitis B core antigen (HB_c Ag)	Measures a core antigen of hepatitis B virus in liver cells, not serum. Used only for research purposes.
Hepatitis B e antigen (HB_e Ag)	Measures the e antigen of the hepatitis B virus. Correlates well with high titers of the virus so used to evaluate infectiousness, particularly in chronic states.
Anti-HB_sAg	Measures antibodies to hepatitis B surface antigen. Demonstrates immunity to hepatitis B virus, except for a few unusual subtypes. Used to demonstrate if vaccine is needed for person at risk for hepatitis B.
Anti-HB_cAg IgM IgG	Measures antibodies to the core antigen of hepatitis B. Appears in the serum later than the anti-HB_sAg so may be used to diagnose hepatitis B in the "window" or convalescent state. IgM indicates *current* infection. IgG indicates past infection and probable immunity. Also can demonstrate if vaccine is needed for person in high-risk group.
anti-HB_eAg	Measures antibodies to the e antigen of hepatitis B virus. Appears late in infection and shows resolution. May be too weak to be detected.

Note: See Gurevich (1983), Jacobs et al. (1984), Tietz (1983), and Wallach (1986) for more details.

■ ANTIBODY SCREENING TEST (INDIRECT COOMBS)

An antibody screen is used to detect Rh antibodies in maternal serum. This test used to be called the "indirect" Coombs because the serum is subjected to several different conditions to detect various antibodies. It is a screening test because it does not directly identify specific antibodies. However, by observing which types of mixtures cause agglutinations, the laboratory can identify specific antibodies indirectly. If there is a positive result from the antibody screening, the laboratory may do more tests to identify the specific antibodies. This test is also done as part of a cross match.

Preparation of Client and Collection of Sample
The laboratory needs 10 ml of venous blood in a red-top container.

Reference Values for Antibody Screen

The antibody screening test should be negative.

MICROBIOLOGIC SEROLOGICAL TESTS

The tests in this section are used for various types of diseases with infectious agents. Table 14–5 provides an overview.

Serological Tests for Hepatitis

The several different forms of viral hepatitis are designated as hepatitis A (formerly called infectious hepatitis), hepatitis B (formerly called serum hepatitis), and non-A/non-B hepatitis. There are at least two different types of non-A/non-B hepatitis. Table 14–6 describes a wide array of tests presently being used to detect hepatitis A and hepatitis B. At the present time, there are no tests to detect non-A/non-B hepatitis.

■ HEPATITIS B SURFACE AND e ANTIGENS (HB$_s$Ag and HB$_e$Ag) AND ANTIBODIES AGAINST HEPATITIS B ANTIGENS

The virus that causes hepatitis B was discovered in 1965 in an Australian man. It was originally named the "Australian" antigen, and early laboratory tests were called HAA for hepatitis Australian antigen. The commonly used test now is called hepatitis B surface antigen (HB$_s$Ag). Because a typical virus has many different antigens, a surface antigen is but one component of the hepatitis B virus. Numerous tests are now available to identify the hepatitis B antigens and antibodies as noted in Table 14–6.

The detection of hepatitis B surface antigen in a person's serum means either that the client is ill with the disease or is a carrier. In either case, the blood is a possible source of infection for other people. Evidently most people do not carry the virus after the disease is over. London (1977) states that in about 90% of hepatitis B clients the antigen disappears from the serum in about 6 weeks. Hepatitis B is spread primarily by blood or blood products. Because the incubation period is 50–180 days, a client who gets hepatitis B from a blood transfusion may not show symptoms for up to 6 months. Thus no one who has had a blood transfusion can donate blood for 6 months. Tests of HB$_s$Ag have become very useful in screening blood donors, many of whom would not be aware that they are carriers. (Note that because blood also transmits non-A/non-B hepatitis, hepatitis is still a possibility after any blood transfusion.)

In addition to testing for the presence of the HB$_s$Ag, the laboratory can also test for antibodies against the hepatitis B antigens. A person who has antibodies against HB$_s$Ag is presumed to be immune to hepatitis B, but not necessarily to other types of hepatitis. Table 14–6 summarizes information about the usefulness of three different antibody tests.

Preparation of Client and Collection of Sample

The laboratory uses venous blood to test for hepatitis B. The exact amount needed depends on the specific test used. Anyone drawing blood for hepatitis B testing should be aware of the danger of hepatitis. When drawing blood, wear gloves and avoid any contact with the blood or contaminated needle. The laboratory specimen should be labeled as "possible hepatitis."

Reference Values for Hepatitis B

A positive HB_sAg indicates either active hepatitis or a carrier state. In either case, the client's blood may be a source of infection.

A positive antibody titer to HB_sAg presumably indicates immunity to hepatitis B.

Both a negative antigen and an antibody test for HB_sAg indicate the person is susceptible to hepatitis B.

POSSIBLE NURSING DIAGNOSES RELATED TO POSITIVE TEST FOR HEPATITIS B

Knowledge Deficit Regarding Spread of Infection

Because hepatitis B is spread by the parenteral route (blood and blood products), nurses must use blood precautions when hepatitis B is suspected or confirmed by testing. They should wear gloves to draw blood, to start an intravenous, or to handle any blood-contaminated articles. Clients must be informed on why these precautions are taken. Nurses in other areas, such as blood laboratories, operating rooms, and delivery rooms, must also be aware of the risk in handling blood. All cuts, skin breaks, or injuries with a needle should be avoided or reported if they do occur. Too many nurses do not report needle injuries (Hamory, 1983) and many may not follow basic needle stick precautions as noted by Scharf (1986). Also clients may share needles and thus spread the infection. Clients who are carriers must be informed of the potential risk to others through blood or contact with other body secretions such as semen. Hepatitis B is also spread by sexual contact.

Bauer (1980) outlines a specific program for regular serologic testing in renal dialysis units because the incidence of hepatitis B is high for both staff and clients. Both clients and staff may be routinely monitored by the HB_sAg test and the HB_sAg antibody test. Clients and staff who are identified as carriers of HB_sAg are then separated from clients who do not have antibodies against HB_sAg.

Knowledge Deficit Regarding Prevention of Disease

Gamma globulin is used to lessen the severity of hepatitis A, but it is not generally used to lessen the impact of hepatitis B. Hepatitis B immune globulin, which differs from the standard gamma globulin, is available (Mar, 1982). A vaccine to protect against hepatitis B has been developed to provide active immunity against hepatitis B (Roche 1981). Education about the vaccine is important for high-risk groups, which in addition to health workers includes drug abusers and homosexual men.

Activity Intolerance Related to Extreme Fatigue
See the discussion under hepatitis A and on bilirubin levels (Chapter 11) and transaminase levels (Chapter 12) for more information on other nursing diagnoses of clients with hepatitis. Hepatitis B tends to be more severe than Hepatitis A.

■ HEPATITIS A TESTS: anti-HAV, IgM, IgG

Hepatitis A is primarily spread by the oral-fecal route. It is often spread by food handlers or by sexual contact. The incubation period is about 15–45 days, which is much shorter than the 50–180 days of hepatitis B. Zuckerman (1979) states that various tests for hepatitis A have shown that hepatitis A is endemic all over the world, that it is not transmitted by blood transfusions, and that there is no evidence of progression to chronic liver disease. Much research is now being done to find out how non-A/non-B hepatitis differs from the clinical entity called hepatitis A. Clinical features cannot distinguish hepatitis A from other types of hepatitis (Koff et al. 1982). As noted in Table 14–6, there are two tests for hepatitis A and many more for hepatitis B. If all are negative, the client is presumed to have non-A/non-B hepatitis (Walach, 1986).

Preparation of Client and Collection of Sample
Collect 2 ml of serum, being careful not to touch the blood. Because some types of hepatitis are spread through the blood products, the laboratory should be warned that the client is suspected of having hepatitis.

Reference Values for Hepatitis A

A positive test for hepatitis A antibodies of the IgM type is good evidence of an acute infection with the virus. Antibodies of the IgG type are indicative of past exposure to hepatitis A. About 7–77% of adults are positive for IgG, depending on geographic location (Tietz, 1983).

POSSIBLE NURSING DIAGNOSES RELATED TO POSITIVE HEPATITIS A TEST

Knowledge Deficit Regarding Spread of Disease
If the test indicates acute infection, the major nursing implication is to initiate enteric precautions so that feces-to-oral transmission of the virus does not occur. Isolation is usually not necessary if the person is a responsible adult who can do thorough handwashing after touching the perianal area. The person should not be allowed to handle or prepare any food for others. The disease can also be transmitted by sexual contact.

Potential for Injury Related to Gamma Globulin Injections
If there is a possibility that the infected person may have infected others by food handling or by intimate contact, the contacts may be offered gamma

globulin. Gamma globulin (Gamastan) is also recommended for persons who plan to travel in areas where hepatitis A is common. Gamma globulin, which can be given up to two weeks after exposure, does not prevent the disease, but it may lessen the severity. The immune serum globulin against hepatitis A comes from human sources. The product information sheet gives the recommended dosages based on weight. Note that anaphylactic reactions, although very rare, can occur (Mar, 1982).

Activity Intolerance Related to Extreme Fatigue

There is no drug to cure hepatitis; the mainstays of treatment are rest and a nutritious diet to promote liver regeneration. For other nursing diagnoses see bilirubin levels (Chapter 11) and transaminase levels (Chapter 12), which are used to monitor the progress of the patient. Gurevich (1983) and Vargo (1984) are excellent resources on nursing needs of clients with hepatitis.

■ ACQUIRED IMMUNE DEFICIENCY SYNDROME (AIDS) TEST: ANTIBODIES FOR HTLV-III OR HIV

A lymphadenopathy associated virus (LAV) known as human T-cell lymphocytic virus (HTLV-III) or human immunodeficiency virus (HIV) is considered to be the likely cause of AIDS, but its exact role has not yet been proven (Bennett, 1985b). Serum antibodies against HTLV-III or HIV can be measured and are the basis of the tests for AIDS at the present time. The laboratory can do both screening and confirmatory tests for the antibodies. Whether or not people who have the antibodies will get the disease is not known, although the appearance of antibodies is of concern. The time between exposure to the virus and the appearance of antibodies (seroconversion) is unknown (Jason et al., 1986). Some authorities believe only about 1 in 5 clients who have positive antibodies will get the disease.

Blood banks began using the test for antibodies against HTLV-III or HIV in 1985. The use of this screening test has very dramatically reduced the risk of transmission of AIDS via blood transfusions. Also in 1985, the U.S. Public Health Service announced establishment of alternative sites for antibody testing so high-risk clients for AIDS could get the test without going to a blood bank. High-risk groups include male homosexuals, intravenous drug users, and hemophiliacs. The risk for hemophiliacs is reduced now because of the screening test but there are an estimated 20,000 hemophiliacs who are already seropositive (Helquist, 1986). The sexual contacts of hemophiliacs positive for the antibodies are also likely to become positive (Mason, 1986). Although heterosexual transmission is less likely than male homosexual activity, AIDS virus transmission is possible from men to women and vice versa (Lederman, 1986).

The establishment of test centers has raised many legal and ethical dilemmas, many of which are not resolved, as indicated by the continuation of many newspaper articles on concerns about the tests. The Centers for Disease Control has conducted

---

Reference Values for HTLV-III or HIV Antibodies

Negative for antibodies to HTLV-III or HIV

---

several seminars in various locations to help health care workers obtain the latest information about the tests used and how to counsel people who do test positive.

POSSIBLE NURSING DIAGNOSIS RELATED TO POSITIVE HTLV-III OR HIV

Alteration in Health Maintenance
Bennett (1985b) lists the ten recommendations to be given to a person who has a positive antibody test for HTLV-III or HIV. The recommendations are to help decrease the possible spread of the virus and to inform the person of good health practices. The reader is encouraged to consult the most current literature to obtain up-to-date information about the AIDS test and the appropriate counseling for those who do test positive. At the present time, transmission of the AIDS virus seems similar to transmission of the hepatitis B virus. (See the earlier discussion on blood precautions.) Much anxiety is generated by the unknown aspects of this disease. Health care workers should be well informed so they can help the public deal with this epidemic of the eighties. As Bennett (1985a) notes, we know how to prevent transmission, but more than 500,000 may already be infected. Morrison (1986) notes that the care of clients with AIDS is nursing's special challenge and hence the *California Nurse* devoted a whole issue to this challenge.

■ SEROLOGICAL TESTS FOR SYPHILIS (STS)

Except for the common cold and flu, venereal diseases are the most common infectious diseases in the United States. Although chlamydia, herpes, and gonorrhea are more common than syphilis, syphilis is the more dangerous if left undetected and thus untreated. (See Chapter 17 for the tests for gonorrhea, chlamydia, and herpes.)

Although the spirochete, *Treponema pallidum,* that causes syphilis may occasionally be identified from a syphilitic sore, or chancre, syphilis is more commonly diagnosed by a serology test. Testing for syphilis may be divided into tests done for screening and those done for a confirmation of a positive screening test. The venereal disease research laboratory (VDRL) or rapid plasma reagin (RPR) are screening tests, whereas the fluorescent treponemal antibody absorption test (FTA-ABS) and the microhemagglutination (MHA) are confirmatory tests for syphilis. The Wassermann test, which used a complement fixation technique, was the first serological test for syphilis, but it is no longer used.

VDRL and RPR

The VDRL is named for the research laboratory that perfected this flocculation test for syphilis. The test measures a globulin complex called reagin that appears early in the course of syphilis. If the globulin complex reagin is present, an aggregation occurs that can be reported as either negative, weakly reactive, or reactive. The RPR rapid plasma reagin uses the VDRL antigen, but it adds some carbon particles so that the flocculation can be seen on a plastic card.

The VDRL and variations of it are indirect tests for syphilis because they are tests for a reaction to a globulin, not to the spirochete itself. Thus a person who is treated for syphilis may still have antibodies in the serum for a time, but they usually decline. A person who has just contracted syphilis may not have had time to build up antibodies against *Treponema pallidum*. The tests usually become positive in three to four weeks after exposure. Because the screening tests react to abnormal globulins, other types of pathology, such as malaria, other infections, and some connective tissue disorders, may cause false positives.

FTA-ABS and MHA-TP

The FTA-ABS is used to confirm an infection with the spirochete that causes syphilis. It tests for the specific antibodies against *Treponema pallidum*. The laboratory prepares a slide and stains it to make the antibodies show up as a yellow-green color under an ultraviolet microscope. Technical difficulties are involved in doing the test, and false positives can occur.

Another confirming test is the microhemagglutination for *Treponema pallidum* (MHA-TP) test. The MHA-TP may be substituted for the FTA-ABS in certain situations to confirm the diagnosis of syphilis. The MHA-TP is easier to perform and costs less than the FTA-ABS. These two confirmatory tests are not appropriate for screening because they remain positive even after treatment.

Preparation of Client and Collection of Specimen

The laboratory uses 4 ml of venous blood for STS. Alcohol may interfere with some tests. Fasting is usually not required but is preferred by some laboratories.

Reference Values for STS

These tests should be negative.

Note that various conditions may cause false positives in the screening test, as explained in the text. Also note that the tests will be the most strongly positive 4–6 weeks after exposure.

POSSIBLE NURSING DIAGNOSIS RELATED TO POSITIVE SEROLOGICAL TEST FOR SYPHILIS

Knowledge Deficit Related to Need for Screening and Follow-up of Sexual Contacts

If not detected in the early stages, syphilis may eventually spread, causing severe neurological problems, blindness, and even death. The treatment of syphilis is extremely easy: penicillin by injection. Other antibiotics are used if the person is allergic to penicillin.

As a communicable disease, syphilis must be reported to the public health department. Venereal disease clinics and public health departments have staffs who follow up the sexual contacts of the person who has a positive STS. Nurses may take an active role in educating the public about the importance of screening people who may have been exposed to the disease. Nurses working with clients who have a positive STS can help impress upon them the importance of early detection and early treatment of their sexual partners. Obviously, nurses need to be nonjudgmental in their approach.

Because syphilis can be passed to a fetus, it is extremely important that a pregnant woman be treated for syphilis. (See Chapter 16 for information about other venereal diseases and pregnancy.) The nurse working in a prenatal clinic can help to explain to clients why a STS is done in early pregnancy.

■ COLD AGGLUTININS OR COLD HEMAGGLUTININS

In some disease states, antibodies cause clumping of the client's blood when the blood is refrigerated at a certain temperature. When a client has a respiratory infection with *Mycoplasma pneumoniae*, there is often an increase in cold agglutinins. Hence this test of cold agglutinins is primarily used to assess for the possibility of primary atypical pneumonia. Mycoplasmal pneumonia is caused by a pleuropneumonia-like organism (PPLO) that has characteristics of both a virus and a bacteria. *Mycoplasma pneumoniae* is also called the Eaton agent (Wallach, 1986). The PPLO can be cultured, but it takes longer, so a rising titer of cold agglutinins helps with the diagnosis sooner. Other conditions, such as severe anemia, congenital syphilis, hepatitis, and cirrhosis, may also cause cold agglutinins. Antibiotic therapy may interfere with the formation of the cold agglutinins.

Preparation of Client and Collection of Sample
The test requires 10 ml of whole blood. The blood is drawn into a warm tube or syringe and immediately put into a 37 °C (98.6 °F) water bath for transportation to the laboratory. The specimen should be hand-carried to the laboratory.

Reference Values for Cold Agglutinins

All groups	Titers over 1:32 are considered abnormal. A rising titer is more significant than one high titer
Pregnancy	May have positive titer
Aged	Titer is higher in older people

POSSIBLE NURSING DIAGNOSIS RELATED TO POSITIVE COLD AGGLUTININS

Potential for Impaired Gas Exchange
Because the client who has cold agglutinins ordered usually has a respiratory infection, general nursing care takes the form of the standard care for the client with pneumonia. Antibiotics, such as erythromycin or one of the tetracyclines, may be ordered for atypical pneumonia by the Eaton agent. Respiratory isolation is needed.

■ FEBRILE AGGLUTININS FOR TYPHOID FEVER, PARATYPHOID, BRUCELLOSIS, AND TULAREMIA

Febrile agglutinins are antibodies that are produced in response to certain bacterial infections that cause fever in the patient. (Although cold agglutinins are tested by cooling the blood sample, febrile agglutinins are not tested by heating the sample.) A specific bacterial cell antigen is mixed with the sample of blood from the client to see if agglutination occurs. For example, the Widal test uses the *Salmonella* antigen to test for typhoid and paratyphoid fever. Two other common tests using specific bacterial antigens are for tularemia (rabbit fever) and brucellosis (undulant fever). With simple slide agglutination techniques for these bacterial infections, the laboratory can easily do the test of "febrile agglutinins." The febrile agglutinins for typhoid and paratyphoid are no longer useful because the laboratory can do more specific cultures and serological tests for these infections (Zuerlein & Smith, 1985).

Preparation of Client and Collection of Sample
The laboratory needs 6 ml of whole blood. At least two samples are needed, one during the acute stage and one during the convalescent stage.

Reference Values for Febrile Agglutinins

A fourfold rise in titer is considered strong evidence of infection with the specific bacteria being tested.

■ INFECTIOUS MONONUCLEOSIS

Heterophil Antibody Titer (HAT)
The heterophil antibody titer (HAT) is a test for infectious mononucleosis, a viral disease. The word "heterophil" refers to an affinity for more than one group or species. Normally humans do not have antibodies against the red blood cells of sheep, but clients with infectious mononucleosis do develop antibodies that agglutinate the red blood cells of sheep.

The test, however, is not specifically diagnostic, because other factors may also cause an increase in heterophile antibodies. For example, allergic reactions, such as serum sickness, cause an increased HAT. Therefore serological tests to measure the titer of antibodies to the Epstein–Barr virus may be needed for confirmation.

Diagnostic Kits for Infectious Mononucleosis
Spot tests for infectious mononucleosis include Monospot (Ortho Diagnostics), Monotest (Wampole), and Monoscreen (Smith Kline & French). The "spot" test uses a saline suspension of antigen derived from horses' red blood cells. The mixture of the test material with a drop of the client's serum causes a coarse granulation if the client has infectious mononucleosis. The spot tests are rapid, specific, and sensitive as screening tests, and they are valuable in supporting a clinical diagnosis of infectious mononucleosis. Yet they do not positively identify the Epstein–Barr virus of infectious mononucleosis and titers may be needed, as discussed earlier. Other criteria

for diagnosing infectious mononucleosis include lymphocytosis and the presence of atypical lymphocytes in the serum. (See Chapter 2 for a discussion of lymphocytes as part of a differential WBC).

Preparation of Client and Collection of Sample
The screening tests require 1–2 ml of blood. A WBC with differential is also ordered.

NURSING DIAGNOSIS FOR A POSITIVE HAT OR SPOT TEST

Activity Intolerance Related to Fatigue
Nursing care for clients with infectious mononucleosis includes providing rest and other general measures to help them overcome a viral infection. There is no drug therapy for the virus. Although infectious mononucleosis is sometimes called the "kissing disease," the exact mode of transmission is unknown. Isolation is not necessary. Large epidemiological studies have demonstrated that 50–80% of people have antibody titers against the Epstein–Barr virus (Bullock & Rosendahl, 1984). Transaminase levels (Chapter 12) and bilirubin levels (Chapter 11) are used to assess the degree of liver dysfunction.

■ STREPTOCOCCI INFECTIONS

Definition and Purpose
Three tests are used to identify a recent infection with group A-beta hemolytic streptococci:

1. Anti-streptolysin-O (ASO)
2. Anti-streptodornase-B or anti-deoxyribonuclease-B (anti-DNase-B)
3. Streptozyme test

Group A-beta hemolytic streptococci produce several substances (antigens) that induce the formation of measurable antibodies in the serum. Because the aftermath of group A streptococci infections may be such diseases as rheumatic fever or glomerulonephritis, one or more of these three streptococcal antigen tests is used to help in confirming that the client did have a streptococci infection in the recent past. Rheumatic fever is becoming rarer because of early recognition and treatment of streptocci infections such as strep throat. In Third World countries rheumatic fever is a major problem (Bullock & Rosendahl, 1984). (See Chapter 16 on the importance of throat cultures to identify strep throat.) In clients with rheumatic fever, 95% show an elevated titer to one or more of the streptococcal antigen tests (Fitzmaurice, 1980). A rising titer suggests a very recent infection, while a stable titer indicates previous exposure to the streptococci antigens.

Anti-streptolysin-O (ASO). The antibodies to streptolysin-O appear about 7 days after an acute streptococcal infection. The antibodies peak two to four weeks later, remaining high for weeks to months. The test may not always be elevated with streptococci infections, and other disease conditions, such as liver disease, may make the test falsely positive.

Anti-streptodornase-B (Anti-DNase-B). Anti-DNase-B measures the antibodies formed against another of the streptococcal enzymes called deoxyribonuclease-B. It may be used in conjunction with the other two tests for streptococci antigens.

Streptozyme Test. This test, a commercial product, is more general than the ASO or anti-DNase-B. It measures antibodies against five different streptococcal enzymes: (1) streptolysin-O, (2) deoxyribonuclease-B, (3) hyaluronidase, (4) streptokinase, and (5) nicotinamide adenine dinucleotidase. This test may be more sensitive than the other tests, but false positives can also occur.

Preparation of Client and Collection of Sample

These tests require venous blood. Make a note on the laboratory slip if the client was on antibiotics, because titers may not increase if the client has been on antibiotics.

Reference Values for Tests for Streptococci Infections	
ASO titers:	
Preschool	1:85
Age 5–18	1:170
Adults	1:85
Anti-DNase-B titers:	
Preschool	1:60
Age 5–18	1:170
Adults	1:85
Streptozyme titers	Less than 100 streptozyme units

■ RUBELLA

Rubella (also called three-day measles or German measles) is usually of no significance unless it occurs in a pregnant woman. Rubella may cause a miscarriage, or it may bring about congenital heart disease, cataracts, deafness, and brain damage in the fetus. Thus, it is important to assess whether women who are to become pregnant have an immunity against rubella.

Reference Values for Rubella
Titers of 1:32 or more indicate immunity (Tietz, 1983)
If tested by EIA, IgG = index greater than 1.2 shows immunity
IgM = index greater than 1.09 is positive for acute infection

The laboratory uses either hemagglutination inhibition (HI) or complement fixation serology tests to assess for the presence of antibodies against the rubella virus. Antibodies appear within a week or less after the rash. Once the person has had the disease, an elevated titer of antibodies persists for many years or perhaps for life. Even a small number of antibodies indicates some immunity from the disease. Women who are not immune to rubella (that is, who have no antibody titer) should be vaccinated before becoming pregnant. The rubella test for antibodies is one of the blood tests necessary to obtain a marriage license.

Preparation of Client and Collection of Sample
The test requires venous blood.

POSSIBLE NURSING DIAGNOSES RELATED TO NEGATIVE TITER

Knowledge Deficit Regarding Need for Vaccine
The lack of a titer to rubella is significant in women who may become pregnant. Since 1969, when the first rubella vaccine was licensed in the United States, there has been a mass immunization program for school-aged children. However, there are still women in their childbearing years who are susceptible to rubella. A single dose of rubella vaccine is recommended not only for children more than 12 months old, but also for any woman who has no antibody titer for rubella and who may become pregnant (Abramowicz, 1979).

Whether some action should be taken may be a very disturbing question for the woman who contacts rubella during her pregnancy. If a pregnant woman is suspected of having contacted rubella, a rise in maternal rubella IgM would be evidence of recent infection. The client needs to confer with the physician about the possible damage to the fetus.

Health care workers must take all measures necessary to prevent susceptible pregnant women from contacting rubella. All health workers who might transmit rubella to pregnant women should also be immunized against the disease. Claypool (1981) describes a program that was used in a health agency to establish rubella protection. The policy at the agency included immunization for all health workers who did not have evidence of a positive rubella titer within the past five years.

Potential for Injury Related to Vaccine
Nurses should be aware that adult women who are given the vaccine should avoid pregnancy for three months. Giving the client information about reliable birth control may be necessary. Also, because the vaccine can cause some joint symptoms, particularly in adults, the possible side effects of the vaccine need to be explained. Women may need to sign an informed consent noting the risks inherent in getting pregnant within 3 months of the injection.

■ TOXOPLASMOSIS (TPM, Toxo)

TPM is caused by an infection with the protozoan *Toxoplasma gondii,* which is found in raw or poorly cooked meat and in the feces of cats. The infection causes fatigue, fever, and lymph gland swelling. The oldest test for TPM is the Sabin–Feldman, which uses a dye to stain the organism. Other tests for TPM use serological tests of antibodies. The immunofluorescent antibody test (IFA) is considered almost diagnostic if one other test, such as the indirect hemagglutination (IHA) or complement fixation (CF), is positive (Lake, 1979). TPM can be treated by certain drugs so that usually the infection is not too serious in an adult unless the host is immunocompromised, such as in AIDS. Toxoplasmosis can be passed to the fetus and cause various types of neurological damage and eye problems.

Preparation of Client and Collection of Sample
Check with the laboratory for the specific type of serological test being used. Most of the tests for toxoplasmosis require about 4 ml of whole blood. Pertinent history includes whether the client has been exposed to cats, may be pregnant, or is immunosuppressed.

Reference Values for TPM

IFA titer of 1:10 is considered almost diagnostic if IHA or CF test is up.

Note that the IFA is falsely positive if the serum contains antinuclear antibodies (ANA), which are discussed later in this chapter.

Infants may have an increased titer due to the transfer of antibodies from the mother. Infants need to be retested later.

POSSIBLE NURSING DIAGNOSES RELATED TO POSITIVE TITER

Knowledge Deficit Related to Danger for Pregnant Women
People should be aware that poorly cooked or raw meat can introduce organisms into the human body. Also the importance of avoiding hand contamination from the feces of cats should be made common knowledge. Because cats are the host, the pregnant woman needs to be careful about handling the feces of a cat and certainly to avoid strange cats. A veterinarian can be contacted about the health status of a house cat.

Anxiety Related to Unknown Diagnosis
The presence of lymphadenopathy (enlarged lymph glands) and vague symptoms in an otherwise healthy person may suggest a viral infection. The client with suspected TPM may also have tests done for infectious mononucleosis. In contrast to infectious mononucleosis, there is no elevated heterophil antibody test. (See earlier in this chapter for the discussion of the HAT.) Until the diagnosis is made by the physician, the client may be afraid that the lymph gland swelling is due to a malignancy and is likely to be very relieved to find out that the problem is an infection with a protozoan. The drugs used for treatment include pyrimethamine, sulfonamide, and sometimes clindamycin (Lake, 1979). In the immunosuppressed client TPM may be a serious or even fatal disease.

■ AMEBIASIS

Entamoeba histolytica is an ameba that causes amebic dysentary and hepatic abscesses. The ameba can be identfed by microscopic examination. (See Chapter 16 for the technique used to obtain a stool culture for ameba.) The stool examination is the most definitive test for ameba, but it is technically difficult to obtain live amebae for direct examination. An indirect hemagglutination technique can identify antibodies to *Entamoeba histolytica,* which are present in 95% of clients with a hepatic abscess due to the ameba and in 70% of clients with an intestinal infection of *Entamoeba histolytica* (Tietz, 1983).

Preparation of Client and Collection of Sample

The test requires venous blood. Check with the laboratory for the exact amount.

Reference Values for Ameba

Fourfold titer increase indicates infection with the ameba. Antibody levels persist for some time after an active infestation.

POSSIBLE NURSING DIAGNOSIS RELATED TO INCREASING TITER

Knowledge Deficit Related to Spread of Disease
See Chapter 16 for the client teaching needed when a patient must be on enteric precautions.

■ CYTOMEGALOVIRUS (CMV) TITERS

CMV, a type of herpes virus found in almost all body secretions, can cross the placenta and be transferred by blood. Many adults have had exposure to the virus and thus have developed immunity. The virus is particularly dangerous for the pregnant woman because of damage to the fetus. The virus can cause cerebral malformation and necrosis of brain tissue (Bullock & Rosendahl, 1984). Immunosuppressed clients are also very susceptible to CMV. At least 50% of renal transplant patients will show positive CMV titers (Tietz, 1983). Clients with AIDS usually have high titers for CMV. Acute infection with the virus in the client with AIDS often leads to eye damage and blindness as well as cerebral damage.

The potential risk to health workers is probably low because healthy people have adequate immune systems. Young et al. (1983) conducted a study to see if CMV was a serious hazard to female staff caring for newborns infected with CMV. The precaution of screening the antibody status of employees, tried for 18 months, did not prove necessary as CMV was not a substantial risk to staff. Standard techniques to avoid contamination with body secretions, including the admonition that babies should not be kissed by nursery personnel, were adequate to protect the staff.

Reference Values for CMV

A fourfold or greater rise in titer between acute and convalescent samples is evidence of infection. A single IgM-specific titer of more than 1:8 is evidence of an acute infection.

■ HERPES SIMPLEX VIRUS (HSV) ANTIBODIES

A primary infection with HSV (either HSV type 1 for oral herpes or HSV type 2 for genital herpes) may produce rising antibody titers. Because exposure to one of the herpes viruses is almost universal in the population, the serological test for herpes is usually not useful for clinical management. However, the titers of HSV are useful in epidemiology studies or for research (Jacobs et al., 1984). Clinical diagnosis of genital herpes is usually made on the basis of history and symptoms. The two specific tests to confirm HSV type 2, the Tzanck test and viral cultures, are discussed in Chapter 16. Diagnosis is particularly important in the pregnant female (Bassing, 1985).

■ TORCH SCREEN

The TORCH screen includes testing for *T*oxoplasmosis, *O*ther (usually hepatitis or syphilis), *R*ubella, *C*ytomegalovirus, and *H*erpes simplex. The TORCH screen is done in newborn infants to evaluate possible congenital infection with one of these viruses. Rubella and CMV are the two most common viruses to infect the fetus (Bullock & Rosendahl, 1984). By evaluating the type of the antibody present in the cord blood, the laboratory may be able to determine if there is passive transfer from the mother (IgG antibodies) or actual congenital infection (IgM antibodies). Because antibody production may not occur early enough in the infection, the TORCH screen is not always useful. TORCH screen is not a substitute for careful clinical examination and Leland et al. (1983) warn that it is usually much better to focus on isolating a specific suspected organism.

■ FUNGAL ANTIBODIES: HISTOPLASMOSIS, COCCIDIOIDOMYCOSIS, AND BLASTOMYCOSIS

By use of the complement fixation (CF) or immunodiffusion techniques, the laboratory can identify antibodies that occur in response to fungus diseases, such as histoplasmosis, coccidioidomycosis, and blastomycosis. Histoplasmosis is particularly found in the Ohio Valley area, and coccidioidomycosis (valley fever or desert fever) is prominent in the San Joaquin Valley of California. Because many people who live in an area where a fungus is endemic may have positive serologic tests from past exposures, one titer is not enough to be diagnostic. A fourfold rise in titer would be evidence of a present infection. Although certain types of fungus are endemic in certain areas, in this age of jet travel, clients with the disease may be far from the origin. A travel history is mandatory when a fungus is suspected (Einstein, 1980).

Skin testing and cultures may also be used to identify the particular fungus causing the systemic infection. (See Chapter 16 for some tips on cultures for fungus.) A positive skin test does not indicate that an infection is currently present, because the antibodies may be from past exposure. More significant is a conversion of a negative skin test to a positive one. Because skin tests can also cause a serological test to become positive, they should be started after the blood is drawn for serological tests for fungus antibodies.

■ FUNGAL ANTIGENS

Tests to identify antigens (rather than antibodies) for various fungi are being developed. Antigen tests are already used for cryptococcosis and are promising for candidiasis, aspergillosis, and histoplasmosis (Wheat et al., 1986).

Preparation of Client and Collection of Sample
These tests require venous blood, which should be drawn before any skin testing is done.

Reference Values for Fungal Antibodies and Antigens

Fourfold rise in antibody titer is evidence of infection. Specific antigens may be found in blood, urine, or cerebrospinal fluid.

NURSING IMPLICATIONS

The nurse should confer with the physician to see if the client presents any danger to other clients or to the staff. Refer to a nursing text for detailed information on the care of clients with fungus disease. Nurses may administer ordered skin tests for fungus. The technique for intradermal injection, the diluent strength of the antigen, and the times to read the results are clearly explained with the product information that comes with the test material.

■ RICKETTSIAL DISEASE: *PROTEUS* OX-19, *PROTEUS* OX-2, AND *PROTEUS* OX-K (WEIL–FELIX REACTION)

The nonpathogenic organism, *Proteus* OX-19, is agglutinated by the serum of people with certain rickettsial diseases, such as Rocky Mountain spotted fever and typhus. This reaction is called the Weil–Felix reaction. Other types of *Proteus,* such as OX-2 or OX-K, may be used to determine other specific types of infection with rickettsiae (Wallach, 1986). Culturing the rickettsiae is possible, but it must be done in a special laboratory. Any laboratory, on the other hand, can do serological testing. So the *Proteus* test is commonly used when a rickettsial disease is suspected.

Preparation of Client and Collection of Sample
The test requires 6 ml of venous blood. Because the Weil–Felix reaction involves a reaction to the *Proteus* antigen, the test is not indicative of rickettsial disease if the client has an infection with certain pathogenic strains of *Proteus.* Note the possibility of any *Proteus* infections. (See Chapter 16 for a discussion of *Proteus* infections of the urinary tract, respiratory tract, and wounds.) Other diseases, such as typhoid, may occasionally cause agglutinations of *Proteus* OX-19 and conditions such as liver disease may cause false positives.

Reference Values for Felix–Weil Reaction

A titer of 1:40 or 1:80 is considered possible evidence of rickettsial disease.

A titer of 1:160 or above is presumptive evidence of infection with one of the rickettsiae.

All rickettsiae are spread by vectors. For example, epidemic typhus is spread by body lice, and Rocky Mountain spotted fever is spread by a tick. The laboratory needs to know of possible exposure to these vectors. Because transmission requires a vector, the client is not infectious to others.

IMMUNOLOGICAL TESTS

The few tests discussed in this section are used primarily to assess for diseases such as systemic lupus erythematosus (SLE), rheumatoid arthritis (RA), or other auto-immune reactions. See Table 14–7 for a list of the common serological tests used in immunology and Appendix A, Table 5 for less common ones.

■ C-REACTIVE PROTEIN (CRP)

The CRP, not normally present in the blood, appears with inflammatory processes or with tissue destruction. It is not elevated in viral infections. Sometimes this test is used to monitor rheumatic fever or RA. Like the erythrocyte sedimentation rate (ESR), the CRP is a very nonspecific test that indicates only an inflammation. The CRP may rise sooner than the ESR, and different clinicians may choose to use either the ESR or the CRP. (See Chapter 2 for the discussion of ESR as the more common test used to monitor RA.) The CRP has been found to be the most reliable predictor of chorioamnionitis, a bacterial infection that can develop following premature rupture of the membranes (Hawrylshyn et al., 1983).

Preparation of Client and Collection of Sample
The test requires 3 ml of venous blood.

TABLE 14–7. COMMON SEROLOGICAL TESTS USED IN IMMUNOLOGY

Test	Description
C-reactive protein	Measures an abnormal protein found in the serum in certain inflammations. Compare to ESR in Chapter 2
Complement activity	Measures activity of the complement system
C_3 and C_4	Specific measurements of the amount of two of the complement factors
LE prep	Examination for a particular type of cell in SLE
ANA	Measures antinuclear antibodies, which are sometimes increased in SLE
Anti-DNA	Other humoral antibodies, which are sometimes elevated in SLE
RF	Measurement of antibodies, which may be elevated in rheumatoid arthritis
Thyroid colloid and microsomal antigen tests	Measurement of antibodies, which may be elevated in certain types of thyroiditis

ANA = antinuclear antibodies; ESR = erythrocyte sedimentation rate; LE = lupus erythematosus; RF = rheumatoid factor; SLE = systemic erythematosus.

Reference Values for C-Reactive Protein

Should be negative except in pregnancy.
Oral contraceptive pills may cause an increase.

■ COMPLEMENT ACTIVITY: C_3, C_4, and C_1 ESTERASE INHIBITOR

The complement system consists of several proteins that are active in producing the inflammatory response sometimes following an antigen–antibody reaction. In the classical pathway, the complement is activated by an antigen–antibody response. In the alternate pathway, polysaccharides, endotoxins, or immunoglobulins activate the complement cascade. The final reaction of the complement system produces a complex protein capable of lysing cell membranes.

The total amount of complement activity may be measured by a hemolytic assay and expressed in units as compared to a normal standard. The test of total complement activity is difficult to do and to standardize because it must use fresh human or guinea pig complement. A much simpler test involves measuring two of the components of the complement system. These two components, C_3 and C_4, as well as the other components of the complement system, are used up in the very complicated series of reactions that follow some antibody–antigen reactions. In certain of the rheumatoid diseases, tests of complement activity help clinicians to judge the number of immune complexes occurring. Immune complexes appear to be the primary mediators of tissue injury in SLE, RA, and polyarteritis nodosa (Koffler, 1979).

C_3 is the preferred test in most clinical situations. C_3 comprises about 70% of the total protein in the complement system and is central to activation of both the classical and alternate pathways (Jacobs et al., 1984). C_4 is utilized only by the classical pathway. Diseases such as hereditary angioedema (HAE) can be screened by C_4. HAE is an autosomal dominant trait that causes a lack of C_1 esterase inhibitor, a serum protein that regulates activation of the first component of the complement cascade (Huber & Calliari, 1985).

Preparation of Client and Collection of Sample
Tests for C_3 and C_4 require 2 ml of serum collected without additives. The C_1 esterase inhibitor test requires 5 ml of clotted blood. The test for total hemolytic activity requires 10 ml of blood sent on ice.

Reference Values for Total Complement, C_3, C_4, and C_1 Esterase Inhibitor

---

Complement, total hemolytic activity	150–250 U/ml
C_3	83–177 mg/dl
C_4	15–45 mg/dl
C_1 esterase inhibitor	13.2–24 mg/dl

Values are lower at birth and slightly higher in the aged (Tietz, 1983).

Clinical Significance. An increase in the total complement activity occurs in some acute inflammatory diseases but depressed levels have more clinical significance.

Decreased serum levels of C_3 and C_4 indicate the presence of immune complexes that have used up the complement factors (assuming no inherited complement deficiencies). Complement deficiencies can be genetic but acquired ones are most common (Fidler, 1983).

Although an increase in the amount of complement activity and a decrease in serum C_3 and C_4 indicate that immune complexes are being formed, the actual diagnosis may be very difficult to establish. These tests are likely to be only part of the assessment needed to help the physician establish a diagnosis of a rheumatoid disease. (See the following discussion on LE prep, ANA, and RF.)

A normal level of serum complement levels does not rule out the possibility of an immune reaction, because some antigen–antibody responses do not cause an activation and depletion of the complement factors. Much research is presently being done on the very complicated picture of immune response. Nurses must read current articles to obtain up-to-date information on the current status of immunological tests. Huber and Calliari (1985) discuss HAE (assessed by the test for C_1 esterase inhibitor) and the nursing diagnoses for the client.

■ LE PREP

The LE prep is a microscopic examination for a particular type of neutrophil that has been changed due to the LE factor in the rheumatoid disease called SLE. The LE factor evidently consists of antibodies that react with the cells. A direct test for antibodies to native DNA and ANA are more sensitive tests for SLE (Koffler, 1979; Jacobs et al, 1984). Not all clients with SLE have a positive LE prep, and clients with other diseases, such as RA, may also have a positive test.

Preparation of Client and Collection of Sample
The test requires 5 ml of whole blood with heparin as an anticoagulant (method I) or defibrinated blood (method II) (Scully, 1986).

Reference Values for LE Prep

The test should be negative.

■ ANTINUCLEAR ANTIBODIES (ANA)

ANA are gamma globulins found in clients with certain types of autoimmune diseases. The test is typically used to rule out SLE because most clients with SLE have a positive ANA. However, the test is not specific for SLE because the test may also be positive in RA, scleroderma, carcinoma, tuberculosis, and hepatitis. Various drugs may also cause an increased ANA.

Preparation of Client and Collection of Sample
The test requires 2 ml of serum, which should be sent to the laboratory immediately.

Reference Values for ANA

Test is considered positive if detected with serum diluted 1:8
Aged   ANA levels seem to increase with age even in people without immune
               diseases

■ ANTIBODIES TO NATIVE DNA (Anti-DNA)

In addition to the ANA test, a test for antibodies to DNA, such as anti-DNA or anti-native DNA, are used to confirm diagnosis of SLE (Tietz, 1983). Consult the current literature to find out more about the recent advances in the use of these tests.

Reference Values for Anti-DNA

Negative at 1:10 dilutions

■ RHEUMATOID FACTOR (RF)

The RF is a test of abnormal proteins found in the serum of many clients with RA. Evidently the RF really consists of different types of IgM antibodies. (See Chapter 10 for the measurement of IgM.) Although the RF is present with other diseases, the highest titers are found in clients with RA. Koffler (1979) states that the RF is present in approximately 75% of clients with RA, but it does not always correlate with the severity of the disease activity. Some "normal" people, particularly the elderly, may have the factor. Clients with tuberculosis, bacterial endocarditis, syphilis, and collagen diseases may have the RF. The RF also commonly occurs in both B and non-B hepatitis (London, 1977).

Preparation of Client and Collection of Sample
The test requires 10 ml clotted blood. A fasting sample is preferred.

Reference Values for RF

Less than 60 IU/ml

POSSIBLE NURSING DIAGNOSIS RELATED TO RF

Alteration in Health Maintenance
The client with RA needs a lot of nursing care both during the acute stages and during remissions. Brown-Skeers (1979) gives some excellent tips on how nurse practitioners can manage clients with RA. The basic triad of treatment includes (1) physical therapy and exercises, (2) emotional and psychological sup-

port, and (3) monitoring of anti-inflammatory drug therapy. The ESR (Chapter 2) is used to follow the disease process. The CRP may also be used to monitor the amount of inflammatory response over time.

■ THYROID ANTIBODIES

In certain types of thyroid disorders, the body produces antibodies against certain thyroid constituents. The end result is inflammation and destruction of the thyroid gland. Although the level of antibodies does not exactly correlate with the severity of the symptoms, identifying the probable cause of thyroid dysfunction is a help. (See Chapter 15 for a complete discussion on hypo- and hyperthyroidism, along with the tests used.) Relatives of clients with thyroid autoimmunity problems may also have high titers of the thyroid antibodies. Because other diseases, such as the collagen diseases, may cause increased titers too, the client may also have other types of antibody tests (see Appendix A, Table 5).

Preparation of Client and Collection of Sample
The test requires 2 ml of serum. Because oral contraceptives may cause titers to become detectable, note whether the client is on birth control pills.

Reference Values for Thyroid Antibodies

Titers should be negative at a 1:10 dilution of serum
Titers increase with age, particularly in some elderly, normal women

---

QUESTIONS

1. Which of the following tests is not routinely done on a unit of donor blood?

    a. HB$_s$Ag (hepatitis B surface antigen)
    b. Coombs (antibody screening)
    c. ANA (antinuclear antibodies)
    d. HTLV-III or HIV antibodies (screen for AIDS virus)

2. Mr. Royal has type AB blood. Theoretically, based on the ABO typing, Mr. Royal could receive any type of blood because he has which of the following?

    a. No A or B antigens
    b. No antibodies against A and B antigens
    c. Only antibodies against O
    d. Only AB antibodies

3. Mrs. Tudor had a hemolytic transfusion reaction, possibly due to incompatible blood. She had fever, chills, and low back pain. The unit of blood was stopped

and returned to the laboratory. The nurse should also save all urine voided for which reason?

a. The urine needs to be checked for free hemoglobin
b. Dehydration must be prevented
c. A bilirubin test should be done stat
d. Circulatory overload may require use of a diuretic

4. Mrs. Sanchez, who is Rh negative, just delivered a healthy 8-lb baby boy who is Rh positive. She was given an injection of RhoGAM. She asks the nurse why she had the shot. Which of the following explanations by the nurse is accurate? "This shot . . .

a. Prevents you from having any problems with any other pregnancies because it eliminates the Rh factor."
b. Gives you temporary antibodies against the Rh factor so that your body won't make any on your own, which could still be present if you have another Rh positive pregnancy."
c. Helps to eliminate any antibodies that you might have gotten from this pregnancy so that the next pregnancy will be normal."
d. Helps your body to manufacture antibodies, so that if you have another pregnancy with a Rh baby there won't be any problems."

5. A positive Coombs test indicates coating of erythrocytes by some type of globulin. Which of the following clinical situations is *not* assessed for by a positive Coombs test?

a. Hemolytic disease of the newborn
b. Autoimmune hemolytic anemias
c. Hemolytic transfusion reactions
d. Administration of gamma globulin

6. Mr. Wayler is a client receiving renal dialysis three times a week. His laboratory test shows a positive report for HB_sAg (hepatitis B surface antigen). Mr. Wayler does not have any symptoms of hepatitis. Based on this data, which precaution should be instituted?

a. None, since he has no evidence of clinical disease
b. Good handwashing technique after contact with Mr. Wayler
c. Use of gloves when any blood-contaminated articles must be handled
d. Administration of gamma globulin to staff who must work directly with Mr. Wayler

7. The school nurse has been asked to provide some information about syphilis to a group of teen-age girls. Which of the following statements is *not* correct?

a. A blood test for syphilis should be done on anyone who had sexual contact with a person who has syphilis
b. Syphilis is treated with a penicillin injection, or with other antibiotics if the person is allergic to penicillin
c. Syphilis is a communicable disease that must be reported to the health department

d. A positive laboratory test for syphilis is always indicative of active infection

8. Mrs. Ritter has an acute respiratory infection. She is to have blood drawn for cold agglutinins, because she may have primary atypical pneumonia due to an infection with a PPLO (pleuropneumonia-like organism). Preparation for the cold agglutinins test includes which of the following?

   a. NPO for 8 hours
   b. Placement of blood sample into a 37 °C bath for transport to the laboratory
   c. No special preparation
   d. Checking the client's temperature and drawing the blood when there is a fever spike

9. Shirley Bowden is a college freshman who has been weak and very tired for a week. She has swollen lymph glands and a slight fever (100.6 °F). The nurse practitioner in the student health service thinks Shirley may have infectious mononucleosis. Which of these laboratory tests is not used to help establish a diagnosis of infectious mononucleosis?

   a. Heterophil antibody test (HAT)
   b. Spot tests for mono
   c. WBC with a differential
   d. C-reactive protein

10. ASO, anti-DNase B, and Streptozyme (the serological tests for antibodies against group A-beta hemolytic streptococci) may be part of the data base for all the following pediatric clients except which?

    a. Carolyn, age 10, who has just been diagnosed as having "strep" throat
    b. Billy, age 8, who has symptoms of possible rheumatic fever
    c. Tommy, age 14, who has acute glomerulonephritis
    d. Barbara, age 9, who has a history of repeated sore throats and joint pains

11. Martha Leahy, age 25, is getting married next week. Her premarital blood test showed a negative titer of rubella antibodies. What should Martha do before she becomes pregnant?

    a. Nothing, because a negative titer shows immunity to rubella
    b. Try to catch rubella by exposure to young children with measles
    c. Consult her physician about receiving the rubella vaccine if she becomes pregnant
    d. Ask her physician to give her the rubella vaccine now and practice some form of birth control for at least three months

12. Ginny Jasper is to have a serology test for toxoplasmosis. Which of the following is a significant factor in her health history in relationship to the test for TPM?

    a. Has had a tick bite
    b. Just moved from the San Joaquin Valley
    c. Has a cat
    d. Likes raw fruits and vegetables

13. In the Ohio Valley area, where the fungus *Histoplasma capsulatum* is endemic, people who have positive skin and serology tests for histoplasmosis are:

a. Highly susceptible to the fungus

b. Always carriers of the fungal disease

c. Always infected with the fungus

d. Showing evidence of some exposure to the fungus

14. The laboratory test, *Proteus* OX-19, is an indirect test for which?

a. *Proteus* infections

b. Rickettsial diseases

c. Protozoan infestations

d. *Entamoeba histolytica*

REFERENCES

Abramowicz, M. (1979). The new rubella vaccine. *The Medical Letter on Drugs and Therapeutics, 21,* 53–54.

Bassing, S. (1985). Saving the baby when mom has herpes. *RN, 48*(10), 35–37.

Bauer, D. (1980). Preventing the spread of hepatitis B in dialysis units. *AJN, 80*(2), 260–261.

Bennett, J. (1985a). AIDS epidemiology update. *AJN, 85*(9), 968–972.

Bennett, J. (1985b). HTLV-III-AIDS link. *AJN, 85*(10), 1086–1089.

Birdsall, C. (1985). How do you avoid transfusion complications? *AJN, 85*(3), 312.

Brown-Skeers, V. (1979). How the nurse practitioner manages the rheumatoid arthritis patient. *Nursing 79,* (6), 26–45.

Bullock, B., & Rosendahl, P. (1984). *Pathophysiology.* Boston: Little, Brown.

Claypool, J. (1981). Rubella protection for maternal child health care providers. *Maternal Child Nursing, 6,* 53–56.

Cozad, J. (1985). Autologous blood recovery. *Ethicon Point of View, 22*(2), 20.

Cullins, L. (1979). Preventing and treating transfusion reactions. *AJN, 79*(5), 935–937.

Einstein H. (1980). Coccidioidomycosis. *Basics of RD, 9*(11), 1–6.

Fidler, R. (1983). Complement assays. *Nursing 83, 13*(3), 65–67.

Fitzmaurice, J. (1980). *Rheumatic heart disease and mitral valve disease.* Norwalk, CT: Appleton-Century-Crofts.

Gillott, A., & Thomas, J. (1984). Clinical investigation involving the use of the haemonetic cell saver in elective and emergency vascular operations. *American Surgeon, 50*(11), 609–619.

Govoni, L., & Hayes, J. (1985). Drugs and nursing implications (5th ed.). Norwalk, CT: Appleton-Century-Crofts.

Gurevich, I. (1983). Viral hepatitis. *AJN, 83*(4), 571–586.

Hamory, B. (1983). Underreporting of needlestick injuries in a university hospital. *American Journal of Infection Control, 11*(5), 174–177.

Hawrylshyn, P., et al. (1983). Premature rupture of membranes: The role of C-reactive protein in the prediction of chorioamnionitis. *American Journal Obstetrical Gynecology, 147,* 240–246.

Helquist, M. (1986). Hemophilia and AIDS. *Focus. A Review of AIDS Research, 1*(6), 3–4.

Huber, M., & Calliari, D. (1985). Hereditary angioedema, the swelling disorder. *AJN, 85*(10), 1090–1092.

Jacobs, D., Kasten, B., DeMott, W., & Wolfson, W. (1984). *Laboratory test handbook with DRG index.* St. Louis: Mosby/Lexi Co.

Jason, J., et al. (1986). HTLV-III/LAV antibody and immune status of household contacts and sexual partners of persons with hemophilia. *JAMA, 255*(2), 212–215.

Kazak, A. (1979). Processing blood for transfusion. *AJN, 79*(5), 931–934.

Koff, R., et al. (1982). Hepatitis A and non-A, non-B viral hepatitis in Sao Paulo, Brazil: Epidemiological, clinical and laboratory comparisons in hospitalized patients. *Hepatology, 2*(4), 445–448.

Koffler, D. (1979). The immunology of rheumatoid disease. *Ciba's Clinical Symposia, 31*(4).

Lake, K. (1979). Lympho-glandular toxoplasmosis: A diagnosis often missed. *Post Graduate Medicine, 65,* 110–117.

Lang, G., & Drozda, E. (1979). Survey of blood ordering practices for 12 elective surgical procedures. *Wisconsin Medical Journal, 78,* 27–31.

Lederman, M. (1986). Transmission of the acquired immune deficiency syndrome through heterosexual activity. *Annals of Internal Medicine, 104*(1), 115–117.

Leland, D., et al. (1983). The use of TORCH titers. *Pediatrics, 72*(1), 41–43.

London, W. T. (1977). Hepatitis B virus and antigen-antibody complex diseases. *NEJM, 296,* 1528.

Mar, D. (1982). New hepatitis B vaccine: A breakthrough in hepatitis prevention. *AJN, 82*(2), 306–307.

Mason, J. (1985). Alternative sites for screening blood for antibodies to AIDS virus. *NEJM, 313*(18), 1157–1158.

Miller, J., et al. (1984). Evaluation of the Directigen Group A Strept test kit. *Journal of Clinical Microbiology. 20*(5), 846–848.

Morrison, C. (1986). Nursing's special challenge. *California Nurse, 82*(4), 1–16.

Ortho Diagnostics (1981). *What every Rh negative woman should know about RhoGAM and MICRhoGAM.* Raritan, NJ: Ortho Diagnostic Systems, Inc.

Querin, J., & Stahl, L. (1983). Twelve sensible steps for successful blood transfusions. *Nursing, 83, 13*(11), 34–43.

Roche, C. (1981). At last! Reliable protection from hepatitis B. *RN, 44*(10), 79.

Scharf, L. (1986). Safe needle disposal: A timely reminder. *RN, 49*(6), 42.

Scully, R. (Ed.). (1986). Normal reference laboratory values. *NEJM, 314*(1), 46–49.

Tietz, N. (Ed.). (1983). *Clinical guide to laboratory tests.* Philadelphia: Saunders.

Vargo, J. (1984). Viral hepatitis: How to protect patients and yourself. *RN, 47*(7), 22–29.

Wallach, J. (1986). *Interpretation of diagnostic tests.* Boston: Little, Brown.

Weinstein, A., & Farkas, S. (1979). Serological tests in infectious diseases: Clinical utility and interpretation. *Medical Clinics of North America, 62,* 1099–1117.

Wheat, L., et al. (1986). Diagnosis of disseminated histoplasmosis by detection of *Histoplasma capsulatum* in serum and urine specimens. *NEJM, 314*(2), 83–88.

Young, A. B., et al. (1983). Is cytomegalovirus a serious hazard to female hospital staff? *Lancet, 1,* 975–976.

Zuckerman, A. (1979). Specific serological diagnosis of viral hepatitis. *British Medical Journal, 2*(6182), 84–86.

Zuerlein, T., & Smith, P. (1985). The diagnostic utility of the febrile agglutin tests. *JAMA, 254*(9), 1211–1214.

15

Endocrine Tests

- Growth Hormone (GH) or Somatotropin
- Prolactin (PRL)
- Adrenocorticotropic Hormone (ACTH)
- Cortisol Plasma Levels
- Urinary Cortisol Levels
- 17-Hydroxysteroids (17-OHCS) (Porter–Silber Test)
- 17-Ketosteroids (17-KS)
- 17-Ketogenic Steroids (17-KGS)
- Urinary Pregnanetriol
- Aldosterone
- Renin
- Saralasin Infusion Test
- Catecholamines, Vanillylmandelic Acid (VMA), and Metanephrines
- Parathormone or Parathyroid Hormone (PTH)
- Thyrotropin or Thyroid-Stimulating Hormone (TSH)
- L-Thyroxine (T_4) Serum Concentration
- Triiodothyronine (T_3) Serum Concentration (T_3-RIA)
- T_3 Resin Uptake (Percentage of T_3 Uptake)
- Free Thyroxine Index (FTI) and Free T_4
- Thyroid-Binding Globulins (TBG) Capacity
- Follicle-Stimulating Hormone (FSH)
- Luteinizing Hormones (LH)
- Estradiol and Other Forms of Estrogen
- Progesterone
- Pregnanediol (Progesterone Metabolite)
- Testosterone and Other Androgens

OBJECTIVES

1. Explain the concepts of negative feedback, circadian rhythms, and ectopic hormone production.
2. Give examples of how laboratory tests are used to assess the relationship of the anterior pituitary gland to other endocrine glands.
3. Determine the appropriate nursing diagnoses for a client with increased or decreased serum cortisol levels.
4. Devise a teaching plan for parents who have a child with adrenogenital syndrome.
5. Identify the characteristic clinical manifestations of increased and decreased levels of serum aldosterone, including changes in renin activity.
6. Explain the purpose of 24-hour urine specimens for vanillylmandelic acid (VMA) and metanephrines.
7. Describe the clinical effect of an increased level of parathormone (PTH) and the major nursing intervention needed.
8. Explain the usefulness of TSH, T_4, T_3, and T_3 resin uptake in evaluating clients with hyper- or hypothyroidism.
9. Determine the appropriate nursing diagnoses for clients with increased or decreased serum thyroid hormones.
10. Explain why infants who may have hypothyroidism (cretinism) need immediate medical evaluation and treatment.
11. Identify the key nursing diagnoses when a client has altered levels of the sex hormones.

The brief discussions of the negative feedback system, circadian rhythms, ectopic hormone production, and other physiological information in this chapter should help the reader to better understand the tests that are done to measure hormone levels. In addition, the techniques for doing radioimmunoassay (RIA) and enzyme immunoassay (EIA) are briefly described because immunoassay methods have made it possible to measure all hormones by direct, rather than by indirect, methods.

Except for ectopic hormone production (discussed later) each hormone is produced by a specific endocrine gland, and each has a very specific function or functions. These functions are briefly discussed in relationship to the tests for each hormone.

Table 15–1 gives an overview of the endocrine glands, the hormones produced by each gland, and how the hormones are tested by specific laboratory tests of blood and urine samples. The releasing factors (discussed in the following section) are not included in this table because they are not normally measured.

BACKGROUND INFORMATION

Releasing Factors That Stimulate Anterior Pituitary

The central nervous system is very closely connected to the endocrine system because some releasing factors from the hypothalamus are carried to the pituitary gland through the venous system that connects the hypothalamus and the pituitary gland. Because hypophysis is another name for the pituitary gland, this venous system is called the *hypophyseal portal system*. These releasing factors from the hypothalamus

TABLE 15–1. COMMONLY MEASURED HORMONES

Source of Hormone	Name of Hormone	Tests Used to Assess Hormone Levels
Anterior pituitary	Growth hormone (GH) or somatotropin (STH)	Serum GH levels
	Adrenocorticotropin (ACTH)	Serum ACTH levels; see section on adrenal gland for ACTH suppression and stimulation tests.
	Thyrotropin (TSH)	Serum TSH levels; see section on tests of thyroid gland.
	Follicle-stimulating hormone (FSH) (one of the gonadotropins)	Serum and urine FSH levels; see section on sex hormones.
	Luteinizing hormone (LH), sometimes called interstitial-cell-stimulating hormone (ICSH) in male (the other gonadotropin).	Serum and urine levels; see section on sex hormones.
	Prolactin (PRL)	Serum prolactin
	Melanocyte-stimulating hormone (MSH)	Serum MSH not usually measured directly; see discussion about increase of MSH with cortisol lack.
Posterior pituitary	Antidiuretic hormone (ADH) or arginine vasopressin (AVP) (Pitressin)	Not commonly measured; see Chapter 4 on serum and urine osmolality.
	Oxytocin (Pitocin)	Not measured as diagnostic test; note that oxytocin is used in obstetrics as drug to induce labor.
Adrenal cortex	Glucocorticoids (cortisol as major one)	Plasma and urine cortisol; 17-hydroxycorticosteroids (17-OHCS) or Porter–Silber test; 17-KGS; see ACTH tests also.
	Mineralocorticoids (aldosterone as major one)	Serum and urine aldosterone levels; tests for renin activity; saralassin test; see Chapter 5 for serum levels of sodium and potassium.
	Sex hormones (androgens, progesterone, and estrogen)	Pregnanetriol in urine; 17-ketosteroids (17-KS) in urine.
Adrenal medulla	Norepinephrine	Catecholamines in urine; metanephrines in urine; vanillylmandelic acid (VMA) in urine; norepinephrine and epinephrine are not commonly measured in serum; pharmacological tests not commonly done anymore (i.e., Regitine).
	Epinephrine	
Parathyroid	Parathormone (PTH)	Serum PTH; serum and urine calcium and phosphate levels; see Chapter 7.

TABLE 15–1. (Continued)

Source of Hormone	Name of Hormone	Tests Used to Assess Hormone Levels
Thyroid	Calcitonin	Calcitonin not commonly measured; see Chapter 7 on serum calcium.
	L-thyroxine (T₄) and triiodo-thyronine (T₃)	T₄; T₃ resin uptake; T₃; free thyroxin index (FTI); TSH levels.
Pancreas	Insulin Glucogen	See Chapter 8 for tests on glucose metabolism.
Testes	Androgens	Serum testosterone; see 17-KS urine test for androgens.
	Estrogen and progesterone in minute amounts	Serum estradiol; see also tests for FSH and LH.
Ovaries	Estrogens	Serum estradiol; serum and urine estriol in pregnancy (see Chapter 18) Serum progesterone
	Progesterone	Pregnanediol in urine.
	Androgens in minute amounts	17-KS for androgens; see also tests for FSH and LH.

stimulate the pituitary to release certain hormones. For example, thyrotropin-releasing factor (TRF) is sent from the hypothalamus to the pituitary gland. The pituitary gland is thus stimulated to release thyroid-stimulating hormone (TSH), which in turns acts upon the thyroid gland to produce thyroxine.

At the present time, the existence of several of these factors has been documented, and it is hypothesized that there is probably some type of hypothalamus control for all the pituitary hormones. Two of the releasing factors have been used diagnostically: the releasing factor for the gonadotropic hormones (FSH and LH) and the releasing factor for thyrotropin (TSH).

Currently, several releasing factors from the hypothalamus are being extensively studied in relation to the effect of various drugs. Locke (1978) names over 30 drugs that may affect the secretion of anterior pituitary hormones. The susceptibility of the hypothalamus–anterior pituitary system to drugs is taking on major clinical importance as more is being learned about the interaction of drugs and hormone levels.

Negative Feedback System for Endocrine Functioning
The anterior pituitary gland secretes hormones that act on specific target organs to cause the release of other hormones. For example, the pituitary releases ACTH, which then stimulates the adrenal gland to produce cortisol. When the cortisol reaches a certain level in the bloodstream, there is a suppression of continued secretion of ACTH from the pituitary. In other words, a high level of cortisol turns off the secretion of ACTH. Conversely, a low level of serum cortisol is a stimulus for the increased production of ACTH. This interplay, in which the increased level of one hormone causes a decrease in the level of the other hormone, is called *negative feedback*. The hormones from the adrenal cortex, thyroid gland, ovaries, and testes all have negative feedback systems with hormones from the anterior pituitary gland. Understanding negative feedback is important because tests for the suppression or stimulation

of hormones are based on this physiological principle that levels of one hormone should change the level of another hormone.

Other Methods to Control Hormone Production

Not all hormones are controlled by a negative feedback system through the pituitary gland. For example, parathyroid hormone (PTH) is regulated by the serum calcium and phosphorus levels (see Chapter 7). A high level of serum calcium causes a suppression of the parathyroid hormone from the parathyroid gland. A decrease in the serum calcium level causes an increased production of PTH.

The intricate balance between too much and too little of a hormone is one of the wonders of the human body. In a healthy state, all hormones are kept within a precise range that can fluctuate as the body needs change. All hormones are interrelated to some degree, so changes in one hormone may affect the level of others, although not in as direct a fashion as in negative feedback.

Circadian Rhythms and Other Rhythms

A change in the levels of a hormone every 24 hours is called a *circadian* (around the day) *rhythm*. For example, cortisol is higher in the morning than in the evening. While cortisol seems to be relatively independent of the sleep pattern, growth hormone is strongly bound to the sleep pattern (Krieger, 1979). Much research is being done to investigate which factors, other than activity patterns and sleep, regulate the normal variations every 24 hours. In addition to cortisol and growth hormone, aldosterone, prolactin, thyrotropin, testosterone, LH, and FSH all vary considerably during each 24-hour period. Because the hormones do fluctuate, more than one blood sample or one urine specimen may be needed to get an accurate reflection of an individual's hormone level.

The female hormones, estrogen and progesterone, are, of course, on another rhythm that must also be taken into account in comparing reference values. Rhythms that are longer than circadian (24-hour) rhythms are termed *infradian rhythms*. In adult women, the menstrual cycle is an infradian rhythm, because the variations in FSH and LH are on a monthly, not a daily, cycle. Besides the sex hormones, other hormones may fluctuate with menstrual cycles. In adult women, therefore, various hormones must be considered in relation to the menstrual cycle.

Ectopic Hormone Production

Most elevations of serum hormone levels are due to an overproduction by the specific endocrine gland. They can also occur if there is production of the hormone from a nonendocrine source. Hormones from nonendocrine sources are called *ectopic hormones* because they come from the wrong place or originate outside the normal pathway. For example, certain benign and malignant tumors are able to manufacture hormones that are very similar to the hormone produced by the endocrine gland. Certain types of neoplasms of the lung can secrete a form of ACTH. ACTH, melanocyte-stimulating hormone (MSH), gonadotropins, antidiuretic hormone (ADH), and PTH are the five most common ectopic hormones. Ryan (1979) lists 17 different polypeptide hormones that can be produced by nonendocrine neoplasms.

In certain malignant states, hormone tests may be done to see if some of the symptoms are due to ectopic hormone production. For example, a tumor that produces PTH may cause symptoms of hypercalcemia. (See Chapter 7 for a discussion of hypercalcemia.) The physician may have to order a variety of tests to determine whether the symptoms of a hormone imbalance are due to a malignancy or to primary dysfunction of the endocrine gland.

Screening Tests and Definitive Tests
for Primary and Secondary Imbalances

In general, screening tests for hormone imbalances are done by measuring the concentration of the hormone in the serum. If the serum level is above or below the reference values, more definitive tests are done to find out whether the problem is in the gland itself. If the disorder is due to a problem in the gland itself, the disorder is called *primary*. If the endocrine imbalance is due to other causes, such as pituitary dysfunction, the endocrine disorder is termed *secondary*. For example, if hypothyroidism is due to the malfunction of the thyroid gland, the disorder is called primary hypothyroidism. If the hypothyroidism is due to pituitary insufficiency, the disorder is called secondary hypothyroidism. Laboratory tests that use drugs to stimulate or to suppress hormone production are useful in determining whether the disorder is primary or secondary (Table 15–2).

The Technique of Radioimmunoassay (RIA)

By being able to identify very small amounts of chemicals, such as hormones or drugs, in the bloodstream, the laboratory technique of RIA has revolutionized the laboratory approach to testing for hormones. Rosalyn Yalow received a share of the 1977 Nobel Prize in Medicine and Physics for the development of the technique. The method is considered very valuable because, before RIA, many substances, such as hormones, could not be detected by chemical means because the amounts in the serum are so small (Holum, 1983). Four elements are required for RIA:

1. An antibody to the hormone to be measured (the antigen)
2. A labeled or radio-tagged hormone
3. A highly purified hormone standard
4. A method to separate the bound from the free hormone (Juebiz, 1979, p. 345)

Antigen. The hormone to be measured in the client's blood is termed the antigen. Any substance can become an antigen if it is in pure enough form to elicit *specific antibodies* from the immune system. Thus drugs are also measured by the technique of RIA (see Chapter 17 on toxicology). The antibodies against the specific hormone (or other substances, such as drugs) are obtained by giving the antigen (hormone or drug) to animals, such as rabbits or guinea pigs.

Radio-Tagged Hormone. In addition to the antibodies to a specific hormone, the laboratory uses a small amount of radioactive material to tag a measured amount

TABLE 15-2. SCREENING AND DEFINITIVE TESTS OF HORMONE FUNCTION

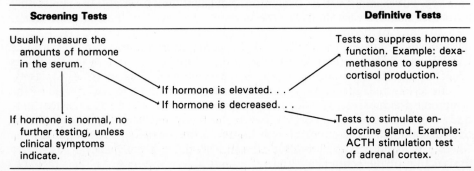

Screening Tests	Definitive Tests
Usually measure the amounts of hormone in the serum.	Tests to suppress hormone function. Example: dexamethasone to suppress cortisol production.
If hormone is elevated. . .	
If hormone is decreased. . .	
If hormone is normal, no further testing, unless clinical symptoms indicate.	Tests to stimulate endocrine gland. Example: ACTH stimulation test of adrenal cortex.

of the antigen. Samples of the antibody and tagged antigen are mixed with a sample of the client's blood. If the client's sample has little of the hormone (antigen), most of the antigen–antibody complex is composed of the radioactive antigen. On the other hand, if the client's blood sample contains a lot of hormone (antigen), this untagged hormone is what reacts with the antibody.So the antibody–antigen complex does not contain much of the radioactive-tagged antigen.

Hormone Standard. The laboratory has then to determine exactly what amount of the antibody–antigen reaction is due to antigens from the client and what amount is due to the tagged antigen. To make that determination the laboratory technician measures the radioactivity of the antibody–antigen complex and compares this with known standards.

Extremely small amounts of hormones or other substances can be detected by RIA. These very small amounts are expressed as nanograms (10^9 g) or picograms (10^{12} g). A picogram is 1/10,000,000,000,000 of a gram. It seems incredible that such a tiny amount can be accurately measured, but with RIA even very minute amounts of an antigen are locked into the antigen–antibody complex.

Enzyme Immunoassay (EIA)

Laboratories may also use enzymes as labels in antibody–antigen reactions. The enzyme is tagged either to the antigen or to the antibody before they are mixed with the blood sample from the client. The use of an enzyme as a tagging agent eliminates the need for a radioactive tag, and the tests are as sensitive to small amounts of the antigen (hormone or drug) as the radioimmunoassay. The enzyme method, as described by Galen (1978), has made it possible to make a test for thyroid hormone part of an automated sysem. Now many laboratories do many tests by EIA.

POSSIBLE NURSING DIAGNOSES RELATED TO PITUITARY DISORDERS

Anxiety Related to the Disease Process

Emotional problems with mood changes are likely to be a significant part of most disorders of the pituitary gland. Some of the symptoms are directly related to the hormonal imbalance whereas others may be brought on by the delay before an accurate diagnosis is made. Cowan (1984) notes that if the client is a female, the symptoms may be labeled as "hysteria." Because it is not unusual for clients to have been misdiagnosed for several years, a sense of bitterness and anger may complicate the efforts to help the person deal with the problems of the disease. After the diagnosis is established, clients and their significant others need help to deal with the surgery or other planned treatment.

Disturbances of Self-concept Related to Change in Body Image

Various pituitary disorders cause physical changes such as acromegaly, dwarfism, or obesity. Clients need help in accepting the physical changes that may or may not be remedied with therapy. For example, acromegaly may necessitate plastic surgery with reconstruction of the bones of the face. The physical changes may also affect sexual functioning, an issue often overlooked (Perez, 1984).

■ GROWTH HORMONE (GH) OR SOMATOTROPIN

Growth hormone (GH), produced by the anterior pituitary, stimulates the growth of bone and other tissue. GH affects metabolism by increasing protein synthesis, decreasing carbohydrate utilization, and increasing fat mobilization. GH is higher in children, but it is present in smaller amounts all through life. GH levels are done to evaluate a lack of growth in the child. For the adult, measurement of GH is done as one assessment of pituitary function. Research (Press et al., 1984) is investigating the importance of GH in mediating the metabolic derangements of diabetes.

Several factors influence the production of GH. Diets low in protein cause an increased production of the hormone. Hypoglycemia also causes an increased surge of GH in the serum, and hyperglycemia causes a decreased production of it. Because GH production is suppressed by hyperglycemia and stimulated by hypoglycemia, tests for GH may involve the administration of a glucose load or an insulin injection. Because exercise and sleep also cause variations in plasma GH levels, the activity of the client and the timing of the specimen are important to note. (For reasons that are still unknown, GH levels increase during sleep.)

Preparation of Client and Collection of Sample
The laboratory needs 1 ml of serum. The activity of the client, including sleep patterns, needs to be normal. A baseline level is done with the client fasting and at rest, although the client should have been on a regular diet before the fasting period.

GH levels may also be drawn after the client has been given L-dopa, insulin, or arginine (Jacobs et al., 1984). Several serum blood samples are drawn after the administration of a drug to see how much the GH increases. The problem with giving a test dose of insulin is that the client may have symptoms of hypoglycemia (see Chapter 8 for symptoms of hypoglycemia).

In clients with GH excess, a glucose load may be given to demonstrate that the GH cannot be suppressed. The procedure may consist of a glucose tolerance test with simultaneous glucose and GH measurement. (See Chapter 8 for the procedure for glucose tolerance tests.)

Reference Values for GH

Adult (fasting and at rest)	Below 5 ng/ml See Appendix A for values after exercise and glucose loads
Newborn	10–40 ng/ml
Children	Over 10 ng/ml

In adults, the usual values may be so low that the hormone cannot be detected by RIA. Stimulation by L-dopa or insulin should increase GH to measurable levels.

With sample drawn at 8 A.M. after normal sleep.

Increased GH Serum Level

Clinical Significance. Severe malnutritional states cause a prolonged elevation of GH. Various types of tumors, either benign or malignant, can cause excess secretion of GH. In children, an abnormal increase of GH causes *gigantism*. Increased GH after puberty brings about a distortion of bony structures because the bones are stimulated to grow. Growth hormone excess in the adult is called *acromegaly*.

POSSIBLE NURSING DIAGNOSIS RELATED TO INCREASED GH

The client with a pituitary tumor may have radiation or surgery to remove the tumor. See earlier discussion of general nursing diagnoses. An important point to remember in relation to increased GH levels is that hyperglycemia may be a clinical problem. An increased level of GH decreases the body's ability to handle glucose. (See Chapter 8 for more discussion of hyperglycemia and appropriate nursing diagnoses.)

Decreased GH Serum Level

Clinical Significance. Lack of GH is due to hypofunction of the pituitary gland, which can result from a tumor, from trauma, or from an unknown cause. In the child, a lack of GH causes *dwarfism*. In the adult, although the lack of GH does not cause clinical symptoms, it may be associated with deficiencies of other pituitary hormones, so symptoms are related to the other deficiencies. Hence a measurement of GH may be used to help in assessing the presence of hypopituitarism in the adult.

Sheehan's syndrome is a type of hypopituitarism that sometimes occurs after a complicated delivery with bleeding and shock. During the postpartum period, a thrombus may occur in the hypophyseal vessels, which causes destruction of the pituitary gland.

POSSIBLE NURSING DIAGNOSIS RELATED TO DECREASED GH

Knowledge Deficit Related to Replacement Therapy

In the child, a lack of GH is treated medically by injections of GH so that the child develops normally. In 1985, the U.S. Food and Drug Administration approved the manufacture of growth hormone (Protropin by Genentech) by gene splicing. (This was the second product of recombinant DNA technology to be approved for human use. The first was insulin approved in 1982.) Parents need detailed instructions about the injections and follow-up care. In infants, a lack of GH may create an immediate problem by causing hypoglycemia (Kaplan, 1979). Older clients with a lack of GH may show symptoms of hypoglycemia only if they are fasting. Adults are not given injections of GH, but they may need replacement of other pituitary hormones, all of which can be replaced by parenteral injection. Also, the hormones from specific glands, such as thyroid, may be given. The nursing implications for specific hormone therapy are briefly covered in the discussion for each hormone. Also see the two general nursing diagnoses discussed earlier.

■ PROLACTIN (PRL)

Prolactin, a hormone from the anterior pituitary gland, is normally increased during pregnancy and the subsequent lactation period. Tumors of the pituitary gland, drugs, or other variables can result in an increased prolactin secretion. Women have an abnormal secretion of breast milk and suppression of menstruation (amenorrhea-galactorrhea syndrome). Some women may not realize they have galactorrhea until a milking pressure is applied to the breast. Other symptoms, such as headaches and weight gain from sodium retention, may occur. In males there may be impotence because excess prolactin has a negative feedback to the pituitary gland, suppressing gonad function.

An enlarging tumor can cause visual problems because of the pressure on the optic chiasm. The impairment of vision is particularly noted in pregnant women who have a pituitary tumor because the pituitary gland normally increases in pregnancy (Cecil, 1983).

If the increased secretion is a result of a tumor, it is usually benign and can be removed surgically. Bromocriptine (Parlodel) is a drug used for short-term therapy (Govoni & Hayes, 1985). Some drugs, such as tranquilizers, can mimic the prolactin tumor syndrome, and thus treatment is elimination of the causative factor. Magnetic resonance imaging (MRI) (see Chapter 21) can be used to evaluate the effect of drug treatment on the size of the tumor (Glaser et al., 1986).

Preparation of Client and Collection of Sample
Test requires 2 ml of serum.

Reference Values for Prolactin	
Adult: Male	Less than 20 ng/ml
Female	Less than 23 ng/ml
	Increases up to 40 ng/ml in luteal phase
Pregnancy	1st trimester: less than 80 ng/ml
	2nd trimester: less than 160 ng/ml
	3rd trimester: less than 400 ng/ml
Newborn	10 times the adult levels (Tietz, 1983)

> ### NURSING DIAGNOSES RELATED TO INCREASE OR DECREASE OF PROLACTIN LEVELS
>
> See the general nursing diagnoses for pituitary disorders discussed earlier.

ADRENAL CORTEX

The adrenal cortex secretes three types of hormones (Table 15–3):

1. The glucocorticoids: The glucocorticoid that is usually measured in the plasma is cortisol, and free cortisol can also be measured in the urine. Also, various metabolites of the glucocorticoids can be measured in the urine as 17-OHCS.

TABLE 15-3. MAJOR EFFECTS OF THREE TYPES OF HORMONES FROM ADRENAL CORTEX

Hormone	Major Effects
Glucocorticoids (cortisol)	Major effects on metabolism of carbohydrates, fats, and proteins. Suppresses immune responses.
Mineralocorticoids (aldosterone)	Major effect on fluid and electrolyte balance. Increased retention of sodium and water. Decreased retention of potassium.
Sex hormones (androgens, progesterone, and estrogen)	Affect secondary sex characteristics but not as significantly as hormones from ovaries and testes.

   2. The mineralocorticoids: The mineralocorticoid that is measured in the serum is aldosterone.
   3. The sex hormones: The sex hormones that are produced by the adrenal cortex include the androgens, progesterone, and estrogen. Both males and females have the male hormones (androgens, such as testosterone) and the female hormones (progesterone and estrogen). A measurement of androgens becomes important when there is hyperplasia of the adrenal gland, which increases the production of the sex hormones. A urine test, 17-KS is one way to determine an increase of sex hormones from the adrenal gland.

ACTH-ADRENAL AXIS

Production of cortisol by the adrenal cortex is controlled by the ACTH-adrenal axis. Because ACTH and cortisol are related by the concept of a negative feedback system, the pituitary is stimulated to produce ACTH when the plasma cortisol level is low. ACTH then causes an increased production of cortisol by the adrenal cortex. The increasing plasma cortisol level becomes the stimulus for the pituitary to discontinue the high levels of ACTH production. Homeostasis is maintained by the increases and decreases of ACTH, which keep a certain balance of cortisol in the serum. ACTH also causes an increased production of the sex hormones by the adrenal cortex, but this effect is usually not significant except in certain adrenogenital syndromes. (Androgen excess is discussed in the section on the clinical significance of decreased cortisol levels.) ACTH has little or no effect on the serum levels of the third type of adrenal cortex hormones, the mineralocorticosteroids, or aldosterone. Aldosterone is controlled by the renin–angiotension system, which is explained under the section on aldosterone.

■ ADRENOCORTICOTROPIC HORMONE (ACTH)

The level of ACTH can be measured directly by RIA. A measurement of ACTH helps to determine whether the lack of serum cortisol is due to hypofunction either of the adrenal cortex or of the pituitary. The administration of certain drugs, such as insulin, dexamethasone (Decadron), and metyrapone, are used to stimulate or to suppress the production of ACTH. Each of these tests is discussed briefly, along with a summary of the clinical significance of the findings.

Preparation of Client and Collection of Sample
The base line specimen for which the laboratory needs 5 ml of plasma, is usually collected in the morning. The specimen should be put on ice and sent to the laboratory immediately. Use EDTA tube only.

Reference Values for ACTH

15–70 pg/ml

ACTH Stimulation Test with Metyrapone
Metyrapone is a drug that interferes with the normal production of cortisol by blocking some enzymatic actions so that compound S is not converted to cortisol. Due to negative feedback, a fall in plasma cortisol level should cause an increase in the level of circulating ACTH. If clients have pituitary insufficiency, however, the ACTH level is *not* increased, even with the blockage of cortisol production by metyrapone. Because several ACTH levels may be drawn after the administration of metyrapone, nurses must check with the individual laboratory for the exact timing of the specimens. Phenytoin (Dilantin) interferes with the test because the drug has a variety of endocrine effects. Estrogen compounds also interfere with the test.

ACTH Stimulation with Insulin
Because a drop in blood sugar normally causes an increased production of ACTH, insulin can be used to stimulate the production of ACTH. Insulin, however, is not used as frequently as metyrapone. One of the problems with using insulin as a test drug is that the patient must be watched carefully so that the hypoglycemia is not too severe. (See Chapter 8 for the symptoms and treatment of hypoglycemia.)

ACTH Suppression Test: Dexamethasone Suppression Test (DST)
Normally, high plasma corticosteroid levels suppress the formation of ACTH (the negative feedback concept again). Dexamethasone (Decadron), which is a potent corticosteroid that suppresses the formation of ACTH, is given as a test to determine whether the client continues to produce large amounts of cortisol after ACTH is suppressed. Clients with a hyperactive adrenal cortex (Cushing's syndrome) do continue to have high serum cortisol levels because the suppression of pituitary ACTH does not affect the hyperactive adrenal gland.

The DST is also used in the psychiatric setting to help evaluate which depressed clients will best respond to somatic interventions. Those with a positive test, i.e. no suppression, are most likely to respond to somatic rather than psychological or social interventions. DST may also be used to decide when to stop antidepressant medications (Harris, 1982).

For screening purposes, 1 mg of dexamethasone is given orally at 11 P.M. (a client who weighs more than 200 lb takes a larger dose) to suppress ACTH formation. A serum cortisol is drawn the next morning at 8 A.M. The plasma levels of cortisol should drop below 5 μg/100 ml. Urine levels of cortisol and other metabolites may be measured too (these tests are discussed later). To confirm the results, the dexamethasone dosage may be increased and given for several days.

Use of ACTH to Stimulate Cortisol Production
Clients with suspected diseases of the adrenal cortex can be given a test dose of ACTH

to determine whether ACTH causes an increased production of cortisol in the serum. A synthetic type of ACTH, called cosyntropin, may be given intravenously, intramuscularly, or, sometimes, infused over a period of hours. The dosages used and the timing of the serum samples vary. Nurses must follow the exact procedure for a particular institution. The administration of ACTH should stimulate the adrenal cortex to produce a plasma cortisol level of at least 30–45 μg/100 ml. A lack of response to ACTH indicates primary hypofunction of the adrenal cortex.

■ CORTISOL PLASMA LEVELS

Cortisol, the glucocorticoid found in the largest concentration in the serum, is the one usually measured to gain information about the functioning of the adrenal cortex. Plasma cortisol has a diurnal variation, its levels being higher in the morning than in the evening. Baseline readings are done in the morning with the client at rest. The timing of cortisol levels with suppression and stimulation are determined by the procedure of the particular laboratory.

Preparation of Client and Collection of Sample
The laboratory needs 1 cc of plasma. The specimen is usually drawn in the morning after the client has been fasting. Evening samples may also require about 3 hours of fasting. Water is allowed. Because activity increases the level, the client needs to be supine for 2 hours before the test. The administration of estrogens in contraceptive pills causes an increase in cortisol levels. Spironolactone (Aldactone) may also cause false positives.

Reference Values for Serum Cortisol

---

8 A.M. (client at rest) 5–25 μg/100 ml

8 P.M. Below 10 μg/100 ml

1. There are no age or sex differences but pregnancy causes an increase. Obese people do have higher levels. Activity also increases levels
2. Dexamethasone suppression (DST) should decrease cortisol levels to below 5 μg/100 ml
3. ACTH stimulation should increase 8 A.M. cortisol levels 30–45 μg/100 ml

---

Increased Serum Cortisol Level

Clinical Significance. An increase in cortisol can be either ACTH-dependent or ACTH-independent. A pituitary tumor can cause an increase of ACTH, which in turn causes an increased cortisol level. This type of cortisol increase is ACTH-dependent, and it is sometimes called Cushing's disease. Increases of serum cortisol from other causes are called Cushing's syndrome. (Cushing was an American endocrinologist who first described the characteristic signs and symptoms of cortisol excess.)

Plasma cortisol levels are increased independently of the pituitary gland when there is hyperplasia of the adrenal cortex. Hypersecreting tumors of the adrenal cortex may be malignant or benign.

Certain nonendocrine malignancies can also secrete ACTH, which can result in increased serum cortisol levels. (Note the earlier discussion on ectopic hormones.) Cushing's syndrome, or high plasma cortisol levels, can also be caused by the administration of corticosteroids over a long period of time. Long-term administration of cortisone causes a suppression of ACTH and an eventual atrophy of the adrenal glands.

The specific medical treatment for elevated cortisol levels depends on the etiology. The client may have a battery of tests to determine whether there is a tumor of the pituitary or of the adrenal gland. If Cushing's syndrome is due to exogenous cortisol administration, the dosage of cortisone may be decreased. However, until the specific treatment is effective, the client may have several problems related to the effects of cortisol excess. Sometimes difficult medical decisions must be made regarding the continuation of cortisone therapy. The problems created by the disease condition must be weighed against the untoward effects of the therapy.

POSSIBLE NURSING DIAGNOSES RELATED TO INCREASED SERUM CORTISOL LEVEL

Potential for Infection
Nurses must recognize that clients with cortisol elevations do not have a normal response to infections. Cortisol impairs antibody production and cellular immunity, qualities that are beneficial in the treatment of abnormal inflammatory responses but detrimental in the face of an infection. Such clients may have little elevation of temperature or other response to a bacterial invasion. So they must be taught to avoid possible sources of infection.

Alterations in Nutritional Requirements
Cortisol stimulates the formation of glucose from other substances, such as protein (gluconeogenesis), and it also interferes with the action of insulin. Clients may thus have problems with hyperglycemia. (See Chapter 8 for nursing implications with hyperglycemia.) Obesity is usually a problem so a typical diet plan for a client with Cushing's syndrome would be a low-sodium, high-protein, low-carbohydrate, and low-calorie diet (Jones, 1982).

Potential for Injury Related to Poor Wound Healing and Possible Fractures
High levels of cortisol cause a reduction in protein stores and, in children, suppression of growth. Wound healing is delayed. If cortisol levels are elevated for more than 6 months, the matrix of the bone may be upset, and calcium is lost, leading to osteoporosis. With their healing diminished, clients need to be protected from falls or wounds.

Potential for Bleeding Related to Development of Gastric Ulcers
Increased cortisol levels cause an increased secretion of hydrochloric acid and pepsinogen. There is also an inhibition of collagen formation and of other protective proteins in the gastric mucosa. The exact cause of gastric ulcers is not known, but ulcers are a risk of high cortisol levels. To protect the stomach mucosa, clients may be given antacids. Any signs of gastrointestinal bleeding should be reported at once. (See Chapter 13 for guaiac for occult gastrointestinal bleeding.)

Alterations in Fluid and Electrolyte Balance
Depending on the level of cortisol increase, clients may have sodium retention and potassium excretion. (See the discussion on the effects of aldosterone.) They may also have elevated blood pressure, weight gain, and edema. (See Chapter 5 for the nursing implications for the client with hypernatremia or hypokalemia.)

Poor Self-esteem Related to Changes in Body Image
Elevated cortisol levels cause a round, full face ("moon face") and a redistribution of fat deposits. Clients may have a buffalo hump on the back. Their trunks are obese, while their wasted muscles make the extremities thin. Females may become masculinized with unwanted hair and acne. All in all, the person is not what is usually considered physically attractive. Treatment helps to correct most of these body changes, but clients need help to cope with their altered body images.

Ineffective Coping of Family Related to Changes in Mood
Increased cortisol levels tend to cause hyperactivity. Clients may need to be cautioned about too much activity. There is an increased stimulation of the central nervous system, which can lead to convulsions. The person may have dramatic mood changes. Euphoria is often present, and psychotic behavior may occur. The family may need help in learning to deal with such wide mood changes. Perez (1984) noted many clients with Cushing's disease have undergone marital disruption which they attribute to the fatigue and depression of the disease process.

Decreased Serum Cortisol Level

Clinical Significance. A subnormal level of cortisol in the plasma is known as Addison's disease. (One way to remember that Addison's disease involves a lack of cortisol is to remember that in *Add*ison's disease, one must *add* some cortisone.) The lack of cortisol in the serum may be due to primary hypofunction of the adrenal cortex, or it may be secondary to hypofunctioning of the pituitary. Infections such as tuberculosis may invade the adrenal cortex. Once the most common cause of adrenal insufficiency was tuberculosis, but now it is idiopathic autoimmune adrenalitis. Adrenal insufficiency can be a complication of AIDS (Green et al., 1984).

Long-term administration of high doses of corticosteroids causes suppression of ACTH production and a resulting inactivity of these clients' own adrenal glands. There is some atrophy of the adrenal cortex so that the glands do not respond normally to the need for more cortisone in stress. The inability of the adrenal cortex to increase production of cortisol during stress may cause a collection of symptoms known as an *Addisonian crisis.* If cortisol drugs are not withdrawn gradually (tapered off), the client may have a lowered cortisol level before the adrenal glands can begin to function normally again. (See the separate section on congenital adrenocortical hyperplasia for an explanation of cortisol lack in newborns and young children.)

Clients with borderline adrenal cortex functioning may not have problems until they are faced with a stressful situation, such as surgery or some other physical or psychologic trauma. Insufficiency occurs when at least 90% of the adrenal glands are destroyed (Adams, 1983). Once the symptoms of a lack of cortisol and aldosterone are recognized and confirmed, replacement therapy is started. Until the hormones are replaced, or when the need is greater than the supply, these clients may have problems related to the lack of cortisol and aldosterone.

POSSIBLE NURSING DIAGNOSES RELATED TO DECREASED SERUM CORTISOL LEVEL

Fluid Volume Deficit Related to Lack of Retention of Sodium and Water
A lack of cortisol and of the mineralocorticoid aldosterone causes low serum sodium levels, which may lead to hypovolemia. Thus clients with a lack of cortisol tend to get dizzy, and they may faint if they are gotten out of bed rapidly (postural hypotension). In more advanced cases, the lack of sodium retention can lead to hypovolemia that is severe enough to cause shock. (See Chapter 5 for the nursing implications for clients with hyponatremia.)

Potential for Alteration in Cardiac Output Related to Retention of Potassium
Cortisol and, even more so, aldosterone cause sodium retention and potassium excretion. So in Addison's disease, when cortisol is low, not only is the serum sodium low, but the serum potassium rises. The serum potassium may or may not be high enough to cause symptoms. Certainly the client should not be given additional potassium. (See Chapter 5 for the nursing implications for hyperkalemia.)

Potential for Injury Related to Hypoglycemia with Fasting States
Clients with a lack of cortisol are less able to maintain a normal blood sugar when there is no continual replacement of glucose. Thus clients with suspected cortisol deficiency may have symptoms of hypoglycemia if they fast. (See Chapter 8 for the signs, symptoms, and treatment of hypoglycemic episodes.)

Ineffective Coping Related to Inability to Handle Stress (Addisonian Crisis)
Clients with slightly low cortisol levels may be asymptomatic until faced with stress: They cannot cope with a crisis. The client needs to be protected not only from physical stress, such as infections, but also from psychological stress, such as high levels of anxiety. In either case, because the adrenal cortex cannot produce enough cortisol and aldosterone, the person has an Addisonian crisis. The symptoms of an Addisonian crisis are the extreme of the problems already described. The clients develop shock from the lack of sodium and water in the plasma, while their serum potassium levels increase. They have pain, nausea, and vomiting. Circulatory collapse and death can occur. Treatment of an Addisonian crisis includes the administration of cortisol intravenously, along with the replacement of sodium, chloride, and water.

Alteration in Self-concept Related to Changes in Body Image
On the whole, a lack of cortisol does not cause as many physical changes as does an excess of cortisol. One characteristic of a lack of cortisol is pigmentation of the skin, because the lack triggers the release of MSH. The exact reasons for the increase in MSH are not well understood. It is hypothesized that the

lowered cortisol triggers the pituitary to produce not only more ACTH, but also MSH. Clients can be told that the darkening of the skin will fade when the cortisol level is brought back to normal.

If the cortisol lack is associated with a lack of androgens, there may not be many changes because most sex hormones are produced by the gonads. However, if only cortisol is lacking, the adrenal cortex may be stimulated to increase the production of androgens. This increase causes a collection of symptoms known as adrenogenital syndrome, which causes the masculinization of females. (See the section on androgen levels.) In infants and children, congenital hyperplasia of the adrenal due to cortisol lack causes many body changes, as described in the section on adrenogenital syndrome.

Knowledge Deficit Regarding the Need for Lifelong Replacement Therapy

Clients with a lack of cortisol are placed on cortisone supplements. The majority of the dose is usually given in the morning because this is in keeping with the normal rhythm of the hormone (Gotch, 1981). They may be taught to take the cortisone replacement with food or antacid. (See the discussion under excess cortisol for the symptoms possible with too high levels of cortisol.)

A mineralocorticoid may also be needed; fluorohydrocortisone (Florinef) is one that is given orally, while desoxycorticosterone (DOCA) is another that is given parenterally. The mineralocorticoid replacement is needed only when clients are deficient in aldosterone as well as in cortisol.

These clients need to carry identification that notes the need for extra cortisone in times of stress. They may also keep parenteral hydrocortisone (Solu-Cortef) for emergency replacement. They may be taught to double their doses for minor stress and triple them for major stress, such as surgery (Burnett, 1980). The adult client needs to know exactly how to recognize the need for more cortisone. Also parents need to know when to give extra medication to children. (See the discussion on congenital adrenal hyperplasia.)

ADRENOGENITAL SYNDROME DUE TO CONGENITAL ADRENOCORTICAL HYPERPLASIA

A congenital lack of certain enzymes can cause a decreased production of cortisol and sometimes of mineralocorticoids. At least six different inherited genetic defects cause a decreased synthesis of cortisol, and some of these defects also cause a lack of mineralocorticoids.

The lack of cortisol causes an increased production of ACTH and hyperplasia of the adrenal gland. Even when the adrenal gland enlarges, it does not produce more cortisone, due to the genetic defect in manufacturing cortisol. However, the adrenal cortex is stimulated to produce more androgens and the precursors of hydrocortisone. In the infant or in the young child, although the increase in estrogens is not apparent, the increase in androgens causes masculinization of the female and signs of early puberty in the male. In addition to the genetic defect that causes a lack of manufacturing of cortisol, there may be an associated inability to produce aldosterone. The children who also lack aldosterone are called *salt losers* because they are unable to retain sodium and water.

Nursery nurses need to examine each newborn's genitalia for any abnormalities. Sometimes the female is incorrectly assumed to be a male. The infant may fail to thrive and have milk intolerances. The salt loser may have a very poor appetite, frequent vomiting, and other symptoms of severe fluid and electrolyte imbalance.

Some children may seem normal at birth but show symptoms of a very early puberty. In these cases, diagnosing the lack of cortisol is important so that the increased androgen level does not create secondary sex characteristics. The female child may need surgery later, to repair an enlarged clitoris or fused vagina. The parents need reassurance that normal sexual functioning can be expected later. The child is tested for serum cortisol levels, which will be low. Urine tests are also done to evaluate the presence of metabolites of the glucocorticoids and the androgens in the urine. (These urine tests are covered next.) Treatment with cortisol and, if necessary, with a mineralocorticoid, reduces the level of ACTH and thus the hyperplasia of the adrenal cortex causing the excess of androgens.

POSSIBLE NURSING DIAGNOSIS RELATED TO CONGENITAL ADRENOCORTICAL HYPERPLASIA

Knowledge Deficit Regarding Emergency Replacement Therapy
Children with a cortisol lack and their parents need careful instruction on how to manage the replacement of cortisol. It is recommended that families always keep a plastic syringe, two needles, and an ampule of hydrocortisone (Solu-Cortef) in their automobiles and homes for emergency injections. Parents are told that a dose of Solu-Cortef, given unnecessarily, does not harm the child, but a delay in giving a dose could be fatal. Older children can be taught to recognize symptoms that indicate a need for more hydrocortisone. Burnett (1980) describes a case study of a child with cortisol lack and how he managed to live with the disease.

URINARY MEASUREMENT OF THE ADRENAL CORTEX STEROIDS

Free urinary cortisol, as well as various metabolites of the adrenal cortex hormones, can be measured by 24-hour urine specimens. In general, the urine excretion of steroids is increased when the serum levels of the steroids are increased and decreased when the steroids are low in the serum. Sometimes creatinine measurements are done on the urine sample too, to ensure that the volume of urine is normal.

Very important is that all urine for 24 hours be saved (see Chapter 3 for details of urine collections). The nurse should check with the laboratory to see if any preservative is needed. The urine specimens are kept cold to decrease bacterial growth. These urine specimens may be ordered as part of the test of ACTH suppression or ACTH stimulation.

■ URINARY CORTISOL LEVELS

This test, which measures cortisol itself rather than the metabolites, has become the usual test for evaluating adrenal hyperfunction or Cushing's syndrome. Various drugs, such as spironolactone (Aldactone) or quinacrine (Atabrine), will interfere with the results. Low values do not necessarily mean adrenal hypofunction.

Reference Values for Urinary Cortisol

20–70 µg/24 hr

Increased in pregnancy and with oral contraceptives

■ 17-HYDROXYSTEROIDS (17-OHCS) (PORTER–SILBER TEST)

This urine test, sometimes called the Porter–Silber test, measures several of the metabolites of both the glucocorticoids and aldosterone. These metabolites are increased in Cushing's syndrome. The administration of ACTH should cause a rise in the 17-OHCS too. These metabolites are decreased in Addison's disease and in the adrenogenital syndrome of lack of cortisol. Abnormal values can be caused by hepatic or renal dysfunctions. Chlorpromazine and related drugs interfere with assay. The specimen should be kept cold. This test is being replaced by urinary cortisol levels.

Reference Values for 17-OHCS

All groups	3–8 mg/24 hr urine specimen
Female	Slightly lower than male due to less muscle mass and body weight

---

■ 17-KETOSTEROIDS (17-KS)

The 17-KS are metabolites of the steroids from both the adrenal cortex and the testes except for the major androgen testosterone (Jacobs et al., 1984). The values for men are considerably higher after puberty. The values are increased in tumors when production of hormones from the adrenal cortex or the testes is increased. These metabolites are also increased in the adrenogenital syndrome. Hypofunctioning of the adrenal

---

Reference Values for 17-KS

	Male	Female
Age 10	1–4	1–4
20	6–21	4–16
30	8–26	4–14
50	5–18	3–9
70	2–10	1–7

---

mg/24 hr urine specimen

gland and certain adrenal adenomas cause a decrease. Meprobamate and many other drugs may make the test invalid. So check for possible drug interferences if the client is receiving any drugs. The urine should be kept cold.

■ 17-KETOGENIC STEROIDS (17-KGS)

The 17-KGS test measures several of the glucocorticoid derivatives, as well as pregnanetriol, which is a precursor in adrenal corticoid synthesis. The 17-KGS are elevated when there is increased production by the adrenal gland, whereas they are low if there is hypofunction of the adrenal cortex. Since 17-KGS include the 17-OHCS, they are reflective of a more complete steroid measurement. This test is being replaced by urinary cortisol levels.

Reference Values for 17-KGS	
All groups	5–20 mg/24 hr

■ URINARY PREGNANETRIOL

Because pregnanetriol is a precursor in adrenal corticoid synthesis, this test is useful in confirming the presence of the adrenogenital syndrome due to a lack of an enzyme to make cortisol. (Pregnanediol is a test of progesterone. See the section on gonadotropins.) Pregnanetriol is also increased with certain tumors of the ovary or adrenal cortex.

Reference Values for Urinary Pregnanetriol	
Adult	4 mg/24 hr urine specimen
Children:	
2 weeks to 2 years	0–0.2 mg/24 hr specimen
Ages 2–16	0.3–1.1 mg/24 hr specimen

■ ALDOSTERONE

Aldosterone, a hormone produced by the adrenal cortex, is a mineralocorticoid. Increases in aldosterone cause an increase in the extracellular fluid volume because aldosterone increases the reabsorption of sodium and chloride by the proximal renal tubules while increasing the excretion of potassium and hydrogen ions.

Aldosterone is not regulated by ACTH, as are the glucocorticoids. A decrease in extracellular fluid causes an increased production of aldosterone through stimulation of the renin-angiotensin system. A decreased flow of blood through the kidney is a stimulus for the production of renin, a hormone secreted by the kidney. Renin, when secreted into the bloodstream, acts on angiotensinogen to form angiotensin. (Angiotensinogen is formed in the liver and circulates in the plasma.) Angiotensin then stimulates the adrenal cortex to increase production of aldosterone. Thus a drop in extracellular volume is corrected by the final action of retaining more sodium and water in the plasma. Conversely, an increased extracellular volume is a signal for less production of renin. Without renin, angiotensinogen is not converted to the active form of angiotensin, so the adrenal cortex decreases production of aldosterone. Less aldosterone means less sodium (and water) retention, and so the extracellular fluid volume is decreased to normal again. See Table 15–4 for a simple diagram of the regulation of aldosterone and the related laboratory tests.

Preparation of Client and Collection of Samples

The client needs to be on a regular diet with the usual intake of sodium and potassium. The client may be put on a specific sodium diet of 10 mEq, 110 mEq, or 210 mEq. With more sodium in the diet, the reference values are lower. The dietician must plan the diet if a specific sodium intake is to be followed before the urine and plasma samples are collected.

The laboratory needs 3 ml of plasma or serum for the specimen. The plasma specimen is taken after the client has been resting in the supine position for at least two hours. Samples may also be obtained in an upright position for comparison (Scully, 1986). The peak concentration of aldosterone is in the early morning sample. A 24-hour urine specimen may also be collected, and it needs to be kept cold. (See Chapter 3 on 24-hour urine collection.)

Reference Values for Aldosterone

Plasma level	107 ± 45 pg/ml
Urinary excretion for 24 hr	5–19 µg

Fasting, at rest, 110 mEq sodium diet. Values differ with various intakes of sodium. See Appendix A, Table 3, for other values. Pregnancy causes increased levels.

Note: In addition to direct measurement of aldosterone levels, serum and urine levels of sodium and potassium are measured too. (See Chapter 5 on electrolyte measurements in serum and urine.)

TABLE 15–4. THE RENIN-ANGIOTENSIN CONTROL OF ALDOSTERONE AND TESTS THAT MEASURE ALDOSTERONE-PRODUCING ABILITY OF ADRENAL CORTEX

Decrease of Na in plasma. (Measure of Na levels.)

↓

Increased production of renin by kidney. (Measure of renin activity.)

Aldosterone causes increase of Na in plasma and decrease in K. (Measure of K levels, aldosterone levels in serum and urine, saralasin test.)

↓

↑

Renin converts angiotensinogen into angiotensin I, which through enzyme action becomes angiotensin II. ⟶ Angiotensin II stimulates production of aldosterone by adrenal cortex.

K = potassium; Na = sodium.
See Cryer (1979) and Larrabee and Hanna (1983) for more detail.

Increased Aldosterone Levels in Serum and Urine (Hyperaldosteronism)

Clinical Significance. Increased levels of the hormone aldosterone can be either primary or secondary. In primary hyperaldosteronism, a tumor of the adrenal cortex causes an increased secretion of aldosterone. The renin level in the serum is low because the increased production of the hormone is not due to the renin–angiotensin mechanism. (The test for renin is discussed next.) Note that oral contraceptives may also cause an increased aldosterone level. (See Appendix D.)

Secondary hyperaldosteronism is a much more common clinical problem (Ryan, 1980). In this type of hyperaldosteronism, the oversecretion of aldosterone is due to the continual activity of the renin–angiotensin system. This constant stimulation of the system occurs when the perfusion to the kidneys is not adequate. For example, clients with congestive heart failure (CHF) often have poor renal perfusion. A lack of pressure in the juxtaglomerular apparatus causes the kidney to secrete more renin because the kidneys interpret the lack of perfusion as a lack of extracellular fluid. Renin activates angiotensin, which stimulates aldosterone production. Unfortunately, in congestive failure, the extracellular fluid is already in abundance. So the increased aldosterone level, as a response to poor renal perfusion, does not correct the underlying problem. With secondary hyperaldosteronism, the renin level is therefore high.

Not all cases of increased aldosterone are so simple. Sometimes drugs, such as oral contraceptives, cause an increase in aldosterone levels, although the exact mechanism is not well understood. Clients with severe liver dysfunction, such as in cirrhosis, tend to have elevated aldosterone levels, too, which are partly related to poor renal perfusion. Also, if a failing liver can no longer detoxify aldosterone, levels of serum aldosterone remain higher for longer periods.

POSSIBLE NURSING DIAGNOSIS RELATED TO INCREASED ALDOSTERONE LEVELS

Potential for Fluid Volume Excess Related to Retention of Sodium
Because aldosterone causes increased sodium and thus water retention, these clients need to have their blood pressure monitored as well as weights and intake and output recorded.

If the increased aldosterone level is due to secondary causes, edema is usually a clinical problem. (See Chapter 5 for a discussion of the nursing implications when a client has edema and needs to be on a restricted sodium diet.) Diuretics may be particularly useful for secondary hyperaldosteronism. The type of diuretic often used is spironolactone because this drug is an aldosterone-blocking agent. Spironolactone (Aldactone) is a steroid compound that presumably acts by competing with aldosterone for cellular receptor sites in the tubules. Thus it promotes sodium and water excretion without a loss of potassium.

Decreased Aldosterone Levels

Clinical Significance. The decrease in aldosterone is often part of a generalized hypofunctioning of the adrenal gland. The causes of Addison's disease were discussed in the section on cortisol deficiencies. In congenital adrenal hyperplasia, the infant lacks an enzyme needed to manufacture cortisol from cholesterol, and this deficiency may or may not be associated with a deficiency of aldosterone. In the most common type of genetic defect that causes a lack of cortisol, about one third of the clients are also deficient in a mineralocorticoid or aldosterone (Burnett, 1980). The lack of aldosterone gives the symptoms of "salt wasting" seen in some genetic defects and in Addison's disease.

POSSIBLE NURSING DIAGNOSIS FOR DECREASED ALDOSTERONE LEVELS

Alteration in Fluid Balance Related to Hyponatremia
Clients with decreased aldosterone levels are unable to maintain normal serum sodium levels. (See the discussion on Addisonian crisis under the section on low cortisol levels.) They must therefore have salt, water, and mineralocorticoid replacement. If they lack aldosterone, they must take fludrocortisone (Florinef) orally or desoxycorticosterone (DOCA) parenterally to ensure mineralocorticoid activity. These medications are continued for life. Because a lack of mineralocorticoid activity may also be part of the adrenogenital syndrome, children who experience salt wasting as part of their congenital problem must have replacement too. Children born with severe lack of mineralocorticoids may die, however, before the defect is recognized (Kaplan et al., 1979).

■ RENIN

Renin is an enzyme produced by the juxtaglomerular apparatus in response to a decreased blood flow through the kidneys. A change from the recumbent position to upright also causes an increased production. A high-sodium diet causes a decrease in renin. Thus diet and the position of the client must be taken into account when using reference values for renin activity. The test for renin is used in the differential diagnosis of hypertension (also see discussion on saralasin).

Preparation of Client and Collection of Sample
Because the values of renin are normally higher in the morning, the test is done early. The client is usually in the supine position when the blood is drawn but upright may also be done as a comparison (Scully, 1986). The laboratory needs 4 ml of plasma, which is put into a tube with EDTA as an anticoagulant (lavender Vacutainer). The specimen should be iced. Diuretics cause changes in the values; so make note of the use of any medications on the laboratory slip. Also note the sodium content of the diet, which should be controlled for several days.

Reference Values for Serum Renin

Supine	1.1 ± 0.8 ng/ml/hr
Upright	1.9 ± 1.7 ng/ml/hr

Note: Low-sodium diets and diuretics cause an increased production of renin activity (see Appendix A, Table 3).

■ SARALASIN INFUSION TEST

Saralasin, a competitive antagonist of angiotensin II, is sometimes used as a clinical bioassay of the renin system (Weber, 1979). A drop in blood pressure is expected if the hypertension is renin-dependent. The saralasin (Sarenin) is given as an intravenous infusion and the blood pressure monitored every two minutes during the 20–30 minutes of the infusion. Larrabee and Hanna (1983) describe the protocol to follow.

■ CATECHOLAMINES, VANILLYLMANDELIC ACID (VMA), AND METANEPHRINES

The adrenal medulla secretes epinephrine and norepinephrine, both of which are essential in assisting the body for the "fight-or-flight" response to stress. These two hormones, called the catecholamines, are usually measured in 24-hour urine samples rather than in plasma samples.

Catecholamines are broken down into intermediate metabolites, which are called normetanephine and metanephrines. Laboratories may also measure these intermediate metabolites in the urine. The main product of catecholamine breakdown is an acid called vanillylmandelic acid (VMA). Since the VMA test is easier to do than the other urine tests for catecholamines, the laboratory may use the VMA as the screening procedure. Some laboratories prefer to use the metanephrines as the screening test for hypertension (Camuñas, 1983). The other tests of metabolites, such as the metanephrines, may be elevated even if the VMA is not. If screening tests are positive then all of the urine tests may be done to confirm a diagnosis of increased catecholamine secretion.

Preparation of Client and Collection of 24-hour Urine Specimen

All the tests for the metabolites of the catecholamines require that the urine remain very acid with a pH of 3 or below. Usually 12 ml of hydrochloric acid (HCl) is added to the 24-hour specimen bottle. Clients should be warned about the strong acid in the bottle. The usual procedure for collecting urine for 24 hours is followed (see Chapter 3).

The client needs to be relatively free of stress. Vigorous exercise causes an elevation of catecholamines. Blood pressure, height, and weight should be recorded on the laboratory slip.

Nurses must validate the need for restriction of certain foods by checking with the specific laboratory doing the test. The client should be on a regular diet because

---

Reference Values for Catecholamines and Metabolites in Urine

Epinephrine	Under 20 μg/24 hr urine specimen
Norepinephrine	Under 100 μg/24 hr urine specimen
Metanephrines	0.3–0.9 mg/24 hr urine specimen
Vanillylmandelic acid (VMA)	Up to 9 mg/24 hr urine specimen

fasting increases catecholamines. Depending on the procedure used by the laboratory, certain foods must be restricted in the diet. For example, coffee, tea, chocolate, bananas, avocados, and anything with vanilla interferes with the VMA results. Newer laboratory methods are not affected by food intake.

A multitude of drugs also lead to confusing results. Drugs that act via the sympathetic nervous system, such as some antihypertensives, and antidepressants, make the test invalid. Ideally, the client should be off all drugs for 3–7 days before the test. Nurses must check with the individual physician to see which drugs can be given.

Increased Catecholamines in Urine

Clinical Significance. Mild elevations of the catecholamines and of their metabolites can be due to stress such as surgery, burns, or childbirth. (Obviously, any endocrine response cannot be effectively evaluated during stress.) A marked increase in the catecholamines has two major causes: The first, a tumor of the adrenal medulla called a pheochromocytoma, causes a marked elevation of the catecholamines. The second comes from certain types of malignancies, called neuroblastomas, which arise from primitive sympathetic tissue (Kaplan, 1979). Other tests, such as scans, help to pinpoint the presence of a tumor.

POSSIBLE NURSING DIAGNOSES RELATED TO ELEVATED CATECHOLAMINES

Anxiety and Alterations in Cardiac Output Related to the Effects of Increased Catecholamines

Clients with elevated catecholamines have symptoms reflective of the stimulating effects of epinephrine and norepinephrine. Often their symptoms are attributed to other causes. Some of the outstanding symptoms are increased blood pressure and pulse. Since clients may feel very jittery and notice heart palpitations, their symptoms may be wrongly ascribed to an anxiety attack. The surge of catecholamines may be intermittent, so that, during an attack, the blood pressure may become very high and the client can have pounding headaches, nausea, and vomiting. The high levels of epinephrine can cause hyperglycemia and glycosuria, and the client may be suspected of having diabetes. (See Chapter 8 on symptoms of hyperglycemia.)

Nurses should carefully monitor the blood pressure and pulse of any client with suspected catecholamine increase due to pheochromocytoma or a childhood neuroblastoma. They need to watch for any symptoms that help to confirm the presence of high levels of catecholamines. A blood or urine sample, taken during or soon after an attack, may demonstrate the presence of high levels of catecholamines.

Knowledge Deficit Related to Drug Therapy and Impending Surgery

Symptoms can be controlled with alpha-adrenergic blocking drugs, but the definitive treatment is surgery. Camuñas (1983) gives detailed information on five types of drugs used and the pre- and postoperative care of clients with pheochromocytoma.

Catecholamine Deficiency

Clinical Significance. Even when the adrenal medulla is hypofunctional or destroyed by disease or surgery, the client does not have any symptoms of catecholamine deficiency because catecholamines are also produced by the autonomic nerve endings (Juebiz, 1979).

■ PARATHORMONE OR PARATHYROID HORMONE (PTH)

PTH is produced by the parathyroid glands—the only hormone secreted by these glands. The parathyroid glands, usually four in number, are located in the vicinity of the thyroid gland. Unlike that of many of the other hormones, the level of PTH is not under the influence of the pituitary gland.

The function of PTH is to control serum calcium and phosphorus levels (Table 15-5). Hence the level of PTH depends on the serum calcium and phosphorus levels. A lowered serum calcium level is a stimulus for the release of more PTH to keep the serum calcium level normal. PTH works various ways to keep a constant serum calcium level and a correspondingly normal phosphorus level:

1. It works in concert with vitamin D to stimulate calcium and phosphorus absorption via the intestinal mucosa.
2. It causes mobilization of calcium from the bone.
3. It also causes increased excretion of phosphorus in the urine.

An abnormal elevation or decrease in PTH always causes changes in the serum calcium and phosphorus levels. (See Chapter 7 for a detailed discussion of the effects of PTH on serum calcium and phosphorus levels. Note that phosphorus is measured as phosphate in the serum.)

Preparation of Client and Collection of Sample
The client does not have to be fasting. Collect a morning sample. The laboratory needs 5 ml of plasma, which should be kept on ice in all cases or, if it must be sent a distance, frozen. (Samples are often shipped because the test is difficult to do in most laboratories.)

Reference Values for Serum PTH

Less than 25 pg/ml

Increased PTH Serum Level

Clinical Significance. Increased PTH levels may indicate primary hyper-parathyroidism. Tumors of the parathyroid, which are usually benign, cause increased secretion of PTH. These clients have symptoms of high serum calcium levels and

TABLE 15-5. EFFECTS OF PARATHORMONE (PTH) ON SERUM CALCIUM AND SERUM PHOSPHORUS

$\uparrow$ PTH causes $\uparrow$ Ca $\downarrow$ P
$\downarrow$ PTH causes $\downarrow$ Ca $\uparrow$ P

---

low phosphate levels (as discussed in Chapter 7). A persistently low serum calcium level or a high phosphate level causes a secondary rise in PTH. Also, malignant tumors from nonendocrine sources can secrete PTH. (See the discussion on ectopic hormones.)

Because an elevated PTH causes an increased serum calcium level and a decreased serum phosphate level, the nursing diagnoses are based on these imbalances. (See Chapter 7 for the nursing implications when a client has hypercalcemia.) If client has an adenoma, surgery will restore the balance.

Decreased PTH Serum Level

Clinical Significance. Decreased levels of PTH can be due to trauma to the parathyroid glands during a thyroidectomy. Infections or other traumas may affect the parathyroid gland. Tumors of the gland usually also cause an increase in hormone production, but some tumors may cause a decreased function of the gland. Since the levels of PTH are normally low in the serum, a low level may not be helpful in diagnosis.

The symptoms and clinical manifestations of a lack of PTH are reflected in low serum calcium levels and in high phosphate levels. Severe hypocalcema causes tetany. (See Chapter 7 for a detailed description of tetany and nursing diagnoses for hypocalcemia.)

A lack of PTH is treated by the administration of vitamin D and calcium salts. (See Chapter 7 on the treatment of low serum calcium levels and possible patient teaching.)

THE THYROID GLAND

The thyroid gland secretes three hormones: triiodothyronine (T_3), L-thyroxine (T_4), and calcitonin. Calcitonin lowers the plasma calcium level by inhibiting mobilization of calcium from the bone. (See Chapter 7 on the role of calcitonin in the regulation of calcium levels.) Calcitonin levels are done only for known or suspected cases of medullary carcinoma of the thyroid. (See Appendix A, Table 3 for reference values.) The other two of these hormones, T_3 and T_4, are forms of thyroxine, and they are usually called the *thyroid hormones*. (The T_3 contains *three* iodine atoms and T_4 contains *four* iodine atoms in a molecule.) An adequate intake of iodine is necessary for the continual formation of T_3 and T_4. As with the other hormones, protein intake must be normal too. In many countries, table salt has been iodized so that people have an adequate intake of iodine.

Most of the thyroid's output is in the form of T_4; only a small amount is in the form of T_3, but T_3 is much more potent than T_4. Both T_4 and T_3 can be measured directly. Also, the amount of T_4 can be calculated by other tests, such as the T_3 resin uptake. Each of these tests is discussed individually later in this section. The thyroid hormones, T_4 and T_3 have several functions:

1. They potentiate the effects of epinephrine and decrease the serum cholesterol level.
2. They are necessary for normal development of the central nervous system.
3. They stimulate growth and normal metabolism in all cells.

Tests to Diagnose Hypothyroidism and Hyperthyroidism

No one diagnostic test can be used alone to diagnose hypo- or hyperthyroidism. (Table 15-6 summarizes changes in various tests of thyroid function.) Also, thyroid tests

TABLE 15–6. TESTS OF THYROID FUNCTION

Test	Hypothyroidism	Hyperthyroidism
TSH (thyroid-stimulating hormone)	↓ or ↑ (see text)	↑ or ↓ (see text)
T₄ (L-thyroxine)	↓	↑
T₃ (triiodothyronine)	Not usually done	↑
T₃ resin uptake	↓	↑
FTI (free thyroxin index)	↓	↑
RAI (radioactive iodine uptake)	↓	↑
Thyroid scans (see Chapter 22)	Used to identify nodules not hypo or hyper states per se.	

Wallach (1986) lists over 20 conditions which cause changes in these tests.

are not useful for several months after I-131 therapy (Soler, 1979). T_4 is considered to be the basic screening test in most cases of suspected thyroid disease. In addition to the T_4, T_3, T_3 resin uptake, and TSH, the client may also have thyroid scans and radioactive iodine uptakes done. Cancer of the thyroid is suggested by cold nodules on a thyroid scan and not by thyroid tests (Guimond & Wilson, 1979).

Because the thyroid hormones increase the metabolism of cholesterol, clients with hyperthyroidism tend to have low serum cholesterol levels, and clients with hypothyroidism tend to have high serum cholesterol levels. (See Chapter 9 on cholesterol tests.) Yet the cholesterol level is not particularly helpful in confirming the presence of a thyroid disorder.

Certain types of thyroid inflammations are associated with increased amounts of antibodies. (See Chapter 14 for a discussion on antobodies against thyroid tissue.)

■ THYROTROPIN OR THYROID-STIMULATING HORMONE (TSH)

The production of T_4 and T_3 is controlled by TSH from the anterior pituitary gland. In turn, TSH is released from the pituitary in response to the thyrotropin-releasing hormone (TRH) in the hypothalamus. Thus, like most of the other anterior pituitary hormones, TSH is sensitive to nervous reponse from the hypothalamus. Measurement of TSH is useful in determining whether hypothyroidism is due to primary hypofunction of the thyroid gland or to secondary hypofunction of the anterior pituitary gland. In sophisticated endocrine work-ups, the TRH from the hypothalamus can be measured too (Juebiz, 1979).

Preparation of Client and Collection of Sample
The laboratory requires 2 ml of serum. The client does not need to be fasting.

Reference Values for TSH

0.5–5.0 μU/ml

Increased or Decreased TSH

Clinical Significance. The purpose of measuring TSH is to evaluate the possibility of pituitary failure as the cause of hypothyroidism. A low TSH is an indication for further investigation of pituitary disorders. Primary hypothyroidism, due to insufficiency of the thyroid gland itself, is a much more common cause of hypothyroidism. In primary hypothyroidism, the TSH level becomes greatly elevated in an attempt to stimulate the failing thyroid gland. In hyperthyroidism, the TSH level is suppressed due to the negative feedback system. Yet this test is not useful as a diagnosis of hyperthyroidism because in some people with normal thyroid functioning (euthyroid) the TSH is barely if at all detectable (Cryer, 1979). The TSH measurement is done on newborns who have low T_4 levels as confirmation of primary hypothyroidism (Fisher et al., 1979).

■ L-THYROXINE (T_4) SERUM CONCENTRATION

T_4, the thyroxine with four iodine atoms, is the most abundant of the thyroid hormones. The test of T_4 measures both free thyroxine and the portion carried by the thyroid-binding plasma proteins. (See the test for thyroid-binding globulins.) The T_4 is the test used most often for screening and follow-up of clients who have been diagnosed as having either hypo- or hyperthyroidism.

T_4 can be measured by radio- or enzyme immunoassay. Radioimmunassay is the more costly of the two methods and it does include a radioactive drug in a several-step procedure. The advantage of the enzyme method is that it can be done by an automated system. The development of an enzyme-based test for thyroxine marked the first time that screening for thyroid disorders could be part of an automatic screening profile done by computer (Galen, 1978). T_4, which can be done with a filter paper, is useful for newborn screening (see Chapter 18).

Preparation of Client and Collection of Sample
The laboratory requires 1 ml of plasma. The sample is not affected by food or iodine ingestion, but, if the client is taking a thyroid preparation, this should be noted on the requisition slip. Note that many drugs, e.g., propranolol, may interfere with the test results.

Reference Values for L-Thyroxine (T_4)

Adult	4–12 μg/dl by RIA Values vary according to different laboratory methods
Pregnancy	Causes an increase, as do birth control pills
Infant and children	Higher ranges. Males experience a gradual decline in T_4 as they mature sexually; females do not (Tietz, 1983)
Aged	Values maintained, but decrease in plasma protein lowers values

---

Decreases and Increases in T_4

Clinical Significance. The hormone is increased in hyperthyroidism and decreased in hypothyroidism. The nursing diagnoses for these two conditions are summarized later in this chapter. In clients with hydatidiform mole, the T_4 may be very elevated. Evidently, there is an increase of some TSH activity from the molar tissue. Another nonthyroid cause of an elevation is liver disease.

■ TRIIODOTHYRONINE (T_3) SERUM CONCENTRATION (T_3-RIA)

The test for T_3 is sometimes called T_3-RIA to denote that the hormone is measured by radioimmunoassay. The use of the letters "RIA" also helps to distinguish this test from the T_3 resin uptake (discussed next). T_3 is more biologically active than T_4, but both hormones have similar actions in the body. T_3 is not usually used in confirming the diagnosis of suspected hypothyroidism because other tests can demonstrate hypofunction of the thyroid gland. Sometimes, however, a client may have clinical signs of thyrotoxicosis with a normal T_4. Measurement of the T_3 is then needed, because T_3 may be elevated in thyrotoxicosis while other thyroid tests are still in the normal range (Soler, 1979).

Preparation of Client and Collection of Sample
The preparation and collection instructions are the same as those for the T_4 test.

Reference Values for Total Triiodothyronine (T_3)

Adult	75–195 ng/dl by RIA
Pregnancy and oral contraceptives	Tend to increase the values
Infants and children have higher values	

A decrease in plasma proteins causes lowered values.

■ T_3 RESIN UPTAKE (PERCENTAGE OF T_3 UPTAKE)

T_3 resin uptake measures the amount of T_4 indirectly by measuring the amount of T_3 that can be attached to the proteins that bind the thyroid hormones. Normally, almost all the T_4 is attached to thyroid-binding globulins (TBG). With a lack of T_4, the TBG are able to absorb more T_3 that is added to a blood sample. With an increase in T_4, the TBG are oversaturated with the T_4 and unable to carry much additional T_3. The resin uptake test does not measure the amount of T_3 taken up by the TBG. Instead, it measures the amount of T_3 left over and thus free to bind to the resin added to the blood sample.

In the T_3 resin uptake, a measured amount of radioactive-tagged T_3 and resin is added to a sample of the client's blood. The resin is put into the test tube to absorb any of the radioactive-tagged T_3 that cannot be taken up by the TBG in the blood sample. In other words, the resin is the "sponge" that takes up all the tagged T_3

that cannot bind with the globulins. Since hypothyroid states create a lot of "vacant" TBG, the tagged T_3 is attached to the TBG and less is taken up by the resin. In hyperthyroid states, the TBG are saturated with T_4; so they have little binding capacity for the additional T_3. Thus the added tagged T_3 must go to the secondary binding site, which is the resin. The laboratory measures the amount of T_3 that is taken up by the resin and reports the results in percentages.

Reference Values for T_3 Resin Uptake

25–35% of the tagged T_3 is taken up by the resin. The rest of the T_3 is assumed to be bound to the thyroid-binding globulins.

Values in hyperthyroidism	There is little room for the tagged T_3, so more T_3 goes to the resin. The resin uptake is above 35%.
Values in hypothyroidism	More of the T_3 can be attached to thyroid-binding globulins, so less tagged T_3 is absorbed by the resin. The uptake by the resin is below 25%.

Note: This test is based on the amount of thyroid-binding globulins. So increases in globulins cause more uptake of T_3 on globulins and less by the resin. The resin uptake seems abnormally low when thyroid-binding globulins are elevated in pregnancy and by drugs such as estrogens.

A decrease in plasma proteins means less binding capacity and thus an increased uptake by the resin. Thus in clients with severe liver disease or nephrosis, the lack of plasma proteins causes an unusually high T_3 uptake by the resin (Hallal, 1977).

The important thing to remember is that any changes in plasma proteins invalidate the results of the T_3 resin uptake. To overcome the problems of unknown changes in the amount of plasma proteins, the T_3 resin uptake can be compared to other thyroid tests. One way to make the tests of T_3 resin uptake and T_4 more accurate is to use these two tests to calculate the free thyroxin index (FTI).

■ FREE THYROXINE INDEX (FTI) AND FREE T_4

The FTI is usually a calculated value based on the results of the T_4 and T_3 resin uptake tests. The calculated value is obtained by multiplying the T_4 by the T_3 resin uptake. This value shows the ratio of total thyroxine (T_4) to the total available binding

---

Reference Values for FTI

1–4 (based on the reference values for T_4 and T_3 resin uptakes in the example in the text)

As explained in the reference values for T_3 uptake, the FTI makes corrections when the plasma proteins are not normal or when there is a change in the binding sites rather than in the amount of thyroxine. High amounts of free thyroxine, as shown by the FTI, are highly suggestive of hyperthyroidism. The clinician must also look at both the T_4 and the T_3 resin uptake as individual tests.

---

sites (T_3 resin uptake). For example, a normal T_4 would be 6 μg and a T_3 resin uptake should be about 25%. So the FTI is:

$$6 \ \mu g \ (T_4) \ \times \ 25\% \ (T_3 \ resin \ uptake) \ = \ 1.5 \ (FTI)$$

Laboratories can also measure the free T_4 directly, but this is more costly and usually gives similar results to the FTI (Jacobs et al., 1984).

Preparation of Client and Collection of Sample
The laboratory needs 2 ml of serum.

Reference Values for Free T_4

1.0–2.6 ng/dl

■ THYROID-BINDING GLOBULINS (TBG) CAPACITY

Some laboratories may do direct measurement of the globulins involved in thyroid binding to check on the validity of other tests done for thyroid function.

Preparation of Client and Collection of Sample
The laboratory needs 2 ml of serum.

Reference Values for TBG

15–25 μg of T_4/100 ml

Elevated Serum Thyroid Levels

Clinical Significance. A diagnosis of hyperthyroidism is made when the client has an elevation of several of the tests discussed in this chapter. (One test alone may not be diagnostic.) Table 15–6 shows which of the common tests of thyroid function are usually elevated in hyperthyroidism, which is also called thyrotoxicosis. An excess of thyroid hormone can result from inflammation, tumors, or autoimmune disorders of the thyroid gland. Often the cause of the hyperthyroidism is unknown (that is, it is idiopathic). A hyperthyroid state associated with goiter and a bulging of the eyes (exophthalmos) is called Graves' disease, which is considered the most fully developed hyperthyroid state and the cause of which is not known. It sometimes follows an infection, physical stress, or emotional crisis. Clearly, TSH is not responsible for the hyperthyroid state (Juebiz, 1979). Hyperthyroidism is rare in infants, but it does occur in children and particularly in adolescents. Hyperthyroidism is much more common in girls than in boys (Heagarty et al., 1980). Once the client is definitely diagnosed as having hyperthyroidism, treatment may include the use of antithyroid drugs, such as methimazole (Tapazole), therapy with radioactive iodine, or surgical intervention. The goal of treatment is to bring the client back to a euthyroid, or normal thyroid, balance. The client needs help from the nurse and from others in learning to cope with the manifestations of thyrotoxicosis.

POSSIBLE NURSING DIAGNOSES RELATED TO ELEVATED SERUM THYROID LEVELS

Potential Alteration in Cardiac Output

In general, most of the symptoms of hyperthyroidism are due to the accelerated metabolism that results from an excess of circulating thyroid hormones. These clients have tachycardia and often arrhythmias, such as atrial fibrillation. Even their resting pulses may be over 90. Extreme thyrotoxicosis can even cause heart failure. The high pulse rate decreases as the thyroid gland is brought under control. However, the pulse rate should be monitored to gauge how well clients can tolerate activity so they are not overtaxed. Clients with symptoms of inadequate cardiac output need bed rest and medical assessment.

Alterations in Nutritional Needs

These clients' increased metabolism make them hungry most of the time. They need a well-balanced diet with extra calories, as well as between-meal snacks. Extra fluids are needed due to the diaphoresis. Stimulants, such as coffee, should be avoided. The client should be weighed periodically to see that weight loss is not continuing. If diarrhea is a problem, the diet should avoid foods that tend to aggravate the hyperactive bowel.

Alteration in Comfort Related to Heat Intolerance or Ineffective Thermoregulation and Sleep Pattern Disturbance

These clients have a heat intolerance, so the room should be kept a little cool. Besides being cool, the environment should not be filled with a lot of noise or confusion. Clients need a quiet and relaxing atmosphere, and perhaps sedatives, to sleep.

Alteration in Self-Concept Related to Exophthalmos

Exophthalmos is an abnormal protrusion of the eye that sometimes occurs with hyperthyroidism when lymphocytes and mucopolysaccharides collect behind the eyeball. This collection may be unilateral or bilateral. The treatment of hyperthyroidism does not seem to have an appreciable influence on the progression or regression of the exophthalmos (Ryan, 1980). The key thing is to prevent trauma to the eyes and to help clients adjust to the altered body image.

Ineffective Coping Related to Inability to Handle Stress

Family, coworkers, and friends may find it hard to understand the actions of a client who has hyperthyroidism symptoms. Nurses may be very helpful in explaining in simple terms why these clients fuss about heat, noise, or whatever. Jenkins (1980) gives a personal account of the frustrations of learning to live with thyrotoxicosis and how this has affected her jobs in nursing. Control of a hormone imbalance is not always achieved in a short time. It may take months to years to gain really adequate balance.

Decreased Serum Thyroid Levels

Clinical Significance. The findings of the several tests used to confirm the suspected diagnosis of hypothyroidism are summarized in Table 15-6. In the adult, the presence of hypothyroidism is called myxedema. The failure of the thyroid gland to produce thyroid hormones is usually a primary dysfunction of the gland itself. However, hypothyroidism can also result from a lack of TSH (as discussed in the section on TSH). Diets deficient in iodine also cause a lack of thyroid hormone and an enlargement of the thyroid gland (goiter). Inflammations and autoimmune responses may cause insufficiency of the gland, but often the hypofunctioning cannot be linked to a causative factor.

In congenital hypothyroidism, the lack of the thyroid hormone can cause cretinism. Lack of thyroid in newborns causes growth failure and mental retardation. The symptoms of hypothyroidism may not be present at birth because the fetus has some thyroid hormones from the mother. Past studies (Fisher, 1979) concluded that T_4 should be a screening device for all newborns, so that congenital hypothyroidism can be detected. (See Chapter 18 on newborn screening.) Hypothyroidism may also develop later in childhood.

POSSIBLE NURSING DIAGNOSES RELATED TO DECREASED SERUM THYROID LEVELS

Alterations in Health Maintenance Related to Need for Lifelong Replacement Therapy

Hypothyroidism in Infants. Nurses must be aware of the symptoms of hypothyroidism in newborns and in adults, because they may be involved in case finding. Case finding in infants is very important because mental retardation occurs if the infant is not treated within two to three months after birth (Heagarty, 1980) and sometimes the effects of lack of thyroid may not be prominent at birth because the fetus has some thyroid hormones from the mother. Some of the outstanding characteristics of a lack of thyroid in a newborn are protruding tongue, a broad, flattened nose, a protruding abdomen with an umbilical hernia, and a generalized muscle hypotonia. The baby has a hoarse cry and may be a very poor feeder. The heart rate is slow.

Once the infant is diagnosed as having hypothyroidism, treatment is begun with thyroid replacement. The medication helps the infant to grow and to develop normally. The parents need careful teaching about the importance of life-long administration of the hormone and normal growth and development patterns.

Older Children and Adults. Symptoms of hypothyroidism, or myxedema, in the person beyond infancy are due to the slowing down of metabolism that occurs with insufficient thyroid hormone. These clients may have only slight symptoms so that the disease may be overlooked. They typically have fatigue, lethargy, and an intolerance to cold. Their hair is coarse and their skin is very dry. They gain weight on a limited diet. Constipation may be a problem. Their blood pressure and pulse are low. They may have memory impairment or a definite slowness in mental ability. Thyroid replacement eradicates these symptoms. The client needs to know the signs of overdosage of the drugs. (See the discussion on the symptoms of hyperthyroidism.) A resting pulse above 90 is an indicator of possibly too much thyroid replacement. Clients should be taught to check their own pulses. Any improvement in the way thyroid is commercially prepared can cause a need for less medication as the drugs become more potent (Stoffer & Szpunar, 1984).

Alteration in Comfort Related to Cold Intolerance and Slowness of Thought

Clients with hypothyroidism have a cold intolerance, so the environment needs to be warm. The nurse can provide extra clothing, such as heavy socks. The environment needs to be warm in the psychologic sense too. These clients may be slower in doing activities, so the nurse needs to let them proceed at their own pace. They may need help to adjust to fast-moving situations. Because inactivity may create more lethargy and dullness, some sensory stimulation is needed. In the home setting, the family may need help in making the environment warm, relaxed, and relatively quiet for the client.

Alteration in Nutritional Needs

These clients may need to be on a diet that is low in calories due to their weight gain. The nurse should see that their diets contain all the essential nutrients and vitamins. Clients can be assured that, when their thyroid level is returned to normal, their excess poundage should be easier to lose. (In fact, thyroid pills have been used as a type of diet pill. Obviously, thyroid intake by a client who is euthyroid is not a physiologically sound way to lose weight.) Plenty of fluids and roughage in the diet helps to decrease the problem of constipation.

Potential for Injury Related to Intolerance for Sedatives and Narcotics

Because these clients have a slower-than-normal metabolism, sedatives and narcotics may have a much more profound effect. So these types of drugs should be used with caution, if at all.

Alteration in Body Image

Clients may be distressed by the rough skin and coarse hair they develop. They may need to use hair conditioners and plenty of skin lotion to keep their skin and hair attractive looking. These skin and hair problems fade as the hormonal balance is restored.

GONADOTROPINS AND THE SEX-RELATED HORMONES

The sex-related hormones include the gonadotropins from the anterior pituitary gland (FSH and LH), along with estrogen, progesterone, and the androgens from the ovaries, testes, and adrenal cortex. Both the ovaries and testes produce progesterone, estrogen, and the androgens but in markedly different proportions in males and females. The sex hormones from the adrenal cortex are in minute amounts in both sexes.

Infertility, the lack of development of secondary sex characteristics, and changes in sexual characteristics or sexual functioning are common reasons for measuring the sex hormones. The gonadotropins are measured directly in the serum and in 24-hour urine specimens. Testosterone, the main androgen, can be measured in the serum. Also, some of the metabolites of the androgens from the testes and from the adrenal cortex can be measured in the urine. (See the 17-KS test in this chapter). Progesterone and estrogen are measured in the serum or as various metabolites in the urine.

Only the more common urine and serum laboratory tests for the sex hormones are discussed in this chapter. The clinical significance of the change in each of the different hormones is beyond the scope of this book. Refer to the references at the end of this chapter for detailed information about various disorders that can cause changes in the sex-related hormones.

■ FOLLICLE-STIMULATING HORMONE (FSH)

FSH from the anterior pituitary gland controls the growth and maturation of the ovarian follicles in the female for ovulation. FSH also controls the secretion of estrogen in the female. In the male, FSH stimulates the testes to produce sperm.

Preparation of Client and Collection of Samples
There is no special preparation of the client. The laboratory needs 5 ml of serum or plasma for the blood test. The same sample can be used for LH.

Reference Values for FSH	
Adult: Male	4–15 mU/ml
Female	4.6–22.4 mU/ml pre- or postovulatory; 13–41 mU/ml midcycle peak
Prepubertal: Male	2–10 mU/ml
Female	3–7 mU/ml
Postmenopausal female	30–170 mU/ml

■ LUTEINIZING HORMONES (LH)

LH is the second gonadotropic hormone secreted by the anterior pituitary gland. In the female, LH, along with FSH, is necessary for ovulation to take place. After ovulation, LH stimulates the ruptured follicle to secrete increasing amounts of progesterone. In males, LH stimulates the production of androgens, which are important in determining the secondary sex characteristics. LH in the male is sometimes referred to as the interstitial cell-stimulating hormone (ICSH).

Reference Values for LH	
Adult: Male	3–18 mU/ml
Female	2.4–34.5 mU/ml pre- and postovulation 43–187 mU/ml, midcycle peaks
Children	2–12 mU/ml
Postmenopausal female	30–150 mU/ml

Preparation of the Client and Collection of Sample
The requirement of 5 ml of blood or plasma for LH is the same as for FSH, and both tests can be done on the same specimen.

Changes in FSH and LH Serum Levels

Clinical Significance. Syndromes of excessive gonadotropins are extremely infrequent, if they exist at all (Cryer, 1979). FSH and LH levels are measured to see whether clients with hypogonadism have a primary gonad problem or a secondary problem of pituitary insufficiency. Pituitary insufficiency may be first manifested by a lack of function of the testes or ovaries. The LH and FSH are low if the gonads' failure is due to pituitary insufficiency (secondary hypogonadism). However, basal levels of LH and FSH in hypopituitarism are often indistinguishable from low normals. The levels of FSH and LH in serum and urine are high if the gonads' failure is primary failure of the ovaries or testes. Drugs, such as clomiphene (Clomid) or gonadotropin-releasing factor (GRH), may be given to see if the level of gonadotropins increases. Increased levels of FSH are also used to verify that a woman is undergoing menopause.

■ ESTRADIOL AND OTHER FORMS OF ESTROGEN

Different forms of the estrogens, including estradiol, estrone, and estriol, can be measured. Estriol is the estrogen present in largest amounts at pregnancy. (See Chapter 18 for the use of estriol as a test of fetal well-being during pregnancy.) Because estrogens are produced not only by the ovaries but also by the adrenal cortex and the testes, estradiol levels may be useful to assess pathology in all three glands.

The level of estradiol is increased in males who have testicular or adrenal tumors. In females, the increased estradiol arises from estrogen-secreting ovarian tumors. Decreases of estradiol in the female, or a lack of increase during a menstrual cycle, can be due either to ovarian failure or to pituitary insufficiency. Other factors, such as anorexia nervosa, may also cause decreases in estradiol. Hepatic and renal failure can cause abnormal increases of estrogens in the serum. Females may show no symptoms when estrogens are increased. Males may exhibit feminizing signs, such as enlarged breasts, when any of the estrogens is increased.

Preparation of Client and Collection of Sample
For estradiol, collect 5 ml in a red-top tube. Include date of last menstrual period (LMP). Values vary considerably as to ranges considered normal. (See Appendix A, Table 3 for other values.)

Reference Values for Serum Estradiol	
Male	20–90 pg/ml
Female	
Follicular phase	20–120 pg/ml
Midcycle	80–300 pg/ml
Luteal phase	60–170 pg/ml
Menopause	Less than 20 pg/ml

■ PROGESTERONE

In the female of childbearing age, progesterone is low during the first part of the menstrual cycle (follicular phase). When LH is increased at the time of ovulation (luteal phase), there is a resulting surge of progesterone for several days. Progesterone remains elevated in early pregnancy. Progesterone levels are used to document the occurrence of ovulation. Progesterone is also secreted by the adrenal glands, so progesterone levels may be elevated in neoplasms of either the ovaries or the adrenals.

Preparation of Client and Collection of Sample
Collect 5 ml of blood in a red-top tube. Include date of last menstrual period (LMP) and trimester of pregnancy. Reference values vary; see Appendix A, Table 3 for other ranges.

Reference Values for Serum Progesterone	
Male	0–1.0 ng/ml
Female	
Follicular phase	0–1.5 ng/ml
Luteal phase	2–30 ng/ml
Postmenopausal	0–1.5 ng/ml
Pregnancy	Peaks in third trimester to as high as 200 ng/ml
	(Tietz, 1983)

■ PREGNANEDIOL (PROGESTERONE METABOLITE)

Pregnanediol is the principle form of progesterone in the urine. (Note that pregnane*tri*ol is another urine test done to evaluate adrenocortical function. See the discussion earlier in this chapter.) In the female, the level of pregnanediol in the urine rises rapidly after ovulation and steadily during pregnancy. The 24-hour urine specimen may be done to evaluate the need for progesterone replacement.

Reference Values for Urinary Pregnanediol	
Children	0.4–1.0 mg/24 hr specimen
Male	0.5–1.5 mg/24 hr specimen
Female	
Pregnancy, 28–32 weeks	27–47 mg/24 hr specimen
Nonpregnant	0.5–7.0 mg/24 hr specimen
Luteal phase	2.0–7.0 mg/24 hr specimen
Postmenopausal	0.3–1.5 mg/24 hr specimen

■ TESTOSTERONE AND OTHER ANDROGENS

The male sex hormones, the androgens, are produced by the adrenal cortex, the testes, and the ovaries. The most powerful of the androgens, testosterone, comes mainly from the testes. Adult males with increased testosterone levels do not have any symptoms. In male children before puberty, there is precocious development of secondary sex characteristics. In females of all ages, there is masculinization. The adrenogenital syndrome, which occurs due to a lack of cortisol and an abundance of androgens, was discussed earlier in this chapter. In the adult male, a lack of testosterone, which can be due to primary failure of the testes or secondary to pituitary insufficiency, causes feminization. To evaluate the impotent male, serum testosterone is ordered before the gonadotropins.

Reference Values for Serum Testosterone

Adult male	300–1100 ng/100 ml
Adult female	25–90 ng/100 ml
Adolescent male	Over 100 ng/100 ml
Some laboratories have 250 ng as the lower limit in adult males	

POSSIBLE NURSING DIAGNOSES RELATED TO IMBALANCES IN SEX HORMONES

Disturbance in Self-concept Related to Changes in Body Image
Hormones are very potent in shaping and maintaining secondary sex characteristics. For example, a female who has an increase of testosterone develops more facial hair, more muscle mass, and a deeper voice. The key nursing implication for clients undergoing sex hormone changes due to pathological conditions is to help them cope with the disturbance in their body images. Alterations in sexual characteristics are corrected if the hormone balance can be established. The mood changes and depression may be due both to hormonal influences and to the effect of the physical changes. Nurses can help these clients play down the unwanted characteristics. Even little details, such as helping the woman find a place to have unwanted hair removed, can mean a lot.

Specific Interventions for Malignancies. Several of the tumors that cause masculinizing features in the female or feminizing features in male are malignant. Nurses must be aware of the specific nursing care guidelines related to the pathophysiology of the tumor. Also, some types of cancer are treated by hormone therapy, which causes an imbalance of sex hormones and permanent changes in the body image.

Sexual Dysfunction Related to Hormone Changes
The person may need professional counseling to deal with problems related to sexual functioning. Hogan (1984) contains a chapter devoted to the nursing implications for the client with different types of impaired hormonal function. The major emphasis for any sex-hormonal change is to help the client deal with a decreased sexual self-concept. If hormone tests are being done as part of an infertility work-up, the nurse needs to be sensitive to the anxiety of the couple who have not been able to conceive a child. (See Chapter 28 for specific diagnoses related to infertility.)

Ineffective Family Coping Related to Precocious Puberty in Children
The problem of mistaken sexual identity in newborns was discussed earlier in

the section on adrenogenital syndrome. (See the section on cortisol.) A masculinization of the female child or precocious puberty in either sex is disturbing for the child and probably much more so for the parents. Endocrine problems in children are usually treated by specialists who can also help the parents deal with the frightening changes in their child. A visiting nurse may be very useful in assessing the adjustment of the child and family to these changes. School nurses can be instrumental, too, in recognizing children who may need counseling to deal with the physical and psychologic problems of early maturity. Sexual precocity is three times more prevalent in girls than in boys (Hogan, 1984). Some girls are capable of reproduction at age 8 or 9.

Altered Health Maintenance Related to Use of Anabolic Steroids for "Sports Doping"

Anabolic steroids are sometimes abused by athletes in order to enhance athletic performances. Therefore laboratory studies may be ordered to evaluate the possible presence of these drugs. Duncan and Shaw (1985) discuss the implications for the nurse practitioner who may be involved in identifying the effect of these drugs on the health of the client.

QUESTIONS

1. Which of the following illustrates the concept of a negative feedback system for control of serum cortisol?

    a. An increase of serum cortisol when ACTH secretion is increased
    b. A decreased level of serum cortisol when ACTH secretion is decreased
    c. A decreased secretion of ACTH when serum cortisol is increased
    d. An increased secretion of ACTH when serum cortisol is increased

2. Mrs. Wu has an elevated serum cortisol level with a tentative diagnosis of Cushing's syndrome due to an adrenal cortex tumor. Which nursing action would be most needed?

    a. Observing and reporting any gastric distress, because gastric ulcers may develop
    b. Assessing for potential renal failure due to high serum potassium levels (hyperkalemia)
    c. Recognizing that an extremely elevated temperature may occur with even minor infections
    d. Encouraging physical activity to counteract the lethargy and boredom

3. Mr. Lee has a lower-than-normal serum cortisol level. Which nursing action would *not* be appropriate for this client with a diagnosis of Addison's disease?

    a. Assuring the client that his increased skin pigmentation will fade when the cortisol hormone replacement is adequate
    b. Checking the urine for sugar because hyperglycemia is a potential problem

    c. Helping Mr. Lee to prevent postural hypotension by teaching him to get out of bed slowly

    d. Encouraging rest and relaxation to decrease physical and physiological stress

4. Bobby, age 5, has been referred to an endocrinologist because he has an enlarged penis and other secondary sex characteristics. His serum sodium was low, and his serum potassium was elevated. A 24-hour urine for 17-ketosteroids (17-KS) was elevated. The increased elevation of serum androgens in adrenogenital syndrome is due to a basic lack of which of the following?

    a. ACTH production   **c.** Gonadatropic hormones
    b. Cortisol production   **d.** Testosterone

5. Mrs. Rodriguez has congestive heart failure with secondary aldosteronism. An elevation of the mineralocorticoid aldosterone may cause all of Mrs. Rodriguez's symptoms except which?

    a. BP of 170/100

    b. Serum potassium of 3.0 mEq/L

    c. Pitting edema of the ankles

    d. Polyuria (urine output of 2000 cc in 24 hours)

6. Urine testing for metanephrine and for vanillylmandelic acid (VMA) are two of the screening tests for tumors of the

    a. Adrenal cortex   **c.** Pituitary gland
    b. Adrenal medulla   **d.** Parathyroid gland

7. An increased level of parathormone (PTH) causes an increased serum level of which?

    a. Sodium   **b.** Potassium   **c.** Phosphorus   **d.** Calcium

8. The test most often used to follow clients with hyper- or hypothyroidism is which of the following?

    a. TSH (thyroid stimulating hormone test)

    b. T_4 (L-thyroxine)

    c. T_3 (triiodothyronine)

    d. T_3 resin uptake

9. Mrs. Graves has been admitted to the hospital because of suspected hyperthyroidism. Her T_4 level was elevated. Which of the following nursing actions would *not* be appropriate in caring for Mrs. Graves?

    a. Seeing that she has between-meal snacks

    b. Keeping her room slightly warmer than usual

    c. Allowing her time to rest between activities

    d. Checking an apical pulse when vital signs are done

10. Mr. Lane has come to the clinic to begin tests for hypothyroidism because symp-

toms were noted by a public health nurse who was visiting the Lane family. Which of the following symptoms is not characteristic of a client with suspected hypothyroidism?

a. Memory impairment   **c.** Intolerance to cold
b. Constipation   **d.** Weight loss

11. Baby Finley, age 2 months, has been diagnosed as having congenital hypothyroidism. The baby has been started on a thyroid preparation. If hypothyroidism is not picked up in early infancy (2–3 months), the infant will develop which of the following?

a. Mental retardation   **c.** Generalized muscle hypertrophy
b. Cardiovascular problems   **d.** Vision abnormalities

12. The most important nursing implication for clients with alterations in their sex hormones is to be aware that they often need help in coping with which of the following?

a. Decreased appetite and weight loss
b. Changes in secondary sex characteristics
c. Changes in energy level
d. Physical stress, such as an infection

REFERENCES

Adams, C. (1983). Pulling your patient through an adrenal crisis. *RN, 46*(10), 36–38.

Burnett, J. (1980). Congenital adrenocortical hyperplasia: The syndrome and nursing interventions. *AJN, 80,* 1306–1311.

Camuñas, C. (1983). Pheochromocytoma. *AJN, 83*(6), 887–891.

Cecil, R. (1983). Amenorrhea-galactorrhea syndrome. *Nursing 83,* 13(10), 87.

Cowan, D. (1984). Prejudices toward pituitary disorders. *Newsletter of Brain and Pituitary Foundation* (Western Chapter), *1*(2), 8.

Cryer, P. (1979). *Diagnostic endocrinology.* New York: Oxford University Press.

Duncan, D., & Shaw, E. (1985). Anabolic steroids: Implications for the nurse practitioner. *Nurse Practitioner, 10*(12), 8, 13–15.

Fisher, D., et al. (1979). Screening for congenital hypothyroidism: Result of screening one million North American infants. *Journal of Pediatrics, 94*(5), 700–705.

Galen, R. (1978). Thyroxine as a routine screening test. *Diagnostic Medicine, 1*(4), 89–90.

Glaser, B., et al. (1986). Magnetic resonance imaging of the pituitary gland. *Clinical Radiology, 37*(1), 9–14.

Gotch, P. (1981). Teaching patients about adrenal corticosteroids. *AJN, 81*(1), 78–81.

Govoni, L., & Hayes, J. (1985). *Drugs and nursing implications* (5th ed.). Norwalk, CT: Appleton-Century-Crofts.

Green, L., et al. (1984). Adrenal insufficiency as a complication of the acquired immunodeficiency syndrome. *Annals of Internal Medicine, 101*(4), 497–498.

Guimond, J., & Wilson, S. (1979). Postirradiation thyroid disorders. *AJN, 79*(7), 1256–1258.

Harris, E. (1982). The dexamethasone suppression test. *AJN, 82*(5), 784–785.

Hallal, J. (1977). Thyroid disorders. *AJN, 77*(3), 418–431.

Heagarty, M., et al. (1980). *Child health: Basics for primary care.* Norwalk, CT: Appleton-Century-Crofts.

Hogan, R. (1985). *Human sexuality: A nursing perspective* (2nd ed.). Norwalk, CT: Appleton-Century-Crofts.

Holum, J. (1983). *Elements of general and biological chemistry* (6th ed.). New York: Appleton-Century-Crofts.

Jacobs, D., Kasten, B., DeMott, W.T., & Wolfson, W. (1984). *Laboratory test handbook with DRG index.* St. Louis: Mosby/Lexi.

Jenkins, E. (1980). Living with thryotoxicosis. *AJN, 80*(5), 956–958.

Jones, S. (1982). Adrenal patient, proceed with caution. *RN, 45*(1), 67–72.

Juebiz, W. (1979). *Endocrinology: A logical approach for clinicians.* New York: McGraw-Hill.

Kaplan, S., et al. (1979). Symposium on pediatric endocrinology. *Pediatric Clinics of North America, 26*(2), 1–247.

Krieger, D. (Ed.). (1979) *Comprehensive endocrinology: Endocrine rhythms.* New York: Raven Press.

Larrabee, P., & Hanna, N. (1983). Saralasin infusion test. *AJN, 83*(12), 1658.

Locke, W. (1978). Control of anterior pituitary function. *Archives of Internal Medicine, 138*(10), 1541–1545.

Perez, C. (1984). Up and coming research. *Newsletter of Brain and Pituitary Foundation* (Western Chapter), *1*(3), 7.

Press, M., Tambarlane, W., & Sherwin, R. (1984). Importance of raised growth hormones in mediating the metabolic derangements of diabetes. *NEJM, 310*(13), 810–815.

Ryan, W. (1980). *Endocrine disorders: A pathophysiologic approach.* Chicago: Year Book Medical Publishers.

Scully, R. (Ed.). (1986). Normal reference laboratory values for special endocrine tests. *NEJM, 314*(1), 42–45.

Soler, N., et al. (1979). Isolated high serum triiodothyronine levels. *Archives of Internal Medicine, 139*(1), 38–39.

Stoffer, S., & Szpunar, W. (1984). Potency of levothyroxine products. *JAMA, 251*(5), 635–636.

Tietz, N. (Ed.). (1983). *Clinical guide to laboratory tests.* Philadelphia: Saunders.

Wallach, J. (1986). *Interpretation of diagnostic tests.* Boston: Little, Brown.

Weber, M. (1979). Saralasin testing for renin-dependent hypertension. *Archives of Internal Medicine,* 139(1), 93–95.

16

Culture and Sensitivity Tests

- Culture and Sensitivity (C&S) Tests
- Minimal Inhibitory Concentration (MIC)
- Minimum Bactericidal Content (MBC) or Minimum Lethal Concentration (MLC)
- Urine Cultures
- Blood Cultures
- Sputum Cultures and Acid-Fast Bacillus (AFB)
- Throat Cultures
- Nasal and Nasopharyngeal Cultures
- Wound Cultures
- Eye Cultures
- Vaginal and Urethral Smears
- Stool Cultures
- Cultures of Cerebrospinal Fluid (CSF) and Other Fluids

OBJECTIVES

1. Describe the classification system used by the laboratory to identify bacteria.
2. Interpret the clinical significance of C&S and MIC reports.
3. Identify the general nursing implications when a client has cultures ordered for a possible bacterial infection.
4. Describe in detail the various ways urine is collected for urine cultures.
5. Explain the procedures used to obtain blood cultures, as well as the timing of preliminary and final reports.
6. Describe what the nurse should teach the client to obtain a useful sputum specimen.

7. Explain why it may be important to do throat cultures for children with sore throats.
8. Describe the correct procedure to obtain a wound culture and what should be taught to the client.
9. Describe how gonorrhea and other sexually transmitted diseases are detected by smears and cultures.
10. Describe the proper procedure for collecting a stool specimen for bacterial culture.

The first part of this chapter provides some background information about the classification of bacteria as well as how the laboratory does cultures and sensitivities on clinical specimens. Specific nursing implications for culture collections are outlined. In addition, the nurse's role in caring for clients with infections is reviewed. The last part of the chapter outlines in detail the purpose, procedure, and preparation of the client for each type of common culture.

CLASSIFICATION OF BACTERIA BY MICROSCOPIC EXAMINATION

Bacteria can be classified into groups according to

1. Whether the bacteria take a gram stain
2. The shape of the bacteria—round (cocci), rod-shaped (bacilli), or spiral-shaped (spirilla)
3. Whether the bacteria thrive with oxygen (aerobic) or without (anaerobic)

The distribution of the cocci in pairs (diplococci), in a string (streptococci), or in a cluster (staphylococci) also helps the microbiologist to classify bacteria. A preliminary stain may not identify the exact bacteria, but it can help to make a presumptive diagnosis as well as rule out what the bacteria are not. For example, if the Gram stain shows gram-negative diplococci, gonorrhea is most likely the causative organism. If the Gram stain reveals gram-negative rods, the infection may be caused by organisms such as *Escherichia coli* or *Pseudomonas*. Table 16–1 shows the classification of some of the *common* bacteria that are identified in laboratory specimens.

The trained laboratory technician also notes other details, such as the number of different bacteria present, to estimate the probability of an infection. Gram stains are scanned for polymorphonuclear leukocytes, which are present in infection and for squamous epithelial cells, which are present in mucosal contamination. The technician is able to note that the specimen is grossly contaminated with "normal" flora, too.

Gram stains may be useful for the presumptive identification of gonorrhea in endocervical smears in women and urethral smears in men and for meningitis in cerebrospinal fluid. Gram stains for stool and urine may or may not be helpful, and in several areas, such as sputum smears, the usefulness of a Gram stain is controversial.

CULTURE GROWTHS

A stain is only a presumptive identification of the bacteria. A culture allows the bacteria to grow and to multiply so that the exact organism can be identified by various methods of analysis. The laboratory usually takes two or more days to make a final

TABLE 16-1. EXAMPLES OF COMMON BACTERIA FOUND IN CULTURES

Organisms	Cultures in Which Commonly Found
Aerobic	
Gram-positive cocci	
Staphylococcus aureus (coagulase, positive)	Blood, wound, sputum
Streptococcus (A-beta hemolytic)	Throat, wound, sputum
Streptococcus pneumoniae (pneumococcus)	Sputum, CSF in adult
Gram-negative cocci	
Neisseria meningitidis (meningococcus)	CSF, throat
Neisseria gonorrhoeae (gonococcus)	Urethra, endocervix, throat
Gram-negative rods or bacilli	
Escherichia coli (many strains)	Urine, blood, wound
Proteus	Urine, sputum, wound
Enterococcus	Blood, sputum, wound
Pseudomonas	Sputum, urine, wound
Salmonella	Stool
Shigella	Stool
Anaerobic	
Gram-positive cocci	
Anaerobic streptococci	Wound, stool, vagina
Gram-positive bacillus	
Clostridium group	Wound, stool
Gram-negative bacillus	
Bacteroides	Wound, stool
Acid-fast bacillus	
Mycobacterium tuberculosis	Sputum, gastric contents, CSF

CSF = Cerebrospinal fluid.
Information compiled from various references. See Hargiss and Larson (1981); Tietz (1983); and Jones (1985). Wallach (1986) contains lists of primary and alternate choice of antibiotic for all common infections.

identification of the organisms present in a specimen. For some specimens it may be 6–10 days. The growth on the culture takes about 24 hours. The laboratory must then use various tests to determine the exact species of bacteria present. Various methods, such as the addition of sugars, are used to identify different strains of a species. These tests to positively identify a specific type of bacteria may take another 24 hours or more.

The amount of growth on the culture varies with the organism. For example, some bacteria, such as *Escherichia coli*, reproduce every 20 minutes. At the other extreme, the organism that causes tuberculosis, *Mycobacterium tuberculosis*, reproduces only about once a day. Thus a final report of a culture for tuberculosis may take 3–8 weeks. See the section on sputum collection for acid-fast bacillus (AFB).

Anaerobic Cultures

Without a specific order to the contrary, bacterial cultures are usually done under aerobic conditions because the majority of disease-causing organisms require oxygen. However, if the client may possibly have an infection with an anaerobic organism, the specimen must be cultured without oxygen. For example, a deep wound may be infected with both anaerobic and aerobic organisms, and thus two culture specimens should be obtained. For an anaerobic specimen, the nurse should call the laboratory to obtain the needed container, which may be a tube filled with carbon dioxide rather than oxygen. The tube can be opened long enough to put in the swab that has the material to be cultured. Because carbon dioxide is heavier than air, it remains in the tube as long as the tube is held upright (Marchiondo, 1979). The specimen should be sent to the laboratory immediately. With blood cultures, the routine is to put the blood specimens into two different containers so that an anaerobic culture can be done as well as an aerobic culture. Two laboratory requisitions should be sent with the two specimens so the laboratory is aware of the need to do both types of culture.

Besides wound and blood cultures, cerebral spinal fluid and feces may also commonly be cultured for anaerobic organisms. The female genital tract can also harbor anaerobic organisms, but this is not a commonly performed culture.

Cultures for Fungus

Cultures for fungus require specific preparations with India ink, KOH (potassium hydroxide) or PAS (periodic-acid Schiff stain). With swabs moistened with saline (dry swabs are used for Gram stains of bacteria), small scrapings may be taken from a lesion. The nurse should consult with the laboratory on exactly how to collect the specimen.

The cultures for fungus take a long time to grow, and they must be handled carefully because the spores from the fungus can get into the air. For most of the systemic fungus diseases, such as histoplasmosis, various serology tests are done. (See Chapter 14 on serology tests.) Skin tests are also used to identify clients who have antibodies against certain fungus infections. (Skin tests for fungus diseases are covered in pharmacology books.)

Cultures for Viruses (Herpes and Others)

The laboratory identification of viral diseases is usually done by serology tests because a culture of a virus requires a living cell culture, which demands the services of a specialized laboratory. Recently some viruses have been identified with the electron microscope, but the positive identification of certain viruses is still done only in large medical centers. So, if a specimen is to be transported elsewhere, the nurse must check with the specific laboratory about how to collect it. Some specimens can be frozen for later analysis. (See Chapter 14 for serology tests for viral diseases.)

■ CULTURE AND SENSITIVITY (C&S) TESTS

Sometimes, in addition to knowing the exact organism causing the infection, it is necessary to demonstrate if the organism is sensitive to a certain antibiotic. In regard to C&S, *sensitivity* refers to the ability of the antibiotic to inhibit the growth of the bacteria. Sensitivity has an entirely different connotation when describing the reaction of a client to an antibiotic. A client who is allergic to a drug is said to be "sensitive" or "hypersensitive" to the drug. Obviously, sensitivity of the *client* to the drug is very undesirable, whereas sensitivity of the *organism* to the antibiotic is essential. If the antibiotic does not inhibit the growth of the bacteria, the organism is said to be "resistant" to the antibiotic.

The most common way that the laboratory checks the sensitivity of organisms to specific antibiotics is to put various disks of paper impregnated with antibiotics in a culture. Laboratories may list the test as a Kirby–Bauer susceptibility test. If the growth of an organism is retarded, the report is an "S" for sensitive or susceptible. If the antibiotic disk does not retard the growth of the specific bacteria in the culture, the report is "R" for resistant. An "I" on a report means that the results are in an intermediate zone or inconclusive of growth retardation. Some laboratories place an intermediate growth into the resistant category. Usually the laboratory uses

TABLE 16-2. EXAMPLE OF SENSITIVITIES REPORT

Drug	Escherichia coli	Pseudomonas aeruginosa
Amikacin	S	S
Ampicillin	R	R
Cephalothin	R	R
Chloramphenicol	S	S
Colistin	S	S
Erythromycin	R	R
Gentamicin	S	S
Kanamycin	R	S
Methicillin	R	R
Penicillin G	R	R
Tobramycin	S	S

S = Sensitive, R = Resistant

only one member of an antibiotic family because sensitivity differences are usually minor. Table 16-2 gives an example of the antibiotics that may be used for antibiotic sensitivity testing.

The purpose of doing a C&S is to ensure that the client is receiving the correct antibiotic for the particular organism causing the infection. For example, suppose a client was receiving ampicillin. If a report came back that showed the organisms to be resistant to ampicillin but sensitive to other antibiotics, the physician must change the antibiotic order. (See Table 16-2 for an example of a C&S report that would necessitate notification of the physician before the next dose of ampicillin was given.) Culture and sensitivities are particularly useful when the client is not responding to therapeutic dosages of antibiotics. A routine sensitivity for every culture may not be needed and could be an unnecessary health cost to the client. The physician must determine if a culture *and* sensitivity are cost-effective in a particular situation.

■ MINIMAL INHIBITORY CONCENTRATION (MIC)

MIC is a report of the amount of concentration of an antibiotic that inhibits the growth of the organism. Venous blood containing the microorganism is put into liquid culture mediums, each containing an antibiotic concentration. Table 16-3 shows the range of testing for some antibiotics. The concentration of antibiotic that inhibits the growth of the microorganism in vitro is then noted. The MIC helps the physician choose antibiotics that are clinically appropriate and cost-effective. For an organism to be considered sensitive to an antibiotic, attainable blood levels should be at least 2-4 times the MIC. For urinary tract infections, the dose of antimicrobial in the urine needs to be ten times the MIC.

For example, if for organism X the MIC is reported as 4.0 for methicillin, one uses the information in Table 16-3 to determine if methicillin would be effective. The table shows that p.o methicillin gives an approximate blood level of 1.5-4.0 μg/ml, not enough to be 2-4 times the MIC of 4.0. For IV methicillin, the obtainable blood levels are much higher (10-40 μg/ml) and thus it would be considered an appropriate antibiotic. Hewitt and McHenry (1978) caution that the MIC that is effective in vitro (test tube) may not always correlate well with the effectiveness in vivo. Blood levels vary, depending on body fat and hepatic and renal functioning.

TABLE 16-3. RANGES TESTED FOR MINIMAL INHIBITORY CONCENTRATION (MIC) BY LABORATORY

Antibiotics (Range Tested)	Representative Adult Dose Grams	Approximate Blood Levels μg/ml	Approximate Urine Levels μg/ml
Clindamycin (.25–16)	p.o. .15–.3 q6h IV .3–6 q6–8h	2–4 4–8	30–90 45–240
Erythromycin (.25–16)	p.o. .25–.5 q6h IV .3 q4–6h	1–4 10–20	(5%)
Methicillin (.25–16)	(Ox p.o. .25–.5 q4–6h) IV 1–2 q4h	(1.5–4.0) 10–40	(30–40%)
Penicillin (.06–4)	(VK .25–.5 q6h) IV 1–2 mil q4h	1.5–4.0 20–40	300–450 3000–5000
Ampicillin (.12–8, gram-pos.) (.25–16, gram-neg.)	p.o. .25–1.5 q6h IV 1–2 q4h	1.5–4.0 15–30	50–100 200–400
Cephalothin (1–64)	p.o. .25–5 q6h IV 1–2 q4h	2–15 25–85	300–1000 800–2000
Gentamicin (.25–16)	IM,IV q8–12h (3–5 mg/kg/d)	5–10	65–300
Tetracycline (.25–16)	p.o. .25–.5 q6h IV .5 q6–12h	1.5–4.0 10–20	200–800 600–1000
Carbenicillin (8–512)	p.o. 1q6h IV 4 q4h	5–10 125–175	350–14,000 2000–10,000
Chloramphenicol (.5–32)	p.o. .25–.5 q6h IV .5–1 q6h	1.5–4.0 10–20	200–700 500–1400
Kanamycin (1–64)	IM,IV 5q12h (15 mg/kg/d)	15–20	100–200
Tobramycin (.25–16)	IM,IV q8–12h (3–5 mg/kg/d)	5–10	65–300
Amikacin (1–64)	IM,IV q8–12h (15 mg/kg/d)	16–21	700–830

Reprinted laboratory report courtesy of Kaiser Hospital, San Francisco, Ca.

■ MINIMUM BACTERICIDAL CONTENT (MBC) OR MINIMUM LETHAL CONCENTRATION (MLC)

The MBC or MLC denotes the concentration of antibiotic needed to actually kill the organism. The technique is an in vitro one as described above for the MIC. End reports for the MBC may note either 99%, 99.9%, or 100% colonies killed. Jacobs et al. (1984) suggest the MBC is most useful for debilitated clients with leukopenia. (See Chapter 2 for decreased white blood cells.)

COLLECTING SPECIMENS FOR CULTURE

General Nursing Implications

Specific information about each type of common culture is covered in the second half of this chapter. This section presents general guidelines for the collection of all specimens for bacterial culture.

Collect Specimens Before Giving Antibiotics. If possible, cultures should be collected before the antibiotic is begun. If the client is already on antibiotics, the laboratory should be notified because techniques to counteract the effect of the antibiotic, such as adding penicillinase, may be done.

Use the Correct Specimen Container. All specimens, except stool, must be collected in a sterile container, and anaerobic specimens must be collected in oxygen-free containers. Some cultures, such as throat cultures, may be transferred to the culture media immediately. The nurse should call the laboratory if there is any doubt about the type of culture medium to be used. For example, the laboratory has specific cultures for blood, and it may be desirable to have the blood transferred to the culture medium as soon as it is drawn. In other settings, the laboratory may prefer to receive blood in tubes and make the transfer to the culture medium in the laboratory. If the specimen is not placed in the correct medium, it may be useless.

Know How Much of the Specimen Is Needed. For example, the laboratory can do a culture on just a few milliliters of sputum, so it would be useless to keep the container longer to try to get a larger amount. Table 16–4 lists the amounts needed for each type of specimen. Information on the amount needed for each type of specimen is also covered under the discussion on the specific test.

Do not Expose Others to the Infectious Material. Meticulous hand washing before and after obtaining a culture is essential. The nurse must make sure that the outside of the specimen container does not get contaminated with the contents inside it. Since the contents are potentially infectious, the personnel handling the container must be protected. If the outside of the container does become contaminated, the nurse can use gloves to transfer the contents to another container. As an alternative, the nurse might also put the container into a bag and note that the outside of the container has been contaminated. Thus laboratory personnel will not touch the outside of the container with their bare hands.

Make Sure that the Specimen Is Properly Labeled. The laboratory requisition must be filled out correctly. A specimen that is not properly identified is useless. If the specimen is for an outpatient, making sure that the home phone of the person is available is very important. Information required on the laboratory slip includes the client's name and other identification, such as medical number, hospital room number, or clinic site. The type and *source* of the specimen, as well as the date and time collected, are essential. Sometimes laboratories receive a yellow liquid marked for C&S. The laboratory cannot assume that this is urine. Even if it is marked urine, the technicians have no idea whether it is from a Foley, a clean catch, or whatever. Other items, such as the need for an anaerobic report or whether the client is on antibiotics, should be noted too.

TABLE 16–4. AMOUNTS NEEDED FOR CULTURES AND TIPS FOR COLLECTION

Type of Culture	Amount Needed	Special Notes
Urine	2–3 ml in sterile container (If also for urinalysis, send 15–30 ml)	Must be clean catch or catheterized specimen so not contaminated by perineal flora
Blood	10 ml by venipuncture. Keep in syringe or put into culture at bedside—5 ml aerobic, 5 ml anaerobic	Be sure not contaminated with skin flora. Special skin cleansing needed
Sputum	2–3 ml in sterile container	Sputum, *not* saliva
Throat	One swab put in prepared culture (Culpak)	Touch back of throat only
Nasopharyngeal	One swab in test tube	Do gently
Wound	One swab in test tube. May do syringe for anaerobic	Clean skin around wound first
Eye	One swab	Be careful not to touch cornea
Vaginal	One swab. If anaerobic, need special container	Need to do cervical for gonorrhea
Urethral	One swab	See text for others ways to detect gonorrhea in males
Stool	One-inch lump (walnut size) or 20 ml if diarrhea	Only culture specimen not collected in sterile container
CSF (pleural fluid; peritoneal fluid)	1 ml—aerobic and anaerobic	Need to notify lab that CSF is coming. CSF, pleural, or peritoneal fluid is collected in other tubes for other types of analysis

CSF = Cerebrospinal fluid.
Information compiled from various references.

Send the Culture to the Laboratory as Soon as Possible. All cultures should be sent to the laboratory immediately, but some specimens, such as urine, can be refrigerated if there is a delay in transporting the specimen. Some commercial kits contain an ampule of transport medium that keeps samples moist for as long as 72 hours. For some specimens, such as a culture of cerebrospinal fluid, the laboratory needs to be called before the culture is sent, so that the personnel are available to begin immediate examination of the fluid when it arrives at the laboratory. In the hospital setting, cultures are not usually collected on the evening or night shift unless the laboratory provides 24-hour service. If specimens are collected in a home setting, the nurse must check with the laboratory to see how the specimen can be transported without causing the death of the organism to be cultured.

GENERAL NURSING DIAGNOSES WHEN CULTURES ARE ORDERED

Potential for Infection
Besides the nurse's most obvious role of making sure that the specimen is collected properly, the nurse should consider several other possible actions when a client has the potential for infection.

Conferring with the Physician about the Possible Need for Isolation Until the Results of the C&S Are Known. Depending on the type of potential infection, putting the client into isolation until the definitive diagnosis is made may or may not be warranted. Hospitals have specific procedures for wound isolation, respiratory isolation, or enteric precautions depending on the type of suspected infection. Some hospitals use a procedure-oriented isolation system which consists of four categories of isolation as outlined by Gilmore et al. (1986). The hospital should also have a written policy on criteria that designate when a client should be isolated. If the policies are written, the nurse is given backing to isolate clients independently, without waiting for a physician's order (Aspinall, 1978). Although unnecessary isolation procedures are costly, as well as potentially upsetting to the client, the decision not to isolate the client until a culture is reported positive may expose other clients, family members, and staff to the risk of a serious infection.

Whatever the level of isolation needed, the client should be taught how to decrease the chances of spreading a potential infection to others. Simple things, such as a paper bag for contaminated tissues, may be overlooked. Or nurses and physicians may handle dressings or wounds without using gloves. Hand washing should be routine after physical care of any client, but staff seem to forget this "obvious" way to prevent the spread of bacteria from one client to another (Mayer et al., 1986). Clients may not be washing their hands after defecating either. Unless the nurse carefully surveys the environmental setting, all these breaks in technique can occur. In the home setting, the other family members need to be taught how to protect themselves from the spread of a possible infection.

Assessing for Signs and Symptoms of Infection. Often the nurse may be the first one to detect that the client may be getting an infection, and thus a culture should be done. For example, a nurse in a nursing home may note that the urine in a drainage bag is cloudy and has a foul odor. A pediatric nurse may note that the lungs of a child are congested and that the child has a fever. A nurse making a home visit may note that a wound appears inflamed and sore to the touch. For fevers of undetermined origin (FUO) other nursing assessments should be made for the presence of respiratory symptoms, gastrointestinal symptoms, or a rash.

Although fever is usually present in infections, in some clients, particularly the elderly, fever may be absent and the WBC count and differential normal. (See Chapter 2 for a discussion of the "shift to the left" as a characteristic sign of a developing bacterial infection.) The elderly who complain of "not feeling good" or who are weak or lethargic may need a complete physical to rule out the possibility of an unnoticed infection (Deal, 1979). In the very young, laboratory reports such as the WBC count may not be elevated, but an increase in the sedimentation rate and the bands (see Chapter 2) may be important in screening for newborn sepsis (Grylack & Scanlon, 1979). If the client has a potential infection, a culture is the diagnostic proof of an infection. The collection of a culture depends on the likely site of the infection, such as blood cultures for possible septicemia or a throat culture for a complaint of a sore throat.

Assisting the Client to Combat Infection. Too often health professionals consider that the administration of antibiotics is the *only* way to treat infections, but a holistic approach to the treatment of an infection includes more. Increased fluids, a diet adequate in protein, and plenty of rest are other ways to help the body combat a bacterial invasion. The adult may need antipyretic drugs to reduce the fever, if the fever is high or the client is uncomfortable. Gurevich (1985) notes it isn't necessarily desirable to decrease a fever, even up to 105 °F in the adult. Pediatric guidelines are different (Thomas, 1985), so treatment may be done for 101 °F. Griffin (1986) suggests tepid baths for fever in adults. Aspirin or acetaminophen (Tylenol, Datril) are two drugs prescribed to reduce fevers in the adult. Aspirin is not used with children because of the association with Reye's syndrome. A moderate increase in temperature is considered useful in helping the body mobilize the defense against bacterial invasion. The natural defenses of the body against infection need to be encouraged along with the proper use of antibiotics and antipyretics. Stress reduction should also be employed, so the body is free to mobilize against the infection.

Preventing Nosocomial Infections. A nosocomial infection is one that is acquired as a result of hospitalization or of treatment received in the hospital. Despite some effective control measures, penicillinase-producing staphylococci (that is, staph resistant to penicillin) continue to be a cause of hospital-related infections. In fact, maybe "staph" infections should be spelled "staff" infections, since too often the staff of a hospital are responsible for the hospital-acquired infection. Another type of hospital-generated infection is due to gram-negative bacilli, which in the past few years have also become resistant to antibiotics (Hargiss & Larson, 1981). Organisms such as *Serratia* have become endemic hospital residents (Bond, 1981). The fungi, especially the *Candida* species, have also become important as a cause of hospital infections. Usually harmless organisms, such as fungus and some protozoans, have also begun to fill the ecological void created by the effects of antimicrobial therapy.

Although nurses are not prescribing antibiotics, they should be aware of the problems so they can teach clients about the proper use of antibiotics. Clients may save antibiotics to take for another infection, or they may demand a penicillin shot for a cold. (Antibiotics are not used for viral infections.) Health teaching about the proper use of antibiotics can help to prevent abuse and misuse of antibiotics. Even more basic to nursing is the fact that nurses can help to prevent nosocomial infections by the use of proper techniques for the care of Foley catheters, the suctioning of tracheotomies, or the care of intravenous equipment. All the nursing measures that decrease the chance of the client's developing an infection mean less need for the physician to resort to antibiotics. Aspinall (1978) gives several specific ways on how nurses can score against nosocomial infections. Basic to any successful prevention of bacterial spread is proper hand-washing technique. Again and again, it must be stressed, all staff must wash their hands before and after caring for all clients.

Recognizing Situations that Allow the Growth of Opportunistic Organisms. Poor techniques by health professionals are not always to blame when clients get an infection in the hospital or nursing home. Always present in our environment are opportunistic pathogens, which do not usually cause an infection unless the resistance of the host is low. (See the discussion in Chapter 2 about the controversy over using isolation procedures to protect the client who is severely immunosuppressed.) Reducing all possible pathogens in an environment may be very difficult. For example, food is not sterile. Salad is a notorious source of organisms, and even pepper has been shown to have potential pathogens (Kuhn, 1978). Opportunistic organisms such as *Pneumocystis carinii* are commonly present but only cause pneumonia in immunosuppressed clients, such as those with AIDS. Clients who are immunosuppressed need extra careful observations for any signs of infection.

■ URINE CULTURES

General Indications
On a routine microscopic urinalysis, the findings that suggest a urinary tract infection (UTI) are the presence of a large number of WBCs and bacteria in the urine. Two screening tests for a UTI, nitrites and leukocyte esterase (LE), are discussed in Chapter 3. If the urine is not grossly contaminated with perineal secretions, these exams, which are much cheaper than a urine culture, may be enough to estabish the presence of a UTI. For nonpregnant women, treatment with antibiotics can be given without a culture if there are no signs suggestive of pyelonephritis, vaginitis, or chlamydial urethritis and the client has not had more than one other UTI in the past year (Komaroff, 1984). If the UTI does not respond quickly to medication, the culture may be needed to determine appropriate therapy. The most common organism causing such infections is *Escherichia coli*. Other gram-negative rods, such as the *Proteus* or *Pseudomonas* group, are occasionally present in UTI.

Females are particularly susceptible to urinary tract infections because of the short distance of the urethra and the possible contamination from perineal organisms. (''Honeymoon'' cystitis often occurs when sexual activity introduces organisms into the urinary tract). Young female children are also much more likely to have UTI than are male children. Catheterization procedures for either sex are very likely to result in a UTI unless sterile technique is used.

Preparation of Client and Collection of Urine Sample
Ideally, urine for cultures should be the early morning specimen because the urine is more concentrated. However, urine can be collected at any time for the culture. In addition to the general requirements for specimens noted earlier, the laboratory slip should note whether the client is on a forced fluid regime. Most laboratories consider a clean catch midstream urine the best method to collect urine for a culture. The laboratory needs only 1 ml to do the culture, so the urine can be transmitted by syringe if it is removed from a Foley. (See discussion on Foley specimens.) If a routine urinalysis is to be done before a C&S, the laboratory needs at least 15 ml.

There are various diagnostic kits for doing urine cultures, such as Microstix (Ames Products), Clinicult (Smith Kline & French), and Uricult (Medical Technology). Clients may be taught to use these at home. (See Chapter 1 for a discussion on diagnostic kits and Chapter 3 for a screening test for nitrites and LE as an indication of a urine infection.)

Clean Catch or Midstream Specimens. The problem in collecting urine for culture and sensitivity is that the urine may be contaminated with the bacteria normally present in the perineal area. Thus the perineal area need to be cleansed thoroughly before the urine is collected. In one study, client instruction with diagrams on how to use iodophor-soaked tissues as a cleanser did reduce the number of nonpathogens that often contaminate a urine specimen (McGuckin 1981). The vulvular area in the female or the tip of the penis in the male must be cleansed well with soap and water and/or a disinfectant, such as an iodine solution.

In addition, the urine is collected midstream so it contains fewer of the bacteria that reside on the perineal surfaces near the urinary meatus. To collect a midstream specimen, the client must be able to stop the urine flow after it is begun and then urinate into a sterile cup or directly onto a dipstick for culture. The female needs to hold the labia separated so that the urinary meatus is clear. If the client is unable to do the cleansing, the nurse can cleanse around the meatus. (A nonsterile glove can be used to protect the nurse who washes the perineal area.) In an uncircumsized male, the foreskin must stay retracted during the procedure.

Collecting Urine by Straight Catheterization. In the past, urine specimens for culture were often done by a straight catheterization to make sure that the specimen did not get contaminated from perineal secretions. For example, if a woman has a heavy menstrual flow, the urine may be contaminated with blood. However, the danger of subsequent infection as a result of catheterization is a reason to try to get urine by clean catch whenever possible. During the menstrual flow, or with vaginal secretions, the client can clean the perineal area, insert a tampon, and then clean around the meatus again before urinating. If, for some reason, catheterizing a client for a urine specimen is necessary, strict aseptic technique must be followed.

Collecting Urine from a Foley Catheter. If the client has an indwelling (Foley) catheter, urine can be collected from it. The Foley catheter must be clamped so that urine can accumulate in the bladder. (Urine taken from a drainage bag is never suitable for a culture because the urine is not fresh.) The Foley catheter drainage tubings have a special sample port for inserting a needle and a syringe to remove a few milliliters of urine for tests. The tubing below the area may be bent back on itself so that urine collects near the port. Some tubings have a special clamp with the tubing. The sample port should be cleansed with alcohol before the needle is inserted. It is important for a microscopic urinalysis to remove the needle from the syringe before emptying the urine from the syringe into the specimen cup. Forcing urine through the needle will break up some of the cells.

Reference Values for Urine Cultures

Urine is sterile in the bladder, but it becomes contaminated with organisms
   normally present in the perineal area. The amount of organisms are counted
   and usually interpreted as follows:

Less than 10,000 organisms/ml	Unlikely UTI, probable contamination
10,000 to 100,000 organisms/ml	Probable UTI, particularly if urine specimen is from a catheter
More than 100,000 organisms/ml	Definite UTI

These numbers exclude the presence of normal genital flora such as lactobacilli.
   In low-grade pyelonephritis, the urine culture may be negative even though bacteria are present in the pelvis of the kidney.
   See Chapter 3 for the nitrite and LE dipstick test as a screening test for UTI.

Collecting Urine in Young Children. For very young children, the perineal area is cleansed and a sterile collection bag is secured around the meatus. Obviously, this procedure is easier for male than for female infants. In older children, the perineal area can be cleansed and a urine specimen collected as for an adult. La Fave et al. (1979) have suggested that screening procedures for urinary tract infections in young children can be done just by having mothers collect a voided specimen in a clean Dixie cup. If doing so is essential, children can also be catheterized to obtain a urine specimen.

POSSIBLE NURSING DIAGNOSIS RELATED TO POSITIVE URINE CULTURE

Knowledge Deficit Related to Preventive and Therapeutic Measures for Urinary Tract Infection

The key measure to assist the client in overcoming a urinary tract infection is to keep the urine as dilute as possible so that bacteria cannot multiply rapidly. Keeping the urine acidic may also be helpful for certain bacterial infections. (See Chapter 3 on the use of cranberry juice to make the urine more acidic.) The client needs to know exactly how much fluid should be consumed each day. Caffeine may irritate the bladder. The physician may prescribe sulfa drugs or antibiotics, such as ampicillin, depending on the causitive organism for the UTI, and the client should know the possible side effects of the drugs. In addition, the nurse should make sure that the client knows ways to prevent infections, in the future by continuing adequate fluid intake. Also, some women are not aware that wiping the perineal area should be frontwards to back so that bowel bacteria are not transmitted to the meatus. Avoiding bubble baths and nylon pants are other preventive measures.

As a general rule, a client who has a UTI has just an infection of the bladder, not of the upper portion of the urinary tract, although an infection can ascend if not properly treated. Symptoms of a lower UTI (cystitis) include frequency of urination and burning, and the urine may smell foul and look cloudy. These symptoms should subside as therapy is begun. Symptoms of flank pain, high fever, and overall malaise may indicate that the UTI has ascended and is now pyelonephritis. Clients need to report any worsening of symptoms.

■ BLOOD CULTURES

General Indications

Blood cultures are ordered when the client is suspected of having septicemia. In many localized infections, a few bacteria may enter the bloodstream (bacteremia), but they are usually not sufficient to cause symptoms of sepsis (septicemia). The client with septicemia is usually severely ill with fever, chills, and other signs of serious infection. The spikes of fever may be related to the release into the bloodstream of more bacteria. So sometimes blood cultures are ordered to be done when the client has another spike in temperature.

Bacteria can enter the bloodstream from infections in soft tissues, from contaminated intravenous lines, such as those used for hyperalimentation, or even from minor surgical procedures, such as a tooth extraction or instrumentation by endoscopes, particularly cystoscopes. Bacteremia in elderly clients can result from pneumococcal pneumonia (Deal, 1979). In adults the most common organisms causing septicemia are gram-negative rods, such as *Escherichia coli* or *Aerobacter* species, which can enter the bloodstream due to UTI or instrumentation of the urinary tract. *Staphylococcus aureus* may also cause septicemia. In newborns, *Escherichia coli* and beta-hemolytic streptococcus are the two most frequent causes of septicemia. In the newborn, sepsis is often a result of prolonged and early rupture of the membranes (more than 24 hours before delivery), maternal infection (proven or suspected), and neonatal aspiration (Grylack, 1979).

Preparation of Client and Collection of Sample

Usually blood samples for blood culture are drawn at least two different times and in both arms to increase the chance of detecting any organisms. For example, the order may read, "Blood cultures now and in three hours. If the client has another temperature spike, draw blood cultures immediately." The physician, nurse, or laboratory technician may draw the blood for the cultures. Solitary venipunctures are preferred, but if the client has very poor veins, blood cultures can be obtained from an arterial line (Pryor, 1984).

Usually 10 ml are obtained from one venipuncture. Half of the specimen (5 ml) is put into a culture for anaerobic bacteria and 5 ml into a culture for aerobic bacteria. Some laboratories have the person who draws the blood add the blood directly to the culture media. Other laboratories prefer that the blood sample be sent directly to the laboratory and that the transfer to culture be made by the bacteriology technician.

The major problem with blood cultures is that the specimen is often contaminated with bacteria from the environment. Hence the drawing of venous blood for blood culture is done under aseptic conditions. The skin is specially prepped before the venipuncture is done. The prep, much like a surgical prep, consists of thorough cleansing with iodine and alcohol solutions. The skin over the vein must not be touched after the prep is completed. If the skin over the vein is probed, the person drawing the blood uses a sterile glove. The transfer of the blood sample for the culture medium must also be done as a sterile procedure. For infants, a heel stick may be done to obtain blood for a culture.

Reference Values for Blood Cultures

Any bacteria in the blood are clinically significant. Yet, because there is always the possibility of contamination from the skin, the bacteriologist may make an interpretation of possible contaminants if certain skin bacteria are present in small amounts. At least three cultures in 24 hours may be ordered to determine if bacteria are actually in the blood. A final diagnosis from a blood culture may take seven to ten days. However, if the laboratory identifies the presence of certain pathogens, even in small amounts, it issues a preliminary positive report so that the physician can order appropriate antibiotics. *Escherichia coli* is a common pathogen in both adults and children. Other pathogens may be *Staphylococcus aureus* and various streptococci. (See discussion under general indications.)

If an intravenous catheter tip is cultured, a count of 15 or fewer colonies is usually not significant. A count of more than 15 colonies on the culture suggests the catheter as the source of septicemia (Hargiss & Larson, 1981).

Culturing of Catheter Tip. Septicemia can result from an indwelling intravenous catheter, particularly a central venous catheter used to deliver hyperalimentation fluids. The high glucose content of hyperalimentation fluids supports bacterial growth. Sometimes when the intravenous catheter is removed, the tip is cut off with sterile scissors and sent to the laboratory for culturing. The tip should not be allowed to touch the client's skin or the bedclothes. A sterile towel can be used to catch the catheter when it is removed.

POSSIBLE NURSING DIAGNOSIS RELATED TO POSITIVE BLOOD CULTURE

Potential for Injury Related to Septic State
Clients with septicemia often have low resistance to infection because they are already critically ill from other causes. So most of the appropriate nursing care is that given to acutely ill clients. Refer to nursing texts for care of septicemia clients. Septic shock may occur and be fatal. Usually clients with septicemia are not a source of infection for others, but this possibility should be carefully assessed. In the infant, hypoglycemia (Chapter 8) and hyperbilirubinemia (Chapter 11) are often concurrent problems with septicemia.

■ SPUTUM CULTURES AND ACID-FAST BACILLUS (AFB)

General Indications
Sputum cultures are often ordered when the client has lung congestion (rales), elevated temperature, and other signs of a probable respiratory infection. Respiratory infections cause an increased secretion of respiratory secretions or sputum. Sputum originates in the bronchi, not in the upper respiratory tract. Different bacteria cause the sputum to be greenish, yellowish, or rust-colored. The sputum may have a foul smell.

Almost all of the bacteria that cause respiratory infections are normally present in the upper respiratory tract in small amounts. In healthy people, these organisms, such as *Klebsiella or Staphylococcus,* do not cause disease because they are present in small amounts. Yet when an organism has a chance to grow quickly due to stagnant respiratory secretions, the client can get pneumonia. Sputum cultures can identify which organism is in abundance and thus the cause of the respiratory problem. If tuberculosis is suspected, a special type of culture for AFB is done. Parasites such as *Pneumocystis carinii* are not easily found in routine sputum. Also, sputum is not reliable for *Legionella* so pleural fluid or lung tissue may be needed if either type of pneumonia is suspected (see Chapter 27 on bronchoscopy)

Preparation of Client and Collection of Sample
The laboratory needs only a few milliliters of sputum for a culture. Sputum, however, is not the same thing as saliva. The sputum specimen must be from the bronchial tree, not just saliva from the mouth. Having clients rinse out their mouths before the sputum is obtained is a good idea, so that the sputum is not contaminated with saliva and mouth bacteria. An early morning specimen is ideal because the sputum

is more concentrated then. Early morning sputum also tends to be plentiful if the client has been sleeping through the night and the secretions have tended to pool. Sometimes the sputum culture is ordered "times 3," which means that three different collections should be made, not three at one time.

Sputum from the bronchial tree can be obtained in several ways. If at all possible, the client should be allowed to cough up the sputum. If the client is unable to cough, suctioning can be done with a special catheter that allows some of the secretions to be caught in a special reservoir. Sputum cultures are also obtained by the use of a bronchoscope.

If the purpose is to determine the presence of the AFB that causes tuberculosis, the culture may be done on at least 3 different days. If no sputum can be obtained, the physician may order a gastric analysis because *Mycobacterium tuberculosis* is acid-resistant and thus not destroyed by the gastric acidity. (Urine may be cultured for AFB, too, if tuberculosis of the kidney is suspected.)

Reference Values for Sputum Cultures

Various organisms, if present in large amounts, can cause acute respiratory infections. The laboratory reports the predominant organism or organisms present in the sputum. Common pathogenic organisms include *Streptococcus pneumoniae, Staphylococcus aureus,* and *Hemophilus influenza.* The first organism is the most common in adults. The other two are more common in children (Frame, 1982). Various gram-negative bacilli may also cause respiratory infections. The culture for these common bacteria is completed in 24–48 hours.

A culture for tuberculosis (AFB culture) grows very slowly. It may take 3–8 weeks to get a final report. Yet sometimes the laboratory is able to report a positive smear for AFB, so treatment can be initiated before the final growth is documented.

POSSIBLE NURSING DIAGNOSES RELATED TO POSITIVE SPUTUM CULTURE

Ineffective Airway Clearance
As with other types of positive cultures, antibiotics are given. Clients need encouragement to do deep breathing and coughing exercises. They may also need intensive respiratory therapy by suctioning or some type of postural drainage. The nurse needs to make sure that hydration is adequate because without adequate fluids the sputum becomes very tenacious. The nurse also needs to teach clients how to safely dispose of sputum that is excreted. If clients are coughing up large amounts of sputum, cleaning an emesis basin is easier if the basin is first lined with tissues. Otherwise sputum tends to become encrusted in the basin.

Knowledge Deficit Regarding Spread of Disease to Others
Teaching clients to cover their mouths when coughing seems common sense, but the nurse may have to remind clients. As a general rule, clients with most types of pneumonia are not put on isolation. However, depending on the type of organism in the sputum, respiratory isolation might be justified.

Coagulase-positive staphylococcal and group A streptococcal pneumonias are two organisms that require isolation.

For a positive AFB culture, the client needs to be on respiratory isolation until cultures become negative, which is usually within a couple of weeks of treatment. However, medication is continued for 9 months to a year.

■ THROAT CULTURES

Throat cultures are the only reliable means for differentiating strep throats from viral sore throats. Most sore throats are caused by viruses; only about 10–15% of them in children are caused by group A beta-hemolytic streptococci. Yet identifying whether the patient has group A beta-hemolytic streptococci is important because rheumatic fever and glomerulonephritis may follow such infections. Streptococci are classified according to the antigens. Some are not considered particularly pathogenic whereas group A beta-hemolytic strep are. (See Chapter 14 on the streptococcal antigen-antibody tests of anti-streptolysin-O, anti-streptodornase-B, and Streptozyme.) Occasionally a throat culture for gonorrhea may be done if the client has been engaging in oral sex with a partner with gonorrhea.

Certain clinical signs and symptoms should alert nurses to the possibility that a sore throat is indeed a bacterial infection rather than a viral one. Wang (1977) noted that usually with bacterial infections:

1. Temperatures are higher than with viral infections.
2. The symptoms usually occur more abruptly and the client seems more ill.
3. Also, the patches on the throat are more distinctive.
4. The WBC is characteristically elevated—not so with viral infections. (See Chapter 2 on the significance of the WBC in bacterial infections.)

Preparation of Client and Collection of Sample
Throat cultures are done with a swab that is immediately placed into a test tube or kit with a special medium for the growth of bacteria. The tongue is depressed with a tongue blade and a flashlight used to visualize the inflamed area of the throat. The sterile swab is rubbed over each tonsilar area and the posterior pharynx without touching the lips or tongue. Any white patch should be cultured. The results of throat cultures take 24–48 hours. Special test kits for strep throat show a positive reading in 7 minutes (as a stat test) or 70 minutes as a batch test. Evaluation of the Directigen Group A strep test kit showed that the kit method is relatively simple to perform, easy to interpret, and provides accurate assessment for the organism with little or no cross reactivity with other beta hemolytic groups (Miller et al., 1984).

Reference Values for Throat Cultures

The diagnosis of strep throat is based on finding group A beta-hemolytic streptococcus with a test kit. Other possible pathogens, *Haemophilus influenzae, Corynebacterium diphtheriae,* gonococcus, or meningococcus, can be identified by culture.

POSSIBLE NURSING DIAGNOSES RELATED TO POSITIVE TEST FOR STREPTOCOCCI GROUP A

Knowledge Deficit Related to Needed Treatment

If streptococci are the cause of the sore throat, the client is put on penicillin, or erthyromycin in the case of penicillin allergy. People sometimes discontinue antibiotics after they begin to feel better. Yet antibiotic therapy for strep throat must be continued for at least ten days as a minimum (Wang, 1977), regardless of how well the client feels. So the nurse may assess to make sure that the parents, or the clients themselves, understand the reason why the antibiotic is to be continued for ten or so days. Either the physician or the nurse may have to explain to the parents that undertreating "strep" throat increases the possibility of the later development of rheumatic fever.

Health Maintenance Management to Reduce Community Spread

Clients with strep throat are not isolated because they are considered noninfectious a few hours after antibiotic therapy is begun. Wang (1977) reports that about half of the siblings and nearly one-fourth of the parents of a child with strep throat have the organism too. Because streptococci are transmitted in the droplets from the respiratory tract, the infected person should not cough or breathe on others. The nurse may become involved with follow-up contacts for other family members. In a school setting, the school nurse or public health nurse can be very effective in both detecting and preventing the spread of strep throat in a population. Preventing strep infections helps to prevent rheumatic fever, of which approximately 100,000 new cases occur in this country each year (Fitzmaurice, 1980). Rheumatic heart disease is the only major form of cardiovascular disease that is potentially preventable at the present time. (See Chapter 14 on the streptococci antigen tests used to assess for previous acute infections with streptococci.)

■ NASAL AND NASOPHARYNGEAL CULTURES

General Indications

Nasopharyngeal cultures are done to screen for *Bordetella pertussis, Candida albicans, Coryne bacterium diphtheriae, Neisseria meningitidis, Haemophilus influenzae,* and others. Nasal cultures may be done to identify suspected carriers of organisms, such as *Staphylococcus aureus,* which are also called coag-positive. The differentiation between carrier state and infection is often difficult because some pathogens do transiently appear in the normal human pharynx (Shelter & Bartos, 1980b). Health workers in such areas as newborn nurseries or operating rooms may have nasal cultures to screen out potential sources of spread once an outbreak has occurred (Jacobs et al., 1984).

Preparation of Client and Collection of Sample

A flexible swab is inserted gently into the nose and rotated against the anterior nares for a nasal culture. A longer flexible swab makes it possible also to culture the posterior pharynx (nasopharyngeal). The swab is placed into a tube of transport medium and sent to the laboratory. Identification of particular strains of staphylococcus may require special laboratory resources not found in all institutions.

Reference Values for Nasopharyngeal Cultures

Pathogens such as streptococcus, pneumonococcus, or *Neisseria meningitidis* may or may not be clinically significant. Coag-positive staphylococcus may be present in 50% of people who have nasopharyngeal cultures done.

POSSIBLE NURSING IMPLICATIONS RELATED TO POSITIVE NASAL CULTURES

If a health worker has a positive culture, the physician must evaluate the importance of the person as a carrier. The health worker who is a potential source of pathogens may be assigned to areas where the risk of infecting others is minimized. The actual danger to others is somewhat controversial because many pathogens are always present to some degree and become disease-producing only when the opportunity arises. These opportunistic pathogens are probably dangerous for the already ill and immunodeficient person (Kuhn, 1978). Many hospitals have an infection control nurse as part of an infection control team. As employees, nurses should seek out information about how their institutions handle the problem of carriers.

■ WOUND CULTURES

General Indications
Normally wounds should not be infected with any organisms. Yet once the integrity of the skin is broken, there is a direct pathway for skin flora to reach tissue. An infected wound is usually obvious even to the untrained eye. The characteristic signs are redness, heat, and swelling. There may also be drainage that contains pus (purulent) and that may have a foul smell. If the wound cannot drain, the infection can cause pain and swelling, such as in an abscess. The wounds of surgical clients should be inspected daily for any sign of infection. Clients with burns, abrasions, or bedsores (decubiti) are also very susceptible to infections of the open skin areas.

Preparation of Client and Collection of Wound Culture
In collecting a specimen for culture from a wound, nurses must not contaminate the specimen with the normal skin flora. The skin around the wound should be cleansed to eliminate any flora present. The swab should be put deep into the wound without touching the skin around the wound, and it should be directed to the area where the purulent drainage is the most profuse. It is permissible, and indeed necessary, to make sure that the swab is in direct contact with the infected area. If the infected area is contained in a pocket or abscess, the physician has to do an incision and drainage (I&D) to obtain material for culturing. (The I&D is also therapeutic in that it allows the infected material to be removed.)

As with the collection of other specimens, nurses must be sure to prevent the spread of the infection. After using the swab to collect the specimen, they should immediately place it into a culture tube. One swab, well soaked with wound drainage, is usually sufficient. If there is the possibility of a fungus infection, a swab should be wet with sterile, normal saline before the culture is done. Swabs made for wound culture have an area above the stopper that can be touched by the nurse. If the swab is not attached to a stopper, the nurse can break off the part of the swab that was touched.

For an anaerobic culture, some wound drainage can be collected in a syringe. All of the air should be expelled from the syringe and the sample sent to the laboratory in the syringe (Marchiondo, 1979).

Reference Values for Wound Cultures

Common organisms found in wounds are *Staphylococcus aureus,* group A streptococci, gram-negative bacilli, and fungi. If the wound is deep and hence not in direct contact with the air, anaerobic bacteria such as *Clostridium* or anaerobic streptococci may also thrive. The culture and sensitivity is most useful in assisting the physician to select an effective antibiotic when wounds have not healed with standard therapy.

POSSIBLE NURSING DIAGNOSIS RELATED TO POSITIVE WOUND CULTURE

Potential for Injury Related to Spread of Infection
If the wound is completely covered and is not draining to the outside, simple wound isolation is needed. In essence, wound isolation means using a gown and gloves when the wound must be dressed. Sometimes staff tend to become careless in using sterile technique when the client has a wound infection. A break in sterile technique is shrugged off as being not too important because "the client already has an infected wound." Obviously this kind of thinking is not justifiable because, no matter how infected a wound may be, adding other organisms to it is still possible. Dressing changes of an infected wound require the same careful sterile technique as do wounds that are not already infected.

If the wound is draining enough so that the dressings become soaked, the client may become a source of infection to others. So more extreme isolation procedures may need to be carried out. Refer to the specific policies of a given institution. Many hospitals now have an infection control nurse who can help nursing personnel decide what level of isolation is required for the hospitalized client with a wound infection. In the home setting, the nurse needs to teach the client how to avoid transmitting the infection to others. Because proper wound healing requires good nutrition, the dietary needs of the client should be assessed. (See the ideas discussed earlier in this chapter about ways to increase a person's resistance to infection.)

■ EYE CULTURES

Though the eye contains a few bacteria, the bathing of the eye with tears usually keeps the actual count of bacteria very low. An infected eye is easy to see even by the lay person. The physician may wish to determine whether an eye discharge is due to a viral or bacterial invasion. Because of the need to treat most eye infections with topical antimicrobials, the laboratory may routinely test the found organisms for susceptibility to drugs such as neomycin, chloramphenicol, etc. on the Kirby–Bauer disk. If the physician plans systemic rather than topical treatment, the laboratory can do the standard MIC, discussed earlier in this chapter.

Preparation of Client and Collection of Sample
A sterile swab is used to collect some of the purulent matter from the eye. The client should be told to look up while the nurse gently pulls down on the cheek. The swab can be placed on the conjunctiva. Not touching the cornea with the swab is important. After the specimen is collected, it is put into a sterile culture tube.

Reference Values for Eye Cultures

Staphylococcus aureus and *Pseudomonas aeruginosa* are two bacteria that may cause eye infections. In the newborn, *Neisseria gonorrhoeae* can be transmitted when the baby goes through the birth canal. To prevent this transmission of gonorrhea, some state laws require delivery room personnel to instill silver nitrate or an antibiotic ointment in every newborn's eyes.

POSSIBLE NURSING DIAGNOSIS RELATED TO POSITIVE
EYE CULTURE

Knowledge Deficit Related to Care for Eye Infection
Clients should be taught not to wipe the infected eye. They must also avoid transmitting the infection to the other eye. Dark glasses may offer some comfort to clients, if they need to be outdoors. They may also need instructions on the proper way to instill eye drops. For example, clients may not know how to put pressure on the lacrimal duct to prevent the drop from entering the nasal cavity.

■ VAGINAL AND URETHRAL SMEARS

The vagina normally contains such bacteria as *Lactobacillus, Staphylococcus, Escherichia coli,* and some yeast. Most commonly, vaginal infections are due to *Trichomonas vaginalis* or to the fungus *Candida albicans.* Smears of the discharge may detect the causative agent. If gonorrhea is suspected in a female, an endocervical smear is done. In the male, smears or cultures of the drainage from the urethra may be done for gonorrhea or other organisms. Also in the male, centrifuged urine may be cultured for gonorrhea. Newer tests for herpes and chlamydia have increased the ability to detect sexually transmitted diseases. (See Chaper 14 for serology tests for syphilis.)

Preparation of Client and Collection of Sample

Vaginal and Endocervical Smears in Females. To obtain a vaginal smear or culture, the swab needs to be inserted well into the vagina. Check with the laboratory regarding any special techniques needed for smears, such as a wet saline swab for *Trichomonas* or KOH for *Candida.* The client or the nurse needs to hold the labia apart so that the swab does not touch the outer lips. If the nurse must separate the lips of the vagina, a nonsterile glove should be used. An endocervical specimen, necessary for suspected gonorrhea, requires the use of a speculum as for other pelvic examinations. Only water is used to lubricate the speculum. Excess cervical mucus is wiped off with a dry cotton ball and then a cotton-tipped swab is inserted in the endocervical canal for 30 seconds to absorb any organisms. Two specimens are put on one special culture medium. (If an anal specimen is collected it is put on a separate culture.)

Urethral Smears in Males. Collection of urethral smears in the male is often done at the time the physician is examining the client for complaints of discharge from the penis. The exudate is collected on a swab, which is rolled, not rubbed, on a slide. A special loop swab can be gently inserted into the urinary meatus to obtain exudate. If the client has no discharge from the penis, a urine specimen may be centrifuged to obtain a smear or culture for possible gonorrhea.

Reference Values for Vaginal, Endocervical, and Urethral Smears

---

The presence of pathogens on a smear is considered diagnostic. A culture may or may not be needed to confirm the identification of certain organisms, such as fungus (*Candida*) or protozoan (*Trichomonas*), that may be causing vaginitis.

Clinical Significance of Positive Smears or Cultures

Gonorrhea. About half of the cases of pelvic inflammatory disease (PID) in women are due to infection with *Neisseria gonorrhoeae.* Although a smear may be diagnostic for men with gonorrhea, women need a culture because the smear may not distinguish between other vaginal flora and gonorrhea (Jacobs et al., 1984). The sample for the culture needs to be taken from the endocervical canal, not from the vagina. Oropharyngeal and rectal smears and cultures need to be done if the person has had oral or anal sex with an infected person. Penicillin is the treatment of choice. Cultures can identify the penicillin-resistant strains of gonorrhea, and other antibiotics can be substituted.

Chlamydia (Lymphogranuloma venereum). *Chlamydia* is a bacteria-like microbe with some of the characteristics of a virus. The disease may have few symptoms and often is found with other sexually transmitted diseases. Unlike syphilis and gonorrhea, chlamydia is not eliminated by penicillin and if left untreated, the disease may cause sterility because of the chronic inflammation in the urogenital tract. A new test, which uses the enzyme immune assay (EIA) method discussed in Chapter 15, can detect chlamydia in about 30 minutes. Older methods required a culture that was difficult to do. Once detected, chlamydia can be successfully eliminated with tetracycline.

Herpes Simplex. The genital type of herpes is caused by a virus called herpes simplex virus type 2 (HSV2). (Herpes simplex type 1 is the virus that causes cold sores in the mouth.) Exudate from the lesions present during an acute episode of herpes can be examined under a microscope. If the lesions are dry, some saline can be added before scraping the lesion with a tongue blade. The smear is spread on a glass slide and fixed immediately with 95% ethyl alcohol. Herpes inclusion bodies may be seen in multinucleated giant cells. A definitive diagnosis may require a viral culture, which takes 2 or more days. (See Chapter 14 for serology tests that also may be done.)

Herpes is treated with topical acyclovir (Zovirax). Clients should use a finger cot or rubber gloves to reduce the spread to other sites, particularly the eye. After an initial outbreak, stress reduction and general good health habits may keep the virus in remission. Bassing (1985) discusses the care of the pregnant woman who has herpes.

Trichomonas. Trichomonas vaginalis is a protozoan that grows optimally under anaerobic conditions. Sometimes a wet smear may be done to detect the active protozoa in a drop of vaginal discharge or in a drop of urine from the male. Culturing of the urogenital discharges can reveal the protozoa even if the direct microscopic examination seem negative. Treatment with antiprotozoal drugs, such as furazolidone or metronidazole, require detailed client instructions about interactions with alcohol and other side effects.

Moniliasis or Other Yeast Infections. Candida albicans and, less frequently, other species of *Candida* may be normally present in vaginal secretions. These yeast-like fungi may become invasive under conditions that favor their rapid growth. Predisposing factors for rapid growth of fungi include long-term antibiotic therapy, pregnancy, oral contraceptives, diabetes, and wearing nonventilating pants. The vaginal discharge viewed under the microscope on a wet mount using a potassium hydroxide (KOH) preparation shows the many budding yeast cells and may be diagnostic. If needed, cultures using rehydrated modified Nickerson (RMN) culture or Microstix-Candida can be confirmatory (Bertholf & Stafford, 1985). Nystatin is an effective antifungal agent.

Toxic Shock Syndrome (TSS). Toxic shock syndrome is a rare disease believed to be caused by toxin-producing strains of the bacterium *Staphylococcus aureus.* Clients suspected of having TSS have blood and urine cultures as well as a vaginal culture to detect a focal staph infection. The use of tampons containing higher absorbency may be linked to an increased incidence, but another rise in 1983 has not been explained (Petti et al., 1986). Because of the possible association with tampon use, manufacturers of tampons now include detailed information about the symptoms of TSS in their product information folders. Early symptoms may be fever and a rash. Abnormal laboratory reports include leukocytosis with pronounced left shift (Chapter 2), elevated BUN and creatinine (Chapter 4), severe acidosis (Chapter 6), hypocalcemia (Chapter 7), hyperbilirubinemia (Chapter 11), elevated CPK (Chapter 12), and thrombocytopenia (Chapter 13). Treatment involves the use of antibiotic therapy and treatment for circulatory collapse that may occur.

POSSIBLE NURSING DIAGNOSES RELATED TO POSITIVE VAGINAL OR URETHRAL SMEAR OR CULTURE

Knowledge Deficit Regarding Sexual Transmission of Disease

Gonorrhea is a communicable disease that needs to be reported to the health department, which employs people to serve as case finders. Although the sexual contacts of these clients need to be examined to do case finding, clients may or may not wish to name their sexual partners. The nurse can be sensitive to their needs and yet also impress upon them the importance of the disease as a public health problem. These clients need clear instructions from the physician or from other health professionals about the restrictions that should be put on sexual contact until the disease is cured. Penicillin is the usual treatment. Repeat smears or cultures (in women) are done 3–5 days after therapy as a test of cure.

Other diseases, such as *Trichomoniasis,* do not require reporting but the spread from person to person is also of concern. The female may keep getting reinfected from a male partner unless he too is cultured and treated (the ping-pong effect). Thus treatment of any infection of the genitourinary tract involves not only the person, but also the person or persons who have been and who will be sexual partners of the client. At the present time, herpes can not be cured, but the person is only infectious when the disease is active. The nurse can help set a climate that is conducive to assisting these clients to help themselves and others. Clients need factual information on how to best proceed as a sexual being (Lutz, 1986). A punitive, noncaring, or hostile environment alienates persons who come to seek help.

Learning Needs Related to Treatment

Female clients may need specific instructions on how to insert vaginal suppositories or to administer douches, if medicine is ordered in these forms. Again, the nurse must foster a climate that helps clients feel comfortable about discussing intimate details.

■ STOOL CULTURES

Many normal bacteria live in the feces. In fact, a large percentage of the weight of feces is from bacteria. Most of the organisms in the bowel are many types of gram-negative bacilli. For example, *Escherichia coli* is a common normal inhabitant in adults. (In children under one year of age, *Escherichia coli* can be pathogenic.) Bacterial cultures for stool are routinely checked for *Staphylococcus aureus, Salmonella, Shigella* and other enteropathogens. If anaerobic organisms are suspected, such as *Clostridium botulinum,* an anaerobic culture is done too. Microscopic examination to detect the presence of fecal blood, leukocytes, and organisms called vibros can be done in 30 minutes. Kuhn (1985) has an excellent flow sheet for the quick evaluation of the 12 most common organisms found in food poisoning.

In addition to cultures for bacteria, stool specimens may also be collected to identify parasites that can be protozoa or worms (helminths). Protozoa are more common in most areas than are helminths, unless there is a history of travel to the tropics or a heavy influx of immigrants (Most, 1984). If the laboratory is checking for protozoa such as *Entamoeba histolytica,* the nurse must collect several specimens over a period of days. Because the protozoan parasites have cyclical life-spans, multiple collections increase the chance of spotting a parasite (Shelter & Bartos, 1980a). (See Chapter 14 for a serologic test done for amebas.) For helminths, a single stool specimen is usually sufficient.

Two other methods of collecting stool specimens for examination involve cellophane tape and a rectal swab. The cellophane tape may be pressed over the perineal area to pick up pinworms, which are very small intestinal worms. Rectal swabs are sometimes done for *Shigella* and for gonorrhea, if this disease is suspected. Yet few organisms live in the rectal wall; the mass of bacteria or parasites is in the feces.

Preparation of Client and Collection of Sample

For bacterial or protozoan cultures, a walnut-sized piece of feces is all that is needed. Diarrhea stool can also be cultured; only about 15–20 ml are needed, the rest of the stool is discarded. The specimen should be sent to the laboratory immediately. Check with the laboratory for the time span permissible.

The client must defecate into a clean bedpan. Urine in the bedpan may kill some of the growth. A tongue blade can be used to transfer the small amount of stool to the stool container. Commercial kits contain small spoons inside a specimen container. When handling the bedpan, the nurse should wear disposable nonsterile gloves. Because parasites or bacteria may often be harbored in mucus or in streaks of blood, some of this material should be included in the sample. The stool specimen is put into a waxed container with a tight-fitting lid. It is important not to contaminate the outside of the specimen container. Clients may collect a stool specimen at home. If so, they need to be taught how to properly collect the specimen and how to properly wash their hands so that the outside of the container is not contaminated. (Enteric diseases are spread by oral-fecal transmission.) A plastic bag or newspaper can be taped under the toilet seat so the person can sit on the toilet.

If a rectal swab or cellophane tape is used to collect material from the rectal area, the nurse should wear a glove when touching the perineal area. A sterile cotton-tipped swab is inserted 1 inch into the anal canal. The swab should be moved side to side and left for 30 seconds for the absorption of organisms. Note on the laboratory slip whether the client is on antibiotics because these drugs can change the flora in the intestines. Also, the use of antacids may change the pH of the stool and affect bacterial growth.

If the fat content of the stool is to be measured due to malabsorption problems, the *entire* stool for one to three days is sent to the laboratory. The client will be on a 100-g fat diet. (See Appendix A, Table 6 for values.)

Reference Values for Stool Cultures

The laboratory may issue a preliminary report of probable findings of *Salmonella* or *Shigella,* so that enteric precautions can be started. Parasites or worms may be immediately identified by examination. The two major protozoan infections in the United States are amebiasis and giardiasis (John, 1981).

POSSIBLE NURSING DIAGNOSES RELATED TO POSITIVE STOOL CULTURE

Knowledge Deficit Regarding Spread of Infection to Others
Depending on the type of pathogen in the stool, the nurse must make sure that the client does not spread the pathogens to others. Isolation is usually not required if clients can wash their hands properly and if the feces can quickly be flushed into the sewage system. Stool precautions are not needed for botulism, *Clostridium perfringens,* or staph food poisoning (Kuhn, 1985). The nurse should be aware that the collection of stool and the focus on the anal area is often a source of embarrassment for the individual. (Saving a stool has been frowned upon since the age of two and the anal stage.) The client should not be made to feel "unclean" because of the extra precautions needed to protect others. Others in the family need to be checked for pathogens too. Children are very prone to spread disease because of poor hygiene.

Knowledge Deficit Related to Effect of Drugs
Once appropriate therapy has been started, clients need follow-up stool samples to evaluate the effectiveness of the therapy. Some of the drugs used for intestinal pathogens cause gastrointestinal symptoms; so it is important that clients know what may be expected from the drug and what may be an indication that therapy is not being effective. Later stool samples may show a second type of pathogen also present.

■ CULTURES OF CEREBROSPINAL FLUID (CSF) AND OTHER FLUIDS

Specimens of CSF are obtained by lumbar puncture. CSF is sterile, and it is collected under sterile conditions. Various organisms may be responsible for meningitis, including *Hemophilus influenzae, Neisseria meningitidis,* and *Streptococcus pneumoniae.* The first is common in infants and the last in adults.

The laboratory does an immediate smear to see if any organisms exist. The laboratory should be notified that CSF is going to the laboratory so that immediate analysis can begin. The specific identifications of the organism may take 48–72 hours. See Chapter 25 on the procedure for lumbar puncture.

Cultures of Pleural Fluid, Peritoneal Fluid, and Joint Fluid
Pleural fluid, obtained from a thoracentesis, can be cultured for possible bacterial growth as can peritoneal fluid from a paracentesis (See Chapter 25). Joint fluid from a joint aspiration may also be cultured. The role of the nurse in carefully marking the specimens and sending them to the laboratory was discussed in the beginning of this chapter. Careful labeling is necessary for *all* specimens. If a urine specimen is not labeled correctly, it is usually possible to obtain another specimen, but it may be much less feasible to obtain a second specimen of any fluid that requires an invasive technique.

QUESTIONS

1. The laboratory reports a large number of gram-negative rods *are* present on the preliminary stain of a urine specimen. Which one of the following organisms could not be present if all the organisms are gram-negative rods?

   a. *Escherichia coli*
   b. *Proteus* species
   c. *Neisseria gonorrhoea*
   d. *Pseudomonas* species

2. Mrs. Siegel's urine was sent to the laboratory for a C&S (culture and sensitivity). The report notes an "S" next to all the listed antibiotics except penicillin, which is marked with an "R." An "R" next to the penicillin indicates what?

   a. Penicillin is the right drug for the urine infection
   b. Mrs. Siegel is resistant to penicillin
   c. Penicillin must be increased to obtain a successful urine level
   d. The organisms in the culture were resistant to penicillin

3. Common bacteria that cause nosocomial infections are staphylococci and gram-negative rods. Which nursing action would be the most effective way to *prevent* these nosocomial infections?

   a. Administering all prescribed antibiotics on time
   b. Emphasizing hand-washing before and after caring for every client
   c. Isolating all clients with fevers of undetermined origin (FUO)
   d. Culturing all open wounds

4. Mrs. Mozian, age 78, has had cultures done of blood, urine, and sputum because of a persistent fever and general malaise. In planning care for Mrs. Mozian, the nurse in the nursing home should do all the following *except* which?

   a. Assess the fluid intake and determine how much p.o. fluids should be taken daily
   b. Consult with the physician to see if there is any need for isolation procedures
   c. Promote periods of rest so that Mrs. Mozian does not become fatigued
   d. Use aspirin p.r.n. to keep the temperature at a normal level

5. Which of the following is a correct statement about the collection of urine for urine cultures?

   a. The meatus of the male requires more cleansing than does the meatus of the female
   b. A disinfectant should never be used to cleanse the genital area before a clean catch is done
   c. A clean catch urine requires that the urine be caught in midstream
   d. Only a catheterized urine specimen is suitable for urine culture

6. Mr. Edwards has been having fever and chills from an unknown cause. He is to have blood cultures drawn three times. The nurse should be aware of which of the following?

a. The skin over the venipuncture site must be prepped with an iodine preparation to reduce contamination by skin flora

b. Two blood cultures can be drawn at the same time if the specimens are put into two different test tubes

c. Blood cultures should not be drawn after a spike of fever or a chill

d. A positive confirmation of a diagnosis can be made in 24 hours

7. Mrs. Solado has had a central venous catheter in place for several days for hyperalimentation. The physician is removing the catheter because of possible sepsis. The catheter is to be cultured. How should the nurse prepare the specimen for the laboratory?

   a. Wrap the entire catheter in a sterile towel and send to the laboratory

   b. Cut off the tip of the catheter with sterile scissors, put the tip into a sterile container, and send it to the laboratory

   c. Cut off the tip of the catheter with bandage scissors, put the tip in a clean test tube, and send it to the laboratory

   d. Put a sterile swab inside the tip of the catheter and then send the swab to the laboratory

8. Mr. McKay is to have a sputum specimen obtained because of lung congestion and fever. Which of the following instructions by the nurse is correct to tell Mr. McKay?

   a. "Save as much sputum as you can in the next 2 hours because the laboratory needs at least an ounce (30 ml) of sputum."

   b. "Discard the first specimen in the morning because the secretions will not be fresh."

   c. "Saliva will be all right for a specimen if it hurts to do a deep cough."

   d. "Rinse out your mouth before obtaining the specimen so bacteria from the mouth will be less numerous."

9. Mrs. Gardeni is to have sputum specimens three times for AFB. If the preliminary report comes back positive, she will be on respiratory isolation to prevent the spread of what?

   a. Tuberculosis   c. Influenza
   b. *Legionella pneumophila*   d. *Pneumocystis carinii*

10. Timmy, age 10, has come to see the school nurse for a "sore throat." The concern for correctly identifying the cause of the sore throat is important because rheumatic fever or glomerulonephritis sometimes occurs after infection with which organism?

    a. A virus called HIV

    b. Group A beta-hemolytic streptococcus

    c. Staphylococcus aureus

    d. Any of the streptococci

11. Mr. Jason has a Penrose drain from an abdominal stab wound. The nurse is to obtain a culture of the wound. Which action by the nurse is *not* appropriate?

  a. Using sterile gloves to obtain the specimen
  b. Cleansing the skin around the drain before obtaining the specimen
  c. Inserting the swab deep into the wound to get the specimen
  d. Obtaining a second culture from the wound after the wound has been irrigated

12. Mr. Rabinowitz has an infected eye. Which of the following actions by the visiting nurse is *not* appropriate?

  a. Using a sterile swab to collect some exudate and putting the swab into culture medium supplied by the laboratory
  b. Lightly touching the cornea with the swab to get the specimen
  c. Instructing the client not to rub his eye with his fingers
  d. Showing the client how to rinse off the exudate without contaminating the other eye

13. Johnny Phillips, age 17, is concerned that he may have gonorrhea. He asks the nurse in the clinic how gonorrhea can be detected. The nurse should explain to Johnny that the test for gonorrhea involves which of the following?

  a. Drawing blood by venipuncture for a serology test
  b. Obtaining some secretions from the end of the penis for a microscopic exam
  c. Both urine and blood tests
  d. Only a fingerstick for a blood sample

14. Mr. Cohen is to have a stool specimen collected because of a possible *Salmonella* infection. He just had a bowel movement in the bedside commode. Which action by the nurse is appropriate?

  a. Send a small portion of the stool in a waxed container to the laboratory
  b. Discard the stool because it was diarrhea rather than formed stool
  c. Use sterile gloves to transfer all of the stool to a sterile container and send it to the laboratory
  d. Send the entire stool in a waxed container to the laboratory

REFERENCES

Aspinall, M. (1978). Scoring against nosocomial infections. *AJN, 78*(10), 1704–1707.

Bassing, S. (1985). Saving the baby when mom has herpes. *RN, 48*(10), 35–37.

Bertholf, M., & Stafford, M. (1985). An office laboratory panel to assess vaginal problems. *American Family Physician, 32*(3), 113–125.

Bond, G. (1981). *Serratia*—an endemic hospital resident. *AJN, 81*(12), 2183–2186.

Deal, W. (1979). Unusual manifestations of infectious diseases in the aging. *Geriatrics, 34,* 77–84.

Fitzmaurice, J. (1980). *Rheumatic heart disease and mitral valve disease.* Norwalk, CT: Appleton-Century-Crofts.

Frame, P. (1982). Acute infectious pneumonia in the adult. *Basics of Respiratory Disease, 10*(3), 1–8.

Gilmore, D., Montgomerie, J., & Graham, I. (1986). Category 1, 2, 3 and 4: A procedure oriented isolation system. *Infection Control, 7*(5), 263–267.

Griffin, J. (1986). Fever, when to leave it alone. *Nursing 86,* 16(2), 58–61.

Grylack, L., & Scanlon, J. (1979). Practical evaluation of historical data and laboratory screening procedures for recognition of newborn sepsis. *Clinical Pediatrics, 18,* 227–231.

Gurevich, I. (1985). Fever: When to worry about it. *RN, 48*(12), 14–19.

Hargiss, C., & Larson, E. (1981). Infection control. How to collect specimens and evaluate results. *AJN, 81*(12), 2167–2174.

Hewitt, W., & McHenry, M. (1978). Blood level determination of antimicrobial drugs. *Medical Clinics of North America, 62,* 1119–1137.

Jacobs, D., Kasten, B., DeMott, W., & Wolfson, W. (1984). *Laboratory test handbook with DRG index.* St. Louis: Mosby/Lexi.

John, R. (1981). Giardiasis and amebiasis. *RN, 44*(4), 53–57.

Jones, I. (1985). You can drive back infection if you know where to make your stand. *Nursing 85, 15*(4), 50–52.

Komaroff, A. (1984). Acute dysuria in women. *NEJM, 310*(6), 368–375.

Kuhn, P. (1978). Opportunistic pathogens; Microbes with a potential for violence. *Diagnostic Medicine, 1,* 80–92.

Kuhn P. (1985). What kind of food poisoning is it? *RN, 48*(6), 39–43.

LaFave, J., et al. (1979). Office screening for asymptomatic urinary tract infections. *Clinical Pediatrics, 18,* 53–59.

Lutz, R. (1986). Stopping the spread of sexually transmitted diseases. *Nursing, 86, 16*(3), 47–50.

McGuckin, M. (1981). Getting better urine specimens with the clean catch midstream technique. *Nursing 81, 11,* 72–73.

Marchiondo, K. (1979). Collecting culture specimens. *Nursing 79, 9*(4), 34–43.

Mayer, J., et al. (1986). Increasing handwashing in an intensive care unit. *Infection Control, 7*(3), 259–262.

Miller, M. et al. (1984). Evaluation of the Directigen Group A Strep test kit. *Journal of Clinical Microbiology, 20*(5), 846–848.

Most, H. (1984). Treatment of parasitic infections of travelers and immigrants. *NEJM, 310,* 298–304.

Petti, D. (1986). The incidence of toxic shock syndrome in northern California. *JAMA, 255*(3), 368–372.

Pryor, A. (1984). A comparison of blood cultures withdrawn from the arterial line and by venipuncture. *Heart and Lung, 13*(4), 411–415.

Shelter, M., & Bartos, H. (1980a). Stool specimens: Key to detecting intestinal invaders. *RN, 43*(10), 50–53.

Shelter, M., & Bartos, H. (1980b). Respiratory tract cultures. *RN, 43*(11), 52–53.

Thomas, D. (1985). Fever in children. *RN, 48*(12), 18–19.

Tietz, N. (Ed.). (1983). *Clinical guide to laboratory tests.* Philadelphia: Saunders.

Wallach, J. (1986). *Interpretation of diagnostic tests.* Boston: Little, Brown.

Wang, R. (1977). Streptococcal sore throat. *AJN, 77,* 1797–1798.

17

Therapeutic Drug Monitoring and Toxicology Screens

- Antibiotics: Aminoglycosides
- Antibacterials: Sulfa Drugs
- Anticonvulsants
  Phenytoin or Diphenylhydantoin, Primidone (Mysoline, Primoline), Valproic Acid (Depakene), Phenobarbital (Luminal), Carbamazepine (Tegretol), and Ethosuximide (Zarontin)
- Antipsychotic Agent: Lithium Carbonate
- Tricyclic Antidepressants
- Bronchodilators: Theophylline Products and Caffeine Levels
- Cardiac Drugs: Digoxin and Digitoxin
- Antiarrhythmic Drugs
  Quinidine, Procainamide or NAPA, Phenytoin, Propranolol, and Lidocaine
- Salicylates: Acetylsalicylic Acid (ASA)
- Urine Testing: Phenistix
- Blood Alcohol
- Barbiturates
- Toxicology Screens in Blood and Urine
  Drugs Other than Barbiturates, Minor Tranquilizers and Propoxyphene, and Opiate Abuse
- Bromide
- Major Tranquilizers: Phenothiazines
- Heavy Metal Poisoning: Lead
  ALA-D Tests for Lead Poisoning and FEP (Free Erythrocyte Protoporphyrin)

OBJECTIVES

1. Discuss nine reasons for monitoring serum or urine drug levels.
2. Describe how plasma peak and trough levels are used to monitor aminoglycoside levels.

3. Name five anticonvulsants that are sometimes monitored by serum levels, and indicate the clinical symptoms of each that may indicate toxicity.

4. Identify the antipsychotic drug that must be monitored by serum drug levels to avoid toxicity.

5. Describe possible nursing diagnoses related to toxicity from antidepressants and other drugs.

6. Identify the two major clinical problems that may develop if a client has a serum theophylline level above the therapeutic range.

7. Identify which cardiac drugs are most commonly monitored by serum drug levels, along with the key nursing implications for each drug.

8. Describe three different clinical situations in which aspirin (ASA) serum levels are useful.

9. Identify the important facts that emergency room nurses should know about blood levels of alcohol and other depressant drugs.

10. Identify the usual medication history of a client who develops bromide toxicity.

11. Identify the major source for lead poisoning in young children.

Clinical toxicology involves the study of drugs that are therapeutic as well as those that are toxic. In clinical practice, the line between therapeutic effects and toxic effects may be narrow. The cardinal principle of experimental toxicology, first expressed by a sixteenth-century physician and alchemist, is that only the *dose* differentiates between a poison and a remedy (Scala, 1978). For example, digoxin in the correct dosage for an individual is therapeutic, but if the dose is increased even slightly the drug may be extremely toxic. Measurements of arsenic, carbon monoxide, or lead (all poisons) are traditional examples of toxicology. Therapeutic drug monitoring, as a type of clinical toxicology, has expanded in the last few years because more and more drugs can be easily measured in the serum. The radioimmunoassay method (RIA) and the enzyme methods (discussed in Chapter 15) have made it possible for the laboratory to detect even very small amounts of a drug or toxic substance in the bloodstream.

Although any drug can be measured in the serum, this chapter focuses on the drugs that are commonly measured and that have clinical significance for the nurse. Some general reasons for monitoring drugs, some of the pitfalls of using drug levels as assessment tools, and the general nursing implications when drug levels are used are discussed at the beginning of the chapter. Tests for specific drugs, along with any needed precautions about collection of the sample and about the specific nursing implications, are listed separately in the second part of this chapter.

PLASMA DRUG LEVELS

Reasons for Monitoring
Richens and Warrington (1979) list seven reasons why plasma drug levels need to be measured. In addition, two other reasons for monitoring are discussed.

When the Rate of a Drug's Metabolism Has a Wide Interindividual Variation. Many drugs are given at about the same dosage for all people because the rate of metabolism does not vary much from person to person. For other drugs, such as theophylline, the rate of metabolism may vary greatly, depending on many metabolic variations in the individual. With regard to theophylline, the Federal Drug Administration has put out specific guidelines for dosage based on weight, age, smoking/nonsmoking, and presence of certain diseases (FDA Bulletin, 1980b). The dosage of theophylline must be tailored to fit the particular individual. For example, if a smoker becomes a nonsmoker, the theophylline dose may need to be decreased. The serum theophylline concentrations can be measured to make sure that the dosage is maintaining the correct serum level.

When Saturation Kinetics Occur. For some drugs, such as phenytoin (Dilantin), an increase in dosage beyond a certain point does not increase the effectiveness of the drug because the body is saturated. The actual pharmacokinetics of a drug may be very complex, and they are used to determine the serum level considered therapeutically effective. On the other hand, for some drugs, the serum level is not at all reliable because the main action of the drug may be in tissues.

When the Therapeutic Ratio of the Drug Is Close to the Toxic Level. If a drug leaves a lot of leeway between its therapeutic effect and its toxic effect, carefully monitoring it by *serum* levels is usually not considered necessary. Lithium, however, is a good example of a drug that has a narrow margin of safety and that must be monitored.

When Signs of Toxicity Are Difficult to Recognize Clinically. Serum levels for certain drugs help to detect or to prevent toxicity that might otherwise not be noticed because of other clinical problems. In way of illustration, an antiarrhythmic drug, such as quinidine, may depress the myocardium and cause symptoms that could be wrongly attributed to a worsening of the underlying cardiac disease, rather than to the toxicity from the drug.

When Gastrointestinal, Hepatic, or Renal Disease Is Present. If gastrointestinal problems are present, any oral medication may have an erratic drug absorption. (Usually the drug would be ordered parenterally to avoid this problem.) If hepatic disease is present, drugs that are metabolized by the liver—and almost all are—are not cleared from the serum normally. (See Chapter 11 for the role of the liver in conjugating drugs and other substances, such as bilirubin.) Finally, because most drugs are excreted in the urine, renal disease means a problem with excretion. For example, the aminoglycoside antibiotics, if given at all, must be carefully monitored by serum levels when renal disease is present. (See Chapter 4 for assessment of renal function.)

When Drug Interactions Result from the Use of Several Drugs. Clients with epilepsy may be on several types of anticonvulsants, most of which can cause central nervous system symptoms, such as lethargy and depression. It may not be at all clear which drug or combination of drugs is causing the toxic effects. A serum level of the drugs helps to pinpoint the culprit.

When Noncompliance Is Suspected. "Noncompliance" means that a client is not taking a drug as ordered. The reasons for not taking a drug can be varied, including such a simple thing as a misunderstanding of the need. Clients who are put on certain drugs may be overly afraid of side effects, so they cut down on the amount of drug that was prescribed or they "forget" to take the pill at certain times. Squire et al. (1984) found many clients on long-term anti-arrhythmics had low serum levels, most likely due to noncompliance. Sometimes, when clients are admitted to the hospital, they develop a toxic reaction to a drug, such as digoxin, because in the hospital they are given it religiously every day as ordered. At home, the administration may not have been on schedule. A community health nurse can be of valuable assistance in visiting clients at home to determine whether noncompliance is a reason for erratic serum drug levels.

When an Overdose of an Unknown Substance or Substances Has Occurred. Therapeutic drugs, such as aspirin or barbiturates, are often taken in toxic amounts either accidentally (poisoning) or deliberately as a suicidal gesture. With drug experimentation, the client may have inhaled, ingested, or injected a variety of different drugs. The laboratory can do screens of serum, urine, and gastric contents to identify the chemicals present. In chronic posioning with heavy metals, such as lead, the laboratory can identify the toxic substances in both the serum and urine.

To Detect Abuse of Drugs for Legal Prosecution. The legal implications of the blood alcohol test are discussed under the section on alcohol tests. Other legal problems are discussed in the section on opiate abuse.

Reasons for Not Monitoring

Although there are many reasons to monitor drugs, there are also reasons not to monitor them. One good reason is cost. If the drug is not particularly toxic, and if the client responds well to the usual prescribed dosage, a serum drug level is unnecessary (Conrad, 1978). The nurse can help to explain to clients in simple terms why drug monitoring either is or is not necessary. For some drugs, the effect of the drug on other laboratory tests is more important than the actual serum level of the drug. For example, if the client is on anticoagulants, either the partial thromboplastin time (PTT) (for heparin) or the prothrombin time (PT) (for coumarin) is used to monitor the dosage of the respective anticoagulants. (See Chapter 13 on tests for coagulation.) If the client is on insulin therapy, blood glucose levels are used to monitor drug effects, not the insulin level per se. (See Chapter 8 on glucose, and Chapter 3 on urine tests.)

Caution in Interpretation

Because serum drug levels reflect only the amount of the drug in the plasma at a given time, the level may not reflect the actual physiologic activity of the drug. Laboratory tests of serum drugs measure both the bound and unbound parts of the drug. A client with less albumin in the serum may thus have a larger amount of "free" drug in the serum. With some tests, the clinician has to take into account the conjugated and unconjugated portions of the drug or the amount of plasma proteins available for binding. (See Chapter 10 on the measurement of albumin.) Also some drugs will affect the serum level of the drug being measured.

Variation in results due to a lack of standardization in different laboratories is also a problem. McCormick et al. (1978) found a wide range of test results when three different laboratories ran tests on standardized samples of digoxin, phenobarbital, and phenytoin. Although laboratory error is not a nursing problem, the potential for laboratory error must be kept in mind when serum drug levels do not correlate well with the clinical picture.

TABLE 17-1. PEAK AND TROUGH LEVELS

Timing of Medication	Peak to Be Drawn 60 Minutes After IV Completed		Trough to Be Drawn 5 Minutes Before Next Dose	
Netilmicin 80 mg in 100 ml of D_5 W q8h intravenously over 1 hour:				
8 A.M.–9 A.M.	Draw sample at	10 A.M.	Draw sample at	7:55 A.M.
		or		or
4 P.M.–5 P.M.		6 P.M.		3:55 P.M.
		or		or
12 midnight–1 A.M.		2 A.M.		11:55 P.M.

Note: Check with individual laboratory for peak time for other drugs. May be shorter than 1 hour (Howard, 1986). Lerner et al. (1983) used the above times in a study on the ototoxicity and nephrotoxicity of tobramycin and netilmicin. See Chapter 4 on serum creatinine levels also used to monitor drug nephrotoxicity.

GENERAL NURSING IMPLICATIONS

Correct Sample Timing: Peaks, Troughs, and Steady States

Serum samples of drug levels may be ordered as peak levels, as trough levels, or after obtaining a steady state. For serum drug levels, *peak* times refer to measurements of the highest level of drug reached in the serum; *trough* times represent the lowest levels. Some laboratories may refer to the trough levels as "residuals."

The *steady state* of a drug refers to the time when the plasma level has been stabilized by a maintenance dose. For some drugs, a steady state is not obtained for several weeks. The client may have periodic samples drawn to check on the exact "steady rate" that is being maintained with a specific dosage level. Howard (1986) suggests that nurses ask the hospital pharmacist to compile a list of optimal sampling times for all drugs being monitored. Each drug has its own distribution time and volume of distribution (VD) to the tissues. Some drugs have a small VD which means they remain in the serum. Other drugs have a large VD which means they are distributed to the tissues.

The trough or residual level is usually drawn just before the next dose of the drug is given. The timing for the peak level drawing is based on the knowledge about when the particular drug is usually at a peak in the serum.

Controversy exists about whether peak or trough levels are better indicators of toxicity for specific drugs. In general, the peak is a determination of the rate of absorption of the drug, while the trough is a measurement of the drug's rate of elimination. A timetable for drawing peak and trough levels for netilmicin is shown in Table 17-1.

Peak and trough levels of serum drug levels are meaningless unless it is known when the drug was given, the amount given, and the route. Knowing what other drugs are being taken by the client is also important, because they may interfere with some tests. If the client is being assessed for a steady state of the drug, make note not only of this information, but also of the daily dosage that has been maintained over a certain period. (Also, question the client and make sure that the ordered dosage was in fact the dosage being taken at home.) In summary, the laboratory needs the following information:

1. The exact timing of the last dose of the drug
2. The exact amount of the drug given
3. The route of the drug (peak times change dramatically between oral and parenteral administration)
4. How long the client has been on a certain dosage (if the client is being assessed for a steady state level)
5. Other medications that may interfere with the specific test (check with the individual laboratory to determine this)

Reason for Tests and Deviations from Reference Values

The information gained by serum drug levels is used primarily by the physician, who readjusts the dosages if needed. Nurses need to be aware of the reference values used in a particular setting, so that deviations from normal can be reported before another drug dosage is given. For example, if a trough level shows a range as high, or nearly as high, as the expected peak, continuing with the drug may be dangerous. Contacting the physician before the next dose of the drug is administered would be wise. Unless the information from the laboratory report is utilized, the serum drug levels are just a costly academic exercise that are of no benefit to the client.

■ ANTIBIOTICS: AMINOGLYCOSIDES

Serum antibiotic levels are not routinely done if the antibiotic is not usually toxic, if the infection is responding appropriately, and if the client does not have liver or renal dysfunction. For example, because penicillin and the cephalosporins have a much wider range between therapeutic doses and toxic doses than do the antibiotics that are classified as aminoglycosides, clients who are on penicillin or the cephalosporins are not routinely followed by serum antibiotic levels.

All aminoglycosides have a central amino sugar—hence the name aminoglycoside (sugar). These antibiotics are used for serious infections with gram-negative bacteria, such as *Escherichia coli* and *Pseudomonas*. (See Chapter 16 on cultures and sensitivities.) The aminoglycosides that are commonly monitored by serum levels are gentamicin (Garamycin), tobramycin (Nebcin, Tobrex) and amikacin (Amikin). A new one, netilmicin (Netromycin), may have less neuro- and nephrotoxicity (Lerner et al., 1983).

POSSIBLE NURSING DIAGNOSES FOR AMINOGLYCOSIDES

Potential for Injury Related to Dizziness or Hearing Loss

The nurse needs to be aware that the aminoglycosides have the potential for nerve damage (neurotoxicity). The eighth cranial nerve is often affected by this group of antibiotics. Impairment may involve both the auditory branch (ototoxicity) and the vestibular branch. Involvement of the vestibular branch causes a lack of equilibrium. The client may complain of a lack of balance and dizziness. If clients are on aminoglycosides for more than ten days without having their serum levels monitored, they may be given hearing tests to check for ototoxicity (Yoshikawa, 1980).

Potential for Alteration in Urinary Patterns

Aminoglycosides may also cause kidney damage (nephrotoxicity). Neurotoxicity is more likely if renal function is not normal. BUN and/or creatinine tests are often used to monitor renal function while the client is on aminoglycosides. (See Chapter 4 on BUN and creatinine.) The client must remain well hydrated and the intake and output record must be carefully maintained. If a client has liver or, particularly, renal dysfunction, the serum levels may be the only way to safely give aminoglycoside antibiotics (Langslet & Habel, 1981).

Preparation of Client and Collection of Sample

The laboratory needs 1 ml of serum. Usually blood samples for peak levels of antibiotics are drawn 45–60 minutes after an intramuscular (IM) injection or 15–30 minutes after completion of an intravenous (IV) antibiotic. The trough or residual level is done immediately before the next dose of antibiotic is due. The nurse should check with the laboratory about exact trough and peak times. Table 17–1 gives an example of the timing of levels for netilmicin. In general, peak levels are used to determine whether the dosage is adequate, whereas trough levels aid in ascertaining whether there is too much drug accumulation.

Reference Values for Aminoglycosides	
Gentamicin (Garamycin) and tobramycin (Nebcin, Tobrex)	Therapeutic, 4–8 µg/ml Peak, below 12 µg/ml Trough, below 2 µg/ml
Amikacin (Amikin) and kanamycin (Kantrex)	Therapeutic, 8–16 µg/ml Peak, below 35 µg/ml Trough, below 10 µg/ml
Netilmicin (Netromycin)	Peak, 6–10 µg/ml Trough, below 2 µg/ml

■ ANTIBACTERIALS: SULFA DRUGS

Sulfa drugs are antibacterials, not antibiotics (which are obtained from living organisms). Sulfa drugs are usually not measured in the serum because the concentration in the urine is usually a more useful assessment of the therapeutic effectiveness (Hewitt & McHenry, 1978). Occasionally sulfa drugs may be measured in the serum if renal function is not optimal.

Preparation of Client and Collection of Sample

The laboratory needs 2 ml of serum or urine.

Reference Values for Sulfa Drugs	
Therapeutic level:	
In serum	5–16 mg/dl
In urine	15–20 mg/ml

■ ANTICONVULSANTS

PHENYTOIN OR DIPHENYLHYDANTOIN

Phenytoin, formerly called diphenylhydantoin, is the most common drug used to treat various types of epilepsy. It may be used alone or in combination with the other anticonvulsants in this section. Phenytoin is also used as an antiarrhythmic for certain types of cardiac irregularities. (See the section on antiarrhythmic drugs.)

Clients may have serum phenytoin levels done to determine the proper dose level for long-term therapy. Since it takes at least a week or two to achieve stable serum phenytoin levels, during this time the clients may have blood samples drawn several times. As with most other serum drug levels, the level per se is not always a prediction of toxicity from the drug.

Serum levels are related to certain side effects. In general, nystagmus (involuntary rapid movements of the eyeballs) appears when serum phenytoin levels are above 20 µg/ml. Gait ataxia occurs at about 30, and constant lethargy if the level is about 40.

Preparation of Client and Collection of Sample

The laboratory needs 1 ml of serum. Note the time of the last dose, the route, and the amount of phenytoin. Intramuscular injection of phenytoin, rather than oral administration, reduces blood levels about 50%. Levels are usually drawn about 3 hours after the last dose. Caffeine, theophylline, probenecid (Benemid), warfarin, and quinidine interfere with the results.

Reference Values for Phenytoin	
10–20 µg/ml	As an anticonvulsant
10–18 µg/ml	As an antiarrhythmic

PRIMIDONE (MYSOLINE, PRIMOLINE)

Primidone is not a barbiturate, but it is closely related, with similar actions. Primidone is used for the control of certain types of epilepsy. Doses higher than the therapeutic range can, however, cause significant ataxia and lethargy. The laboratory needs 1 ml of serum.

Reference Values for Primidone	
Therapeutic level	4–12 µg/ml

VALPROIC ACID (DEPAKENE)

Valproic acid is a relatively new anticonvulsant that is given orally. Because valproic acid has a short biological half-life, the time of the last dose and the time of the sampling must be considered carefully when judging the clinical effect from a certain concentration. A short half-life means that it is cleared from the serum in a short time. A steady state of valproic acid is reached in about 40 hours. The laboratory needs 1 ml of serum.

Reference Value for Valproic Acid

Therapeutic range	50–100 μg/ml

PHENOBARBITAL (LUMINAL)

Phenobarbital is a long-acting barbiturate (see later discussion of barbiturate panel) that is sometimes used in conjunction with other anticonvulsants. Phenobarbital is also given as treatment for neonatal bilirubinemia (see Chapter 11) and as a treatment for increased intracranial pressure.

Preparation of Client and Collection of Sample

The laboratory needs 1 ml of serum. The dose, the time of the last dose, and the time of the sampling should be noted. Because phenobarbital is long-acting and cumulative, the client's daily dose should also be noted. Clients can develop a tolerance to high levels of phenobarbital if the increase is gradual. Valproic acid may raise the phenobarbital level (Howard, 1986).

Reference Values for Phenobarbital

Therapeutic range	For anticonvulsant control 15–50 μg/ml
Newborn	Levels over 40 μg may cause apnea

CARBAMAZEPINE (TEGRETOL)

Carbamazepine is used for seizure control but can itself cause seizures if the serum level is above the therapeutic range. The most widely feared side effect is bone marrow depression (Jacobs et al., 1984). Clients need monitoring with a CBC (Chapter 2) and platelet counts (Chapter 13). It takes about two weeks for the drug to reach the steady state. Many drugs interfere with this test.

Reference Values for Carbamazepine

Therapeutic range	4–12 μg/ml (some laboratories use 2–10)

ETHOSUXIMIDE (ZARONTIN)

Ethosuximide is used to treat petit mal seizures. Toxic effects include gastrointestinal disturbances, headaches, dizziness, and fatigue. A rarer side effect is a lupus-like syndrome. Peak or trough levels can be measured as the drug has a fairly constant serum level.

Reference Values for Ethosuximide	
Therapeutic range	40–100 μg/ml

POSSIBLE NURSING DIAGNOSIS FOR ANTICONVULSANT THERAPY

Potential for Injury Related to Gait Disturbance and Seizure Activity
As noted above, most of the anticonvulsants in higher-than-therapeutic levels in the bloodstream can lead to ataxia, gait disturbances, dizziness, and/or drowiness. Attention to safety needs is warranted. And if the anticonvulsants are in the lower-than-therapeutic range, the client may be vulnerable to a return of seizure activity. However, if there are no side effects, long-term monitoring may not be needed. Over the years there is less of a tendency for fully controlled seizures to return, and it is likely lower serum levels will continue to be effective (Troupin, 1984).

■ ANTIPSYCHOTIC AGENT: LITHIUM CARBONATE

Lithium (Lithane, Eskalith, Lithonate) is a psychotherapeutic agent used to treat manic clients with certain types of bipolar depression (manic depressives). When the dosage is being adjusted, blood samples are done one to two times a week. Blood for the serum level may be drawn 8–12 hours after the dosage is given. After a therapeutic dosage level has been established, the client may have serum lithium levels done on a monthly basis. Newman (1979) has suggested that red cell lithium levels may be more reliable indicators of incipient toxicity than serum levels. Electroencephalograms (EEG) may also be done to evaluate the neurotoxicity from lithium.

Preparation of Client and Collection of Sample
The laboratory needs 1 ml of serum. Lithium samples are drawn 8–12 hours after the dosage. Note the amount, the route, and the time of the last dosage on the laboratory request.

Reference Values for Lithium	
Therapeutic range	0.5–1.5 mEq/L

POSSIBLE NURSING DIAGNOSIS FOR LITHIUM LEVELS

Potential Injury Related to Toxicity or Adverse Reactions

Lithium toxicity is a very serious problem. In some clients, particularly the elderly, neurotoxicity can develop even with normal serum levels. Hence clients must be assessed for such symptoms as diarrhea, vomiting, muscle weakness, and incoordination. An important nursing implication is to make sure that these clients have normal amounts of salt because lithium toxicity may be greater if serum sodium levels are low. (See Chapter 5 on diets with high sodium content.) Hypothyroidism (Chapter 15) is one of the chronic adverse reactions (McDermott, 1983).

■ TRICYCLIC ANTIDEPRESSANTS

Jacobs et al. (1984) note that the tricyclic antidepressant drugs represent a frequent and serious problem in both unintentional and intentional overdosage. These drugs may take up to a month to relieve depression, and needed dosage adjustments vary from person to person. The steady state is obtained after one week of a dose schedule. Many drugs interfere with the test results.

Reference Values for Antidepressants

Imipramine (Tofranil)	75–250 ng/ml
Desipramine (Norpramin)	150–300 ng/ml
Amitriptyline (Elavil)	125–250 ng/ml
Nortriptyline (Aventyl)	50–150 ng/ml
Doxepin (Sinequan)	75–300 ng/ml

POSSIBLE NURSING DIAGNOSIS FOR ANTIDEPRESSANTS

Potential for Injury Related to Possible Adverse Reactions of Antidepressant Drugs

The client on antidepressant drugs needs careful assessment for adverse reactions, which can include cardiotoxicity and orthostatic hypotension. Clients receiving these drugs are suffering from clinical depression, so usual client teaching may be difficult. Significant others must be educated about ways to decrease potential problems from long-term use. Govoni and Hayes (1985) list three pages of nursing implications for imipramine (Tofranil), the prototype for this classification of drugs. Boehnert and Lovejoy (1985) found that serum drug levels failed to identify clients with the toxic effects of ventricular arrhythmias or seizures. The prolongation of the QRS duration, noted by ECG, was a better predictor (see Chapter 24 on electrocardiography).

■ BRONCHODILATORS: THEOPHYLLINE PRODUCTS AND CAFFEINE LEVELS

Theophylline and its derivatives, such as aminophylline, dyphylline, and oxtriphylline, are all used as bronchodilators. For example, theophylline or a theophylline derivative is usually the primary drug for the treatment of asthma. There are many brand names for theophylline and the derivatives: Aminodur, Theo-Dur, Choledyl, Bronkodyl, Elixophyllin and various others. Consult a pharmacology text for peak times and durations of the various products. The timing of the serum samples varies with the exact form of theophylline or theophylline derivative used. For example, because aminophylline is 85% theophylline, aminophylline causes different theophylline levels than do other theophylline products.

If theophylline products are being given in high doses for an acute asthmatic attack, serum level monitoring is crucial. Because high serum levels of theophylline can result in life-threatening cardiac arrhythmias and seizures, the Federal Drug Administration recommends that the safest approach to individualize dosages of theophylline or theophylline products is to monitor serum levels (FDA Drug Bulletin, 1980b). For clients who are on chronic theophylline therapy, measurement of trough levels as well as peak levels should be made. Clients who have abnormal liver function, who have congestive failure, or who are very young or very old may need very close monitoring of serum theophylline levels. Caffeine levels are sometimes ordered by neonatologists treating infants with theophylline because neonates quickly metabolize theophylline to caffeine.

Preparation of Client and Collection of Sample

The laboratory needs 3 ml of serum. The dose, the route, and the time of the last dose should be entered on the requisition. Note the specific times to draw peak and trough levels, which vary depending on the theophylline product being monitored. Because both theophylline and caffeine are xanthines, the client should not have coffee, colas, tea, chocolate, or any other sources of caffeine for several hours before the serum specimen is drawn. Cimetidine, erythromycin, and propranolol may raise serum levels. In rare instances, ranitidine can raise serum theophylline to toxic levels (Gardner & Sikorski, 1985).

Reference Values for Theophylline	
Therapeutic range	10–20 μg/ml
Risk of toxicity	Over 20 μg/ml

POSSIBLE NURSING DIAGNOSIS FOR THEOPHYLLINE LEVELS

Potential for Alteration in Cardiac Output and Anxiety
Nurses should be aware of early clinical symptoms of theophylline overdose. Because theophylline is a xanthine, as is caffeine, some of the early symptoms

of theophylline toxicity resemble a "coffee jag." Clients may have tachycardia with skipped beats. They may also be very nervous and jittery, with tremors of the hands. The dosage of theophylline must be readjusted to prevent further development of lethal cardiac arrhythmias and/or seizures.

■ CARDIAC DRUGS: DIGOXIN AND DIGITOXIN

Digoxin (Lanoxin) is a cardiotonic used to prevent or to treat congestive heart failure (CHF). Digoxin is also used to treat various types of atrial arrhythmias, such as atrial fibrillation (AF). Digoxin and the other forms of digitalis, such as digitoxin, are all cumulative in action, and thus serious toxicity can occur over time.

Preparation of Client and Collection of Sample
The laboratory needs 1 ml of serum. The dosage of digoxin or digitoxin, the route, and the time of the last dose should be included on the requisition. (Digoxin is given only orally or intravenously because the intramuscular route has an erratic absorption rate.) The serum level is usually drawn at a minimum of 16 hours after either an oral or intravenous dose because it takes at least this long for the drug to equilibrate in the tissues. Falsely elevated levels are caused by drugs such as spironolactone (Aldactone) and prednisone. Nifedipine, verapamil and quinidine can increase serum digoxin levels and barbiturates and cholestyramine can increase serum digitoxin levels (Howard, 1986).

Reference Values for Digoxin and Digitoxin

Therapeutic range	
Digoxin, with dosage of 0.25 mg/day	0.8–1.6 ng/ml
Digoxin, with dosage of 0.5 mg/day	1.1–1.9 ng/ml

Some sources give a wider range of 1–3 ng/ml, with much emphasis on clinical data to substantiate toxicity.

POSSIBLE NURSING DIAGNOSIS FOR DIGOXIN

Potential for Injury Related to Development of Digitalis Toxicity
To prevent digitalis toxicity, the key nursing implication is to monitor the client's pulse before digoxin is given. Digoxin, or other digitalis products, should be withheld and the doctor notified if the adult's pulse is below 60. Usually a pulse below 70 is the guideline for children, but this criterion varies depending on age. Clients should be taught to take their own pulses because, once digoxin is begun, it is usually continued on a long-term basis. Other symptoms of digitalis toxicity—such as nausea and vomiting, diarrhea, headaches, and visual disturbance—are also sometimes relied upon to signal digitalis toxicity. An electrocardiogram (ECG) also helps the clinician determine whether there is a toxic effect from digoxin. However, the symptoms of mild toxicity from digoxin may not be readily noted by clinical assessment or ECG data. A measurement of

serum levels of digoxin therefore aids in determining whether symptoms are due to a higher-than-necessary digoxin level.

Other laboratory tests that are important in assessing for potential digitalis toxicity are the serum potassium and the serum calcium levels. The nurse needs to be aware that a low serum potassium or a high serum calcium level tends to increase the risk of digitalis toxicity, even though the serum digoxin levels are not high. (See Chapter 5 on potassium and Chapter 7 on calcium levels.) Because digoxin is excreted by the kidneys, clients with poor renal function are also more prone to develop digitalis toxicity. (See Chapter 4 for tests of renal function, BUN and creatinine.)

■ ANTIARRHYTHMIC DRUGS

QUINIDINE

Quinidine (Quinaglute, Cin-Quin, Quinidex, Cardioquin, and others) is an alkaloid obtained from the bark of the cinchona tree. Hence toxicity from quinidine products is sometimes referred to as cinchonism. Since quinidine depresses the excitability of the heart, it is used as an antiarrhythmic drug. It can be given intravenously for acute states or orally as a long-term maintenance drug. Serum quinidine levels help the clinician to adjust the dosage to the correct amount for the individual client. In fact, quinidine is the antiarrhythmic drug that is most often monitored by serum levels. Because the toxicity from chronic use may not be readily apparent or may be attributed to other causes, peak and trough levels can be used to ascertain whether clients are in a therapeutic range.

Preparation of Client and Collection of Sample
The dosage, the time of the last dose, and the route should all be noted on the lab requisition. The peak level for quinidine occurs about 2 hours after the dose. The laboratory needs 1 ml of serum. Concurrent use of phenytoin or barbiturates may lower serum quinidine level.

Reference Values for Quinidine

Therapeutic range	1.2–4.0 μg/ml
Toxic range	5–6 μg/ml

POSSIBLE NURSING DIAGNOSIS FOR QUINIDINE

Potential for Alteration in Cardiac Output and Other Adverse Reactions
Nurses should be aware that quinidine, particularly in the intravenous form, can cause severe bradycardia and hypotension. Hypersensitivity reactions, gastrointestinal upsets, and central nervous system effects, such as tremors or even coma, can occur with quinidine toxicity. When a dosage schedule is being started, these clients need to have their pulses and blood pressures closely monitored.

PROCAINAMIDE OR NAPA

Procainamide (Pronestyl) is usually given orally for long-term prevention of arrhythmias. As with quinidine products, serum peak and trough levels help to prevent toxicity such as myocardial depression. Some laboratories measure N-acetyl procainamide (NAPA), the active metabolite of procainamide.

Preparation of Client and Collection of Sample
The dosage, the route, and the time of the last dose should be noted on the laboratory request. The level is usually drawn about 3 hours after the last dose.

Reference Values for Procainamide and NAPA	
Procainamide therapeutic level	4–10 μg/ml
NAPA therapeutic level	2–8 μg/ml

PHENYTOIN

Although phenytoin (Dilantin) is more commonly used as an anticonvulsant, it is also sometimes used to control cardiac arrhythmias, such as those caused by digitalis toxicity. It is not, however, as commonly used as procainamide or quinidine for long-term prevention of arrhythmias. (See the reference values under anticonvulsant drugs.)

PROPRANOLOL

Propranolol (Inderal) is used for the treatment of certain arrhythmias because it is a beta-adrenergic blocker. Because propranolol decreases the rate and the force of heart contraction, hypotension and bradycardia are serious side effects. Propranolol is used in combination with other drugs for the treatment of hypertension.

   Serum levels of propranolol may occasionally be drawn, but doing so is not a common practice because a wide range is included in the therapeutic index (Conrad, 1978).

Preparation of Client and Collection of Sample
The dosage, the route, and the time of the last dose should be noted on the laboratory slip. Check with the laboratory on the timing of the sample, which is usually drawn 4 hours after the last dose of this beta-blocking agent.

LIDOCAINE

Lidocaine (Xylocaine) is given intravenously for the immediate control of premature ventricular contractions (PVCs). Because lidocaine is usually given only on an intermittent basis when the need arises, lidocaine levels are seldom measured. If clients have a continuous lidocaine drop, there may be a need to monitor serum levels. Cimetidine and propranolol may cause increased serum levels of lidocaine.

Reference Values for Propranolol	
Therapeutic range	100–300 ng/ml

Includes bioactive 4-OH metabolite.

Preparation of Client and Collection of Sample
Note the concentration of the drug and the rate of intravenous administration on the laboratory request.

Reference Values for Lidocaine	
Therapeutic range	1.5–6 μg/ml

■ SALICYLATES: ACETYLSALICYLIC ACID (ASA)

Acetylsalicylic acid, or aspirin, is used as an analgesic, as an anti-inflammatory agent, and as an anticoagulant. ASA is a component of many over-the-counter (OTC) pain relievers, such as Anacin, Bufferin, Excedrin, and others. Aspirin poisoning is the most common type of poisoning in children. Adults may also take ASA or ASA-containing drugs in a suicidal gesture. In an overdose case, the laboratory can do a screen of a serum sample to see whether ASA is the culprit. (If an overdose has occurred, gastric contents and urine specimens should also be sent to the laboratory, if available.)

Mild intoxication, or salicylism, causes a ringing in the ears (tinnitus) and gastric upsets. Because ASA acts as a respiratory stimulant, the hyperventilation that may result from aspirin overdose can cause respiratory alkalosis. (See Chapter 6 on acid-base balance.) Large doses of ASA may also cause gastrointestinal bleeding, which is due to the irritant effect on the gastric mucosa and to the interference with coagulation factors.

With its anticoagulant properties, ASA is sometimes used as a regular medication for clients who have a high potential for thromboembolic episodes. Serum ASA levels may be done to prevent ASA toxicity.

ASA is also commonly used in high doses for clients who may benefit from the anti-inflammatory properties of ASA. For example, clients with rheumatoid arthritis may be on large doses of ASA over a long period of time. It may take 12–20 grV aspirin tablets to keep the serum level around 20 mg/dl. Serum ASA levels may be done periodically to aid in maintaining the client in a therapeutic but not a toxic range. Sometimes clients are afraid to take enough ASA to really ever achieve therapeutic benefit. Serum levels may be used to evaluate whether they are complying with the plan.

Preparation of Client and Collection of Sample
The laboratory needs 2 ml of plasma, collected in a heparin (green top) or EDTA (lavender top) tube. In the case of an overdose client, urine, any vomitus, or gastric lavage should be saved for laboratory analysis, too. For a routine assessment of salicylate level, the total daily dosage of ASA should be noted, as well as the time and amount of the last dose. Note exactly how many *tablets* the client says he or

she takes a day. Do not rely on what the physician has ordered and assume that the client has followed this dose at home.

Reference Values for Salicylates

Therapeutic range (3 hours after dose)
    Children to age 10   25–30 mg/100 ml
    Adult   20–25 mg/100 ml
Toxic range
    Children and adult   Over 30 mg/100 ml
    After age 60   Over 20 mg/100 ml
Lethal range may be around 60 mg/100 ml

■ URINE TESTING: PHENISTIX

Phenistix (Ames Product Information, 1980) are reagent strips used primarily to test for phenylketones in the urine. (See Chapter 18 for a discussion on PKU.) However, metabolites of aspirin, other salicylates, and phenothiazines also cause color changes in Phenistix. The color chart used to detect salicylates or phenothiazines shows tan for small amounts and brown for large amounts. (The color change for PKU uses a different color chart.) Phenistix can be used as a screening device of urine to check for overdose with aspirin or phenothiazines. (Phenothiazine testing is covered later in this chapter.)

■ BLOOD ALCOHOL

Ethanol, or grain alcohol, is the type of alcohol in alcoholic beverages. Ethanol, undoubtedly the most commonly abused drug, may often be one of the drugs involved in an overdose. As part of a toxicology screen, the laboratory may do an alcohol panel that, in addition to ethanol, includes methanol (wood alcohol), isopropyl (rubbing alcohol), and acetone (an alcohol-related compound). A serum osmolality test (Chapter 4) may also be used to screen for ethanol or methanol. Alcohol and related toxic compounds may be ingested by drinking undrinkable solutions, such as cleaning fluids, shaving lotions, or disinfectants. Methanol is particularly dangerous because it can result in convulsions, blindness, and possibly death.

In addition to determining the cause of a coma, blood alcohol tests are also used to determine whether a driver was intoxicated at the time of an accident. The drawing of the blood specimen must be done in a medically suitable environment according to the legal requirements of the state. (Breath analyzers are used at the scene of the accident, so nurses are not involved in obtaining samples.) Nurses who are trained in venipuncture may draw the blood for alcohol blood samples when the client is brought to the emergency room for medical treatment. George (1976) noted that many hospitals do not permit nurses or technicians to obtain specimens at the request of the police. The reluctance to involve hospital staff in drawing blood for legal evidence is based on the facts that the persons drawing the blood may not know the exact legal ramifications of the procedure and that they will probably be subpoenaed to testify in a court case. Although it is permissible for qualified nurses to draw blood for the alcohol test, it is important that they understand the legal ramifications of the procedure and the policy for nurses in a particular institution. Blood may be drawn without consent in some states if the blood is drawn in a legally and medically accepted manner (Buley, 1986). A refusal to allow blood to be drawn may have legal consequences.

Legal Definitions of Intoxication

Each state determines the exact blood alcohol level that is considered legally permissible for driving. Levels over 0.10% are considered proof of intoxication in the majority of states. A few states have higher levels (0.12 to 0.15) and a few as low as 0.08. Some people may not be sober with very low blood alcohol levels, but the exact line for sobriety is disputable. Holum (1983) notes that as little as 0.05% means the person is no longer sober and that the risk of an auto accident for a driver with 0.20% alcohol in the blood is a hundred times higher than for the sober driver.

With regard to the legal meaning of a blood alcohol level, the recommendation of the National Safety Council on alcohol and drugs is:

1. Less than 0.05%: No influence by alcohol within the meaning of the law.
2. Between 0.05% and 0.10%: Alcohol influence is usually present, but courts of law are advised to consider the person's behavior and the circumstances that led to the arrest.
3. Above 0.10%: Definite evidence of being "under the influence."

Relationship of Alcohol to Other Laboratory Tests

In addition to the usual symptoms of alcohol intoxication, the client with alcohol abuse may have severe hypoglycemia, because alcohol tends to inhibit the formation of glucose. (See Chapter 8 for symptoms and treatment of hypoglycemia.) Alcohol-induced hypoglycemia carries a high mortality if not identified and corrected. The mortality is particularly high for children (Dipp, 1978). High blood alcohol levels are also a major cause of secondary hyperlipidemia. (See Chapter 9 on serum triglyceride levels.) High alcohol levels in the pregnant woman are of grave concern because of the fetal alcohol syndrome (Ouellette, 1984).

Reference Values for Serum Alcohol

Ethanol or Ethyl (Grain) Alcohol	
0.00%–0.05%	Sobriety is presumed
0.05%–0.01%	"Gray zone"
0.10%–0.15%	Legal limit, depending on state law (a few states have as low as 0.08)
0.30%–0.40%	Marked intoxication
0.40%–0.50%	Severe toxic effects with alcoholic stupor
0.50%–over	Coma and death possible
Methanol or Methyl (Wood) Alcohol	
25 mg/dl	Toxic level
80–115 mg/dl	Lethal

Preparation of Client and Collection of Blood Sample

The client should give consent for a blood specimen, but blood may be drawn without consent in some states if the blood is drawn in a legally and medically accepted manner, as noted earlier. Be aware of the legal ramifications, state requirements, and the individual hospital's policy. No alcohol, such as alcohol wipes, should be used to obtain the blood specimen. Iodine or an aqueous germicidal solution such as benzalkonium, can be used. Tinctures should not be used, because they have an alcohol base. The laboratory needs 2 ml of blood in an oxalated tube (black top). The specimen should be refrigerated if it cannot be sent to the laboratory immediately.

■ BARBITURATES

The barbiturates are used as anticonvulsants, as sedatives, and as hypnotics. The most severe effect of overdosage with barbiturates is respiratory failure followed by circulatory collapse. Because the various barbiturates are often used in overdoses, the laboratory runs a barbiturate panel when clients are comatose from an unknown cause. The barbiturates usually measured include:

1. Short-acting ones—pentobarbital (Nembutal) and secobarbital (Seconal)
2. Intermediate-acting ones—amobarbital (Amytal,) butabarbital (Butisol, Butacaps) and aprobarbital (Alurate)
3. Long-acting ones—phenobarbital (Luminal) and mephobarbital (Mebaral)

A smaller amount of the short-acting barbiturates, as opposed to a larger amount for the long-acting barbiturates, causes coma. A toxicology screen for barbiturate overdose also includes an analysis of urine samples and gastric contents. So any vomitus or gastric lavage products should be saved for laboratory analysis.

Preparation of Client and Collection of Blood Sample

The laboratory needs 5 ml or less of serum depending on the method used. Note any drugs that the client may have taken. Theophylline, for example, can cause a false elevation of the barbiturate level as can valproic acid.

Reference Values for Barbiturates

Short-acting barbiturates   Coma level at about 1–3 mg/dl
Long-acting barbiturates   Coma level at about 9–10 mg/dl
See the section on anticonvulsants for the measurement of therapeutic levels of
  phenobarbital.

■ TOXICOLOGY SCREENS IN BLOOD AND URINE

DRUGS OTHER THAN BARBITURATES

In addition to barbiturates, many other sedative/hypnotic drugs have the potential for overdosage through drug abuse. Laboratories screen for these sedative/hypnotics when the cause of the overdose is not known. Three common hypnotic drugs that can cause coma are glutethimide (Doriden), methyprylon (Noludar), and ethchlorvynol (Placidyl).

The following drugs may be tested for in urine screening:

1. Narcotics (codeine, morphine, methadone, etc.)
2. Phenothiazines (prochlorperazine, chlorpromazine, etc.)
3. Tricyclic antidepressants (imipramine, amitriptyline, etc.)
4. Stimulants (amphetamines, methylphenidate, etc.)
5. Antihistamines (diphenhydramine, chlorpheniramine)
6. Phencyclidine (PCP)
7. Cocaine (as benzoylecgonine metabolite)
8. Other drugs, such as acetaminophen.

Preparation of Client and Collection of Sample

A urine sample of 50–100 ml is needed for complete toxicology screen. Check with the individual laboratory. Only a small amount is needed if screening for a special drug, such as cocaine. Consult current literature for the legal status of requiring urine screens for employees.

MINOR TRANQUILIZERS AND PROPOXYPHENE

Three minor tranquilizers or antianxiety agents may be associated with drug abuse. These three minor tranquilizers are diazepam (Valium), meprobamate (Equanil, Miltown, and others), and chlordiazepoxide (Librium). For several years, diazepam (Valium) has been the most frequently prescribed prescription drug. Reports from the Drug Abuse Warning Network (FDA Drug Bulletin, 1980a) show that, in 1978, diazepam ranked second only to alcohol as the drug most often combined with other drugs in drug abuse episodes treated in emergency rooms.

Propoxyphene (Darvon) is a prescription analgesic that is often associated with drug deaths. Many of these deaths are in association with alcohol and tranquilizers. Clients at particular risk of propoxyphene-associated deaths include adolescents and young adults who engage in multidrug abuse. Also, clients with chronic pain and depression are likely to use propoxyphene in deliberate overuse or abuse (FDA Drug Bulletin, 1980c).

OPIATE ABUSE

Opiates, such as morphine or methadone, can be measured in the urine as well as in the serum. Opiates are measured in the serum to see if they are present in a high enough level to be the cause of coma. Narcotic antagonists can then be used to reverse a narcotic coma. For detecting chronic abuse, urine tests may be used. Detecting opiate abuse by laboratory methods is difficult because clients may refrain from drugs if they are to have testing done. Recently, the analysis of human hair by radioimmunoassay (RIA) has been developed as a way to detect opiate use (See Chapter 15 for the RIA method). Baumgartner et al. (1979) discuss the impact of the test (Abuscan I-123 by Roche Diagnostics) that can detect morphine content for the life of the hair. Obviously, many legal and ethical considerations come into play when clients who are not comatose are tested for suspected drug abuse. Refer to current literature for the legal issues in dealing with the complex problem of suspected or known drug abuse. Employers may wish to screen all their employees, and this has created much controversy.

POSSIBLE NURSING DIAGNOSIS RELATED TO ELEVATED DRUG LEVELS, INCLUDING ALCOHOL

Alterations in Sensory Perception
The focus for nursing interventions is to promote a sense of reality by explaining environmental stimuli and also reducing those stimuli. Because the altered perceptions may be frightening, the client needs reassurance of safety and protection by health care workers (Carpenito, 1985). Long-term management for drug abuse would necessitate other nursing diagnoses based on the individual client's needs and coping methods.

■ BROMIDE

Bromide is an ingredient in several OTC drugs that are used as sleeping aids and "nerve tonics." Too often, the clients and the health professionals consider all OTC drugs as harmless. Bromide, a central nervous system depressant, in large doses can cause toxicity, which is called bromism. Clients with inadequate renal function are particularly susceptible to bromide overdosage.

The symptoms of bromism are nonspecific, but they usually include signs and symptoms of central nervous system toxicity, such as muscle incoordination and impaired intellectual functioning. The patient may have vomiting and a rash. A public health nurse or clinic nurse may detect clients with symptoms of bromism. A health history should contain a list of all OTC drugs that these clients take.

Preparation of Client and Collection of Sample
The laboratory needs 3 ml of serum. All medications that contain bromide should be noted. Iodine will falsely elevate levels. (Also high levels of bromide will falsely elevate the chloride levels [Jacobs et al., 1984].)

Reference Values for Bromide	
Toxic level in serum	Above 17 mEq/L

■ MAJOR TRANQUILIZERS: PHENOTHIAZINES

Phenothiazines are used in high dosages as antipsychotic agents. The phenothiazine most often used for schizophrenic clients is chlorpromazine (Thorazine). Other phenothiazines commonly used as major tranquilizers include fluphenazine (Prolixin), trifluoperazine (Stelazine), thioridazine (Mellaril), and promazine (Sparine). Serum levels of phenothiazines are usually not used to regulate dosage because the serum levels do not correlate well either with toxic or with therapeutic effects of the drugs. Phenothiazines are occasionally monitored in the urine, and, in the case of a suspected overdose, the laboratory can screen the urine for the presence of phenothiazines. (See the discussion on urine testing with Phenistix, which is a quick method to screen for phenothiazines.)

■ HEAVY METAL POISONING: LEAD

Heavy metal poisoning can result from the ingestion or inhalation of zinc, mercury, arsenic, or lead that is used in paint, in insecticides, or in other substances. To discover the presence of a heavy metal, laboratories do screening tests of urine.

Among children, lead toxicity is second only to malnutrition as a major public health problem in the United States. Anders (1985) reports that the Centers for Disease Control estimate 675,000 preschoolers suffer some degree of lead poisoning. Exposure to lead is also an occupational hazard for some adults. The person usually has a variety of chronic symptoms, such as abdominal pain, weakness, and eventually neurological dysfunction, with the potential for permanent brain damage. Because lead interferes with the normal synthesis of red blood cells, clients have anemia and characteristic changes in the peripheral blood smear (see Chapter 2).

Preparation of Client and Collection of Sample
The laboratory needs 2 ml of blood. It is very important that all the blood drawing equipment be free from lead or lead particles. Special collection tubes have brown tops to notify they are lead free. A complete history is needed concerning the client's exposure to toxic chemicals, etc. Most public health surveys will have a definite assessment guide that is to be followed when interviewing clients. The possible exposure of other people in the client's environment must be considered, too. Industrial pollution can be a major public health problem.

Reference Values for Serum Lead

Centers for Disease Control (1985) consider levels above 25 μg/100 ml toxic for lead.

ALA-D TESTS FOR LEAD POISONING AND FEP (FREE ERYTHROCYTE PROTOPORPHYRIN)

Laboratories may do screens for lead poisoning by enzyme testing of ALA-D (aminolevulinic acid-delta), an enzyme that is increased after lead exposure. The free erythrocyte protoporphyrin (FEP) is another screening test that requires only a drop of blood on a filter paper. The Centers for Disease Control (1985) recommends that children be screened by this test. Enzyme levels and porphyrins may also be measured in the urine. The actual confirmation of lead toxicity may be difficult when the exposure to lead is either too small or not current enough to change serum lead levels. (See Chapter 3 for a discussion on the 24-hour urine specimen for ALA-D and porphyrins.

Reference Values for FEP

Toxic level less than 35 μg/dl (Centers for Disease Control, 1985)

POSSIBLE NURSING DIAGNOSIS FOR LEAD POISONING

Impaired Health Maintenance Related to Unhealthy Environment
In the past few years, nurses have been involved in doing lead screening for children who may have chronic lead poisoning. The child most likely to get lead poisoning is a preschool child who lives in a poorly maintained house. Lead was banned as an ingredient in interior paint in 1977, but older houses that have not been repainted may still contain lead paint. Lead screening programs have been done by the government in areas where the prevalence of lead poisoning is great. Croft and Frenkel (1975) report about the lead screening and treatment program for children in a southern city, describing in detail the role of the nurses in a community survey.

The treatment of lead poisoning is a process called *chelation*. For deleading by chelation, the client is given the calcium salt of a chemical called EDTA. Lead replaces the calcium, and the lead-EDTA is excreted in the urine. (Note that other heavy metal poisoning may also be treated with various types of chelating products.)

QUESTIONS

1. Serum levels of drugs may be needed when the risk of toxicity from a drug is increased. Factors that increase the toxicity of most drugs include all *except* which?

    a. Increase in dosage
    b. Use of intravenous rather than intramuscular or oral route
    c. Hepatic dysfunction
    d. Increased urine output due to increased intake of fluids

2. Mr. Telerechio is having blood drawn for peak and trough serum antibiotic levels. The nurse should be aware that the type of antibiotics that are commonly monitored by serum levels are the:

    a. Penicillins
    b. Cephalosporins
    c. Aminoglycosides
    d. Tetracyclines

3. Bobby, age 13, is an epileptic whose seizures are controlled by phenytoin (Dilantin). A serum phenytoin level drawn today was 23 μg/ml. Because he is

slightly above the therapeutic range of 10–20 μg/ml, he may begin to show a symptom of early phenytoin toxicity, which is:

a. Severe lethargy

b. Cardiac arrhythmias

c. Gait ataxia

d. Nystagmus (involuntary rapid movements of the eyeballs)

4. Molley Faber is a psychiatric client being observed in a mental health clinic. Which of the following antipsychotic drugs requires monitoring by serum levels?

a. Chlorpromazine (Thorazine)   c. Fluphenazine (Prolixin)
b. Lithium carbonate (Lithane)   d. Thioridazine (Mellaril)

5. Johnny, age 8, is receiving aminophylline 20 mg an hour via the intravenous route for treatment of an acute asthmatic attack. Because aminophylline is a theophylline derivative, serum theophylline levels have been measured. His latest level of 30 μg/ml is considerably higher than the desired therapeutic range of 10–20 μg/ml. The nurse needs to make assessments of the client and be prepared for potential:

a. Cardiac arrhythmias and seizures   c. Renal and hepatic failure
b. Bronchospasms and dyspnea   d. Hypertension crisis and stroke

6. Johnny has recovered from his acute asthmatic attack. He is being discharged with instructions to take a theophylline suspension (Elixophyllin 50 mg) every 6 hours. Johnny and his parents need to be taught that early symptoms of overdose from this drug may be similar to which of the following?

a. Deep sleep   c. Another asthmatic attack
b. Overuse of coffee   d. Cold or flu

7. Mr. Gardener is a 78-year-old man who is on digoxin 0.25 mg/day due to congestive heart failure (CHF). He is being visited by a community health nurse. Which of the following information in Mr. Gardener's health history should alert the nurse to the fact that this client should be closely watched for digoxin toxicity?

a. Large intake of sodium in the diet, refusal of visit from dietician

b. Slightly low-serum calcium level caused by a possible endocrine problem, work-up in progress

c. Poor renal function as evidenced by increased serum creatinine

d. History of noncompliance with physician's orders

8. Mrs. Ramos has a serum quinidine level of 4 μg/ml, which is higher than the therapeutic range of 1.5–3 μg/ml. Because there may be possible toxic effects from the quinidine, the nurse should assess and record which of the following?

a. Level of consciousness every 2 hours

b. Blood pressure and pulse every 2 hours

c. Lack of appetite or other gastrointestinal symptoms

d. Hourly urine output

9. Serum aspirin (ASA) levels may be part of the necessary clinical assessment for all of the following clients *except* which?

   a. Mr. Fink, who uses ASA p.r.n. for a headache

   b. Sally, age 2½, who was found in the bathroom playing with an empty bottle of Bufferin

   c. Mrs. Catalina, who takes ASA gr X q.i.d. for treatment of rheumatoid arthritis

   d. Mr. Weber, who is on ASA gr X b.i.d. for an anticoagulant effect and who is complaining of ringing in his ears (tinnitus)

10. In relation to blood alcohol levels, the emergency room nurse should know that all of the following are true *except* which?

    a. Alcohol should not be used to wipe the skin before the blood specimen is drawn

    b. A blood alcohol over 0.15% is usually considered legal evidence of intoxication, but this criterion may vary from state to state

    c. The client's permission should be obtained for a blood specimen according to legal requirements

    d. The person who draws the blood may be subpoenaed to testify in a court case

11. Mrs. Gearhart is a 78-year-old woman who uses various over-the-counter (OTC) sleeping medications and nerve tonics. Mrs. Gearhart's niece reports to the home care nurse that her aunt has become very forgetful and irritable since she increased her nerve tonic. The niece thinks her aunt is taking "too much nonprescribed medicine." After looking at the ingredients in the OTC medicine, the nurse may need to refer Mrs. Gearhart for a medical evaluation of possible:

    a. Salicylism (aspirin toxicity)   c. Plumbism (lead poisoning)

    b. Cinchonism (quinidine toxicity)   d. Bromism (bromide toxicity)

12. A public health nurse should be aware that the major source for lead poisoning in young children is which of the following?

    a. Contaminated food   c. Polluted water

    b. Lead-based paint   d. Fumes from industrial plants

REFERENCES

Anders, M. (1985, November 10). The silent epidemic of lead poisoning. *San Francisco Examiner,* p. E-4.

Ames Product Information. (1980). *Phenistix reagent strips.* Elkhart, IN: Ames Co., Miles Laboratories.

Baumgartner, A., et al. (1979). Radioimmunoassay of hair for determining opiate abuse histories. *Journal of Nuclear Medicine, 20,* 748–752.

Boehnert, M., & Lovejoy, F. (1985). Value of the QRS duration versus the serum drug level in predicting seizures and ventricular arrhythmia after an acute dose of tricyclic anti-depressants. *NEJM, 313*(8), 474–477.

Buley, D. (1986). When the burden of proof falls on you. *Nursing 86, 16*(2), 41.

Carpenito, L. (1985). Altered thoughts or altered perceptions? *AJN,* (11), 1283.

Centers for Disease Control. (1985). *Preventing lead poisoning in young children.* Atlanta: Department of Health and Human Services.

Conrad, K. (1978). Measurement of drug levels in clinical practice. *Arizona Medicine, 35,* 747–748.

Croft, H., & Frenkel, S. (1975). Children and lead poisoning. *AJN, 75*(1), 102–104.

Dipp, S. (1978). Metabolic effects of alcohol. *Arizona Medicine, 35,* 651–652.

Federal Drug Administration. (1980a). Prescribing minor tranquilizers. *FDA Drug Bulletin 10,* 2–3.

Federal Drug Administration. (1980b). Dosage guidelines for theophylline products. *FDA Drug Bulletin 10,* 4–6.

Federal Drug Administration. (1980c). Propoxyphene prescriptions. *FDA Drug Bulletin 10,* 11.

Gardner, M., & Sikorski, G. (1985). Ranitidine and theophylline. *Annals of Internal Medicine, 102*(4), 559.

George, J. (1976). Blood alcohol tests. *Journal of Emergency Nursing, 2,* 7.

Govoni, L., & Hayes, J. (1985). *Drugs and nursing implications* (5th ed.). Norwalk, CT: Appleton-Century-Crofts.

Hewitt, W., & McHenry, M. (1978). Blood level determinations of antimicrobial drugs. *Medical Clinics of North America, 62,* 1119–1137.

Holum, J. (1983). *Elements of general and biological chemistry* (5th ed.). New York: Wiley.

Howard, P. (1986). A crash course in serum drug monitoring. *RN, 49*(4), 20–25.

Jacobs, D., Kasten, B., DeMott, W., & Wolfson, W. (1984). *Laboratory test handbook with DRG index.* St. Louis: Mosby/Lexi.

Langslet, J., & Habel, M. (1981). The aminoglycoside antibiotics. *AJN, 81*(6), 1144–1146.

Lerner, A., et al. (1983). Randomized, controlled trial of the comparative efficacy, auditory toxicity, and nephrotoxicity of tobramycin and netilmicin. *Lancet, 1,* 1123–1125.

McCormick, W., et al. (1978). Errors in measuring drug concentrations. *NEJM, 299*(20), 1118–1121.

McDermott, J. (1983). Your patient on lithium. *Nursing 83, 13*(8), 45–48.

Newman, P. (1979). Lithium neurotoxicity. *Postgraduate Medical Journal, 55,* 701–703.

Ouellette, E. (1984). The fetal alcohol syndrome. *Contemporary Nutrition, 9*(3), 1–2.

Richens, A., & Warrington, S. (1979). When should plasma drug levels be monitored? *Drugs, 17,* 488–500.

Scala, R. (1978). The duty to report hazards: A toxicologist's view. *Bulletin of New York Academy of Medicine, 54,* 774–781.

Squire, A., et al. (1984). Long-term antiarrhythmic therapy: Problem of low drug levels and patient noncompliance. *American Journal of Medicine, 77,* 1035–1038.

Troupin, A. (1984). The measurement of anticonvulsant agent levels. *Annals of Internal Medicine, 100*(2), 854–858.

Yoshikawa, T. (1980). Proper use of aminoglycosides. *American Family Physician, 21,* 125–130.

18

Tests Done in Pregnancy and the Newborn Period

- Urine Pregnancy Tests
  Biological Tests for Pregnancy and Immunological Tests for Pregnancy
- Serum HCG Levels
  HCG Qualitative Pregnancy Test and HCG Quantitative Test
- Alpha-Fetoprotein (AFP)
- Sickle Cell Anemia
- Thalassemia (Cooley's Anemia)
- Tay–Sachs Disease
- Estriol Levels
- Phenylketonuria (PKU)
- Hypothyroidism
- Galactosemia
- Sweat Test for Cystic Fibrosis (CF)

OBJECTIVES

1. Identify how a normal pregnancy changes the values of common laboratory tests, as compared with the women's prepregnancy values.
2. Explain the basic immunological principle of tests for pregnancy.
3. Explain which of the autosomal recessive genetic diseases are commonly tested by screening programs for certain ethnic groups.
4. Explain why PKU, galactosemia, and hypothyroidism are done as routine screening tests for newborns even though the infants appear healthy.
5. Describe the new screening test for cystic fibrosis.
6. Describe the appropriate nursing functions for a community health nurse who is following a family that has a child with a genetic defect.

Previous chapters have described some tests important in pregnancy (Table 18–1). Appendix D summarizes the expected changes in laboratory values in a normal pregnancy and some of the changes that occur with oral contraceptives. Appendix B highlights some expected changes in newborns. Although integration of content from all clinical settings is stressed in this book, some tests pertain *only* to the pregnant or to the newborn state. This chapter, therefore, focuses on common laboratory tests that are unique in maternal-child health settings.

Interwoven with all these advanced methods of testing is the nurse's involvement with the client as a person. The premise of this chapter is that pregnancy and childbirth should be joyous and healthy events for a couple. If tests must be used for a pregnancy, then the health professionals need to make sure that such tests are as unthreatening as possible. So the focus can be on what is normal about the pregnancy, not what may be abnormal.

PREGNANCY TESTS

Although pregnancy has early presumptive signs and symptoms, such as amenorrhea, nausea and vomiting, and skin changes, the positive signs are rarely present until a few months of pregnancy. Any one of the following signs is both legal and medical proof of pregnancy: (1) fetal heartbeat, (2) palpation of fetal outline, (3) recognition of fetal movements by someone other than the mother, and (4) ultrasonographic demonstration of the fetus.

In today's modern world, few, if any, women are willing to wait a few months to know for sure if they are pregnant. The desire to know as soon as possible is strong,

TABLE 18–1. ROUTINE TESTS DONE DURING PREGNANCY

Name of Test	Assessment	Location in Book
Hb–Hct	Anemia	Chap. 2 on CBC
Microscopic urinalysis (or nitrites and leukocyte esterase)	Possible urinary tract infection (UTI)	Chap. 3 on routine urinalysis, nitrites, and LE
Urine for protein	Possible toxemia	Chap. 3 on proteinuria
Urine for glucose	Possible diabetes	Chap. 8 for diabetes and pregnancy
Rh typing and unexpected antibody screen	Possible hemolytic disease of newborn (HDN)	Chap. 14 for Rh factor in pregnancy
STS	Possible congenital syphilis	Chap. 16 on syphilis and pregnancy
Rubella titer (done *before* pregnancy)	Immunity to 3-day measles	Chap. 14 on why rubella titers are done *before* pregnancy
Sickle cell (for black clients)	Also need to test father	Chap. 28 on follow-up

Note: Other tests, which are not routine, such as those for cytomegalovirus (CMV), AIDS, herpes (Chap. 14), and gonorrhea (Chap. 16), may be done if the pregnant woman is at high risk for these diseases, which will harm the fetus. Also see TORCH in Chapter 14.

both for the woman who desires a child and for the woman who may choose to terminate the pregnancy if it is present. A pregnancy test is also very important if the client is thought to have an ectopic pregnancy, as immediate surgical intervention is needed. Ectopic pregnancies are increasing as pelvic inflammatory disease increases (Devore & Baldwin, 1986).

All the pregnancy tests are based on detecting the presence of human chorionic gonadotropin (HCG) in the urine or serum of the pregnant woman. HCG, produced by the trophoblast cell component of the fetal placental tissue, can be measured as subunits of alpha and beta. The alpha subunit is identical with that of the luteinizing hormone (LH), follicle-stimulating hormone (FSH), and thyroid-stimulating hormone. The beta subunit is unique for HCG and thus is a more sensitive test for pregnancy (Jacobs et al., 1984). HCG is present in the serum within 6–10 days after implantation, peaks in 12–14 weeks, and remains elevated all during pregnancy. HCG is also produced by certain types of tumors of the testes or placenta. (See the quantitative test for HCG.) Although HCG can be measured directly in the serum to detect pregnancy (see the qualitative test for HCG), most pregnancy tests rely on indirect measurements of the amount of HCG in the urine.

■ URINE PREGNANCY TESTS

BIOLOGICAL TESTS FOR PREGNANCY

The older pregnancy tests used animals to test for pregnancy: Some of the woman's urine was injected into mice, rabbits, or frogs, and various changes in the animals were evidence that HCG was present. For example, HCG in the injected urine causes ovarian changes in rabbits. (Friedman test) and in mice (Achheim-Zondek [AZ] test). In frogs (Galli-Mainini test), sperm are found in the frog's urine if the injected urine contains HCG. With the advent of immunological techniques, these older, biological tests for pregnancy are only of historical interest.

IMMUNOLOGICAL TESTS FOR PREGNANCY

Pregnancy tests now use monoclonal antibodies specific for HCG. A solution containing these antibodies is mixed with a small amount of urine. The presence of HCG causes a change of color in the urine. Urine pregnancy tests which use an older agglutination-inhibition technique are about 80% sensitive, whereas the immunoenzymetric assay with monoclonal antibodies is 100% sensitive.

Home Pregnancy Tests

Kits that can be used at home to detect pregnancy were introduced in 1976. Various manufacturers make the tests, which are widely advertised for the public. Some of these tests can detect pregnancy as early as the first day after the expected period. Some are done 9 days after the missed period. Although each manufacturer claims a high degree of accuracy, each also acknowledges that false readings can occur.

Each kit has very specific directions. With these home pregnancy tests it is important to follow the directions exactly and determine whether the technique being used means that agglutination is a positive or negative result. Most require two drops of urine. A first voided morning sample is ideal because it is concentrated. One kit used to boast that the result was ready in 1 hour rather than the 2 hours for the other tests. Now some tests give results in 20 minutes. All the tests recommend a second test if the first test is negative and if menses does not begin within a week. A second test may be needed because the urine did not have enough HCG yet, or because the woman may have miscalculated her period. If the test is positive, the woman can call her physician or clinic to have definite confirmation of the pregnancy.

All the kits stress the fact that the kit does not replace the advice or care of a physician. If repeated tests are negative, the woman has saved the expense and time of consulting the health care system. Advertisements for the kits also make the point that a pregnancy test at home provides a way for a couple to discover the good news together. A test done at home means no waiting for appointments and no suspense in waiting for an answer. A home pregnancy test may be a way for a woman to establish right from the beginning that the baby belongs to her—not to a health professional. On the other hand, health professionals express concern that a woman may not do the test correctly and thus function under the false assumption that she is not pregnant, continuing to take medicines that could be dangerous to the fetus. (Valanis and Perlman (1982) found about one fourth of their clients had a false-negative report because they did not follow instructions.) Various drugs such as aspirin may make the test invalid.

■ SERUM HCG LEVELS

HCG QUALITATIVE PREGNANCY TEST

The laboratory can use radioimmunoassay to detect small amounts of HCG in the serum. (The technique of radioimmunoassay is described in Chapter 15.) There is some cross sensitivity with LH, and other pituitary hormones if the total HCG is measured. To reduce cross sensitivity the laboratory measures the beta subunit of HCG.

Preparation of Client and Collection of Sample
The test requires 0.5 ml of serum.

Reference Values for HCG Pregnancy Test

The laboratory reports either positive or negative for pregnancy.

HCG QUANTITATIVE TEST

HCG can be increased due to certain tumors, such as a hydatidiform mole (a benign adenoma) of the placenta, a choriocarcinoma (malignancy) of placenta-like tissue, or certain types of testicular carcinoma. If any of these conditions is suspected, the beta subunit of HCG helps to confirm a diagnosis. Serial HCG levels are also used to monitor the response to surgical therapy or chemotherapy. In certain cancers of the testes, the beta subunit of HCG can be used as a tumor marker as can alpha fetoprotein (Bullock & Rosendahl, 1984). For some types of testicular cancer (seminomatous) there will be only a small elevation of HCG but never of AFP (Ostchega & Culnane, 1985). For these pathological conditions, it is not enough to just know whether HCG is present. The physician needs to know whether the levels are increasing or decreasing.

Preparation of Client and Collection of Sample
The test requires 0.5 ml of serum.

Reference Values for HCG Quantitative

Less than 5mIU/ml	Not significant
5–40 mIU/ml	Possible cross reaction with LH[a]
Above 40 mIU/ml	Significant for tumors

---

[a]Postmenopausal women or women who have had their ovaries removed may show positive HCG due to the cross reaction with LH. (See Chapter 15 for a discussion about LH, the luteinizing hormone and how this hormone increases at menopause.) Measurement of the beta subunit eliminates the problem of cross sensitivity.

■ ALPHA-FETOPROTEIN (AFP)

Alpha-fetoprotein is made by the liver of the embryo. If the fetus has a neural tube defect the protein leaks out to the amniotic fluid. Between 16 and 20 weeks of pregnancy, AFP may be measured in the mother's blood. Presently, a maternal blood test for AFP is the *only* screening test that can be done of the pregnant woman's blood as a check for genetic defects in the child. (Table 18–2). In some states laws require that pregnant women be offered the test.

Unfortunately, high levels of AFP in pregnant women do not always indicate a problem with neural tube defects because the fetal age may be incorrectly estimated, the woman may be bearing twins, or the rise could be due to other reasons that are not yet well understood. If the AFP blood screening test is abnormal, a repeat is done. If the test is positive on the second blood sample, the woman has an ultrasonogram. If there is still doubt about the possibility of a defect, an amniocentesis is done. (See Chapter 28 for a detailed discussion on screening for neural tube defects. See Chapter 10 for discussion of AFP as a tumor marker.)

Low values of AFP may also be significant as less AFP is present when the fetus has Down's syndrome (Cuckle et al., 1984). However Knight et al. (1986) warn that low values obtained with commercial test kits are not correlated with Down's syndrome.

Reference Values for Maternal Serum

Week 19–21	2.1–9.6 µg/dl
31–33	8.4–34.4 µg/dl
37–40	6.3–16.5 µg/dl (Tietz, 1983)

TABLE 18-2. COMMON GENETIC DISEASES THAT MAY BE DETECTED BY SCREENING

Defect	Types of Screening				Comments
	Detected in Carrier State by Blood Samples of Both Parents	Screening of Maternal Blood after Woman Is Pregnant	Amniocentesis[a]	Fetal Blood Sampling (Research Studies)	
1. Sickle cell anemia	X		X	X	Most common in black families. May be difficult to accurately diagnose in fetus or newborn, but new tests on cord blood are being tried.
2. Tay–Sachs disease	X		X		Most common in Jewish families of Eastern European origin. Wide-scale testing is done for Jewish populations.
3. Neural tube defects (alpha-fetoprotein tests)		X	X		At the present time, only genetic defect that can be screened for in maternal blood. Can occur in any pregnancy.
4. Cystic fibrosis					No prenatal tests. See sweat test. More common in Caucasians.
5. Galactosemia			X		Tests of newborns required by law in some states.
6. Hemophilia			(See comment)	X	Sex-linked gene. Amniocentesis cannot determine if disease present, but can do so indirectly by determining sex of fetus.
7. Down's syndrome			X		Incidence increases with maternal age. Most common reason for amniocentesis is to check for Down's syndrome.
8. Thalassemia (beta)	X		X	X	Most common in families of Mediterranean descent. Screening of carriers not commonly done on large-scale basis.
9. PKU	X				Screening of carriers not common. More common in Caucasians. Almost all states require newborn screening.

Note: Updates on genetic disease are available from the National Maternal and Child Health Clearinghouse, 38th and R Sts., N.W., Washington, D.C. 20057.
[a]See Chapter 28 for a discussion on amniocentesis and on newer technique of chorionic villi biopsy.

TESTS TO SCREEN CARRIERS OF GENETIC DEFECTS

Laboratory tests can be done to detect whether parents are carriers of certain autosomal recessive genetic defects. If both parents are carriers, the fetus has a one-in-four chance of having the genetic defect. (Table 18–3 shows the probability when each parent has an autosomal recessive gene for a specific disease.) For the fetus to have the defect, both parents must contribute the recessive gene. This one-in-four chance refers to autosomal recessive traits, not to sex-linked recessive traits or to dominant traits. At the present time, two common tests are done to identify carrier states for sickle cell anemia and Tay–Sachs disease, both of which are predominant in specific ethnic groups. Intermarriage eventually changes the gene pool for various ethnic groups. Two other tests for carrier states are sometimes done, namely thalassemia and PKU, but not on wide-scale screening. See Table 18–2 for common genetic diseases detected by screening.

■ SICKLE CELL ANEMIA

Sickle cell anemia results from an autosomal recessive gene that produces an abnormal type of hemoglobin called *hemoglobin S*. (See Chapter 2 for tests on hemoglobin.) Hemoglobin S does not function as normal hemoglobin. The red blood cells have a sickle form, particulary when they are exposed to low oxygen concentrations or if the person is dehydrated. The abnormal cells are hemolyzed at an increased rate. Also, the capillaries can become occluded by these sickled cells.

A person can either be a carrier or have the disease. If the person has only one recessive gene for sickle cell, the person is a carrier who has the sickle cell trait. The person with sickle cell trait usually has no symptoms, although exposure to very low oxygen concentrations may cause minor symptoms. However, the effect of the trait, if any, is being studied at the present time because in the past some people with the trait were denied jobs, such as piloting planes. If only one person is a carrier, there is no difficulty. If both parents are carriers, they face the one-in-four risk, for each pregnancy, that their child will have the disease. As shown in Table 18–3, the risk

TABLE 18–3. PROBABILITY OF AUTOSOMAL RECESSIVE GENETIC DISEASES WHEN BOTH PARENTS ARE CARRIERS

Mother ↓ ND	Father ↓ ND	
NN	**DD**	**ND** **DN**
1:4 have two normal genes, so no disease or carrier state.	1:4 have two defective genes, so have disease.	2:4 (or 1:2) have one normal and one defective gene, so will be carriers of the trait.
(25%) of all children born to couples who are carriers.	(25%) of all children born to couples who are carriers.	(50%) of all children born to couples who are carriers.

N = Normal gene, D = Defective gene
Note: autosomal recessive diseases discussed in the chapter include: 1. PKU; 2. Cystic fibrosis; 3. Sickle cell anemia; 4. Tay–Sachs; 5. Thalassemia (Cooley's anemia).
Sex-linked recessive traits occur in different patterns. See the text for a discussion of hemophilia, which is transmitted by X chromosome.

is also one-in-four that the child will not receive the trait from either parent, and the chance is one-in-two that the child will be a carrier. The carrier state is estimated to be present in about 10% of American blacks and the disease to be present in about 1 in 625 blacks. (Wallach, 1983).

Prospective black parents can be given the screening test for sickle cell anemia. The quick screening tests for sickle cell trait (Sickledex, Ortho Diagnostics) do not distinguish whether a person has the trait or the disease. So the actual diagnosis of sickle cell anemia is made with hemoglobin electrophoresis. In recent years, prominent black people have done a lot to see that the test is made available to all who desire it. For example, a traveling van in San Francisco, sponsored by Sickle Cell Anemia Research and Education, Inc. (SCARE), goes to neighborhoods to educate the community and to identify carriers of the disease. *Mandatory* screening of children is potentially harmful if a careful follow-up is not done to explain about the meaning of the trait. The addresses of regional centers for sickle cell anemia testing are available from the Department of Health and Human Services.

In the newborn period, the amount of fetal hemoglobin present makes it technically difficult to determine whether the disease is present. New techniques being developed are making it possible to identify sickle cell anemia from samples of cord blood in the newborn and also in the fetus (see Chapter 28 on amniocentesis and chorionic biopsy). In New York a test for sickle cell is one of eight of the tests required for all newborns (Grover et al., 1983).

■ THALASSEMIA (COOLEY'S ANEMIA)

Thalassemia, like sickle cell anemia, is transmitted by autosomal recessive genes. Several variations of the defect can occur. Both the carrier state (thalassemia minor) and the presence of two recessive genes (thalassemia major) can be detected by hemoglobin electrophoresis (see Chapter 2). Thalassemia major is a chronic disease that causes severe anemia and mongoloid faces. Thalassemia minor is characterized by mild to moderate hemolytic anemia. Thalassemia is most common in children of Mediterranean origin (McCormack, 1979). The disease can be detected by fetal sampling (see Chapter 28.)

POSSIBLE NURSING DIAGNOSES

Ineffective Coping Related to Chronic Illness
Both sickle cell anemia and thalassemia major are chronic conditions for which there is no cure. The child and the family need a lot of help in coping with the disease. Families who have one child with the disease may greatly fear another pregnancy. See the discussion at the end of this chapter.

Activity Intolerance Related to Anemia
Children with hemolytic anemias have lowered hemoglobin and hematocrit counts, elevated reticulocyte counts, and, in some cases, abnormal red blood cells on a peripheral smear. (See Chapter 2 for a discussion on activity intolerance and other nursing diagnoses for a client with anemia.) Children with hemolytic anemias also have elevated *indirect* bilirubin levels. (See Chapter 11 for a discussion on indirect bilirubin as an indicator of hemolytic disease.)

■ TAY–SACHS DISEASE

Tay–Sachs, another inherited autosomal recessive condition, is most commonly found in Ashkenazi Jews who are of Eastern European origin (McCormack, 1979). As with all other recessive diseases, both parents must have the gene to produce a child with the disease. Tay–Sachs causes mental retardation and eventual death of the child by around age 3 or 4. There is no cure at the present time. It is evidenced by an absence of the enzyme hexosaminidase A.

There is a simple blood test to screen for carriers of Tay–Sachs, and it requires only a venous blood sample. The carriers of the recessive gene have lowered levels of the enzyme hexosaminidase A. The Tay–Sachs test is done on Jewish couples to see whether both are carriers. If needed, the Tay–Sachs test can then be done on amniotic fluid (see Chapter 28 on amniocentesis). Unless both parents have the gene, however, there is no need to test the amniotic fluid because the infant will not have the disease. Although the rate of Tay–Sachs is much lower in the non-Jewish population, Tay–Sachs can be done for non-Jewish couples who are concerned about all possible risks. Mass screening programs are planned for Jewish populations who may need to know if the trait is in their family. For example, in San Francisco, various synagogues, in conjunction with the genetic counseling center at the University of California at San Francisco, offer mass screenings for a nominal fee.

TESTS TO MONITOR FETAL WELL-BEING

■ ESTRIOL LEVELS

During pregnancy, the fetus and the placenta function as a unit to produce estrogens, of which estriol (E_3) is the major estrogenic compound. (See Chapter 15 for a discussion on other tests of estrogen compounds.) Estriol levels begin to increase about the eighth week of pregnancy and continue at high levels to term (Tietz, 1983). Consistently high levels of estriol indicate a normally functioning fetal–placental unit. Measurement of estriol may be done on either the plasma or the urine of the pregnant woman.

Toxemia, suspected intrauterine growth retardation (IUGR), chronic hypertension, diabetes, and postmaturity are the common reasons for monitoring a pregnancy through estriol levels. To recognize a trend, however, there must be more than one serum or urine estriol. A decrease over two or three samples, either as a slow downward trend or as an abrupt drop, is evidence of potential fetal distress because the placenta is not functioning normally. Some authors suggest a baseline should be done at 26 weeks for women who are high risk. Diabetic women may have weekly estriol levels after 30 weeks gestation, biweekly after 34 weeks, and every other day after 36 weeks (Schuler, 1979). See Chapter 28 for other tests of fetal well-being such as the nonstress test.

Preparation of Client and Collection of Sample
If the urine levels are to be monitored, the client must collect all urine for 24 hours. (See Chapter 3 for the key points to tell a client about a 24-hour urine specimen.)

If the estriol level is to be monitored by serum levels, there is no special preparation of the client. The test requires 2 ml of venous blood. Due to the ease of collecting the blood sample, serum levels may be a more desirable way to monitor the high-risk pregnancy. However, urine levels are more commonly done.

Reference Values for Estriol

Plasma	Varies with time of gestation. Level continues to rise during pregnancy up to 350 ng/ml by week 40.
Urine (24-hr specimen)	In the last 6 weeks of pregnancy, the average excretion is between 10–24 mg/day, with a mean of 16 mg. (Diamond, 1979). Interpretation of the values for an individual client must be done on a series of tests to see whether there is a downward trend. Decrease of more than 40% of previous value suggests that the fetus is at risk (Tietz, 1983).

POSSIBLE NURSING DIAGNOSIS RELATED TO HIGH-RISK PREGNANCY

Lack of Knowledge About Needed Health Maintenance
High-risk clients need detailed instructions about how to ensure a favorable outcome for the pregnancy. Aukamp (1984) has fully developed this diagnosis for all the common high-risk pregnancies.

NEWBORN SCREENING

For many newborns, the symptoms of serious inborn errors of metabolism are evident at birth. Nurses who work with newborns need to be on the alert for any symptoms or signs that require medical assessment. Some of these characteristics may also be noted by the parents. McCormack (1979) has listed nine clinical hints for the diagnosis of inborn errors of metabolism:

1. Unexplained metabolic alterations in electrolytes with acidosis or dehydration
2. Progressive downhill course with central nervous system deterioration
3. Unexplained renal or cardiac failure
4. Unexplained large viscera
5. Abnormal urine odor
6. Marked change in features, large tongue, coarse features
7. Thrombocytopenia, neutropenia, or anemia
8. Renal colic or calculus
9. Idiosyncratic or unusual reaction to drugs

Different inborn errors of metabolism, of course, cause different symptoms. For example, the only symptom of PKU is a musty odor of the urine, which may not be noticed. Several other inborn defects give urine an odor that has been described as smelling like rotten cabbage, sweaty feet, stale fish, or burned sugar.

Although some genetic diseases have symptoms at birth, others do not. Some of these "hidden" defects can cause serious damage if treatment is not begun early. Many tests can be done to detect genetic abnormalities in the newborn, but doing a large number of screening tests on all apparently healthy newborns is simply not feasible. A few genetic diseases are common enough, however, to warrant mass screening for all newborns. For a test to be used as a screening device in healthy newborns, the test must be accurate and highly reliable, it must be easy to do in mass volume, and it must measure a genetic disease that is common enough to warrant the cost of mass screening and for which treatment is available.

For example, at the present time, there is no screening test for cystic fibrosis, which is an autosomal recessive genetic disease, or for the carrier state. But if cystic fibrosis is suspected, the physician will order a sweat test. The sweat test is expensive and technically difficult to interpret, but it is warranted for specific cases. (A more recent screening test for cystic fibrosis is discussed at the end of this chapter.)

Another newborn test that is not done routinely is a test for a lack of an enzyme to manufacture cortisol, which is called the adrenogenital syndrome. If a physician suspected the disease, she or he would order tests for various enzyme defects. (See Chapter 15 for a detailed description of the tests for adrenogenital syndrome.)

Newborn Screening Tests Required by Law

Different states may require one or more tests for newborns as a general screening program. For example, one of the most recent tests being considered for wide scale screening is biotinidase deficiency (Nyhan, 1985). Since the 1960s, most states have required a test for phenylketonuria (PKU). Any *mandatory* tests for newborn screening must be not only accurate and suitable for mass screening, but they must also detect diseases that can be controlled if early treatment is begun. For example, California requires three screening tests for newborns: galactosemia and hypothyroidism, besides PKU. All three diseases can be treated successfully. All three use capillary blood placed on a filter paper. The hospital is also authorized by state law to charge a fee for the tests. An information sheet is given to all new parents that explains in lay terms the reason for the three tests. If the parents do not wish their child to have the tests, they must sign a statement relieving the physician and hospital of any liability for damages that may result from the lack of early detection of the three disorders (Cunningham, 1980). Parents are told that if they refuse the tests now, they can request the tests from a physician or a public health nurse later. The nurse can often be useful in further explaining how these tests are very beneficial in helping the newborn get off to the best start possible. The reader is encouraged to discover what screening tests are mandatory in a particular state. Legal liability and quality assurance have become issues, as noted by Andrews (1985).

■ PHENYLKETONURIA (PKU)

Phenylalanine is an amino acid found in all protein foods. The infant with PKU has a buildup of phenylalanine in the serum due to the lack of an enzyme needed for the normal metabolism of this amino acid. Because the phenylalanine spills into the urine, the condition is called phenylketonuria. PKU is dangerous because the high levels of phenylalanine in the serum can cause brain damage and mental retardation. Originally, screening tests for PKU were done on the urine, but the blood test (Guthrie test) is more valuable. PKU is much more common in Caucasians.

Serum PKU Levels

Preparation of Client and Collection of Sample. The serum level may be abnormally elevated within 24 hours after the infant begins a milk diet. If the infant is not taking milk well, the test should be delayed. (See the discussion on the urine test that can be done later at home.) The laboratory needs to know the date and time of birth, as well as the date and time of the first milk feeding.

The usual procedure is to do the PKU on the third day. If the baby is breast feeding, a second PKU may be done after the milk supply is abundant. A screening test for PKU can be done on capillary blood drawn from a heel stick. (Chapter 1 describes the procedure for heel sticks for infants.) Serum levels are followed if there is a positive first test. Some babies may have increased phenylalanine levels due to immaturity of the liver.

Reference Values for Phenylalanine

Serum phenylalanine   1–3 mg/dl

Urine PKU Levels (Phenistix)

Although PKU is better detected through the Guthrie blood test, urine can be used when blood testing is not feasible. The child's urine can be tested by a dip and read stick (Phenistix by Ames). Because the recommended times for urine checks for PKU are during the second, fourth, and sixth weeks of life (Ames Product Information, 1980), the urine screening may detect cases missed by too early blood screening in the hospital. Any positive discoveries, indicated by a green color, should be followed up with serum testing. (Urine should not be collected from disposable diapers as there may be chemical interference.) Urine tests may also be used to monitor the effectiveness of dietary management of PKU when it is not feasible to do serum levels.

Because the Phenistix also detect the presence of p-aminosalicylates (PAS), they are used to monitor clients who are taking PAS as treatment for tuberculosis. (A special color chart is used if the Phenistix are used to see if the client is taking PAS.) Phenistix will react with aspirin metabolites and with phenothiazines, therefore may be of value in revealing or checking for the presence of aspirin or phenothiazines in cases of possible drug overdosage. (See Chapter 17 for more information on toxicology testing.)

Preparation of Client and Collection of Sample

Phenistix may be used on any urine specimen either by dipping the stick into the urine or pressing it against a wet cloth diaper. Because salicylates and phenothiazines also cause positive reactions to the test, these drugs invalidate Phenistix as a test for PKU.

POSSIBLE NURSING DIAGNOSES

Alteration in Nutritional Requirements
The treatment for PKU consists of limiting the intake of phenylalanine to a level that is appropriate for each child. (There are several varieties of PKU.) Commercial products, such as Lofenalac, contain the essential amino acids with only a small amount of phenylalanine.

A restricted diet, tailored to the serum levels of phenylalanine, makes it possible for the child to develop normally without any mental retardation. The nurse may have a major role in helping the family to meet the dietary needs of the child with PKU. Reyzer (1978), a nurse, and a mother of a boy with PKU, has explained in detail how to plan diets that contain a precise amount of phenylalanine. The National Foundation of the March of Dimes gives a free copy of a *Low Protein Cookery for Phenylketonuria* to any family with a child with PKU. Some researchers believe PKU children can stop the diet when they reach school age; others feel that it is wise to continue the diet (March of Dimes, 1984). Holtzman et al. (1986) have findings which suggest children should continue on the diet even after age 8 and that females should not terminate the diet until their reproductive career is finished.

Anxiety Regarding Future Pregnancies

PKU is an autosomal recessive genetic disease. So if a couple have one child with the disease, they have a one-in-four chance of having another child with the disease (refer to Table 18–3). At the present time, PKU cannot be detected by amniocentesis. Parents may opt for a second child, however, even with the known risk, if they see that a first child is progressing well on dietary control. People who have a history of PKU in their families can also be tested for the carrier state because a diet high in phenylalanine causes higher-than-usual serum levels in people who have the one recessive gene. See the discussion on genetic counseling at the end of this chapter.

Knowledge Deficit Related to Danger of PKU for Newborn

When a woman who has PKU becomes pregnant there is great danger that her infant will be retarded unless she goes back on her PKU diet before and during pregnancy. If a woman becomes pregnant without planning to, the damage may be done before the diet takes effect. Also some women may have forgotten they were ever on a special childhood diet or were never told the reason why. Therefore, all women who have PKU need to be educated about the problems of maternal PKU and referred to a PKU clinic.

■ HYPOTHYROIDISM

The pilot program for screening for hypothyroidism in newborns began in North America in 1972. The screening of over 1 million infants resulted in the recommendation to use the T_4 filter paper test for screening and a follow-up of thyroid-stimulating hormone (TSH) for the 3–5% of low T_4 results (Fisher et al., 1979). The T_4 filter paper test requires only a drop of capillary blood. (See Chapter 1 for the discussion about heel sticks of infants.)

The tests used for hypothyroidism are discussed in Chapter 15. See the sections on hypothyroidism of the newborn for the symptoms of the disorder, on the medical treatment, and on the nursing implications.

■ GALACTOSEMIA

The urine test used to screen the inborn metabolism of galactose is discussed in detail at the end of Chapter 8 where the treatment of the disease and the nursing diagnoses are also covered. Like PKU and hypothyroid tests of the newborn, galactosemia tests can be done via a heel stick to obtain capillary blood for a filter paper. (Chapter 1 discusses heel sticks of infants.) Lack of the enzyme RBC galactose-1-phosphate uridyl transferase establishes the diagnosis. A measurement of galactose 1-phosphate is used to monitor therapy and restrict dietary galactose to maintain a level at 4 mg/g of hemoglobin (Wallach, 1983).

■ SWEAT TEST FOR CYSTIC FIBROSIS (CF)

Cystic fibrosis is a hereditary disease, caused by an autosomal recessive gene that affects the exocrine glands of the body. Because in this disease the mucous glands produce very thick mucus, its other name is mucoviscidosis. The thick mucus is the most troublesome in the lungs. The other major problem in CF is the partial destruction and malfunction of the exocrine glands in the pancreas. Although CF occurs in 1 of every 1500 to 2000 live births in most Caucasian populations (Kruger et al., 1980), there is no genetic screening test for CF at the present time. Because CF also affects exocrine glands, such as the sweat glands, the tests for its detection are based on determining the amount of sodium (Na) and chloride (Cl) in the sweat. The volume of sweat is not increased, even though the Na and Cl content is increased. A screening test involves the use of a paper patch test with a small battery powered stimulator. The test is easily done in the clinic or office (Coury et al., 1983). If the paper patch test is positive a quantitative pilocarpine iontophoresis test (QPIT) is conducted (Yeung et al., 1984).

Preparation of Client and Collection of Sample
A screening test is done with gel pads containing pilocarpine. The small portable generator, easily applied with a Velcro strap, performs the sweat stimulation. (The pilocarpine in the gel pads causes some tingling.) The sweat is collected in a fill tab. High chloride levels cause a color change on the sweat tab.

Reference Values for Sweat Test (Quantitative, Not Screening)	
Children	40 mEq of Na or Cl is the upper limit of normal
Adult	May have up to 60 mEq/L (Scully, 1986)

POSSIBLE NURSING DIAGNOSIS

Ineffective Airway Clearance
For a child with CF, the malabsorption problems may be partially overcome by the use of oral preparations of pancreatic enzymes. The problem with mucus in the lungs requires diligent and daily respiratory care. Refer to a pediatric text for details on nursing care.

HELPING THE FAMILY WITH A GENETICALLY DEFECTIVE CHILD

GENERAL NURSING DIAGNOSES

Normal Grieving Related to Loss of "Ideal" Infant

The family who has a child with a genetic defect needs help and encouragement to adjust to the changes that the disease requires. Because hypothyroidism can be controlled by the administration of thyroid, and galactosemia and PKU by diet restrictions, the family can be assured of a normal healthy child. Still, the family needs time to mourn the "loss" of the perfect child.

Potential for Ineffective Family Coping Related to Chronic Illness

In the case of other defects, such as sickle cell anemia and CF, parents have no assurance that the child will be normal and healthy. When a child is born with any disorder treatable or not so treatable, nurses are in a key position to focus their attention on the total needs of the family unit. They can, for example, be part of a team that does follow-up studies of the family. Johnson (1980) describes how nurses can be involved in self-instruction for the family who has a child with CF. Kruger et al. (1980) studied the reaction of families to CF and summarized five methods of assistance used by nurses and other health professionals to help families cope. These five measures are:

1. Offering support, including the role of a listener
2. Guiding the parents, which involves use of available resources
3. Teaching so that all family members really understand the disease
4. The physical care during bouts of illness
5. Providing an environment that promotes personal development to meet the demands of the situation

As nurses take on expanded roles, they may be able to do more and more of this type of care. Surely the development of nursing needs to progress to match the technical advances that make it possible for children with defects to receive sophisticated medical interventions. Medical technology has certainly made it possible to increase the quantity of life. Nurses surely have a role of helping to improve the quality of life.

Knowledge Deficit Related to Risk of Future Pregnancies

One final important point in helping the family to adjust to the birth of a child with a genetic defect is the availability of genetic counseling to help the couple make a decision about future children. Tishler (1981) has stated that, during the presentation of genetic information, families often first experience denial of the problem, followed by anger and blame. The desirable final phase is integration and insight into the problem. The couple can then make their own decision about future pregnancies. See Chapter 28 on amniocentesis and chorionic villi biopsy.

QUESTIONS

1. Mrs. Fannin is 6 months pregnant. Which one of these following laboratory reports is *not expected* in a normal pregnancy? (Increases or decreases refer to her pre-pregnancy values.)

   a. An increase of the neutrophils on a WBC
   b. A slight increase in both Hgb and Hct levels
   c. A decrease in P_{CO_2} levels
   d. An increase in serum alkaline phosphatase levels

2. The month after Mary had a hysterosalpingogram, she missed her period. When menses still had not occurred after 2 weeks, Mary bought a home pregnancy test kit of the direct agglutination type. If Mary is pregnant, then:

   a. The human chorionic gonadotropin (HCG) in her urine will react with sensitized cells in the test sample
   b. The test will be negative because it is only 14 days after an expected period
   c. The HCG antibodies in her urine will agglutinate the HCG in the test sample
   d. The gonadotropins LH and FSH may cause a false *negative* result because the test is the direct agglutination type

3. A quantitative HCG measurement may be used to follow all of the following conditions *except* which?

   a. Hydatidiform moles   c. Choriocarcinoma
   b. Testicular cancer   d. Normal pregnancy

4. All of the following are tests for carrier states of specific autosomal recessive genetic diseases. Which one is done as a screening test for Jewish people who are of Eastern European origin?

   a. Sickledex for sickle cell anemia   c. Tay–Sachs blood test
   b. Thalassemia blood test   d. PKU urine test

5. Mr. and Mrs. Green are both carriers of the autosomal recessive genes for sickle cell anemia. They have one child who has sickle cell anemia. What is the probability that a second pregnancy will produce a child who does not receive the defective gene from either parents (i.e., no sickle cell anemia or even sickle cell trait)?

   a. One-in-four chance
   b. One-in-two chance
   c. All children will have the trait
   d. Risk cannot be stated because one child has the disease

6. Mrs. Sommers is pregnant and 2 weeks past her due date. She is having serial determinations of serum estriol levels. A consistently high level on several samples would be evidence of which of the following?

   a. No congenital defects in the fetus
   b. Possible fetal distress

    c. An intact and functioning fetal–placental unit

    d. Maturity of the fetus

7. The rationale for doing PKU, galactosemia, and hypothyroid screening on all newborns is based on all the following principles *except* which?

    a. Mass screening tests for all three disorders are accurate, technically easy to do, and considered cost-effective

    b. All three genetic defects cause mental retardation if treatment is not begun within weeks or months after birth

    c. All these diseases may cause symptoms within a day or two after birth

    d. All three diseases can be effectively controlled by either dietary restrictions or hormone replacement

8. Phenistix (Ames Products), urine dip sticks, are used for all the following purposes *except* which?

    a. Detecting salicylate overdosage

    b. Detecting phenothiazine overdosage

    c. Confirmatory diagnosis of PKU

    d. Assessment of the effectiveness of a low phenylalanine diet

9. Which of the following is not an appropriate role for the home care nurse who is following a family that has a child with a genetic defect?

    a. Helping the family find and use available community resources

    b. Teaching the family about the effects of the disease

    c. Encouraging the family not to risk having another child

    d. Assisting with some physical care if the child is ill

REFERENCES

Ames Product Information. (1980). *Phenistix, semi-quantitative dip and read test for phenylketones in urine.* Elkart, IN: Ames Laboratories.

Andrews, L. (Ed.). (1985). *Legal liability and quality assurance in newborn screening.* Chicago: American Bar Association.

Aukamp, V. (1984). *Nursing care plans for the childbearing family.* Norwalk, CT: Appleton-Century-Crofts.

Bullock, B., & Rosendahl, P. (1984). *Pathophysiology.* Boston: Little, Brown.

Chedd, G. (1981). The new age of genetic screening. *Science, 81*(1), 32–40.

Coury, A., Fogt, E., Norenberg, M., & Untereker, D. (1983). Development of a screening system for cystic fibrosis. *Clinical Chemistry, 29*(9), 1593–1597.

Cuckle, H., et al. (1984). Maternal serum alpha–fetoprotein measurement: A screening test for Down's syndrome. *Lancet, 1,* 926–929.

Cunningham, G. (1980). *Important information for parents* (Letter given to all parents of newborns). Sacramento, CA: Maternal and Child Health, Branch of Department of Health Services.

Devore, N., & Baldwin, K. (1986). Ectopic pregnancy on the rise. *AJN, 86*(6), 674–678.

Diamond, F. (1979). High-risk pregnancy screening techniques. *JOGN, 7,* 15–19.

Fisher, D. et. al. (1979). Screening for congenital hypothyroidism: Results of screening one million North American infants. *Journal of Pediatrics, 94*(5), 700–705.

Grover, R. et al. (1983). Current sickle cell screening program for newborns. *American Journal of Public Health, 73*(3), 249–252.

Holtzman, N., et al. (1986). Effect of age at loss of dietary control on intellectual performance and behavior of children with phenylketonuria. *NEJM, 314*(10), 593–597.

Jacobs, D., Kasten, B., Demott, W., & Wolfson, W. (1984). *Laboratory test handbook with DRG index.* St. Louis: Mosby/Lexi.

Johnson, M. (1980). Self-instruction for the family of a child with cystic fibrosis. *Maternal Child Nursing, 5*(5), 345–348.

Knight, G., et al. (1986). Maternal serum alpha–fetoprotein: A problem with a test kit. *NEJM, 314*(8), 516.

Kruger, S., et al. (1980). Reactions of families to the child with cystic fibrosis. *Image, 12*(10), 67–72.

McCormack, M. (1979). Medical genetics and family practice. *American Family Physician, 20*(9), 143–154.

March of Dimes. (1984). *Public health education: Information sheets on sickle cell anemia, PKU, and thalassemia.* White Plains, NY: Birth Defects Foundation.

Nyhan, W. (1985). Neonatal screening for inherited disease. *NEJM, 313*(1), 43–44.

Ostchega, Y., & Culnane, M. (1985). Tumor markers. *Nursing 85, 15*(9), 49–51.

Reyzer, N. (1978). Diagnosis: PKU. *AJN, 78*(11), 1895–1898.

Schuler, K. (1979). When a pregnant woman is diabetic: Antepartal care. *AJN, 79*(3), 448–452.

Scully, R. (Ed.). (1986). Normal reference laboratory values. *NEJM, 314*(1), 49.

Tietz, N. (Ed.). (1983). *Clinical guide to laboratory tests.* Philadelphia: Saunders.

Tishler, C. (1981). The psychological aspects of genetic counseling. *AJN, 81*(4), 733–734.

Valanis, B., & Perlman, C. (1982). Home pregnancy testing kits: Prevalence of use, false-negative rates, and compliance with instructions. *American Journal of Public Health, 72*(9), 1034–1036.

Wallach, J. (1983). *Interpretation of pediatric tests.* Boston: Little, Brown.

Yeung, W., et al. (1984). Evaluation of a paper-patch test for sweat chloride determination. *Clinical Pediatrics, 23*(11), 603–607.

Part II

CASE STUDIES

19

Practice Interpretation of Laboratory Data

Introduction

The following four case studies are presented:

- Mrs. Rita Rios, age 38
- Sally Jamison, age 14
- Mr. Jack Lee, age 77
- Max Goldstein, age 2½

These case studies give the reader an opportunity to practice interpreting laboratory data and using the data to formulate possible nursing diagnoses. The reader may select from the nursing diagnoses presented with each case study, although this is not meant to be an exclusive list of possibilities. (Reference values for the laboratory tests are found in Appendix A.) A discussion of the laboratory data follows each case presentation. Interpretation of each test is done and some suggested nursing diagnoses are given. Also, page numbers are listed in the discussion so the reader can refer quickly to the text for further elaboration on each test and possible nursing diagnoses.

■ RITA RIOS

Rita Rios, age 38, was admitted last evening with possible pneumonia. She had completed a course of chemotherapy last week for cancer of the pancreas. She appears malnourished and states that she has no appetite. She is being maintained on intravenous fluids of D_5 0.45 NaCl with 20 mEq KCl/150 ml/hr. Her urine is orange in color and her skin is slightly jaundiced. Present vital signs are: BP 130/80, P 130, R 28, T 102°F. Night nurse reports that Mrs. Rios keeps removing O_2 cannula. The current laboratory results are:

1. Hb 8 g; Hct 25%; RBC 3 million mm³
   MCV and MCH both low

2. WBC 4000 mm^3 with 30% neutrophils (absolute count of neutrophils is thus 1200)
3. Platelets 30,000 mm^3
   PT 50%, 20 seconds (control 12 seconds)
4. Urinalysis: Positive for nitrites, leukocyte esterase, glucose, and bilirubin
5. BUN and serum creatinine WNL (within normal limits)
6. Lytes: K 3.0 mEq/L
   Chlorides slightly elevated, 115 mEq/L
7. ABGs: pH 7.52; P_{CO_2} 30 mm Hg; P_{O_2} 60 mm Hg; and bicarbonate 20 mEq/L
8. FBS 190 mg/dl
9. Bilirubin: Total 5 mg/dl; indirect 0.5 mg/dl; direct 4.5 mg/dl
10. Alkaline phosphatase 150 U/L; GGTP 135 U/L

What Are the Priority Nursing Diagnoses for This Client?

- Ineffective airway clearance?
- Ineffective breathing pattern?
- Anxiety?
- Activity intolerance?
- Sensory perceptual alterations?
- Potential for injury? Infection? Bleeding?
- Alterations in nutritional requirements?
- Fluid volume deficit? Actual or potential?
- Alteration in cardiac output?
- Alteration in comfort?

Discussion on Laboratory Data for Rita Rios

1. The values for Hb, Hct, and RBC indicate anemia, most likely related to the malignancy and her malnourished state. The anemia is not just from acute blood loss because the low MCV and MCH are indicative of a microcytic, hypochromic anemia (see Chapter 2, p. 33). Chronic blood loss and iron deficiency are common reasons for changes in these two erythrocyte indices. Possible nursing diagnoses related to this chronic anemia would be an *alteration in the nutritional requirements of iron and protein,* potential for *activity intolerance, potential for infection,* and a possible *alteration in comfort* related to feeling chilly. If Mrs. Rios is put on iron supplements later, she may have a *knowledge deficit* regarding side effects (see Chapter 2, p. 30).
2. Mrs. Rios has neutropenia, not an unexpected side effect of chemotherapeutic drugs. The priority nursing diagnosis related to a lack of neutrophils is the *potential for infection* (Chapter 2, p. 46 discusses neutropenia).
3. Mrs. Rios has thrombocytopenia, also as a possible side effect of the chemotherapy. The PT time is increased and the percentage is decreased; both show a lack of some of the coagulation factors manufactured by the liver. The changes in the PT may be due to the obstructive jaundice (see the bilirubin levels) or to liver dysfunction from metastatic disease. For whatever the reason, these abnormal coagulation tests indicate that Mrs. Rios has a *potential for bleeding* (see Chapter 13, p. 286 on PT tests).
4. Positive tests for nitrites and leukocyte esterase are usually indications of a urinary tract infection (see Chapter 3, p. 71). The *potential for infection*

is a high priority as the glucose in the urine increases the risk of urinary tract infections and perineal abscesses. The spilling of sugar in the urine also alerts the nurse for *potential fluid volume deficit,* although other data do not suggest that this is an actual problem at the present time, probably because she is on intravenous fluids (see Chapter 3, p. 68 on glycosuria).

5. A normal BUN and creatinine indicate no renal dysfunction from the chemotherapeutic drugs. Also, a normal BUN is evidence of no significant fluid volume deficit at the present time (see Chapter 4, page 82 on BUN measurements).

6. The low potassium level may be due to a loss from vomiting and/or a lack of intake. Hypokalemia is also found in alkalotic states. The chlorides are slightly elevated because another negative ion is slightly low (see Chapter 5, p. 119 on the electrolyte changes in acid–base imbalances). Because of the hypokalemia, Mrs. Rios has an *alteration in nutritional requirements.* The physician should be notified so additional potassium can be given, probably IV at the present time, and oral supplements or dietary intake, including salt substitutes later on.

7. By looking at the ABGs one can see that Mrs. Rios is in respiratory alkalosis. The most likely cause for the respiratory alkalosis is the hypoxia. The reason for the hypoxia is not immediately evident. The *impaired gas exchange* may be due to the pneumonia or even to metastatic disease. The hypoxia might also be due to *ineffective airway clearance* related to mucus plugs or fluid in the lungs. *Anxiety* and an elevated temperature may be contributing to the hyperventilation and thus an *ineffective breathing pattern.* Certainly, the present method of oxygen delivery is not satisfactory. A thorough respiratory and neurological assessment needs to be done to determine the best way to raise the PO_2 (see Chapter 6, p. 144 for possible nursing diagnoses related to hypoxia). In addition to the restlessness and anxiety from hypoxia, Mrs. Rios may also have *alteration in comfort* related to the neuromuscular irritability found in alkalotic states (see the symptoms of alkalosis on p. 139). In this case study sedation would be appropriate given these blood gas values, but not with case study 3.

8. The elevated blood glucose levels, in the absence of hyperalimentation, is an indication of a lack of enough insulin to transfer glucose into the cells. The beta cells in the pancreas may have been damaged by the pancreatic tumor. The physician may need to order insulin if hyperglycemia persists. Also Mrs. Rios may be a candidate for hyperalimentation if nutrition continues to be a problem. A continued hyperglycemia will lead to a potential for *fluid volume deficit* and increase the *potential for infection* (see Table 8-2, p. 185 on the effects of hyperglycemia).

9. The elevation of the direct bilirubin is an indication of obstructive jaundice. Direct bilirubin is the conjugated bilirubin that is increased in the bloodstream when the normal biliary pathway is blocked (see Table 11-2, p. 238 on the types of prehepatic and posthepatic jaundice). For Mrs. Rios, the obstruction is most likely due to the pressure of the pancreatic tumor on the biliary tree. The dark orange urine with a positive test for bilirubin is further evidence that conjugated bilirubin, which is water soluble, is being eliminated by the urine rather than through the intestinal tract. (The urine would foam if shaken.) If the obstruction is complete Mrs. Rios' feces will become clay colored. Obstruction in the biliary tract will also decrease the absorption of fat soluble vitamin K needed for the manufacture of prothrom-

bin and other coagulation factors. Thus Mrs. Rios has the *potential for bleeding* (see Chapter 11, p. 246 on the relationship of obstructive jaundice to the prothrombin time). Because of the biliary obstruction Mrs. Rios will have an *alteration in nutritional requirements* due to the inability to tolerate fats in the diet. As mentioned earlier, hyperalimentation may be needed during this acute phase, until the obstruction is relieved by successful chemotherapy or surgical interventions. The need to increase her nutritional status will be a long-term goal. Two other nursing diagnoses related to the elevated direct bilirubin may be an *alteration in comfort* due to the pruritis from bilirubin deposits in the skin and *alterations in body image* related to the appearance of the jaundice (see Chapter 11, p. 247 for further discussion of the care of the client with obstructive jaundice).

10. The markedly elevated alkaline phosphatase and GGTP give further evidence that Mrs. Rios has biliary obstruction (see Chapter 12, p. 258 on enzymes used to assess for biliary obstruction). Needless to say, Mrs. Rios has many serious problems. She needs a caring, knowledgeable nurse to devise an individualized care plan. Mrs. Rios and her family have the *potential for ineffective coping* as they decide what further treatments, such as surgery or chemotherapy, are wanted as palliative, or less likely, curative measures.

■ SALLY JAMISON

Sally Jamison, age 14, was just admitted because of uncontrolled diabetes mellitus. She responds to questions, but is drowsy if not stimulated. Her skin is flushed and dry. Her eyeballs are soft and she complains of blurred vision.

Vital signs are: BP 106/88, P 128, R 32, T 100°F. Her physician is writing orders now. Her sister states that the client has been under a great deal of strain due to a family conflict. The admission laboratory results show:

1. Hct 59%; RBC 5 million mm³; Hb 14 g
   Erythrocyte indices WNL
2. WBC 15,000 mm³. No shift to the left
3. Platelets normal
4. Urinalysis: SG 1.040; sugar 2%; acetone moderate
5. Serum osmolality 316 mOsm
   Urine osmolality 1400 mOsm
6. BUN 40 mg/dl. Serum creatinine normal at 1.0 mg/dl
7. Lytes: K 5.8 mEq/L
8. ABGs: pH 7.30; Pco_2 30 mm Hg; Po_2 98 mm Hg; and bicarbonate 15 mEq/L
9. Random blood sugar 450 mg/dl
   Plasma ketone 4+ in 1:1 diluted sample

What Are the Priority Nursing Diagnoses for This Client?

- Anxiety?
- Alterations in nutritional requirements?
- Potential for injury? Infection? Bleeding?
- Alterations in urinary patterns?
- Fluid volume deficit? Actual or potential?
- Knowledge deficit?

- Ineffective coping? Individual or family?
- Ineffective breathing pattern?
- Activity intolerance?
- Alterations in cardiac output?
- Noncompliance?

Discussion on Laboratory Data for Sally Jamison

1. The elevated Hct is an indication of a *fluid volume deficit*. The increase could be due to polycythemia (see Chapter 2, p. 25) but all the other laboratory data indicate fluid volume deficit. Normal erythrocyte indices indicate no apparent abnormalities with the size or amount of Hb content of the erythrocytes.

2. The elevated WBC indicates that the body is responding to stress or infection. There is no shift to the left. Therefore there may not be a bacterial infection yet (see Chapter 2, p. 44 on the meaning of the shift to the left). Sally is vulnerable because of her diabetes; therefore *potential for infection* is a priority.

3. A normal platelet count indicates no potential problem with bleeding due to thrombocytopenia.

4. The elevated specific gravity is due to the presence of glucose in the urine and also is reflective of an *actual fluid volume deficit* as supported by other laboratory data. The urine osmolality is a better indicator of fluid imbalance because it is not affected by glucose. The moderate acetone level in the urine indicates that Sally has progressed from hyperglycemia to ketoacidosis.

5. The elevated serum osmolality is reflective of the *fluid volume deficit* and the hyperglycemia that has made the serum very hypertonic. The elevated urine osmolality is reflective of *actual fluid volume deficit* (see Table 4–4, p. 91 on serum and urine osmolality).

6. The elevated BUN with a still normal creatinine is indicative of a *fluid volume deficit*. The ratio is 40:1 rather than the normal ratio (see Chapter 4, p. 83). The other factor that could elevate the BUN, but not the creatinine level would be a marked increase in protein intake or gastrointestinal bleeding, but the Hct shows no evidence of blood loss.

7. The hyperkalemia is expected because of the acidotic state (see Chapter 5, p. 113). Sally has the potential for *alterations in cardiac output* related to the development of arrhythmias. When the acidotic state is corrected she will become hypokalemic unless her fluid and electrolyte balance is carefully monitored (see Table 6–6, p. 130 on usual electrolyte changes with acid–base imbalances). As Sally becomes able to resume oral intake she may have an *alteration in nutritional requirements* related to the need for electrolyte replacement as well as other diet modifications for her diabetes.

8. The ABGs indicate that Sally is in metabolic acidosis. The test for the plasma ketones indicates that the acidosis is ketoacidosis. She does not have an ineffective breathing pattern even though her respiratory rate is 32. These rapid and deep respirations (Kussmaul's respirations) have lowered the PCO_2 so that there will be less carbonic acid to match less bicarbonate (see Table 6–3, p. 128 on the carbonic acid–bicarbonate ratio). Her acidotic state can lead to the *potential for injury* due to a change in her perceptual awareness and level of consciousness. Her weakness and fatigue will cause *activity intolerance*.

9. The hyperglycemia is due to the uncontrolled diabetes mellitus. These levels of glucose and ketones are consistent with moderate ketoacidosis (see Table 8–3, p. 186). In addition to the other nursing diagnoses identified, others will become appropriate as Sally's diabetes is controlled. Does she have a *knowledge deficit* regarding the balance of food, insulin, and exercise? Or is the basic problem one of *noncompliance* that could be due to many factors? Her sister noted that there is a family conflict. Is there *ineffective individual and/or family coping?* What kind of referrals may be needed?

■ JACK LEE

Jack Lee, age 77, was admitted 4 days ago because of increased difficulty in breathing. He has had several previous admissions related to his chronic obstructive lung disease. He is on 0.25 mg digoxin and a mild diuretic.

Vital signs are stable now. He states that he is ready to go home today. He lives. alone and has no close relatives. The most recent laboratory tests are:

1. Hct 60%; Hb 19.8 g; RBC 7.1 million mm^3
   Erythrocyte indices WNL
2. WBC normal
3. Platelets 450,000 mm^3
   PTT 28 seconds (control 34 seconds)
4. Urinalysis negative except for 2+ proteinuria and consistently low urine osmolality
5. BUN 45 mg/dl; creatinine 2.9 mg/dl
6. Lytes: K 4.0 mEq/L; Cl 90 mEq/L; bicarbonate 35 mEq/L
7. ABGs: pH 7.35; PCO_2 58 mm Hg; PCO_2 60 mm Hg; and bicarbonate 35 mEq/L
8. FBS 128 mg/dl
9. Serum digoxin 1.2 ng/ml

What Are the Priority Nursing Diagnoses for This Client?

- Activity intolerance?
- Impaired gas exchange?
- Ineffective airway clearance?
- Potential for Injury? Thrombophlebitis? Infection? Bleeding?
- Alterations in urinary patterns?
- Anxiety?
- Impaired home management maintenance?
- Potential for fluid volume deficit or fluid volume overload?
- Knowledge deficit?

Discussion on Laboratory Data for Jack Lee

1. The elevated Hct, Hb, and RBC are expected in response to chronic hypoxia. There are no laboratory data to support a fluid volume deficit which would be another reason for an elevated Hct as noted in the second case study. Although Mr. Lee's erythrocytosis or polycythemia is most likely secondary to his hypoxia, he could have polycythemia vera because his platelet count is also elevated. The actual medical diagnosis is the puzzle to the physicians.

From a nursing point of view, the presence of polycythemia or erythrocytosis should alert the nurse to the fact that this client has a *potential for injury* because the increased viscosity of his blood can lead to venous thrombi. Mr. Lee may have a *knowledge deficit* regarding ways to decrease the chance for deep vein thrombosis (see Chapter 2, p. 26 for appropriate nursing instructions about fluids and exercises).

2. A normal WBC indicates that Mr. Lee is unlikely to have any current problems related to infection. However, elderly clients may not always have an increased WBC as a response to infection; therefore careful assessment for any other signs of a potential infection would be warranted (see Chapter 16, p. 399 on infections in the elderly).

3. Mr. Lee's elevated platelet count could be due to many factors including polycythemia, as discussed earlier. Compared with the normal (the control), the PTT time is decreased. A decreased PTT can also be caused by many factors (see Chapter 13, p. 293). The decreased PTT gives additional data to suggest that Mr. Lee has a *potential for injury* due to the formation of venous clots. There is no evidence that his platelet count showed abnormal type of platelets; if it had, bleeding could be a potential problem (see Chapter 13, p. 296).

4. The proteinuria indicates some renal dysfunction as verified by the other laboratory reports. The consistently low urine osmolality is evidence that the kidneys have lost the ability to concentrate urine. A urine osmolality is much more precise than a specific gravity in evaluating renal function (see Chapter 4, p. 92).

5. Elevations of both the BUN and the serum creatinine indicate that Mr. Lee does have renal insufficiency (see Table 4-1, p. 84). Because of this limited renal reserve there is a *potential for injury* or a worsening of his renal function due to infection, stress, fluid volume deficits, and some drugs. The use of contrast media for x-ray procedures could be dangerous, too. (See Chapter 20, p. 488.)

6. Mr. Lee has no problem with hyperkalemia because his renal disease is not severe. Also the diuretic has not caused hypokalemia, which could be dangerous with the digoxin. His other electrolytes are consistent with his compensated acid–base imbalance. The bicarbonate is elevated to balance the increased PCO_2 as noted in his ABGs. Because bicarbonate, a negative ion, is elevated, another negative ion, namely chloride, is decreased in the serum to maintain an electrical neutrality (see Chapter 5, p. 102 on electrical neutrality).

7. Mr. Lee's ABGs show that he is in compensated respiratory acidosis. Note that his pH remains within the normal range even though his PCO_2 is quite elevated. The PCO_2 level increased very gradually; therefore the kidneys have had time to retain enough bicarbonate to keep the bicarbonate–carbonic ratio at 20:1 (see Tables 6-3 and 6-4, pp. 128). Although Mr. Lee is stable with regard to his chronic obstructive lung disease, his laboratory data suggest that he could have severe *impaired gas exchange* if he gets a respiratory infection or is given high doses of oxygen or narcotics (see Chapter 6, p. 135 on the potential danger of oxygen therapy and drugs). He may have some *activity intolerance* and thus must learn how to conserve energy.

8. Mr. Lee is not diabetic. This is important to know in an elderly client who already has several other problems common in the aged population. The elder-

ly client does have a FBS slightly higher than young adults (see Chapter 8, p. 178).

9. This serum digoxin level is within the usual therapeutic range for a dose of 0.25 mg/day. Because of Mr. Lee's renal insufficiency, however, he does have the *potential for injury* related to his inability to excrete drugs at a normal rate (see Chapter 17, p. 433 on digoxin toxicity). Mr. Lee may have a *knowledge deficit* regarding how he can check his own pulse and watch for other symptoms related to adverse reactions to his medications. Mr. Lee is stable now, and anxious to go home; an astute nurse would recognize that Mr. Lee may have *impaired home maintenance management* unless he is aware of the health concerns discussed above. Perhaps a nurse should do a follow-up home visit?

■ MAX GOLDSTEIN

Max Goldstein, age 2½, was brought to the emergency room an hour after he took an unknown number of his grandmother's pills. She had hydrochlorothiazide (50 mg), furosemide (Lasix) (40 mg), and aspirin on a shelf in the bathroom. On the advice of a neighbor, Max's father gave Max 3 teaspoons of Ipecac syrup, but no pills were noted in the emesis. Admitting vital signs included pulse rate 160 and respiration 54. Max was drowsy and resisted further examination. He kept putting his hands over his ears. Initial laboratory results showed:

1. Hct 60%; RBC 6.5 million
2. Urinalysis positive for salicylates, SG 1.030, negative for glucose and acetone
3. BUN 35 mg/dl; creatinine 1.0 mg/dl
4. Electrolytes: Na 130 mEq/L; K 2.6 mEq/L; Cl 90 mEq/L
5. ABGs: pH 7.30; PCO_2 25 mm Hg; PO_2 100 mm Hg; and bicarbonate 18 mEq/L
6. Serum salicylates 45 mg/dl (toxic level in children is above 30 mg/dl)

What Are the Priority Nursing Diagnoses for This Client?

- Potential for bleeding?
- Fluid volume deficit?
- Ineffective breathing patterns?
- Impaired family coping?
- Alterations in nutritional requirements?
- Knowledge deficit related to safety needs of toddlers?
- Alteration in cardiac output?
- Anxiety?

Discussion on Laboratory Data for Max Goldstein

1. As in the second case study, the elevated Hct and RBC are reflective of a severe *fluid volume deficit* (see Chapter 2, p. 27).
2. The urine specific gravity also supports a *fluid volume deficit*. Young children cannot concentrate urine as well as adults (see Chapter 3, p. 57 on specific gravity). The positive salicylate is expected given the finding in the serum.
3. The elevated BUN and the normal serum creatinine level are further evidence

of a *fluid volume deficit* (see Chapter 4, p. 83 on BUN–creatinine ratio).

4. The low values for electrolytes are evidence of a massive diuresis. Note that even with a fluid volume deficit, the sodium and chloride levels are low and even with acidosis the potassium is low (see Chapter 6, p. 130). Hypokalemia is probably the greatest concern because of the potential *alteration in cardiac output* related to the development of arrhythmias. The fluid volume deficit may also lead to shock and an *alteration in tissue perfusion* as well as decreased *cardiac output*. Medical interventions are needed to restore fluid and electrolyte balance. Later on, Max may have an *alteration in nutritional requirements* as he may still need oral electrolyte replacements.

5. The ABGs for Max indicate metabolic acidosis. The salicylates are acid products that have used up the bicarbonate in the serum. The low PCO_2 is most likely a compensatory mechanism for the acidotic state. Aspirin is a respiratory stimulant and can cause respiratory alkalosis in the first stage of poisoning, particularly in adults (see Chapter 6, p. 140 on types of acidosis). In very young children the metabolic acidosis occurs very rapidly. The *potential for injury* due to sensory-perceptual alterations and loss of consciousness should be considered. The *anxiety* levels of Max and his parents would also be a high priority.

7. The effect of aspirin on the acid–base balance has been discussed. Large doses of aspirin may also cause gastrointestinal irritation and a decrease in clotting factors. Hence, Max should be monitored for the *potential for bleeding*. As various medical interventions are used to stabilize Max, the nurse needs to keep in mind the potential for *ineffective coping by the family* related to their fear and possible guilt over the accident. After Max's condition is stabilized, attention may need to be focused on any *knowledge deficit* of the parents regarding the safety needs of toddlers.

Part III

DIAGNOSTIC PROCEDURES

20

Diagnostic Radiological Tests

- Chest X-Rays
- Plain Films of the Abdomen: Flat Plates, Three-way Films, and KUB
- Bone or Skeletal X-Rays, Including the Skull
- Upper GI Series, Cardiac Series, and Small Bowel Series
- Barium Enemas (BE)
- Oral Cholecystogram (OCG) or Gallbladder Series
- Cholangiograms: Intravenous, Operative, Transhepatic, and via Endoscope
- Intravenous Pyelograms
- Bronchograms
- Arteriograms
- Venograms
- Lymphograms
- Hysterosalpingogram
- Mammograms
- Myelograms
- Arthrograms

OBJECTIVES

1. Describe the difference between fluoroscopy and routine x-ray films.
2. Explain how the four densities of air, fat, water, and bone are represented on x-ray film.
3. Identify three methods to reduce the hazards of radiation from exposure to x-rays.
4. List several important points to teach clients on how to protect themselves from unnecessary x-ray exposure.
5. Identify possible nursing diagnoses for clients going to x-ray for radiological study.

6. Identify possible nursing diagnoses when clients return from radiological study.
7. Identify radiological tests that require dye or a contrast medium, and explain how the dye adds additional nursing implications.
8. Name specific nursing actions appropriate in assisting the x-ray technician to get a better portable chest x-ray of a client in bed.
9. Compare the diagnostic tests covered in this chapter, and identify those tests that cause pain, which often require the use of analgesics.

The first part of this chapter briefly describes the three ways in which x-rays are used in diagnostic testing and how the hazards of radiation can be reduced when diagnostic x-rays are needed. The second part discusses the general nursing diagnoses to prepare a client for x-ray studies and to take care of the client after the x-rays are completed. The last part of this chapter gives a description of each of the common x-ray studies and the key nursing implications in caring for the client before and after each specific test. Although the specific preparation for each test is outlined in this book, the reader is advised to consult with the radiology department regarding the exact protocol to be followed at that particular institution, especially the guidelines given for pre- and posttest care. Most radiology departments have printed guidelines on the preparations needed for each test. The nurse should never hesitate to consult with members of the radiology department if a question arises about what is or is not necessary before a test. In addition, the nurse may need to consult the radiology department when several different tests are ordered for a client. For example, a radioactive iodine uptake (RAI) test must be done before x-rays with iodine contrast medium. Also, barium studies may make it impossible to do other abdominal tests for a day or two.

Although rare, some radiology departments have a nurse as part of the staff. If a nurse is employed by the radiology department, she or he may have several roles, including: (1) extended temporary floor nurse and guardian, (2) teacher, (3) consultant on how to deal with intravenous bottles, chest tubes, and so on, (4) liaison with the clinic staff, (5) team helper for intensive care unit (ICU) nurse who accompanies the client to x-ray (Maphet, 1981; Ordronneu, 1980).

In specialized areas, such as an ICU or a small emergency room, nurses may be the first professional to see a person's chest film. Obviously the interpretation of x-rays requires a skilled clinician (see Tinker [1976] and Wilson [1977] for written material to help nurses recognize some of the major abnormalities revealed by chest films). The purpose of this chapter is to prepare nurses for the care of clients undergoing x-rays: therefore, there is little emphasis on the interpretation of the findings of x-rays. However, some general information about the clinical significance of a particular type of x-ray is given with each test.

HOW X-RAYS ARE USED IN DIAGNOSTIC TESTS

X-rays were discovered in 1895 by the German physicist Roentgen, who received the first Nobel Prize in Physics (1901) for his discovery. By 1896, the first x-ray machines were in use. Since that time, much has been learned about both the benefits and risks of x-rays or roentgenological studies. X-rays are electromagnetic radiation of very short wavelengths, which are commonly generated by passing a current of high voltage (from 10,000 volts up) through a Coolidge tube. X-rays can penetrate most substances, including human tissues, by strongly ionizing the tissue through which they pass. They cause certain substances to fluoresce and affect photographic plates, qualities extremely useful for diagnostic tests. They are, however, harmful to living tissue. X-rays can alter cells so they cannot reproduce. Consequently, radiation therapy is used to treat various types of cancer. (See Chapter 22 for further examples of diagnostic and therapeutic use of radiation in the form of radioisotopes.)

At the present time, there are three major ways x-rays are used as diagnostic tests: (1) x-ray films or roentgenograms, (2) fluoroscopy, and (3) tomography. Tests using the first two methods are discussed in this chapter, tomography in Chapter 21.

Roentgenograms or X-Ray Films

Roentgenograms, or x-ray pictures of body structures, are like negatives of photographs. X-rays that go through the body and the x-rays that reach the film positioned on the other side of the body turn the film black. X-rays penetrate air easily; therefore, areas filled with air or gas appear very dark on the film. For example, lungs, which contain a lot of air, appear very dark on a plain x-ray film. In contrast, bones or the dyes used as contrast media appear almost white on the film because the x-rays cannot penetrate these substances to reach the sensitive x-ray film. Organs and tissues appear as various shades of gray because they have more mass than air but not as much as bone. For example, heart tissues contain a lot of water and the heart appears lighter on film than say fatty tissues. From the blackest to the whitest the four densities of x-ray are:

1. Air—blackish
2. Fat—dark gray
3. Water—lighter gray
4. Bone—whitish

Fluoroscopy

In this method of using x-rays for diagnostic purpose, the client is put in front of an x-ray tube and a fluoroscopic screen is held over the body part to be examined. Recall that x-rays have the ability to make certain substances, such as those used to coat the screen, fluoresce or give off light. As with the roentgenograms, different structures of the body allow different amounts of x-ray beams to project on the fluoroscopic screen. The image remains on the monitor for continuous observation; therefore, any movements in the body can be monitored. For example, as a client swallows barium, the flow of barium can be monitored on a fluoroscopic screen. Fluoroscopy is also very valuable in cardiac catheterizations to help the physican see the exact position of the catheter in the heart. (See Chapter 26 on cardiac catheterization.) Fluoroscopy is done in the dark so that images of the various densities are seen in sharper outlines. Before fluoroscopy is done the physician puts on goggles with red lenses, which help the eyes adjust to the dark. Fluoroscopy prolongs the time of exposure to radiation; therefore it is only used when it is deemed very important to observe the change in position or some movement in the body. Videotapes of the fluoroscopic procedure (cineradiography) enable the movements to be studied at later times. Cineradiography is also valuable as a teaching tool.

Tomograms and Computerized Axial Tomography Scans

A tomogram, also called laminagram or planogram, is a special type of x-ray film that is taken with both the x-ray tube and film kept in motion during exposure. The x-ray takes pictures of several different planes of tissues. With each change in the position of the camera, a slightly different level of tissue is in focus. Computerized axial tomography (CT) uses computers, scanners, and tomography to obtain a three-dimensional, cross-sectional view of any body structure. The CT scan is the newest method of using x-rays for diagnostic purpose. (Tomography and CT scans are discussed in Chapter 21.)

REDUCING THE HAZARDS OF RADIATION EXPOSURE

Probably the most important point for the nurse to remember about radiation is that exposure to any type of radiation is cumulative. The nurse must be aware of the serious risks to clients or personnel who are repeatedly exposed to radiation. Some of the risks associated with cumulative doses of radiation are (1) increased chances of developing cancer or genetic damage, (2) sterility, (3) alterations in the makeup of individual cells, and (4) depression of the production of bone marrow. In addition, leukemia and skin cancer are more common in people who use radioactive substances in their occupations (Henry, 1982). Certainly the amount of radiation in one x-ray is not enough to cause these major problems, but radiation exposure must always be as limited as possible.

The effect on humans of any kind of radiation, natural or synthetic, is measured in a unit of quantity called rems (*roentgen equivalent for man*). A millirem is 1/1000 of a rem. Most references estimate that the average American receives 100–200 millirems of radiation a year from the sun, cosmic rays, television sets, and diagnostic x-rays. Medical irradiation is probably between 50 and 70 millirems per person per year. For x-rays, one rem is equivalent to one rad (radiation absorbed dose). X-ray exposure is designated as so many millirads. Berger and Hübner (1983) list the high, moderate, and low doses of x-rays in relation to the gonad dose and the bone marrow dose. For example, x-ray of the lower gastrointestinal tract has a high gonad dose (over 100 mrad) and a high bone marrow dose (400–2000 mrad).

The exact amount of radiation allowed for the general public cannot be expressed as so many millirems. The general guide of the National Council on Radiation Protection and Measurements is that all radiation exposure should be held to the lowest practicable level. The permissible levels of radiation incurred under occupational circumstances is 5 rems or 5000 millirems per year. (NCRP Report 48, 1976). The allowable amount for workers in nuclear plants or in radiology or nuclear medicine departments, however, is not just a simple numerical rule. The formulas used to calculate the allowable radiation exposure for these workers takes into account the lifetime exposure of workers. People who work with radiation must wear badges to monitor the exact amount of exposure to ensure that these limits are not exceeded. Nurses do not need to wear badges because they are not routinely exposed to radiation sources. Because radiation is cumulative through life, however, it is reasonable for the nurse to limit exposure to as little as possible, in all situations where radiation is being used. For example, see the discussion in Chapter 22 on handling urine when radionuclides are used for diagnostic tests. The nurse should also help make sure that clients have maximum protection.

Some readers may remember the fluoroscopy machines used in shoe stores before the 1950s. A parent could see, with delight, that the child's shoe was a perfect fit. Yet the risk of this procedure far outweighed the benefit.

At one time, dental x-rays were frequently used for screening purposes. Consumers were later advised that one should refuse to allow routine dental x-rays every six months, especially for children (Mongeau & Poirier, 1979). When dental x-rays are needed, one should ask if the machine has a focusing adaptor, which restricts the beam size. Also, the public needs to be taught that lead aprons should be worn even for dental x-rays.

Communitywide use of chest x-rays has been used to screen for tuberculosis and cancer. Routine chest x-rays for tuberculosis are not commonly done anymore, unless there is a reason to suspect the disease. Thus, chest x-rays once required yearly of employees are no longer done routinely (Health and Human Services, 1984). In 1984, the House of Delegates of the American Nurses Association passed a resolution that the ANA educate its constituents about the new criteria for chest x-rays and the role of the nurse in preventing unnecessary chest x-rays.

The annual chest x-rays, which used to be recommended for early detection of lung cancer, are not deemed worthwhile either. Even with early detection, lung cancer is still very resistant to cure. Reducing questionable chest x-rays helps eliminate unnecessary radiation exposure. The American Cancer Society (ACS) feels that more attention to the prevention of smoking is a better way to attack the problem of lung cancer. The newest guidelines for breast x-rays are covered in the ACS 1983 report on mammograms. Mammograms were widely used in the early 1970s, but again, the use of x-ray as a screening device has been reevaluated in terms of benefits versus risks. (See the discussion on mammograms later in this chapter.)

Wilson (1977) has suggested three questions that need to be asked before a client is exposed to x-rays:

1. Is the x-ray clearly necessary for the client's well-being?
2. Are there previous x-rays available or other tests that would serve the same purpose?
3. If x-rays are necessary, is everything being done to assure the lowest possible radiation dose?

Time, distance, and shielding are three ways to offer radiation protection. For example, the time of exposure to x-rays should always be as short as possible. Fluoroscopy is not done if a simple x-ray film will suffice—exposure is shorter with a traditional x-ray. Keeping a distance from the x-ray machine is a second way to avoid radiation exposure. Thus, all personnel should leave the x-ray room when x-ray studies are being done. California law states that only individuals required for the radiographic procedure shall be in the radiographic room during exposure; and except for the client, all such persons shall be equipped with appropriate protective devices (Henry, 1982). Occasionally, a nurse may be asked to help with some x-ray procedure being done at the client's bedside. (See the discussion on portable chest x-rays.) If the nurse must be involved in the procedure, then shielding is important. Shielding, (the third method of protection from radiation) involves the use of lead as a barrier to the x-rays, e.g., lead aprons and sometimes lead gloves. The walls of the x-ray room are also shielded with lead, as are containers for radioactive materials.

It is sometimes difficult for health personnel to remember that x-rays are present because they cannot be seen, heard, or felt. There is a type of monitor that gives an audible beep when the wearer is exposed to a certain level of exposure. The use of an audible beeper has helped new radiology residents and other health workers gain an immediate awareness of radiation safety in clinical areas (Gray, 1979).

Teaching Clients About X-Rays
The government has joined in the effort to reduce the risks and cost of unnecessary x-rays. The U.S. Department of Health and Human Services will send a free x-ray

and vaccination card on request.* This x-ray record card is wallet-size and can be carried to the physician, clinic, or hospital. The card should be filled in each time an x-ray is taken, including the date, type of examination, address where the x-rays are kept, and the name of the referring physician. Other tips for the public from Health and Human Services (1984) are:

1. Don't decide on your own that you need an x-ray.
2. Don't insist on an x-ray as part of a routine physical.
3. If your doctor orders an x-ray, ask how it will help with the diagnosis.
4. Tell your doctor about any similar x-rays you have had.
5. Ask if gonad shielding can be used for you and your children. (A lead apron should be routinely provided.)
6. Tell your doctor if you think you are pregnant.

Pregnant and Potentially Pregnant Women: The 14-Day Rule

Ideally, a woman in her childbearing years should only be x-rayed during her menses or 10–14 days after onset, to avoid any exposure to a fetus. The routine use of lead aprons will offer some protection to the fetus of the woman who is unaware that she is pregnant. The NCRP Report 54 (1977) gives guidelines to help the clinician schedule or postpone *elective* x-ray examinations of the pregnant or potentially pregnant woman. This report also notes that the original recommendation was that women who might be pregnant should be x-rayed only up to 10 days after onset of menses (10-day rule). However, later recommendations changed the rule to up to 14 days after onset of menses (14-day rule). The 14-day rule is a tentative recommendation from the NCRP. A few hospitals have formal procedures about scheduling in relation to menses. Thus, nurses working with clients in the childbearing years should be aware of the 14-day rule for x-rays. However, many times the enforcement of the rule is not practical.

Benefit Versus Risk Including Costs

Only recently has the public become aware of the health risks of unnecessary x-rays. Certainly the controversy about nuclear plants has caused an increased awareness by the public of the potential dangers from radiation. In addition to the potential health hazards from overuse of x-rays, the cost of unnecessary x-rays should also be considered. The cost of x-rays may be paid by insurance companies, but the cost is ultimately passed on to the consumer. As more stringent criteria are used to control insurance payments, consumers are now becoming aware of costs. Sobel and Ferguson (1985) in a book for laypeople note the usual cost of all the common diagnostic procedures including laboratory work and x-rays. If consumers can take more responsibility for avoiding unnecessary x-rays, there may be a financial gain as well as a decreased risk of illness or mutations from radiation exposure.

The point does need to be emphasized that if the client needs an x-ray for diagnostic purposes, the benefit will far outweigh the risk and cost is not a deciding factor. It is beyond the scope of nursing practice to evaluate the usefulness and safety of specific tests ordered for a client. If the nurse encounters a client who is refusing an x-ray because of a fear of radiation, it would probably be better to have the radiologist or physician explain the benefits of the test in comparison with any small

---

*To obtain more information write for 6516 to the Consumer Information Center, Pueblo, Colorado 81009 or to Training Resource Center, CDRH, HFZ-265, Rockville, MD 20857.

risk of radiation. An informed public can cooperate with health professionals to reduce the possible risks and increased costs from x-ray tests. When x-rays are done, the client should feel confident that the benefit of a specific test far outweighs the risk. The nurse can be instrumental in educating the public to have a healthy respect for x-rays as diagnostic tools. Jankowski (1986) is an excellent reference for putting the risks of radiation in perspective for the pregnant client.

PRETEST NURSING DIAGNOSES RELATED TO X-RAY PROCEDURES

Knowledge Deficit Regarding Test Procedures

When radiology tests are necessary for a client, the physician is responsible for informing the client why the tests are needed and the benefits and risks associated with the specific tests. If an x-ray is part of an invasive test, a special permit will have to be signed (see Chapter 25). Most radiology departments have printed material that gives information about how the test is done and what is necessary for client preparation. The role of the nurse is primarily to clarify the information the client has received and follow up on anything that seems unclear. If there are no printed instructions or if the client is unable to read, the nurse will have to explain the information. If the client does not speak English, an interpreter will be needed. The nurse must understand enough about the test to be able to give simple, accurate information to the client. (Key points about specific tests are covered later in this chapter.)

Anxiety Related to Unknown Sensations of the Procedure

Often the client may be more concerned about what the test "feels like" than a technical explanation of the test itself. Hartfield and Cason, (1981) studied the effects of procedural information, sensation information, and no information on the anxiety levels of clients having barium enemas. Clients who received sensation information reported less anxiety than the other groups. Nursing research for the past several years has suggested clients cope better with discomfort and pain if they are told what sensations to expect (Johnson & Rice, 1974).

Based on nursing research about preparing clients for painful procedures, McHugh et al. (1982) have suggested several guidelines:

- Physical sensations should be described, but not evaluated.
- Clients should be told what causes the sensations (i.e., dye causes flushing), so they will not conclude something has gone wrong.
- Clients should be prepared for those aspects of the experience that are noticed by the majority of clients.

Anxiety Related to Possible Findings of Test

The nurse can often relieve much of the client's anxiety by making sure that the client has received all the information he or she needs about the test, including any preparations that are needed. However, even with adequate information many clients are anxious about x-rays. In addition to the fear of pain and discomfort from some x-rays, there is often a certain amount of worry about what might be found. The nurse must not overlook the psychological needs of the client when focusing on the physical preparation. Clients may be relieved to find a nurse who not only listens but actively encourages them to ventilate any feelings they have about the upcoming test. Specific questions about the interpretation of the test should be referred to the physician who is diagnosing the problem. The nurse may help the client think of those specific questions that should be answered.

Alteration in Comfort Related to Lack of Preparation for the Procedure

A study done in an English hospital identified four major factors that clients labeled as being stressful during barium x-ray studies (Barnett-Wilson, 1978): (1) waiting time in the x-ray department, (2) moving about on the hard x-ray table, (3) darkness and noise during the screening, and (4) enemas or suppositories that made the clients sleepless and exhausted before the test. An awareness of the physical factors likely to cause stress during x-ray studies should help the nurse plan care that is nurturing and supportive both before and after what many clients may experience as an ordeal.

The waiting time in the x-ray department may be very exhausting to some clients. The nurse can alert the x-ray department's personnel that the client is confused or incontinent or in a great deal of pain so that the client with a major problem is not left waiting for a long time. If a very weak client must wait, a stretcher should be used for transportation rather than a wheelchair. If permissible, pain medications may be given before the trip. Because a number of x-ray tests require lying or moving about on a hard table, the client should be well-rested. Enemas or suppositories should be done early enough so that the client can rest awhile before going to x-ray. If possible, the nurse can promise to let the client rest once the x-ray is finished. For some clients, the waiting time in x-ray causes boredom. The nurse can encourage the client to take some reading material or other activity, such as knitting, to help pass the time.

The nurse should see if the client is ready for x-ray. Glasses, dentures, and hearing aides should not be removed before the x-ray if needed. X-ray personnel should be informed that a client is hard of hearing or has other communication problems. The client needs to empty his or her bladder. A robe should be worn for privacy and warmth, as well as slippers if the client is to stand during the test.

These suggestions for ensuring client comfort are basic and thus often not mentioned. However, unless the nurse attends to these details, the x-ray experience may be more uncomfortable than necessary. If the x-ray is being done on an outpatient basis, the nurse can give the client tips on how to come prepared for x-ray. It is also important the client know the approximate time for the x-rays so business or home affairs do not present problems.

Potential for Fluid Volume Deficit Related to n.p.o. Status

The nurse must make sure that the client understands when he or she is not allowed to eat or drink before a test (n.p.o.). If feasible, having the client drink eight glasses of water for a day or two before the test will decrease the potential for a fluid volume deficit. With some tests, a light breakfast or clear liquid may be allowed. Clients may need clarification that clear liquids means just that. Orange juice, milk, and so on are not clear liquids—one cannot see through them. Because of dehydration, especially in the very young or the elderly, the nurse must find out if the test requires strict n.p.o. or if clear liquids are permissible. Most hospital put an n.p.o. sign in the kardex and on the door, but

TABLE 20-1. SUMMARY OF CRITERIA NEEDED FOR BOWEL PREPARATION[a]

1. Restriction of diet to clear liquids (check for times)
2. Hydration of the client by adequate clear liquids (check for amounts)
3. Use of an evacuant that stimulates the small intestine (check for laxative ordered)
4. Use of an evacuant that stimulates the colon (check for laxative or suppositories ordered)
5. Use of an enema as an additional cleansing method (check for orders for tap water enemas or small medicated enemas)

[a]See text for more details on specific preps for various procedures. Note that Golytely may replace these bowel preparations.

a well-informed client is the best guarantee that the client will observe n.p.o. status, if necessary. For children the restrictions on n.p.o. status may only be for 3 hours rather than the usual 6 to 8 hours for adults.

Alteration in Elimination Pattern Related to Need for Bowel Preparations

X-ray studies that involve structures in the lower abdomen may require a "bowel prep" before the x-ray. Table 20–1 summarizes the criteria needed to maximize bowel preparation. Note that clients with ileostomies are not given enemas or laxatives as a bowel preparation. The preparation may be accomplished by cleansing enemas, cathartics, or suppositories. For example, a client may be given a bisacodyl tablet (Dulcolax) or castor oil the night before the x-ray and a suppository the next morning. It is very important for the nurse to assess the effectiveness of the bowel preparation. If the method used did not cause an evacuation of the bowel, other methods may be needed before the client is sent to x-ray. A poorly prepared client may mean that the x-rays have to be repeated.

A newer bowel preparation involves a total gut irrigation with Golytely, a mixture of electrolytes and polyethylene glycol. The glycol prevents transfer of electrolytes into or out of the solution and also prevents production of gas in the intestine (Tuttobene, 1984). The client must drink the chilled solution at a rate of 1.2–1.8 L/hr until the rectal effluent is clear. The procedure usually takes 2–4 hours.

Children and Elderly. A series of cleansing enemas or strong cathartics or repeated suppositories may be very taxing to elderly, frail clients. Also, the irrigation method with an electrolyte solution results in many trips to the bathroom. The nurse should question "standard" orders for bowel preps when the client is very small or frail. Perhaps smaller doses will be sufficient. Cathartics or enemas may be contraindicated if the client has had severe diarrhea or bleeding. Children under 1-year old are usually not given any suppositories as bowel preparations. Children ages 1 to 9 may be given a half suppository. Any dose of laxative must be calculated on the basis of the weight of the child.

Teaching at Home. When bowel preps are to be done in the home, the client must be taught exactly what to do if the procedure does not clean out the bowel. Also, the client needs to be shown exactly how to insert the suppository or how much fluid may be needed for the irrigation method. Often what is "obvious" to the health professional may not be to the client. Written instructions are standard, but a time for verbal interaction is often needed and much appreciated.

Potential for Injury due to Adverse Reactions to Contrast Medium

Many of the dyes used as contrast media contain iodinated compounds, which have the potential to provoke allergic reactions (Table 20–2). Some newer agents do not contain iodine but are more expensive. The radiology department should be notified if the client has any allergies to iodine substances. The nurse should ask the client if he or she has any other allergies. For example, an allergy to seafood may be due to an allergy to iodine.

Clients with any preexisting renal problems have a risk of nephrotoxicity from the dye (Marinelli-Miller, 1983). A BUN and/or creatinine may be done to assess renal function (see Chapter 4). Acute renal failure following use of contrast medium is limited to clients with complicating factors and is usually reversible (Cruz et al., 1986). Development of newer agents may lessen this danger.

Except for the oral tablets used for a gallbladder series, all administration of dyes are done in the radiology department. Before the radiologist injects the dye intravenously, the client will again be questioned about possible allergies. Many of the dyes have an antihistamine in the preparation, but the radiologist still watches carefully for any signs of allergy, such as nausea, vomiting, palpitations, dyspnea, and dizziness. Radiology departments are always equipped with drugs (epinephrine, antihistamines, and corticosteroids) and equipment to treat anaphylactic shock, which can result from the dye. The IV radiographic contrast material can also cause a vagus reaction marked by profound bradycardia and hypotension. Treatment for a vagal response includes IV atropine (Bush et al., 1985).

Clients need to understand that normally the dye causes a flushed warm sensation when it is injected intravenously. The dye may also cause a salty taste in the mouth. Some references suggest to use the term contrast medium rather than dye when explaining tests to the client. The word "dye" may give the impression that the material permanently changes body color, which it does not.

TABLE 20–2. NURSING IMPLICATIONS WHEN CONTRAST MEDIUM OR DYE IS USED FOR X-RAY TESTS

Examples of Common Radiologic Tests Using Iodine Contrast Medium or Dye
1. Gallbladder series (oral tablets)
2. Intravenous cholangiograms (IVC)
3. Intravenous pyelograms (IVP)
4. Arteriograms

Pretest	Posttest
Assess for allergy to iodine	Assess for any allergic reactions
Instruct on sensations of dye	Encourage fluids
	Do not use urine tests, specific gravity, etc., for 24 hours
	Assess for phlebitis at injection site

Note: In addition to allergic reactions, a vasovagal reaction may occur during instillation of dye. See text for details.

The after-effects of the dye are covered in the next section. The section on diagnostic products in the Physician's Desk Reference (1986) gives detailed information on all the common contrast media used in x-ray exams. Dosages of the dye are based on the client's weight.

POSTTEST NURSING DIAGNOSES RELATED TO X-RAY PROCEDURES

The nurse needs to know exactly what type of procedure was done because specific implications are related to specific tests. (Care after a test is detailed under the description of the test later in this chapter.) Some hospitals may have a mini-recovery room for clients who need special observation, such as neurological checks (Maphet, 1981). More commonly, clients are returned to their rooms as soon as the procedures are finished. Also many clients have the x-rays on an outpatient basis, therefore the client or a significant other needs careful instruction on possible complications.

Potential for Injury Related to Use of Contrast Medium

Usually if the client is allergic to the dye, or contrast medium, an immediate allergic reaction will occur in the radiology department, but delayed reactions are possible; consequently, any symptoms such as urticaria, nausea, vomiting, or dyspnea should be reported immediately. Oral antihistamines or corticosteroids may be ordered for allergic reactions not acute enough to require epinephrine. Occasionally, the vein used for the dye injection may become inflamed. Any local tissue reactions should be reported. Warm compresses may be used for phlebitis.

Alteration in Fluid and Food Requirements

Dyes given intravenously for x-ray diagnostic tests are excreted in the urine. The dye acts as an osmotic diuretic. Thus, if other conditions permit, the client who has a dye injection should be given extra fluid to replace the fluid lost with the excretion of the dye. Some clients may complain of some bladder irritation or burning on urination caused by the dye. As noted earlier, the dye poses a risk of nephrotoxicity in clients with preexisting renal problems. The dye is not visible in the urine but it does elevate the specific gravity of the urine. (Note dye does not change the osmolality of the urine so a urine osmolality test would be a valid test of fluid balance (see Chapter 4).

The contrast medium of barium sulfate, used for studies of the gastrointestinal tract, may cause constipation, therefore fluids need to be encouraged after these x-rays. The barium is visible in the stool as white streaks.

The client may be very hungry or thirsty from being on n.p.o. status for a long time. If allowed and tolerated, a cup of tea or some milk will be most appreciated until more solid food can be obtained. The liquids can help eliminate the dehydration, which may develop from the extended n.p.o. status.

For many people, food is more than just physically satisfying. Food can be a symbol of love and care. Concern about the client's lack of food may be interpreted by the client as a very tangible sign of warmth and caring. (One of the cornerstones of professional nursing is nurturing.) It becomes very routine for the nurse to withhold food and fluids because of diagnostic procedures. It is not routine for the client to go without food or fluids, and mere acknowledgment of this deprivation may be satisfying to the client.

Alteration in Comfort Related to Pain After Procedure

Waiting in the radiology department and the test procedures themselves may be exhausting. Clients should, therefore, be allowed to rest and only be disturbed for necessary procedures, such as checking vital signs and inspecting dressings for bleeding. Lying on a hard table will cause a backache for some people. A backrub will often be appreciated. A heating pad may also be helpful if muscles or joints hurt from the positioning during the test. (A physician's order is needed for heat applications.) Some procedures cause pain severe enough to require the use of analgesics. The nurse must assess whether the pain is the expected type for the procedure. For example, pain at the site of arterial puncture would be expected, whereas pain in the foot may be a symptom of an embolus from the puncture site.

After diagnostic tests, an outpatient may need to rest before going home. (Monitoring may also be needed for a couple of hours.) If advisable, clients should be told in advance to have someone available to drive them home. The client should be informed about the level of pain to be expected. For example, hysterosalpingogram may cause severe abdominal pains a few hours after the procedure. The client should be alerted that if the pain is not relieved by analgesics, she should notify the clinic or physician because pain can be a sign of a complication, such as a perforation. Arthrograms are another type of x-ray that can cause considerable pain posttest. The manipulation of the joint entailed in the procedure can cause severe pain when the local anesthetic wears off. Instruction on the use of warm compresses or sitz baths to relax the tense, tired muscles from the painful x-ray session may be helpful. Mild analgesics may be needed.

Anxiety Related to Waiting for the Results of the Test

Interpretation of the test results is usually not ready until the next day or later. The client may be concerned about the results of the test. The nurse can act as a sounding board and help the client formulate questions to ask the physician. The nurse can also let the client vent feelings about any pain or discomfort experienced during the test.

Nursing Implications for Future Care

By listening to the client's personal account of the test, the nurse not only helps the client put the experience in perspective but learns something that might help in preparing the next client for a radiological test. As noted earlier, clients should be prepared for sensations experienced by the majority of clients undergoing a specific diagnostic procedure. McHugh and co-workers (1982) suggest that nurses make lists of all aspects of a client's experience. Then using the list, the nurse can interview clients to discover what aspects of the experience are noticed by at least 50% of the clients. The nurse will also discover what words are most often used to describe the sensations. Clients' descriptions are usually less technical and complex than nurses'.

■ CHEST X-RAYS

Description. Chest x-rays are not only done in the radiology department but also at the client's bedside, if the client cannot be transported to the radiology department. However, bedside, portable chest x-rays are not of as good a quality as those in the radiology department. In the radiology department, the client stands 6–9 feet from the x-ray machine; whereas, the smaller, portable chest x-ray must be at most 3 feet from the client. In the x-ray department, the standard chest film is a posterior–anterior (PA) view because the client stands with the anterior part of the body next to the film. The portable chest x-ray only gives an anterior–posterior (AP) view because the film is behind the client's back. In describing positions of the client, the first term refers to the site of entry and the second term to the exit of the x-ray beam, which is captured on the film. Note the basic working principle: the part that needs to be studied should be next to the film (Felson, 1980). Chest x-rays may be lateral views or oblique views as well. If there is a question of free pleural fluid, the film is taken with the client supine or in a lateral decubitus position, so that the fluid will pool. (Decubitus means a lying-down position; hence, a decubitus ulcer results from a lying-down position.) If air is suspected, the client is kept sitting up. For most chest films, the client is asked to take a deep breath and hold it so that the lungs are fully expanded and the diaphragm is descended.

Purposes. X-ray films of the chest are used to identify various abnormalities of the lungs and structures in the thorax. In addition, the size of the heart and abnormalities in the ribs or diaphragm can be determined. The three most common abnormalities seen in chest films are pneumonia, atelectasis, and pneumothorax. Unfortunately, in early stages of tuberculosis or asthma the client may have a normal chest x-ray. Also in chronic obstructive lung disease the chest x-ray may not correlate with the clinical status. Expiration films are used to detect a small pneumothorax or to demonstrate alterations in ventilation due to emphysema or partial bronchial obstructions. Tumors of the lung can be identified by chest x-rays, but tomograms may give more information about the exact location in the tissue. (See tomograms in the next chapter.) As discussed earlier, chest x-rays are not done as routinely as they were because of the concern about too much radiation exposure for too little benefit.

Client Preparation

A chest x-ray done in the radiology department requires no special preparation. The client should not wear jewelry or any metal around the neck or on the hospital gown. Most clients are very familiar with the chest x-ray and realize that there is no pain or discomfort.

Nurse's Role with Portable Chest X-Rays

If a portable chest x-ray is used at the client's bedside, the nurse may have a more active role in preparing the client. For example, chest electrodes need to be temporarily removed so the metal will not interfere with the picture. Intravenous tubing and arterial lines, may cause shadows; thus, nothing should be lying on top of the client's chest. The client's back needs to be in even contact with the film holder. If the client is slumped in bed, the picture may be of very poor quality. Sometimes the nurse may be asked to hold the client during the x-ray. California law states that no individual occupationally exposed to radiation shall be permitted to hold clients during exposures except during emergencies, nor shall any individual be regularly used for this service

(Henry, 1982). If it is absolutely necessary for someone to help hold the client in a position, the helper should wear a lead apron. (Lead gloves may also be used for protection.) As discussed earlier, although the radiation from one chest x-ray is minimal, the nurse must remember that radiation exposure is cumulative over a lifetime. Pregnant nurses should definitely not be exposed to any x-rays being done on clients. Nurses who could be pregnant should follow the 14-day rule discussed earlier (i.e., radiation only up to 14 days after onset of menses).

POSTTEST NURSING IMPLICATIONS

There are no special implications for nursing care after a chest x-ray. If the x-ray film shows atelectasis, the client will need vigorous pulmonary toilet for potential ineffective airway clearance.

■ PLAIN FILMS OF THE ABDOMEN: FLAT PLATES, THREE-WAY FILMS, AND KUB

Description. Plain films, or scout films, of the abdomen may be done as the first step in assessing a variety of abdominal problems. They may be done with the client lying down flat, turned to the left, and upright. These three positions are called a three-way abdominal x-ray. If the main focus is on the *k*idneys, *u*reters, and *b*ladder, the x-ray is called a KUB.

Purposes. Abdominal x-rays can detect loops of dilated bowel, patterns of gas, and possible obstructions. Stones and calcified areas in the pancreas, biliary system, or urinary system may be detected but films with contrast medium are needed for diagnosis. Perforations in the gastrointestinal tract will result in the escape of air into the peritoneal cavity, which will cause an elevation of the diaphragm on the affected side. The elevated diaphragm will be seen on the plain film.

Client Preparation
In abdominal trauma, the flat plate x-ray will be ordered as a stat procedure. If there are questionable abdominal injuries, there will not be any attempt to clear the bowel of feces and gas. In nontraumatic conditions, however, the client may need a bowel preparation before the x-ray is done. (See the introductory remarks on types of bowel preparation that may be done.)

NURSING IMPLICATIONS

There are no special nursing implications related to a flat plate x-ray of the abdomen. However, the nurse should be aware that the client may be scheduled for other x-rays that involve the use of a contrast medium to identify particular structures. The nurse should also assess and record the exact nature of any abdominal pain and absence or presence of bowel sounds which could be useful in the differential diagnosis of acute abdominal problems.

■ BONE OR SKELETAL X-RAYS, INCLUDING THE SKULL

Description and Purpose. Skeletal x-rays are routinely used to detect fractures. They may also be used to detect tumors of the bone, but scans are more useful. (See Chapter 22 for the use of bone scans with radionuclides to detect tumors.) Simple x-rays are useful in assessing skull fractures; however, the presence or absence of a skull fracture does not correlate with the possible severity of any underlying brain damage. (The CT scan discussed in the next chapter is extremely valuable in detecting soft tissue injuries.) Skeletal x-rays are also used to assess arthritic conditions and to detect osteomyelitis.

Client Preparation

Skeletal x-rays require no special preparation. If the x-rays are being done to assess a possible fracture, the client should be treated as having a fracture until it is ruled out. The client needs careful handling and immobilization of the affected part. Pain relief may be needed before transportation. If skull x-rays are required, the client should have a neurological assessment before transportation to the radiology department. If any drainage is present a check with Tes-Tape will reveal if the fluid is cerebral fluid. Glucose in cerebral fluid makes the test positive. Mucus contains no glucose. The nurse should notify the members of the x-ray department of any instability in the client's vital signs, so that the x-rays are done immediately and the client watched carefully.

NURSING IMPLICATIONS

See the precautions noted in the preparation before bone films regarding care of potential fractures. If the client is having skeletal x-rays because of arthritis, the client may need warmth to the joints and some analgesic after the manipulation.

■ UPPER GI SERIES, CARDIAC SERIES, AND SMALL BOWEL SERIES

Description and Purposes. Barium swallows are used for x-rays of the upper gastrointestinal (GI) tract and to outline the cardiac border. The client drinks barium sulfate, which is a chalky radiopaque substance. Its nonwater soluble quality prevents it from being absorbed by the gastrointestinal tract. If there is a possibility of a leak or an obstruction, the radiologist will use a dye, meglumine diatrizoate (Gastrografin), which is water soluble. Fluoroscopy during the barium swallow will outline the esophagus and any structural defects. If the barium swallow is being done to outline the borders of the heart, the size and contour of the heart will be revealed. Several different views of the heart can be photographed, called a "cardiac series." Esophageal varices may also show on the film.

The swallowed barium coats the stomach walls so that defects, such as tumors or ulcers, are seen as dark areas with a white background of the dye. The upper GI series is the definitive test for stomach and duodenal ulcers. The time it takes for the barium to empty out of the stomach will be important in some cases because duodenal ulcers may cause some degree of pyloric obstruction or gastric outlet obstruction. As the barium goes through the small intestine another series of x-rays may be taken, called a small bowel series.

An upper GI series takes about 45 minutes. If a small bowel series is done, it may take up to 5 hours to complete the x-rays. Also, a follow-up x-ray may be taken in 24 hours.

Certain drugs may be given during an upper GI series. For example, glucagon may be given to relax the intestinal tract. Drugs may also be used to accelerate the passage of barium through the stomach and small bowel to promote better visualization of the jejunum and ileum. Metoclopramide (Reglan by Robbins) is such a pro-motility agent. These drugs are given intravenously after the client is in x-ray.

Client Preparation

The client usually has a light diet the evening before the x-ray and has n.p.o. status from midnight until the test. Food or medicine in the gastrointestinal tract will interfere with the barium coating the walls. Sometimes oral medications may be continued until 2 hours prior to the scheduled examination, if gastric emptying is normal. However, any administration of medications should be cleared by the physician. Some parenteral medications, such as antibiotics, are continued; others may not be, for example, regular insulin would be withheld while a longer acting insulin may be given. Because narcotics and anticholinergic drugs, such as atropine, slow down the mobility of the intestinal tract, the radiologist should be notified if these drugs have been given to the client. Sometimes atropine might be ordered before an upper GI series if the client has a hyperactive bowel. The client should be told that fluoroscopy is done in the dark and that the x-ray table is tilted to help the flow of barium. If a small bowel series is to be done, the client needs to know that it is a lengthy procedure requiring a couple of trips to the x-ray department. The client should also be told that the barium has a chalky taste. Many radiology departments use flavored barium sulfate (e.g., peppermint or chocolate), but most clients still find it rather unpleasant to drink.

POSTTEST NURSING IMPLICATIONS

The client may be returned to the unit to wait for a second series of x-rays to be taken. Food and water should not be allowed until the radiologist completes the test. If the client has an ulcer, the lack of food in the stomach may have aggravated the abdominal pain, so food or antacids should be resumed as soon as possible. The client should be informed that his or her stool will be light-colored due to the barium being excreted. For some clients, the barium may be constipating. Thus, the nurse should note that the client is well-hydrated, that there is adequate roughage in his or her diet. Laxatives or enemas may be needed. Barium in the intestine will interfere with other abdominal tests, so they should be scheduled first; otherwise, the client may need an enema so that other structures can be visualized by these other tests.

■ BARIUM ENEMAS (BE)

Description. For examination of the lower colon an enema of barium sulfate is given. This is done in the radiology department. The client must retain the barium while a series of x-ray pictures are taken. After the barium is excreted a final x-ray of the bowel is taken. Sometimes air is put into the empty colon afterwards for a double contrast examination. The introduction of air may cause slight discomfort. A BE takes about 1–1½ hours to complete.

Purpose. The BE is commonly used for any kind of suspected lower intestine or colon problem. Tumors, strictures, polyps, and diverticulum can all be well visualized by this method. Sometimes the BE is also therapeutic; it may reduce an obstruction if caused by intussusception or telescoping of the bowel.

Client Preparation

The lower colon must be prepared by the bowel preparation used in a particular setting. As noted in Table 20–1, bowel preparations may include enemas, laxatives, electrolyte irrigations, or suppositories. It is essential that there be no fecal matter in the lower colon. The client may be given a cleansing enema early the morning of the x-ray. Some institutions do not schedule enemas the day of the x-ray. If the client has a severely inflamed bowel or active bleeding, strong cathartics or other bowel preparations are contraindicated.

A liquid diet may be ordered for the day before the examination. Clients are given a light breakfast the day of the examination because the food will not reach the large intestine by the time of the examination. However, if there is any question about complications, food may be withheld. Perforation of the colon is a very unlikely complication, but it can occur if the bowel is diseased and friable. In the case where there may be complications, it is always better that the client not have a full stomach. Adequate ingestion of liquids is important so that the client is well-hydrated. An example of client instructions for use with outpatients is shown in Table 20–3.

If the client is unable to retain the fluid of the enema, the nurse needs to inform the radiology department so a special tube can be used to instill the contrast medium. The client who can retain the enema fluid can be spared this extra discomfort. Most people can retain the amount of fluid used for the barium enema, but it is often a concern for the client.

A barium enema can be administered through a colostomy. Usual bowel preparations are done that would include irrigation of the colostomy before the procedure. Arnell and Nassberg (1981) describe, in detail, the techniques used to instill barium via a colostomy. Alterescu (1985) notes that mechanical bowel cleaning differs for clients with ileostomies because enemas and laxatives are not used.

POSTTEST NURSING IMPLICATIONS

A barium enema can be exhausting physically and psychologically. It is embarassing to many people to be given an enema in the radiology department and then to be asked to assume awkward positions in front of other people. If the client did not retain the barium well, a bath may be in order. Although most clients do expel the barium in the x-ray department, some, particularly the elderly, may become constipated from barium still in the intestines. Fluids should be encouraged, 2000 ml a day for the adult, unless contraindicated. Cleansing enemas or laxative may be given if there is a problem with defecation. If the barium was instilled via a colostomy, irrigations can rid the bowel of the residual barium. As mentioned earlier, the client's first stool will be a light color or will have white streaks.

TABLE 20-3. INSTRUCTIONS FOR BARIUM ENEMA

THE SENOKOT SUPPOSITORY AND X-PREP LIQUID MUST BE PURCHASED AT THE PHARMACY. (*Senokot* and *X-prep* are brand names for senna preparations; bisacodyl (*Dulcolax*) may also be used.)

ON THE DAY BEFORE YOUR APPOINTMENT—EAT AND DRINK ONLY THE FOLLOWING:

LUNCH   This meal may include clear broth, white chicken meat sandwich (no butter, lettuce, or other additive), or two hard boiled eggs, strained fruit juices, Jello or gelatine (not including fruits or nuts), coffee or tea (without cream or milk), or carbonated beverages.

3 P.M.   Take 2½ oz of the prescribed laxative and drink one full glass of water.

SUPPER   Limit your evening meal to liquids without milk products. This meal may include clear broth, strained fruit juices, Jello or gelatine (not containing fruits or nuts), coffee or tea (without cream or milk), or carbonated beverages.

10 P.M.   Insert one unwrapped *Senokot* or other suppository into your rectum.

ON THE DAY OF YOUR APPOINTMENT:

BREAKFAST Limit to coffee or tea (without cream or milk), strained fruit juices, dry toast or bread.

Two (2) hours before your scheduled examination, insert one unwrapped *Senokot* or other suppository into your rectum.

PLEASE REPORT TO THE X-RAY DEPARTMENT ON _____ AT _____

WHAT IS THE BARIUM ENEMA?

This is the x-ray examination of the large intestine. For this study it is most important to clean the bowel of all retained fecal matter. A tube will be placed into your rectum, and the barium liquid will flow easily into your bowel. The radiologist will study the bowel under the fluoroscope, and have several x-rays taken.

NOTE: If you have severe diarrhea or considerable rectal bleeding, consult your physician before taking the laxative or suppository requested above. If you have any questions, or require a change of appointment, please call the x-ray department.

Courtesy of Kaiser Permanente Medical Group, San Francisco, California.

■ ORAL CHOLECYSTOGRAM (OCG) OR GALLBLADDER SERIES

Description. For an oral cholecystogram (OCG), six dye tablets are taken orally one or two nights before the x-ray. The tablets contain iodinated compounds, such as iopanoic acid (Telepaque) or sodium ipodate (Oragrafin). The radiopaque dye or contrast medium is excreted via the liver into the biliary system and concentrates in the gallbladder. Dye is not given if the client has any liver dysfunction. For example, a bilirubin above 3 or 4 mg/dl would be a contraindication for a gallbladder (GB) series. (See Chapter 11 on bilirubin levels.)

Purposes. The GB series is used to determine if a gallbladder can fill, concentrate, and empty bile properly. The presence of stones will be seen as light shadows in the gallbladder. If the gallbladder is not visualized on the x-ray film, the test may be repeated with a double dose (12 tablets) of dye. If the gallbladder is still not visualized, this may indicate an obstruction in the biliary tree or a diseased gallbladder. The client may be given a fatty meal after the OCG and more films may be later taken to see how well the gallbladder empties. (Note that the use of ultrasound is a newer diagnostic test for gallstones [see Chapter 23], as is radionuclides [see Chapter 22].)

Client Preparation

Most radiology departments start client preparation 2 days before the examination. On the first evening, the client is given a high-fat meal (milk, eggs, and bread with butter), followed by dye tablets. The next evening, a normal meal without fats is given, followed by a second dose of six tablets. This double dose of tablets may eliminate some cases of nonvisualization of the gallbladder, which are due to lack of dye and not gallbladder disease.

Because the oral tablets contain iodine, the client must be checked for any sensitivity to iodine compounds. The six tablets are taken after the evening meal, one every 5 minutes with water. After the six tablets are taken, the client is placed on n.p.o. status. The tablets may cause nausea, vomiting, and diarrhea in some clients. If the client vomits the tablets, the test will have to be rescheduled. Diarrhea will not cause loss of the dye. If the client cannot swallow the tablets, a contrast medium can be given intravenously in the radiology department. However, the intravenous cholangiograms are usually used to assess the condition of the ducts, not the concentrating ability of the gallbladder (see the next section). A bowel preparation of enemas or suppositories may be ordered to clean out the bowel. If the client has received morphine sulfate, the radiologist should be notified because morphine may cause spasm of the sphincter of Oddi.

POSTTEST NURSING IMPLICATIONS

As mentioned earlier, the client may be given a fatty meal if more films are planned to see how well the gallbladder empties. Otherwise, the client can resume whatever diet is tolerated. Actually, a fat-restricted diet is often needed because of the client's fat intolerance due to an obstruction of the biliary system. (See Chapter 11 for the nursing diagnoses when a client has an obstruction of the biliary system.)

■ CHOLANGIOGRAMS: INTRAVENOUS, OPERATIVE, TRANSHEPATIC, AND VIA ENDOSCOPE

Description and Purposes. A cholangiogram is an x-ray of the biliary tree using contrast medium so the cystic, hepatic, and common bile ducts can be visualized. Note that the oral cholecystogram, discussed above, is used to assess the ability of the gallbladder to concentrate and excrete the dye.

IVC. When the dye is given intravenously (IVC), the liver excretes the dye into the biliary tree. X-ray pictures are taken at intervals after the dye is injected. The dye begins to appear in the biliary tree about 10 minutes after the intravenous administration. It takes about 4 hours but sometimes 8 hours for the dye to be totally excreted, so the client may be in the radiology department for several hours.

Via T-Tubes. Cholangiograms are also done during surgical procedures to check for stones in the common bile duct, which might not be seen or felt. With the operative method, the dye is injected directly into a drainage catheter (T-tube), placed in the common bile duct during surgery. X-ray films are taken immediately after the dye is instilled. A cholangiogram via the T-tube may also be done several days post-operatively to evaluate the patency of the biliary tree. Clients with exploration of the common bile duct have T-tubes for bile drainage until the edema in the common bile duct is gone.

Transhepatic. Transhepatic cholangiograms are done via a percutaneous insertion of a needle into the common bile duct. The insertion is done with the aid of fluoroscopy. After the needle is in the common bile duct, dye is injected.

Endoscopic. A fourth way to inject dye into the biliary system is with the use of an endoscope passed down the gastrointestinal tract through the sphincter of Oddi into the biliary tract. (See Chapter 27 for a discussion about endoscopic procedures.)

Client Preparation

Of the four procedures described above, IVC is most commonly used. The client is kept on n.p.o. status for 6–8 hours before the test. A bowel preparation will be ordered to clear the intestinal tract. The IVC is done in the radiology department and is not particularly uncomfortable except for the sensation of dye being injected intravenously.

If cholangiograms are part of an operative procedure, the client receives the routine preoperative preparation. A percutaneous transhepatic cholangiogram is done in the radiology department. Because this is an invasive procedure, the physician must explain the specific risks to the client. The endoscopic procedure is also invasive and entails certain risks; consequently, institutions will have special protocols to follow regarding permission. (See Chapter 25 for nursing implications for invasive tests.) Because obstructions in the biliary system tend to increase bleeding, the client usually has a prothrombin time done before any type of invasive procedure of the biliary tree. If the prothrombin time is increased, vitamin K must be given parenterally before traumatic tests are done. Gastrointestinal absorption of vitamin K, a fat soluble vitamin, is hampered when there is a biliary obstruction and thus a lack of bile salts for fat absorption. Chapter 11 discusses laboratory tests used to assess for biliary obstruction and the nursing diagnoses for clients with elevation of direct bilirubin (obstructive jaundice).

POSTTEST NURSING IMPLICATIONS

The aftercare for the client who has had dye instilled via an IVC would be the routine nursing diagnoses discussed in the beginning of this chapter.

See Chapter 25 for the nursing implications when a client has had an invasive procedure that may cause bleeding. Frequent checking of vital signs and bed rest for a certain amount of time is important. Just as in a liver biopsy, complications such as leakage of bile into the peritoneal cavity can occur when a needle is put into the common bile duct. Any abdominal pain, which could mean bile peritonitis, should be called to the attention of the physician. Chills and fever may be due to inflammation of the bile duct.

■ INTRAVENOUS PYELOGRAMS

Description. Sodium diatrizoate (Hypaque) or meglumine diatrizoate (Renografin) are dyes used for pyelograms because they are excreted by the urinary system. Another name for an intravenous pyelogram (IVP) is an excretory urography because it demonstrates the ability of the entire urinary tract to excrete dye. After the dye or contrast medium has been injected intravenously, x-ray films are taken every minute for 5 minutes, allowing visualization of the cortex of the kidney. Approximately 15 minutes later, x-ray films are taken as the dye collects in the pelvis of the kidney and is excreted via the ureters into the bladder. The dye outlines the bladder in about 45 minutes. The client is asked to void, and a postvoiding film is taken to see how well the bladder empties. The entire set of x-rays takes about an hour. If the dye is not well excreted a 24 hour follow-up x-ray must be done.

Purposes. Structural defects or tumors can be observed when the urinary system is outlined with dye. A retrograde introduction of dye, through ureteral catheters, to outline the urinary system is done via a cystoscope. (See Chapter 27 for endoscopic procedures.) Note that renograms done with radionuclides (Chapter 22) can be done if clients are allergic to the contrast medium used for IVP.

Client Preparation

The client is given a light meal the evening before the test. Different radiology departments may have different instructions regarding n.p.o. status. Some radiologists prefer that the client not take in any fluids so the dye will not be diluted. Other radiologists want the client to be given clear liquids so that the client is not dehydrated before the examination. A lack of normal renal function may make it hazardous for the client to receive dye that is excreted via the kidney; therefore, serum creatine and BUN levels are assessed before the test is begun (see Chapter 4). The bowel preparation for an IVP needs to be thorough. A cathartic as well as suppositories the evening before and the morning of the examination may be necessary. Enemas may be necessary if the client has had barium studies in the preceding 48 hours.

The client should be instructed about the feeling of the dye being injected. (See the general implications about contrast medium discussed earlier in this chapter.) There may be more than one venipuncture. The only other discomfort will result from lying in one position during the series of films. Voiding in the x-ray department may be embarassing for clients who must use a urinal or bedpan if they cannot go to the bathroom.

POSTTEST NURSING IMPLICATIONS

See the general implications for dye use, including a fluid intake of 2000–3000 ml of fluids. The client should be observed for any signs of urinary problems, such as difficulty voiding or bladder irritation. Note that the serum creatinine levels and/or creatinine clearance tests may be used to assess any loss of renal function.

■ BRONCHOGRAMS

Description. A bronchogram, an x-ray picture of the bronchial tree, is almost always done in conjunction with a bronchoscopy. (See Chapter 27 for the nursing implications when a client has a bronchoscopy.) An iodine dye is instilled by an atomizer or other means into the bronchi. X-ray films are made to show the outline and structure of the bronchial tree and lungs. Bronchograms have almost become obsolete because the flexible bronchoscope leaves few lesions inaccessible to direct vision. Also, CT scans and MRI scans offer great details of lung structure (see Chapter 21).

■ ARTERIOGRAMS

Description. *Angiogram* is a broad term meaning visualization of blood vessels that are either arteries or veins. *Arteriogram* is a more precise term designating visualization of an arterial vessel or vessels. The most common site of dye injection for an arteriogram is the femoral artery. Arterial catheters are positioned, using a guide-wire to advance the catheter to a certain spot in the arterial tree. Because the arterial catheter is radiopaque, movement of the catheter is noted by fluoroscopy. After the correct placement is obtained, dye is injected into the catheter to outline a certain portion of the artery. In this way the circulation in the lower extremity can be visualized. Also, the catheter can be threaded, via the femoral artery, into the abdominal aorta to the level of the renal arteries for renal arteriograms. The arteries of the gastrointestinal tract can be visualized if the dye is instilled in the celiac axis. The brachial artery can be used for upper extremity visualization. Carotid arteriograms may also be done, but can disrupt atherosclerotic plaques, which can become cerebral emboli. Therefore, the carotid arteries are usually visualized by a catheter threaded through other arteries.

Purposes. Arteriograms are extremely valuable for observing the blood flow to a part of the body and to detect lesions, which may be amenable to surgery. The catheter used to confirm the diagnosis of a suspected kidney or liver lesion may also become a vehicle for the selective delivery of chemotherapeutic drugs or drugs to stop bleeding (Athanasoulis, 1980). Catheters in arteries are also used to remove atherosclerotic plaques in a procedure called percutaneous transluminal angioplasty (PTA).

Client Preparation
The client must sign a special permit form. At some hospitals it is routine to discuss the possibility of angioplasty and get informed consent at the time a client signs a consent form for the arteriogram because the therapeutic maneuver may immediately follow the diagnostic procedure (Willard, 1985). After premedication is done, the client cannot legally consent to another procedure not on the original consent form. (See Chapter 25 for the nurse's role in preparing clients for invasive procedures.) Because this test involves the use of an iodinated dye intravenously, the implications for dye use should be considered. The client's weight is used to determine the dose of the dye. (See the discussion on dyes in the beginning of this chapter.) The client is kept on n.p.o. status for 6–8 hours before the procedure; some institutions do allow liquids before an arteriogram. There may be an order to shave an area, but usually any preparation of the puncture site is done in the radiology department.

POSTTEST NURSING IMPLICATIONS

The client is kept on bedrest for a minimum of 6–8 hours, to decrease the possibility of bleeding from the puncture site; some institutions may keep the client on bedrest for 24 hours. The nurse should make an observation of the puncture site as soon as the client returns from the radiology department, which will serve as a baseline comparison if there is any later bleeding on the dressing or some swelling around the site. There may be more than one site if one puncture was not successful. The pressure dressing, on the site, should not be removed. An icebag may also be placed on the site to decrease the possibility of bleeding or hematoma formation. Vital signs should be taken every 15 minutes for the first hour and then every 2–4 hours as ordered or deemed necessary. Frequent temperature checks are not necessary, but should be noted every 4 hours, to detect a beginning septicemia or a reaction to the dye. Pulses distal to the arterial puncture must also be checked along with the vital signs. Thrombus formation, emboli release, nerve damage, or spasms of the artery are all possible complications. Pain at the puncture site is not uncommon and may require analgesics, but pain distal to the puncture site may indicate an embolism. A false aneurysm, a cysticlike mass that communicates with the damaged arterial wall may develop immediately after the trauma or develop weeks later (Fahey & Finkelmeier, 1984).

Femoral Arteriogram. For a *femoral* arteriogram the pedal pulses are checked. (See Chapter 23 for the use of the Doppler instrument to assess arterial pulses.) The client may not have had detectable pulses before the arteriogram; this must be taken into account. The color, sensation, and warmth of the foot examined should be compared with the other foot. Any pain in the foot or leg should be carefully assessed and compared with the pain before the arteriogram.

Brachial Arteriogram. If a *brachial* arteriogram is done, there is concern not only for spasm, embolism, or thrombus formation but also nerve compression. Pain or numbness in the fingers or hand should always be reported immediately. Blood pressure readings should not be taken on the examined arm because they temporarily compromise arterial circulation in the lower arm.

Carotid Arteriogram. For a *carotid* arteriogram, both temporal pulses should be checked. In addition, the client should be assessed for any signs of transient ischemic attacks (TIA), such as facial weakness, visual disturbances, or slurred speech. The client's head should be kept elevated about 30 degrees. A light ice collar may be used to reduce swelling. Pressure on the carotid arterial site should be avoided, this can cause a vagal reponse that can slow the heart. Tracheal obstruction can result from swelling, so the client should be observed for any difficulty in breathing or swallowing. A tracheostomy set should be near by.

Renal Arteriogram. If a *renal* arteriogram is done, hypotension may result from a decrease in the formation of renin for a short time. Renal function needs to be closely monitored. BUN and/or serum creatinines may be ordered (Chapter 4). Fortunately, all of these complications from arteriograms are rare occurrences, but the nurse who makes skilled assessments may detect a problem before it becomes major.

■ VENOGRAMS

Description. A dye or contrast medium can be injected into a vein by a venipuncture or by a cutdown to view the venous system of particular organs or to evaluate flow to a particular area, for example, x-ray films taken as the dye goes through the venous system of the leg. Dye may be injected into a catheter in the femoral vein or inferior vena cava, and the catheter can be threaded to various organs to inspect details in the venous supply of the organ.

Purposes. Venograms may be useful in detecting deep vein thrombosis (DVT) or to assess other venous abnormalities, such as congenital abnormalities or incompetent valves. Venograms only show structure and flow. Radioisotopes (see Chapter 22) are sometimes injected into veins to assess for the presence of DVT.

Client Preparation
Food and fluids may be withheld for 4 hours before the test. A consent form is needed (see earlier discussion on contrast medium).

POSTTEST NURSING IMPLICATIONS

There are no restrictions on eating. The client is usually not confined to bedrest, as with an arteriogram. If the client has DVT, bedrest would be maintained and anticoagulants used. (See Chapter 13 for tests for heparin regulation.) And there are fewer complications from venous puncture as compared with arterial puncture. However, the nurse should carefully assess vital signs and check for any signs of hematoma formation. Phlebitis may result and warm compresses can be used to ease the pain of an irritated vein. The implications for the use of a dye must be noted as discussed earlier in this chapter. If a cutdown was necessary, the area must be assessed for potential infection.

■ LYMPHOGRAMS

Description. Visualization of the lymph system can be achieved by an injection of dye or contrast medium into the lymph system of an arm or leg. A dye (Evans blue) is first injected into the web of skin between the first and second toes or between the fingers. The blue dye is picked up by the lymph system. After approximately 30 minutes the lymph system is outlined, and a lymph vessel is then dissected and a small catheter inserted for the injection of an iodine dye (Ethiodol). X-ray films are taken after the iodine dye is injected and again 24 hours later. Other x-ray pictures may be taken later because the lymph nodes retain the contrast medium for several weeks, even months.

Purposes. Enlarged and diseased lymph nodes can be identified on the films. Also, the lymphogram can show not only the extent of the disease, such as a lymphoma or Hodgkin's disease, but also the effectiveness of therapy.

Client Preparation

The client may be kept on n.p.o. status or may be allowed to eat. Consent form is signed and precautions for use of contrast medium noted. The client shoud be prepared for some discomfort when the hand or foot is given a local anesthetic. The hardest part of the procedure may be lying still for the extent of the procedure, which may be up to 3 hours. Because of the long waits during the test, the client may need reading material or other quiet diversions.

POSTTEST NURSING IMPLICATIONS

To prevent edema, the client should keep the affected limb elevated for 24 hours. Vital signs should be checked to detect any signs of bleeding, infection, or adverse reactions to the dye.

The site of the dissection may become painful as the local anesthetic wears off, and mild analgesics may be needed for the incisional pain. Any numbness in the extremity distal to the incision should be reported immediately because of possible nerve damage. The site will have a few stitches, which need to be removed in 7–10 days. The site should not get wet for a day or two. The site should be examined for any sign of infection and warm compresses applied to ease any discomfort from inflammation. If dye travels to the lung, via the thoracic duct, the client may develop pneumonia. Thus, respiratory problems should be evaluated by the physician. Skin discoloration from the blue dye will fade in a few days. Stool and urine will also show some discoloration. The client may even note a bluish tint in vision (Sobel & Ferguson, 1985).

■ HYSTEROSALPINGOGRAM

Description. The client is placed in the lithotomy position, and a vaginal speculum is inserted. Dye (Ethiodol or Salpix) is injected through the cervix into the uterus and fallopian tubes. The client is awake during the procedure. There is likely to be some abdominal discomfort from the pressure of the dye, even though only about 10 ml are used. The examination is scheduled within a week to 10 days after the client's menstrual period, to ensure that the client is not pregnant. The test takes about half an hour.

Purposes. The test is used to detect blocked fallopian tubes. Other abnormalities in the uterus, such as fibroids, will also be demonstrated on the x-ray. This is one of the tests done as part of an infertility workup. (See Chapter 28 for a discussion on the five basic tests for infertility.) Occasionally, the injection of the dye may also be done to evaluate the success of a tubal ligation.

Client Preparation

A hysterosalpingogram is often done on an outpatient basis. There are no restrictions of food or fluid. The client should have finished a menstrual period within the preceding 7–10 days. The client will need to void right before the procedure. Although some institutions have the client take an enema or suppository before the examination, no special bowel preparation is usually necessary. The client must remove her clothes from the waist down. Some clients are given a mild sedative. (See Chapter 25 on ways nurses can help prepare clients to cope with painful procedures.)

POSTTEST NURSING IMPLICATIONS

A few hours after the procedure, the client may have severe uterine cramps that require analgesia. Warm sitz baths may be soothing, too. Although rare, perforation of the uterus can occur, so any severe cramping or profuse bleeding should be called to the attention of the physician or clinic. The client may have some vaginal spotting for a day or two so she should be informed about the possible need of sanitary napkins. There is a slight chance of infection. Very rarely a pulmonary emboli could result from the entrance of the oil-based dye into the bloodstream.

■ MAMMOGRAMS

Description. A mammogram is an x-ray of the breasts to detect the presence of tumors too small to be discovered by palpation. Mammograms may include the injection of a dye into the mammary ducts, but routine screening procedures do not include the use of a contrast medium. Dye is useful in identifying intraductal papillomas. During the x-ray, the client lies or sits with breasts pushed against the film holder. An inflated rubber cushion is used to decrease the discomfort of the flattened breasts against the film holder. The procedure takes about 20–30 minutes to complete. It is usually done on an outpatient basis as a screening device for women susceptible to the development of breast cancer. For example, a mobile van sponsored by the radiology department of the University of California, San Francisco, remains in one location for a week at a time. Women need the approval of their physicians as the results are mailed to the physicians.

Purposes. Because breast cancer is the leading cause of cancer in women, mass screening for this disease is needed. Mammograms became popular in the early 1960s as a tool to detect early breast cancer. In the late 1970s, however, concern about radiation risks caused a reevaluation of whether mammograms should be done routinely (Gorringe, 1978). The American Cancer Society issued a statement in 1980 and revised it in 1983 to state that in addition to self-breast examinations and regular medical examinations, a baseline mammogram should be done between age 35 and 40. From age 40 to 49 mammograms should be done every year or two. After age 50 a yearly mammogram is recommended. (High-risk clients may need more frequent checks at younger ages.) Xeromammography, which uses a special kind of aluminum plate, subjects the client to less radiation exposure than mammograms done with conventional roentgen film. Hall (1986) notes that widescale screening can lead to overinterpretation of results and needless biopsies. Second opinions should be sought for questionable findings.

Client Preparation
The client should not use deodorant, perfume, or powder on the day of the test; these chemicals may interfere with the x-ray picture. The client should wear clothing easy

to remove from the waist up. The client should be prepared for some physical discomfort, related to the manipulation of the tender tissue, particularly if the breasts are pendulous. Caffeine may make the breast more tender, therefore some guidelines suggest avoiding caffeine for 2 weeks before the test (Kaiser-Permanente Medical Group, 1986). Otherwise, the test is not physically painful, but it may be traumatic to be exposed. The potential diagnosis of cancer may also create much anxiety. A mammogram may be done to place a needle or wire marker in the lump as a guide to subsequent biopsy.

POSTTEST NURSING IMPLICATIONS

There are no specific nursing implications; however, the nurse should assess if the client knows how to do a self-examination of the breast. (See Chapter 25 on breast biopsies for follow-up of lumps in the breast.)

■ MYELOGRAMS

Description. A myelogram is an x-ray film of the subarachnoid space of the spinal column, in which air or dye may be used as a contrast medium. The dye may either be an oily contrast or a water-soluble medium. The water-soluble dye, metrizamide (Amipaque) is most often used and is suitable for both inpatient and outpatient procedures (Godwin, 1985). If an oil-based dye is used, it is removed at the end of the procedure. The water-soluble dye is not. The dye or air is injected via a lumbar puncture. The client will be on a tilted table to allow the dye to flow into different parts of the spinal column.

Purposes. X-ray films, taken after the contrast medium is instilled, can show distortions of the spinal cord due to tumors or changes in the bone structures. Herniations or protrusions of intervertebral disks can also be visualized. Note that the use of the computerized axial tomography (CT scanning) or magnetic resonance imaging (MRI) may give more details (see Chapter 21).

Client Preparation
The client's allergy history is important if iodine is being used. He or she should be on n.p.o. status for 4–6 hours, and a bowel prep may be ordered. Intravenous fluids may be used to hydrate the client. The client should be prepared for the positioning necessary for a lumbar puncture. (See Chapter 25 on lumbar punctures.) Sedatives may be ordered. Phenothiazines are not used because they lower the seizure threshold. Consent forms are needed.

POSTTEST NURSING IMPLICATIONS

If an oil-based dye is used, the client should be kept flat in bed 6–8 hours after it is removed (Maphet, 1981). If the water-soluble dye was used, the head should be kept elevated for at least 8 hours to keep the dye from irritating the cerebral meninges. The client may need analgesics if headache, pain, and stiffness in the neck occur. About 20% of clients will experience headaches, nausea, and vomiting after the test. Less than 1 in 1000 will have a seizure (Sobel & Ferguson, 1985). If conditions permit, fluids should be encouraged to at least 2000 ml for the adult, to help with the production of adequate cerebral spinal fluid. The motor and sensations of the lower extremities should be assessed to make sure there was no nerve damage. The voiding pattern of the client should be assessed because urinary retention may be a problem in the first 24 hours.

Outpatient clients are monitored for at least 2 hours and accompanied home by a family member.

■ ARTHROGRAMS

Description. For an arthrogram, dye is injected into a joint, usually the knee and sometimes a shoulder or other joint. The procedure is done under local anesthesia in the radiology department. After the needle is inserted into the joint space, some fluid is usually aspirated for analysis. Then the dye, and sometimes air, is injected. The client may be asked to run in place to spread the dye around the knee joint. Also, the joint will be manipulated to spread the dye. (Some clients find the movement of the joint rather uncomfortable.) X-rays are taken with the joint in various positions.

Purposes. Arthrograms help evaluate suspected joint damage such as tears in the cartilage of the knee. If surgery is anticipated, an arthroscopy may be done in place of the arthrogram. The arthroscopy allows the physician to directly examine the joint and even do minor repairs (see Chapter 27). On the other hand, the arthrogram shows a detailed picture of the entire knee.

PRETEST NURSING IMPLICATIONS

Precautions related to the use of contrast dye should be noted. If the procedure is being done on an outpatient basis, and many are, someone else will have to drive the client home.

POSTTEST NURSING DIAGNOSIS

Alteration in Comfort Related to Knee Manipulation

Mild-to-moderate discomfort may be present after the procedure. The joint should rest for about 12 hours. The knee may be wrapped in an elastic bandage for 12–24 hours. Ice bags can be used to reduce swelling and mild analgesics may be needed. Some slight grating may be present for a day or two after the procedure. Strenuous activity, such as jogging, should not be resumed until advised by the physician. Exercises to strengthen the knee may be prescribed depending on the results of the examination. Two possible complications after arthroscopic surgery are hemorrhage and thrombophlebitis, but incidence of either is quite low.

QUESTIONS

1. The three methods to provide radiation protection when x-rays are used as diagnostic procedures include all the following *except*

    a. Scheduling x-rays a few days apart so there is a time interval between exposures
    b. Shielding the client with lead aprons to protect uninvolved areas
    c. Having all personnel maintain distance when the x-ray machine is in use
    d. Making the exposure of the client as short as possible

2. The American Cancer Society's recommendation (1983) for the use of mammograms as screening devices for breast cancer is that all women have *annual* mammograms after age

    a. 35   c. 50
    b. 40   d. 60

3. All of the following are ways for consumers to protect themselves from unnecessary x-ray exposure *except*

    a. Asking for a lead apron to be used if dental x-rays are needed
    b. Carrying a card that lists all the x-rays that have been done of the person
    c. Asking the physician to explain how x-rays will help with the diagnosis
    d. Requesting x-rays to validate any unexplained symptoms

4. Factors that clients have identified as being stressful for barium x-ray studies include all *but*

    a. Moving about on a hard x-ray table
    b. Being rushed through the x-ray procedure
    c. Darkness and noise during fluoroscopy
    d. Enemas or suppositories given before the tests

5. General nursing implications for clients going for any type of radiological test include all *except*

    a. Helping the client prepare for waiting by giving a magazine or other diversion
    b. Making sure that the client has slippers if he or she must stand during the test

    c. Instructing the client about any restrictions on food and fluids

    d. Listing the complications that may occur

6. General nursing implications when a client returns from a radiological test include all *but*

    a. Offering a back rub to relieve the discomfort from lying on a hard table

    b. Encouraging extra fluids (if pathophysiology allows) when dye was used as a contrast medium

    c. Finding out if the client can eat, and if so, offering some food as soon as possible

    d. Keeping the client on bedrest for 4–6 hours

7. The specific gravity of urine will be higher than usual after a client has had all the following x-ray tests *except*

    a. KUB   **c.** Arteriograms

    b. Cholangiograms   **d.** IVP

8. Nursing actions that are routine to help the x-ray technician get a better portable chest x-ray of the client in bed include all but

    a. Helping the client sit up as straight as possible before the x-ray is done

    b. Removing electrodes from the chest before the x-ray

    c. Helping the technician place the film holder behind the client's chest

    d. Holding the client in a fixed position while the x-ray is being done

9. Sally is an adolescent who has a history of severe epigastric pain relieved by food or milk. Which of these nursing actions is not routine when Sally has an upper GI series (barium meal)?

    a. Keeping Sally on n.p.o. status before the examination

    b. Telling Sally that when fluoroscopy is done (as the barium is swallowed) the room will be dark

    c. Giving an enema to Sally after the x-rays are completed

    d. Informing Sally that the barium sulfate will make the stools light-colored

10. Mr. Somorini is having a barium enema because of slight rectal bleeding. Which of these nursing actions is not routine for the client having a barium enema?

    a. Administration of cathartics or suppositories the evening before the examination

    b. Informing Mr. Somorini that he will need to hold the barium in the colon while a series of x-rays are taken

    c. Giving a light diet the evening before the x-ray examination

    d. Withholding food when Mr. Somorini comes back from x-ray because a second set of pictures are done in 3–4 hours

11. Mrs. Rigaletti is scheduled for a GB series tomorrow morning. Which of the following preparations is not routine the night before a GB series or OCG?

    a. Oral ingestion of six tablets, which contain the contrast medium or dye

    b. Low fat diet for evening meal

    c. A skin test for sensitivity to iodine

    d. n.p.o. after evening meal

12. Mr. Leonard has just returned to his hospital room after a femoral arteriogram. Which nursing action would be inappropriate?

    a. Allowing him to stand if he cannot void in bed

    b. Checking vital signs every 15 minutes for the first hour then every 2 hours if vital signs are stable

    c. Keeping an ice bag on the puncture site

    d. Checking pedal pulses and the color and warmth of the feet when vital signs are done

13. Pain that often requires the use of analgesics is an expected occurrence after all these radiological procedures *except*

    a. Mammograms   **c.** Myelograms

    b. Arthrograms   **d.** Lymphograms

REFERENCES

Alterescu, K. (1985). What about special procedures? *AJN, 85*(12), 1363–1367.

American Cancer Society. (1983). *Mammography: Two statements of the American Cancer Society. Professional education publication.* New York: A.C.S., Inc.

Arnell, I., & Nassberg, B. (1981). Administer a barium enema through a colostomy. *Nursing 81,* (11),81–83.

Athanasoulis, C. (1980). Therapeutic application of angiograms. *NEJM, 302*(20), 1117–1125.

Barnett-Wilson, J. (1978). Patients' responses to barium X-Ray studies. *British Medical Journal,* 1:6122.

Berger, M., & Hübner, K. (1983). Hospital hazards: Diagnostic radiation. *AJN, 83*(9), 1155–1159.

Bush, W., Mullarkey, M., & Webb, D. (1985). Adverse reactions to radiographic contrast material. *Western Journal of Medicine, 132*, 95.

Cruz, C., et al. (1986). Contrast media for angiography: Effect on renal function. *Radiology, 158*(1), 109–112.

Diagnostic Product Information. (1986). In *Physician's Desk Reference,* 40th ed. Oradell, NJ: Medical Economics Co.

Fahey, V., & Finkelmeier, B. (1984). Iatrogenic arterial injuries. *AJN, 84*(4), 448–451.

Felson, B. (1980). The chest roentgenologic workup. *Basics of R.D., 8*(5), 1–5.

Godwin, C. (1985). Outpatient myelography. *Nursing 85, 15*(12), 57.

Gorringe, R. (1978). The mammography controversy: A case for breast self-examination. *Journal of Obstetric Gynecologic and Neonatal Nursing, 7*, 7–12.

Gray, J. (1979). Radiation awareness and exposure reduction with audible monitors. *American Journal of Roentgenology, 133*, 1200–1201.

Hall, F. (1986). Screening mammography. Potential problems on the horizon. *NEJM, 314*(1), 53–55.

Hartfield, M., & Cason, C. (1981). Effects of information on emotional responses during barium enema. *Nursing Research, 30*, 151–155.

Health and Human Services. (1984). *Are routine chest x-rays really necessary?* (HHS Publication (FDA) 84-8205). Washington, DC: U.S. Government Printing Office.

Henry, T. (1982). Radiation exposure and margins of safety. *California Nurse, 78* (11), 5–7.

Jankowski, C. (1986). Radiation and pregnancy. Putting the risks in proportion. *AJN, 86*(3), 261–265.

Johnson, J., & Rice, V. (1974). Sensory and distress components of pain. *Nursing Research, 23*, 203–209.

Kaiser-Permanente Medical Group. (1986). *Patient instruction sheets for diagnostic x-rays.* San Francisco, CA: Kaiser-Permanente Medical Group.

McHugh, N., et al. (1982). Preparatory information: What helps and why. *AJN, 82* (5), 780–782.

Maphet, M. (1981). Radiology: What it means for your patients. *RN, 44,* 1B–1C.

Marinelli-Miller, D. (1983). What your patient wants to know about angiography. *RN, 46*(11), 52–54.

Mongeau, S., & Poirier, H. (1979). X-rays and cancer. *World Press Review, 26*(12), 50.

NCRP Report 54. (1977). *Medical radiation exposure of pregnant and potentially pregnant women.* Washington, DC: National Council on Radiation Protection and Measurements.

NCRP Report 48. (1976). *Radiation protection for medical and allied health personnel.* Washington, DC: National Council on Radiation Protection and Measurements.

Ordronneu, N. (1980). Helping patients in the radiology department. *AJN, 80*(7), 1312–1313.

Sobel, D., & Ferguson, T. (1985). *The people's book of medical tests.* New York: Summit.

Tinker, J. (1976). Understanding chest x-rays. *AJN, 76*(1), 54–58.

Tuttobene, S. (1984). A bowel prep that's easy to swallow. *RN, 47*(3), 52.

Willard, P. (1985). Percutaneous transluminal angioplasty. *Point of View, 22*(3), 4–6.

Wilson, P. (1977). Evaluating chest films. *Nurse Practitioner, 2*(1), 6–13.

21

Tomography and Body Scans

- Tomograms of the Lungs and Other Structures
- Computerized Axial Tomography (CT Scans) or EMI Scanner
- Positron Emission Tomography (PET)
- Magnetic Resonance Imaging (MRI) or Nuclear Magnetic Resonance (NMR)

OBJECTIVES

1. Compare the usefulness of body scans to older diagnostic tests.
2. Discuss the basic disadvantages of the various types of body scans.
3. Compare and contrast preparations needed for infants, children, and adults for CT brain scans.
4. Describe the usual preparations for CT scans of various parts of the body.
5. Describe how PET (position emission tomography) allows clinicians to examine metabolic functions in a totally new way.
6. Describe the needed preparations for MRI scanning.
7. Identify the priority nursing diagnosis when a scan is completed.

Tomography is a method of body section roentgenography. A specially designed x-ray machine and film holder moves around the client in an arc, focusing at various angles, each with a slightly different depth. With each change in the angle of the tomography, a selected body plane becomes sharply defined, while the areas above and below the focal point become slightly blurred.

The computerized axial tomographer uses the principle of tomography with the addition of detectors, computers, and a scanner, which make possible a three-dimensional cross-sectional view of the head (CT head scanner) or of other body parts

(CT body scanner). Tomograms, also called planigrams or laminagrams, give two-dimensional views.

Cormack, an American physicist, and Hounsfield, an English research engineer, working independently did the research that culminated in the development of the CT scan; they shared a 1979 Nobel Prize for Physiology or Medicine. The Nobel committee acknowledged that no other method of x-ray diagnostics had led to such remarkable success in such a short time. Another type of body scanner, which uses a magnetic field and no radiation, the magnetic resonance imager, has become the newest success story of the eighties.

ADVANTAGES AND DISADVANTAGES

Tomograms and the much more sophisticated scans are noninvasive tests, requiring a skilled technician to operate the machine. Much research is being done to compare the advantages and disadvantages of scans with invasive procedures (Chapter 25), with sonograms (Chapter 23), and with radionuclide scans (Chapter 22) for assessing various pathophysiological conditions. The major advantage of the scans is the exquisite detail of the images.

If a contrast medium is used in conjunction with the tests, as is sometimes done with CT scans, there are risks associated with the dye injection. (See Chapter 20 on nursing precautions when dye is used.) Magnetic resonance imaging does not usually require contrast medium.

A CT scan does have two disadvantages. One is the cost of the test, which must be considered if other less expensive tests can provide satisfactory results. Although CT body scans cost approximately 400–800 dollars per scan, this may be less than the combined charges of the tests replaced (Sobel & Ferguson, 1985). The second disadvantage of the CT scan is the time of exposure to radiation. Although the amount of radiation is very small, all radiation exposure is cumulative through life. (See Chapter 20 for a detailed discussion on the role of the nurse in relation to the radiation hazards of repeated diagnostic tests.) Yet, when wisely used, the CT scan is a marvel. A newer type of tomography, positron emission tomography, is also costly and has some radiation exposure. The newest scan of all, magnetic resonance imaging, has no radiation exposure, but it is also costly (600–1000 dollars) and clients with some artificial devices cannot be scanned.

■ TOMOGRAMS OF THE LUNGS AND OTHER STRUCTURES

Description and Purposes. As mentioned earlier in this chapter, a tomogram (also called planigram or laminagram) is a special type of x-ray, which takes pictures at various depths of tissue to obtain a cross-sectional view of the body. The procedure takes about 30 minutes, but can be longer for a tomogram of a complete area. Lung tomograms are useful in identifying the exact location of a tumor. (Although ultrasound (Chapter 23) is increasingly being used to identify tumors and fluid in many tissues, it is not effective for tissues with a lot of air, such as the lungs.) Other structures, such as the skeletal system, the sinuses, and various organs, may be effectively viewed by tomograms.

PRETEST NURSING IMPLICATIONS

There is no special preparation of the client. As with any x-ray, all jewelry or other metal must be removed. The procedure does not cause any discomfort, other than that of lying still on the x-ray table. Some clients, however, may be bothered by the noise of the machine.

POSTTEST NURSING IMPLICATIONS

Clients having tomograms do not require any special aftercare. (See Chapter 20 for ways the nurse can help relieve the anxiety that is often present after diagnostic testing.)

■ COMPUTERIZED AXIAL TOMOGRAPHY (CT SCANS) OR EMI SCANNER

Description. CT, CAT scan, and EMI scans all refer to the use of computerized axial tomography. The EMI scanner was developed by the *E*lectrical and *M*usical *I*ndustries, a British based group of international companies (Seeram, 1976). Thus, British (Kreel, 1977) and Canadian literature are more likely to use the term EMI scanner. American companies making scans use the term CT. CT is usually used, rather than CAT.

Computerized axial tomography uses an x-ray machine that rotates 180 degrees around the client's head or body. Detectors read the amount of radiation each body tissue or organ absorbs. A computer processes these readings and converts them to a picture shown on a screen, which is stored on discs. The resulting pictures show a three-dimensional cross section of all body parts. The CT scan divides each area of tissue being viewed into an area 3 mm square and 13 mm thick. The results are available in a few minutes. The CT scanner can distinguish almost all types of tissues except nerves. In the older scans of the head, the client's head was fitted in a rubber bag so there was no cushion or air between the hair and scalp. This is not necessary with the newer scans.

The CT scan, a noninvasive procedure, causes no pain. The client just lies still while the machine goes around the body. As emphasized before, no risks are entailed, other than being exposed to a small amount of radiation. The procedure takes from 15–30 minutes. If a contrast medium is used, the procedure takes 30–60 minutes, and there are the usual risks associated with an iodine contrast medium.

Purposes. Around 1972, the first CT scans were used for identifying brain abnormalities and head injuries. The CT was found to be much more valuable in diagnosing problems in the brain than the older x-ray tests such as pneumoencephalograms or cerebral arteriograms. The details available by a CT scan are remarkable. For example, a CT scan can clearly show if a brain abscess is becoming smaller after treatment with antibiotics. CT scans are also used to locate foreign objects in soft tissue, such as the eyes. For example, a piece of metal lodged in an eyeball can be precisely mapped out so the surgeon has to do much less probing. Intracranial lesions, such as neoplasms or hematomas, can be located without a craniotomy. The surgeon thus has a much better understanding of the location and extent of brain pathology before surgery is done.

Body scanners, which were marketed later than head scanners, in 1976, had a less dramatic and, some would say, a debatable impact. Controversy arose about how many CT scanners are needed in one community and if each hospital needs a machine. There was also a debate about whether the body scan offers more diagnostic help than other less costly diagnostic tests (van Dyk et al., 1980). This debate has often been carried out in the public press (Saltas, 1979).

Certainly, CT scans of the body were first very useful in research studies. For example, at the University of California at San Francisco, researchers used the CT body scan to determine the minimum dose of estrogen that will prevent bone degeneration (Hales, 1980). Now there are many exciting ways that CT body scans are being used for both diagnostic and research purposes.

PRETEST NURSING DIAGNOSES

Knowledge Deficit Related to Needed Preparation for a Head Scan
Unless a contrast medium is to be used, the client does not have to maintain n.p.o. status. Some clinicians may even allow clear liquids if a dye is to be used (Bubb, 1981). Wigs and any objects in the hair, such as bobby pins, are removed. The client can be assured that the procedure is not painful and is much like putting one's head in a hair dryer (Stone, 1977). Note that although the CT is not painful, the thought of having one's head immobilized can be frightening. The person must lie still during the procedure. A two-way intercom allows communication with the x-ray personnel. See the discussion on claustrophobia in the section on magnetic resonance imaging.

Radiopaque dye may be given intravenously to outline the cerebral vessels; if so, the client may need preparation for this. (See Chapter 20 on how to prepare for potential reactions to dye, which include flushing and possible allergic reaction.)

Potential for Ineffective Coping of Children
Mills (1980) has developed a booklet to prepare children and their parents for a scan. One suggestion is to encourage the child to play at home by lying still with the head flexed toward his or her chest. The parent can dim the lights in the room and move an arm around the child's motionless head. By humming softly, the parent gives the child an idea of the sounds he or she will hear during the test. The child should be taught that he or she can open and close the eyes but not move the head. This preparation may work for children over three. Infants will sleep during the procedure if kept awake and then fed just before the test. The greatest problems will be with toddlers (and confused adults): sedation may be required. Mills (1980) describes, in detail, the procedure for sedation used at the University of Colorado Hospital. Chloral hydrate is usually used, although a mixture of meperidine (Demerol), promethazine (Phenergan), and chlorpromazine (Thorazine) may sometimes be needed. In rare instances, diazepam (Valium) is given intravenously. (See Chapter 27 for a discussion on adverse reactions to sedatives.)

Knowledge Deficit Related to Needed Preparation for CT Body Scans
Scans of the thorax or pelvic regions may or may not require special preparation. The nurse must ask the radiologist what specific preparations are required. A tampon may be used as a vaginal marker. The client may be required to have a full or empty bladder (van Dyk et al., 1980). A contrast medium may be given to outline various organs. Low density barium solutions and dilute water-soluble iodinated contrast materials are used (Ball et al., 1986). The client must be assessed for allergies and prepared for a flushing sensation (see Chapter 20). However, some of the newer contrast mediums made for CT scans contain less than 10% of the iodine found in older products. The client may be on a low residue diet for a few days before the examination. Bowel preparations vary in importance with the various parts of the body being scanned. Contrast medium can be given by an enema. Drugs may be used to decrease peristalsis during the test, including propantheline and glucagon. Synthetic cholecystokin (Sincalide) may also be given to increase peristalsis to cause filling of the GI tract with swallowed contrast medium (Ruijs, 1979). These medications are given during the procedure and will require an intravenous injection. If a biopsy is planned, guided by the scan, the general nursing implications (discussed in Chapter 25) for invasive procedures, should be heeded.

POSTTEST NURSING IMPLICATIONS

There are no specific nursing implications related to the scanning procedure. If a radiopaque dye has been given, the nursing implications about dye should be followed. (See the general nursing diagnoses discussed in Chapter 20.) The nurse must be aware of any sedatives or other drugs given as part of the procedure because untoward effects from drugs are always possible. (See the discussion on the side effects of medications used for endoscopic procedures in Chapter 27.) And if invasive measures were done, vital signs and the other assessments described in Chapter 25 would be appropriate.

■ POSITRON EMISSION TOMOGRAPHY (PET)

Description. PET became popular in the early 1980s (Toufexis, 1981). For PET studies, the client is injected with a biochemical substance tagged with a radionuclide, which emits positively charged particles. When these radioactive particles combine with the negatively charged electrons normally found in the cells of certain tissue, they emit gamma rays that can be detected by a scanning device. The PET scanner translates the emissions into color-coded images. For example, radioactive glucose can be used to map biochemical activity in the brain (Friedman, 1981). Isotopes used for cardiac studies include oxygen-15, nitrogen-13, and carbon-11 (Ter-Pogossian, 1981). The half-life of the isotopes used is very short so there is very little radiation dosage. The radiation is usually less than a quarter of that received from a CT scan. Theoretically, any physiological substance can be tagged and traced as it is metabolized in the body. Much research is being done to make these theoretical possibilities realities.

Emission scanners are sometimes called ECT scans (emission computed tomography) or emission CT scans. They were found only in major medical centers, but the number is rapidly growing in the United States, Europe, and Japan. PET is often limited to institutions with access to a cyclotron for the production of the isotopes; however, some tracers used for emission studies can be shipped prior to use. For example, technetium-99m, thallium-201, and gallium-67 are used in PET scans, as well as in routine nuclear medicine tests (Kirsch et al., 1981). See Chapter 22 for more information on conventional radionuclide imaging done routinely in most hospitals.

For PET scanning of the brain, two intravenous lines are used: one for injection of the radioisotope and the other for serial blood samples. The client must lie still for as long as 60–90 minutes while scans are being recorded. Blindfolds and cotton earplugs are used to reduce external stimuli to the brain. The client is asked to recite certain things such as the pledge of allegiance. Intellectual tasks are performed to see how the brain activity changes for reasoning or remembering.

Purposes. PET, as a measure of brain activity, is used to study the effects of stroke, epilepsy, migraine headache, Parkinson's disease, and other disorders such as schizophrenia. PET can help differentiate between types of dementia and is shedding light on some aspects of Alzheimer's disease (Marchette & Holloman, 1985). The reader is encouraged to consult the current literature on the use of PET scans for both research and clinical practice.

PRETEST NURSING DIAGNOSIS RELATED TO PET

Knowledge Deficit Regarding Needed Preparation
The client must refrain from alcohol, tobacco, and caffeine for 20 hours before the test. Food should be consumed in a normal pattern. Fluids are permitted, but the bladder should be empty as the test lasts up to 1½ hours. No sedative or tranquilizer should be given because the client needs to follow commands for certain mental activities. The client should be prepared for the sensation of the intravenous and the use of the blindfold.

POSTTEST NURSING IMPLICATIONS

See Chapter 22 for the discussion on general nursing implications for intravenous radioisotopes such as (1) observing the IV site for phlebitis, (2) relieving anxiety, and (3) encouraging fluids to hasten urinary excretion of the isotope.

■ MAGNETIC RESONANCE IMAGING (MRI) OR NUCLEAR MAGNETIC RESONANCE (NMR)

Description. Magnetic resonance imaging is a new type of body scan that uses a huge magnet and radio waves to create an energy field that can be transferred to a visual image. An older term is nuclear magnetic resonance (NMR). The word nuclear may be frightening to clients because it may conjure up a vision of the nuclear fission of the atomic bomb. Nuclear in the sense of NMR just refers to the dense core of the atom. Not only is the test not related to atomic bombs, it does not involve any kind of radiation hazard. Clark (1983) noted that maybe NMR should stand for No More Radiation. The richness of detail of the images without the use of contrast medium and the lack of radiation hazard are advantages the MRI has over the CT scans discussed earlier in this chapter.

The huge magnet in the scanner creates a magnetic field. The magnetic field causes atoms in the tissues and more particularly the nuclei of the hydrogen ions to line up in a parallel fashion. When the technician pushes a switch, radio waves are sent into the magnetic field and the lined up ions pick up some of this energy. When the radio wave is switched off, the atoms revert back to their lined up fashion influenced by the magnet. The change in the energy field is sensed and converted to a visual display on a computer screen.

The entire MRI machine must be enclosed in a room to protect the scan from interference with outside radio signals. The magnetic field around the scanner is always present and will stop watches, erase credit cards, and even pull stethoscopes out of pockets (Sobel & Ferguson, 1985). If the client has an intravenous, the MRI disrupts some intravenous drip regulators, but others may not be affected (Engler & Engler, 1986). At the present time, special emergency equipment such as monitoring devices are being developed which can be used in a MRI room, but the present equipment is likely to malfunction and may be projectile so clients must be moved out of the room for resuscitation.

The client is put on a moving pallet that is pushed into the large cylinder that contains the magnet. As the radio signals are switched off and on the client hears a variety of noises. The sound has been described as initially like the slow beat of an Indian drum and then with abrupt stops and starts like a muffled jackhammer (Osaki et al., 1985). Ear plugs are available if the client wishes them. MacPhie (1983) noted the sounds as dull and lulling and then sometimes as thunderous bombardments, but at no time unbearable.

Purposes. Although these scans are relatively expensive (600–1000 dollars), the detailed scan may be well worth it. In March, 1985, Blue Shield of California approved payments for MRI scans and thus paved the way for Medicare to also consider the test as no longer only an experimental or research tool. The MRI can do some things the CT scan cannot. For example, MRI not only clearly defines internal organ structure, it also detects changes in tissue such as edema or infarcts. Blood flow patterns and detailed information on blood vessel integrity can give an earlier warning than ever before of developing atherosclerotic disease (Marchette & Holloman, 1985). Because of the lack of bone artifacts, MRI scans can identify tumors in the pituitary gland (Glaser et al., 1986). The MRI scan does not require an intravenous contrast medium as may the CT head scan.

PRETEST NURSING DIAGNOSES RELATED TO MRI

Knowledge Deficit Regarding Needed Preparation
Watches, tapes, and credit cards will be damaged by the magnetic field, therefore, clients must shed these items. Clients must also remove jewelry, clothing with metal fasteners, and hair clips. Objects containing ferrous metal will create artifacts. Also, the movement of the object could be detrimental. For example,

clients who have metal implants such as surgical clips, heart valves, or ortho-pedic clips cannot be scanned by MRI because the magnet may move the ob-ject within the body. Artificial joints which are not ferrous present no problems. Clients should also be asked about any injuries that could have left some metal embedded in a sensitive place such as an eye. Any movement of even a small fragment could cause permanent eye damage. Clients may get odd sensations from dental work in their teeth if a filling or bridge contains ferrous material. The machine can deactivate pacemarkers so clients with pacemakers are excluded.

No food or beverage restrictions are necessary. However, because the pro-cedure may take 60 or more minutes, the client should have an empty bladder. For some organ studies the client may need to drink a tasteless, waterlike con-trast substance. Geritol, which contains iron, is sometimes used as a marker. Glucagon may be given to decrease persistalsis.

Anxiety Related to Feelings of Claustrophobia

Huricak and Amparo (1984) found a 1-5% incidence of claustrophobia in adults undergoing MRI and that using the prone position so the client could see out reduced the claustrophobia. Other measures to decrease claustrophobia are visualization of peaceful scenes or other relaxation techniques. One nurse re-called prepared childbirth exercises and thus was able to overcome her initial claustrophobia and anxiety (Marchette & Holloman, 1985).

Osaki, Tesler, and Higgins (1985) did a descriptive study to assess the perceptions of 45 children and their parents of the MRI experience. Some parents were concerned about claustrophobia. Both children and their parents stressed the benefit of sensation information and liked that there were no shots or intra-venous lines (some injectable sedation may be used for the young). Having the parent present was another big plus for the procedure. Parents may read or talk to the child as there is no risk of radiation from the procedure (parents must be debriefed about watches, credit cards, and such, which may be damaged by the magnet).

Because clients must lie still for a long time, young children and very anx-ious adults may need sedation. Drugs do not interfere with the test.

POSTTEST NURSING IMPLICATIONS

There is no special aftercare of the client. (See the discussion in Chapter 20 on the anxiety related to waiting for results which may take a couple of days.) Although there are no known hazards from the test, clients with tumors may be concerned about any possible effect on the tumor (MacPhie, 1983).

QUESTIONS

1. Which of the following is the major disadvantage of CT scans as compared with MRI or ultrasound procedures?

    a. The number of personnel needed to run the machine

    b. The amount of preparation required for the client

    c. The amount of radiation exposure to the client

    d. The lack of detailed images

2. The priority nursing intervention after a client is finished with a body scan is to assess

    a. Vital signs because of possible adverse effects, such as bleeding

    b. Level of anxiety related to potential outcome of procedure

    c. Pain level due to the procedure

    d. Effects of radiation, such as nausea

3. Preparation for a CT head scan for a 3-year-old child is likely to include all the following *except* (no contrast dye is being used)

    a. n.p.o. status for 3–4 hours before the examination

    b. Use of sedation 30 minutes before the test

    c. Removal of bobby pins or other items in the hair

    d. Have the child practice keeping his or her head still while a humming noise is made

4. Certain types of computerized tomography scanning may require specific client preparations. Which of the following types of CT scan requires the most physical preparation of the client?

    a. Brain scans   b. Pelvic scans   c. Thoracic scans   d. Abdominal scans

5. Nursing implications related to the use of intravenous radioisotopes are appropriate for the client receiving a

    a. MRI scan

    b. PET

    c. CT scan

    d. Tomogram

6. Mr. Lagerquist is scheduled for a MRI scan today. Which of the following is an essential part of pretest teaching?

    a. Mr. Lagerquist will have an intravenous started before the examination

    b. Any objects containing ferrous metal will interfere with the test

    c. Food and fluids are withheld for 4–6 hours before the test

    d. Mr. Lagerquist may turn side-to-side during the scan but he must not sit up

7. Clients undergoing a MRI scan may experience all the following sensations *except*

    a. A strange feeling around tooth fillings

    b. Slight redness of the skin

    c. A variety of noises, some rather loud

    d. Claustrophobia or a closed-in feeling

REFERENCES

Ball, D., et al. (1986). Contrast medium preparation during abdominal CT. *Radiology, 158*(1), 258–260.

Bubb, D. (1981). Teaching patients about ultrasound and CAT brain scans. *RN, 44*(12), 64–65.

Clark, M. (1983). NMR = No more radiation? *AJN, 83*(9), 1371–1372.

Engler, M., & Engler, M. (1986). Hazards of magnetic resonance imaging. *AJN, 86*(6), 650.

Friedman, E. (1981). Imaging technology approaches the frontiers of physics. *Hospitals, 55,* 76–82.

Glaser, B., et al. (1986). Magnetic resonance imaging of the pituitary gland. *Clinical Radiology 37*(1), 9–14.

Hales, D. (1980). High tech in medicine: Worth the cos⁺? *UCSF Magazine,* 3, 3–14.

Haughey, C. (1981). What to say and do when your patient asks about CT scans. *Nursing 81, 11*(12), 72–77.

Hricak, H., & Amparo, E. (1984). Body MRI: Alleviation of claustrophobia by prone positioning. *Radiology, 152*(3), 819.

Kirsch, C.M., et al. (1981). Characteristics of a scanning multidetector, single photon ECT body imager. *Journal of Nuclear Medicine, 22,* 726–731.

Kreel, M.D. (1977). Computerized tomography using the EMI general purpose scanner. *British Journal of Radiology, 50,* 2–14.

MacPhie, C. (1983). Apudoma, NMR imager and me. *California Nurse, 79*(6), 8.

Marchette, L., & Holloman, F. (1985). A first-hand report on the new body scanners. *RN, 48*(11), 28–31.

Mills, G. (1980). Preparing children and parents for cerebral computerized tomography. *Maternal Child Nursing, 5,* 403–407.

Osaki, L., Tesler, M., & Higgins, S. (1985). Children's and parents' perception of the magnetic resonance imaging (MRI) examination. *Abstracts for National Symposium of Nursing Research.* Stanford, CA: Stanford University.

Osaki, L., Proctor, E., & March, V. (1985). *The ABC's of your child having a MRI.* San Francisco, CA: University of California Department of Radiology (brochure for client teaching).

Ruijs, S. (1979). A simple procedure for patient preparation in abdominal CT. *American Journal of Roentgenology, 133,* 551–552.

Saltas, R. (1979, November 4). Scanners: Too many of a good thing? *San Francisco Chronicle and Examiner.*

Seeram, E. (1976). The EMI brain scanner. *Canadian Nurse, 72*(11), 40–42.

Sobel, D., & Ferguson, T. (1985). *The people's book of medical tests.* New York: Summit.

Stone, B. (1977). Computerized transaxial brain scan. *AJN, 77*(10), 1601–1604.

Ter-Pogossian, B. (1981). Positron-emission tomography in cardiac evaluation. *Hospital Practice, 16,* 93–101.

Toufexis, A. (1981, September 4). A brainy marvel called PET. *Time, 118,* 74.

Van Dyk, J., et al. (1980). On the impact of CT scanning on radiotherapy planning. *Computerized Tomography, 4,* 55–65.

22

Diagnostic Tests Using Radionuclides or Radioisotopes

- Bone Scans
- Brain Scans
- Gallium Scans
- Indium Scans
- Gallbladder Scans
- Liver and Spleen Scans
- Lung Scans
- Cardiac Scans
- Renal Scans
- Thyroid Scans
- RAI Uptake
- Other Organ Scans Including Fibrinogen Uptake
- In Vitro Sampling: Compatability and RBC Survival
- Blood Volume Studies
- Schilling Test

OBJECTIVES

1. Differentiate between the use of common radionuclides for diagnostic testing and for therapy.
2. Compare and contrast the procedures used for in vitro and in vivo testing.
3. Explain why pregnant women and children are advised not to have radionuclide studies if other nonradioactive tests can suffice.
4. State the general nursing implications for preparing a client for any organ scan with technetium (Tc-99m).
5. State the major use of a bone scan done with radionuclides.
6. Explain the purpose of doing a gallium scan in a client with a fever of undetermined origin.

7. Plan a teaching program for a client who is to have a radioactive iodine uptake in a couple of weeks.
8. Explain the purpose of administration of potassium iodine before an iodine-125 (I-125) fibrinogen uptake for deep vein thrombosis.
9. Describe the nursing functions when a client has a Schilling test.

All of the tests covered in this chapter are done in the nuclear medicine department. The terms radionuclide and radioisotope are both used to describe the radio-pharmaceuticals that are used for diagnostic tests in the nuclear medicine department. Often in general practice, the older term radioisotope is still used. However, recent literature uses the more precise term radionuclides, and this term will be used in this chapter. The term radionuclide implies that the element has a nucleus that has been made radioactive.

In diagnostic nuclear medicine, the radionuclide is given to the client and the radiation emitted from a particular organ is measured. The basic rationale for the use of radionuclides is to observe the function of an organ—not the structure.

RADIONUCLIDES AS RADIOACTIVE ELEMENTS

Radiation occurs where there is a lack of stability in the nuclei of atoms. As the atom spontaneously disintegrates, radiation is emitted in the form of alpha, beta, and gamma rays. Some of the synthetic radionuclides are purified so that only gamma rays are emitted. About 50 of the roughly 350 isotopes of all elements in nature are naturally radioactive (Holum, 1983). Isotopes of an element are slightly different molecular forms of the same chemical element. The discovery that certain natural elements were radioactive was made in 1896 by Becquerel, who was working with uranium compounds. In 1903, Becquerel shared a Nobel prize with Marie Curie and Pierre Curie, who discovered another naturally occurring radioactive substance, radium. The unit used to measure the activity of radionuclides is the microcurie named in honor of the Curies.

In the early part of this century, scientists discovered that it was possible to make naturally nonradioactive elements radioactive by bombarding the nucleus with sub-atomic fragments to make it unstable. The invention of the cyclotron (atom smasher) in 1931 made it possible to make many elements radioactive. Some of these synthetic radionuclides, such as iodine-131 (I-131), have been used extensively for therapy and diagnostic testing. Therapy with I-131 for cancer of the thyroid was begun in 1943; a time when both peaceful and war uses of nuclear products were being explored. The use of I-131 for cancer of the thyroid was dubbed the "atomic cocktail" (Myers & Wagner, 1974). Because of the length of its half-life, I-131 is infrequently used for diagnostic tests. Newer shorter-lived substances have replaced I-131, as discussed later.

USE OF RADIONUCLIDES AS THERAPEUTIC AGENTS

This chapter focuses on the use of radionuclides for diagnostic tests, but it should be pointed out that radionuclides are also used frequently in therapy. Two commonly used radionuclides are I-131, used to treat some cases of thyroid cancer and hyperthyroidism, and phosphorous-32 (P-32), used to treat certain malignancies that create pleural and peritoneal effusions (Brunner & Suddarth, 1984). P-32 is also used to treat polycythemia vera.

METHODS OF DIAGNOSTIC TESTING WITH RADIONUCLIDES

In Vitro Testing

With in vitro testing (sample testing), the radionuclide is given intravenously or orally, and at a later date, samples are taken from the blood and/or urine. Blood volume studies, red blood cells studies, and Schilling test are all examples of tests that use samples, not scans, to measure radionuclides. Sample tests are covered at the end of this chapter, with specific points about nursing implications. Although radioactive iodine uptake (RAI) may also involve the collection of urine samples, it is primarily an in vivo test because the radioactivity of the thyroid gland is measured with a counter. Table 22–1 lists in vitro sampling tests.

In Vivo Testing

The in vivo method (organ scan or scintogram) of measuring the amount of radionuclide in the body is done by organ scanning. Table 22–2 lists in vivo tests. The scan of an organ is referred to as a scintogram because a scintillation camera is used to make a scan or picture. The scintillation camera, which became available in 1964, has made testing with radionuclides a very useful method of diagnostic testing. The client is given a radionuclide compound (radiopharmaceutical) intravenously, orally, or by inhalation, depending on the organ to be scanned. Minutes or hours later, or sometimes the following day, the scintillation camera takes a radioactivity reading from the target organ and feeds these readings into a computer. The computer translates these readings into a two-dimensional image or scan. The scintogram is

TABLE 22–1. IN VITRO SAMPLING TESTS

Test	Example of Radionuclide Used	Timing of Test After Dosage	Special Preparation
Red blood cells Compatibility	Cr-51	1 hr	Blood drawn from client, then reinjected after tagged
Survival and sequestration	Cr-51	3–4 wk	Blood samples drawn 2–3 times a week
Blood volume studies			Blood drawn from client, then reinjected after tagged
RBC Plasma volume	Cr-51 Radioiodinate serum albumin (RISA)		Record height and weight Must have normal hydration
Schilling test (test for absorption of B_{12})	B_{12} tagged with Co-57 (oral)		n.p.o. status before test; urine saved for 24 hr; see text for other details, such as administration of B_{12} IM by nurse

TABLE 22-2. IN VIVO TESTING (ORGAN SCANS OR SCINTOGRAMS)

Scan	Examples of Radionuclides Type and Route	Timing of Scan after Dosage	Special Preparation
Bone	Tc-99m tagged phosphate compounds (IV)	Immediately and 2–4 hr (takes 1 hr to scan entire body)	Push fluids 2–4 hr before Void before ?Bowel preparation
Brain			
Perfusion	Tc-99m pertechnetate (IV)	Immediately	None
Static views	Tc-99m glucoheptenate (IV)	Immediately 15 min 1–4 hr	None
	Radioiodinated human serum albumin (RIHSA) (IV)	18–48 hr	None
Cardiac			
For infarction	Tc-99m pyrophosphate (IV) (Th-201) (IV)	90 min–3 hr	See text
Perfusion scan	(Th-201) (IV)	3–5 min; also in 3–6 hr	
Ejection/ fraction studies	Albumin or RBCs tagged with Tc-99m	Immediate with first pass analysis	
Gated-cardiac pool imaging	Same as above	Continuous over 2 hr	See text
Hepatobiliary			
Liver and spleen (reticulo-endothelial cells)	Tc-99m sulfur colloid	10–15 min	None
Gallbladder	Tc-99m with HIDA or PIPIDA (IV) Tc-99m DISIDA (IV) (Hepatolite)	Immediate and intervals to 24 hr	n.p.o. status for 2 hr before Fat restriction during time of test
Lung			
Perfusion	Tc-99m with albumin (IV)	15 min	None
Ventilation	Xe-133 (inhalation) Kr-85 (inhalation)	Immediate Immediate	None None
Deep vein thrombosis	Fibrinogen I-125 (IV)	4 hr and for several days afterward	Potassium iodide, as ordered, before scan and a few days afterward
Renal[a]			
Perfusion	Tc-99m DTPA, DSMA Glucoheptanate (IV #1)	Immediate (20 min)	Hydrate as ordered
Static views	As above	Up to 4 hr	
Function	I-131 or I-123 tagged to ortho-iodohippurate (IV #2)	Immediate and up to 1 hr as continual scan	Hydrate as ordered Potassium iodide solution as ordered

TABLE 22-2 (Continued)

Scan	Examples of Radionuclides Type and Route	Timing of Scan after Dosage	Special Preparation
Thyroid screening	Tc-99m pertechnetate (IV)	30 min	n.p.o. status 8 hr before and 2 hr posttest
	I-123 (oral)	24 hr	No iodine for 4 wk pretest
RAI (radioactive iodine uptake)	I-123 or I-131 (oral)	2 hr, 6 hr, 24 hr	As above; see text
Total body scans Inflammatory lesions and neoplasms	Gallium citrate, Ga-67 (IV)	4–6 hr and 24–72 hr or longer (up to 5 days)	Usually needs bowel preparation before
Inflammatory only	Tagged leukocytes with In-111 (IV)	4–24 hr	None

[a]A triple renal study uses two intravenous injections to obtain perfusion, static views, and excretory function of the kidney.

printed in a gray scale so there is more variation than in a black-and-white picture. These varying shades of gray show the relative distribution of the radionuclide in the different parts of the organ. Although the scan is viewed by the human eye, there is little discrepancy among observers in interpreting the variations of gray (Chang & Blau, 1979). Very dark spots of the scintogram are called "hot spots" because more of the radionuclide was deposited in that spot. Parts of the tissue that do not pick up the radionuclide are seen as light colored areas. Spots without radionuclide uptake are cold spots or cold nodules. Interpretation of the scintogram is done by a physician trained in nuclear medicine, and a verbal report of the scan is put in the client's chart. Some common findings on scintograms will be discussed for each specific scan covered in this chapter. In general, imaging with radionuclides is most useful where there is disturbance of function rather than a structural defect.

See Chapter 21 for a discussion on positron emission tomography (PET), which combines the use of radionuclides with tomography to study in a very sophisticated way both the structure and the function.

Types of Radionuclides Used in Diagnostic Testing

In the past, I-131 was used not only for diagnosis and therapy for thyroid disorders, but also as a radioactive tag carried to other organs. For example, rose bengal can be tagged with I-131. When the rose bengal is excreted by the liver into the biliary tract, the radioactive substance outlines the hepatobiliary system. Other forms of iodine are also used as radionuclides, including I-123, which has a half-life of 13 hours compared to a half-life of 8 days for I-131. (The significance of half-life will be discussed in the section on hazards.) Other radionuclides, such as gallium and thallium, are used for certain types of scanning. Sodium chromate (Cr-51) is used to tag red blood cells, and cobalt (Co-57) is used to tag vitamin B_{12} for the Schilling test. Although various radionuclides are useful for certain tests, technetium (Tc-99m) is the most commonly used for nuclear medicine diagnostic testing (Pollycove, 1985; Shore & Hendee, 1986).

Technetium. There are several isotopes of technetium, and all are naturally radio-active. A very unstable form of technetium, Tc-99m, has a half-life of only six hours (Valk et al., 1976). Technetium-99m is combined with various compounds, which carry the radionuclide to various target organs. For example, bone uses most of the phosphorous in the body, so Tc-99m combined with pyrophosphate is used for a bone scan. Technetium-99m combined with albumin is used as a lung scan because the radio-tagged albumin disperses in the pulmonary precapillary arterioles. Other compounds can carry Tc-99m to other specific organs, such as the hepatobiliary system, thyroid, or brain. If Tc-99m is given without another compound (straight), it is excreted in the urine and in the saliva. Thus, straight Tc-99m can be used to study the parotid glands or immediate flow through the cerebral vessels. Technetium-99m is always administered intravenously. The timing of the scans after the administration of the radionuclide will depend on the target organ to be viewed. Some organs may take up the substance in a few hours so scans will be done relatively soon whereas others may not be done for 24 hours or longer. Red blood cells can be tagged with Tc-99m to help diagnose gastrointestinal bleeding (Pollycove, 1985).

RADIATION HAZARDS FROM RADIONUCLIDES

The radiation hazard from radionuclide diagnostic testing is very slight because the doses used are usually very small. Also, duration is brief because of the short half-life of the radionuclides used. It was mentioned earlier that the curie (Ci) is the unit used to measure the activity of radionuclides. The curie is based on the radioactivity of a standard gram of radium. The dosages used in therapy are in millicurie levels (1/1000 of a curie). In contrast, dosage levels for the radiopharmaceuticals used for diagnostic testing are in microcurie levels (1/1000 of a millicurie). Thus, the radiation from diagnostic testing is roughly a thousand times less than with therapy (Rummerfield & Rummerfield, 1970). When millicurie levels are being used for therapy, other clients and personnel should be protected from the radiation in the client. The National Council on Radiation Protection and Measurements (1976) has specific guidelines that the hospital *shall* follow when therapy is being done with radionuclides. The guidelines for diagnostic procedures are less complicated than those for therapeutic procedures; however, nuclear medicine personnel must take precautions in handling samples. If urine or fecal matter must be saved for sample testing, the worker should wear waterproof gloves when putting the samples in containers or in cleaning bedpans. If urine can be disposed of by diluting it in the sewage system, then no special precautions are needed. Thus, from a nursing point of view, the usual precaution with urine is not to touch the urine, and if samples need to be obtained, waterproof gloves should be worn to handle the sample. (See the discussion under Posttest Nursing Diagnoses.) Exposure to other clients or personnel is not a major problem when radionuclide testing is done. If clients who have had radiopharmaceuticals administered are to remain in the nuclear medicine department, there must be a separate waiting room provided and children should not be allowed as visitors in this room (NCRP Report 48, 1976). Because the dosage of the substance is very small and half-life short, there is usually no problem in having a client come back in the unit to wait for later scans.

Waste Disposal for Diagnostic Testing Materials

The minimal radiation hazard from radionucline diagnostic testing is brief because the half-life of most diagnostic radiopharmaceuticals is very short. Half-life is the time in which it takes a radioactive element to lose half of its radioactivity. An unstable radioactive element continuously disintegrates but some take much longer than others to "physically decay." Iodine-123 has a half-life of only 13 hours, compared to 8 days for I-131. Technetium-99m has a half-life of only 6 hours and disposal is not a problem. In dramatic contrast, radium has a half-life of 1590 years (Holum, 1983). In addition to less exposure for the client, the shorter the half-life, the less the problem of waste disposal. For nuclear medicine diagnostic testing, the waste disposal problem is not acute because wastes can be held until physical decay occurs.

Radionuclides as Low Level Radioactive Wastes

Because radiation from any source is cumulative, it should always be kept at a minimum for clients, personnel, and the general public. The Nuclear Regulatory Commission grants a license to a physician or an institution to do research, therapy, or diagnostic testing with radioactive material. Specific standards must be maintained, and they are the responsibility of a person designated as the Radiation Protection Officer.

Problems with a Long Half-Life. Large research centers may conduct research that involves the use of carbon-14, which has a half-life of 5750 years. Radioactive waste that has a very long half-life is picked up by private carriers and taken to specified sites for dumping in several states. (Nuclear plants have their own waste disposal systems.) These dumping sites may not be enough as more radionuclides are used in testing. For example, when the Washington site was temporarily closed, research centers such as Harvard had to curtail studies that used radioactive materials with long half-lives (*Dump slump,* 1979). The Nuclear Regulatory Commission is currently working on plans to open up dumping sites in other states for the use of hospitals and other producers of low-level radioactive wastes. The nurse as a health professional, and as a concerned citizen, should keep abreast of what regulations the government provides for all nuclear wastes because the health of entire communities may be threatened when rigid controls are not followed.

Radionuclide Diagnostic Testing during Pregnancy and Childhood

Radiation destroys or alters cells as they go through the dividing stages of growth. In the fetus, and to a lesser degree in the child, cell growth is rapid; thus, many of their cells are vulnerable to alteration by radiation. (This of course is why radiation is used as a therapeutic agent for cancer cells, which are dividing and growing at an increased rate.)

As a general rule, radionuclides are not used for diagnostic testing during pregnancy if other tests can suffice. Although the amount of radioactivity in diagnostic testing is very small it is considered prudent to protect the fetus from any radiation whenever possible. As with x-rays, elective diagnostic tests using radionuclides should be done during menses or within 10–14 days after onset of menses for women who could become pregnant (NCRP, 1977). Children should also be protected from radionuclide testing if at all possible. When children have scans the dosages are calculated to give maximum results with minimum amounts of the radiopharmaceutical (Shore & Hendee, 1986). Nursing mothers should not nurse a child during the time of the testing. The risks and benefits for a specific individual are determined by the client's physician. Eymontt and Eymontt (1977) state that technetium is considered safe for children and for pregnant women. The limits of conservatism may vary in different settings and are sometimes controversial. Jankowski (1986) compares the risk of radiation to other risks of pregnancy and notes that low levels of radiation used for scanning are negligible risks. The pregnant woman should empty her bladder frequently after the test to flush out the radionuclide.

More Recent Techniques for Radionuclides

A technique to make radionuclides even safer is a method called fluorescent excitations analysis (FEA), developed at the Lawrence Livermore Radiation Laboratory in conjunction with the University of California at San Francisco (Hales, 1980). This technique uses radionuclides that are "excited" or turned on to emit signals only when the radionuclides reach the target organ. The radioactivity is only emitted for a short time. With the conventional radionuclide there is a small amount of radiation to the circulatory system as it goes to the target organ and to the bladder as the radionuclide is excreted. Although the radiation from diagnostic radionuclides is very small, it is part of the cumulative amount for the individual. Fluorescent excitations analysis and other methods are being researched to make diagnostic radionuclides as safe as possible.

PRETEST NURSING DIAGNOSES

Knowledge Deficit Regarding Test Procedure

The nurse should be familiar with the particular procedure being used for the test so that the client's questions can be answered. If the client is not sure why the test is needed, the nurse can help the client obtain the correct information from his or her physician. The nurse can assure the client that the scans do not hurt. The nurse should also inform the client that he or she will have to lie still during the scan, but the positioning is usually not uncomfortable. The scans may take from 30–60 minutes. The machine makes clicking noises at times. Some scanners can be brought to the client's bedside, but usually it is preferable to do the scan in the nuclear medicine department. Because there is no radiation hazard from the scan, a mother can accompany her child. Some clients may need a sedative or pain medication before the scan, but this is not a common practice. Sedatives do not interfere with the test. Most of the radionuclides are given intravenously so the client should be told that a venipuncture will be done in the nuclear medicine department. All of the Tc-99m compounds used for organ scans are given intravenously. Iodine compounds may be given orally or intravenously, depending on the test. If radioactive iodine is being used for studies other than of the thyroid, potassium iodide is given before and after the scan to block uptake by the thyroid gland. For some lung studies, the radio-tagged substance is inhaled.

Anxiety Related to Timing of Scans

The length of time between the administration of the radioisotope and the scan varies, depending on the type of scan (see Table 22–2). A member of the nuclear medicine department notifies the nurse of the specific time the client should return for the scan, or if the client is to remain in the nuclear medicine department for the entire time of the test. Clients should know if they are to stay in the nuclear medicine department for an extended length of time so they can bring reading material or handwork. For ambulatory care, the client may be given the radiopharmaceutical and told when to return for the scan. Specific written instructions should be given.

Anxiety Related to Possible Effects of Radiation

The nurse needs to fully understand the standard procedures for diagnostic radionuclide testing in a specific setting so the client is not confused about inconsistencies. (See the discussion under posttest care for some variations in the methods of waste disposal.) The nurse can reassure the client that the dose of radiation used for diagnostic testing is very small and all necessary precautions for safety are being taken. It may also be helpful to point out that only the radioisotope is radioactive. The scintillator acts as a detector of the radiation emitted *from* the client as opposed to a regular x-ray machine, where radiation is emitted from the machine to penetrate through the body. Thus, the long time, sometimes as much as an hour, spent in front of a scintillator does not cause any radiation effects as would long exposure to an x-ray machine. The clicking sound of the scintillator reflects only measurements of radioactivity already present. (Even health workers may need education about the relative safety of procedures done in the nuclear medicine department.)

POSTTEST NURSING DIAGNOSES

Potential for Injury

Major assessments are not needed after most scanning procedures for there is no risk for most of the procedures. If a stress test was done as part of a thallium scan for coronary perfusion, there are specific posttest considerations (see Chapter 26 on stress tests). If the radionuclide was given intravenously, and almost all are, the site of the needle puncture should be assessed for inflammation. Warm packs can be used for any phlebitis that develops. The medications used for testing are unlikely to cause any side effects.

Anxiety Regarding Test Results

As discussed in Chapter 20, the nurse is often able to act as a "sounding board" for the client who has anxiety about his or her condition. The results of the scan are not usually available for a day or two, so the nurse can help the client formulate specific questions to ask the physician. For example, if a liver scan was done to assess for possible metastasis, the person will be very anxious while awaiting the results. The nurse can help the person ventilate feelings and identify the major areas of concern regarding choices about treatments.

Alteration in Fluid Requirements Related to Need to Excrete Isotopes

As noted in the pretest preparations, most of the scans do not require any restrictions in diet, either before or after the scan. If there are no contraindications, the client should be encouraged to drink extra fluids to help expedite radionuclide excretion. This is particularly advised for pregnant clients.

Disposing of Urine

Although the amount of diagnostic radionuclide excreted in the urine is very low, urine should not be used for any laboratory tests. Clients should be told to flush the toilet three times after voiding. Rubber gloves are recommended if the urine must be handled (NCRP Report 48, 1977). The nuclear medicine department must supply the information about the timing of the precautions with urine, based on the half-life of the radionuclide used.

Some hospitals have developed specific guidelines and appointed safety advisors for personnel who care for clients confined to bed and who are undergoing nuclear medicine diagnostic procedures. Infants also pose a problem for disposal of wastes because the nurse must handle the urine. At San Francisco General Hospital (1980) the following guidelines were instituted:

1. Wear disposable gloves (not sterile ones) when handling wastes
2. Flush the toilet three times after excreta is discarded
3. Rinse reusable containers twice before doing general cleaning
4. Rinse disposable containers twice before discarding in the general waste
5. Wash hands with gloves on. Remove gloves and wash hands again. Dispose of gloves in general waste
6. For infants and incontinent clients use disposable diapers, wear disposable gloves when changing diapers, and discard gloves and waste as above

The reader is encouraged to talk to nuclear medicine personnel in a specific setting to obtain accurate up-to-date inforamtion about guidelines used for clients undergoing tests with radionuclides. The nurse should not unduly alarm clients. If some urine is accidentally spilled or touched, this is not an emergency. Immediate disposal of the waste is not of the same urgency as when clients have therapy with radioactive substances. The nurse should act in a prudent manner so that any and all exposure to radiation is minimized. (See Chapter 20 for more discussion on the radiation hazards for health workers.)

■ BONE SCANS

For a bone scan, Tc-99m pyrophosphate is given intravenously. In 2–4 hours, the radionuclide will concentrate in the bone tissue. It takes about an hour for the scintillation camera to scan the entire body, front and back. If there is increased bone activity, the bone tissue will take up more of the radionuclide. The scan will outline areas of osteoblastic and osteolytic processes in the bones, such as malignant tumors or osteoporosis.

Purposes. A bone scan is most often done to check for silent metastasis to the bone. A metastatic lesion in the bone will show up on a scan about 6 months earlier than on a regular x-ray (Robinson, 1979). Bone scans may be done on a routine basis after detection of malignancies of the breast or prostate because bone metastasis is a strong possibility with these malignancies. A bone scan may reveal the reason for an elevated alkaline phosphatase (ALP), an enzyme associated with bone activity (see Chapter 12).

NURSING IMPLICATIONS FOR BONE SCAN

The client must void before a bone scan so the pelvic bones can be seen. Also, the client may need an enema or laxative. Fluids should be pushed for 2–4 hours before the test to ensure that the client is well hydrated and thus will quickly eliminate the radionuclide not absorbed by the bones.

■ BRAIN SCANS

Brain scans are done as perfusion scans and static views of the brain tissues. A cerebral perfusion scan is done 30 seconds after the intravenous injection of Tc-99m. If straight Tc-99m is used, some of it will be excreted in the saliva; the client must not touch the saliva and then put his or her hands near his or her head. Technetium-99m pertechnetate static scans of the brain are done at intervals, such as 15 minutes, 1 hour, and 24 hours. Potassium perchlorate in solution or capsule form may be given 30 to 60 minutes before the procedure to prevent uptake by saliva and other tissues. If a lesion has damaged the blood–brain barrier, the radionuclide will localize in that area. The blood–brain barrier is a complex system of membranes and fluid spaces, which keep substances in the blood from diffusing into the brain tissue. Tumors and other lesions destroy this protective barrier; consequently, more of the radionuclide diffuses into the brain tissue. Radioiodinated human serum albumin (RIHSA) may also be used to evaluate changes in the blood–brain barrier. If CT scans or MRI scans are available these may be more useful than a brain scan (see Chapter 21).

■ GALLIUM SCANS

Gallium citrate (Ga-67) is useful in diagnostic scanning because gallium localizes in inflammatory lesions and in certain neoplastic tumors (Pelosi et al., 1980). A gallium scan may be used to detect a hidden abscess or metastatic nodules. Ultrasound (Chapter 23) may show the presence of a pelvic mass, but is not useful in determining if a mass is benign or malignant. A gallium scan can be a complementary procedure in studying the nature of a mass found by other diagnostic means. Gallium scans may be done 2–3 days after the administration of the Ga-67 to assess neoplasms. For inflammatory lesions, the initial scan is done in 4–6 hours.

A dual isotope scanning can be done with Ga-67 and Tc-99m to enhance the specificity of the scan. Otherwise the interpretation of the scan is limited by the complex distribution of Ga-67 (Karl et al., 1985).

NURSING IMPLICATIONS FOR GALLIUM SCAN

Enemas or laxatives are sometimes given before a gallium scan to empty the gastrointestinal tract. The intestinal tract collects gallium and confusing results may occur if there are shadows in the gastrointestinal tract. Not all institutions require bowel preparation and the dual isotope scanning reduces the amount of confusing results.

■ INDIUM SCANS

Indium (In-111) is used to label leukocytes, which then go to infected areas of the body. In contrast to gallium, In-111-labeled leukocytes are taken up by neither neoplastic lesions nor by noninfected wounds that are healing (Thakur, 1981). Any infected area in the body can be visualized in 4–24 hours. Indium is also used to label platelets and red blood cells for other types of studies. There is no special preparation of the client.

■ GALLBLADDER SCANS

The older technique to screen the biliary tract used rose bengal or BSP dye tagged with I-131. These substances are excreted by the liver into the biliary tree and concentrate in the gallbladder. I-131 rose bengal is still used in neonates with jaundice being evaluated for biliary atresia (Brunner & Suddarth, 1984). The newer method of evaluating biliary function is with Tc-99m combined with chemicals, such as HIDA and PIPDA (Eikman, 1979). These scans are done immediately, every 5 minutes for 30 minutes, and at intervals over a 24-hour period.

When information about organs adjacent to the gallbladder is not desirable, the radionuclide scan of the hepatobiliary tree may become the first procedure done to evaluate acute cholecystitis (Whalen, 1979). Hepatobiliary scans are also done in conjunction with ultrasound (Chapter 23) and x-ray studies of the gallbladder (Chapter 20) for chronic cholecystitis or for assessment of obstructive jaundice (see Chapter 11 on bilirubin).

NURSING IMPLICATIONS FOR GALLBLADDER SCAN

The client is kept on n.p.o. status for a few hours before the test. Sometimes clear liquids are allowed. The client may eat after the initial scan but fats are restricted during the 24-hour test period to decrease rapid emptying of the gallbladder.

■ LIVER AND SPLEEN SCANS

Hepatobiliary scans are used primarily to note biliary function; however, liver function is assessed, too, because the agents used to outline the biliary tree are excreted by the liver. Many different radiopharmaceuticals can be used for specific liver scans to assess the reticuloendothelial system or the structural changes in cirrhosis. A liver scan is a common procedure for clients where liver metastasis is suspected. Technetium-99m is combined with a sulfur colloid to assess for neoplasms in the liver (Snow et al., 1979). Liver scans may also be useful in assessing trauma to the liver or the presence of an abscess. The spleen is visualized simultaneously, if desired. The scan is done 10–15 minutes after the radionuclide is injected intravenously. No special preparation is needed.

■ LUNG SCANS

Lung scans may be done either as perfusion studies or as ventilation scans. Perfusion studies use macro aggregated albumin (MAA) tagged with Tc-99m, which disperses in the pulmonary precapillary arterioles. Perfusion lung scans are used to evaluate the possibility of pulmonary embolisms (Brunner & Suddarth, 1984). Ventilation lung scans are done with radioactive gas. The client inhales a bolus of xenon-123. The lungs are then scanned for about five minutes to determine how much gas enters each lobe of the lung and how long it takes the gas to be expelled. Krypton is another radioactive gas used for ventilation studies (Robinson, 1979). Radionuclide perfusion studies and ventilation studies are usually correlated with other pulmonary function tests (see Chapter 24) and blood gas studies (see Chapter 6). A recent chest film, within the last 24 hours, is usually needed. The lung scan is inappropriate when searching for a tumor, which is almost always more evident on a chest film—unless the tumor has invaded pulmonary vessels (Silberstein, 1980). There is no special preparation of the client. Some clients may be a little anxious about using a mask for the ventilation study.

■ CARDIAC SCANS

Infarction Scans. A test for detecting myocardial infarction uses Tc-99m pyrophosphate (the same compound used in bone scans). If there is an infarction in the myocardium, there will be an increased uptake of the radionuclide in this "hot" spot. The scan of the myocardium is done 1½–3 hours after the intravenous injection of the radionuclide. The test can be done at the client's bedside to prevent exertion on the part of the client. This test is reported to be more than 90% accurate in diagnosing transmural infarctions. For diagnosing subendocardial infarctions the test is 60–70% accurate (Disch, 1980). The hot spot myocardial imaging test is most helpful 1–3 days after the infarction. This test may be useful in cases where the more traditional ways of diagnosing myocardial infarction, cardiac enzymes (Chapter 12), and ECG readings (Chapter 24), have not given enough information.

Perfusion Scans. A thallium scan is also useful for evaluating coronary perfusion. Thallium is a physiological analogue of potassium in regards to distribution in the myocardium. A thallium scan may show the site of an old infarction or demonstrate partial obstructions to coronary blood flow. Poorly perfused regions of the myocardium will show up as low levels of thallium uptake (Disch, 1980). These "cold" spots may be seen in both acute and old infarctions. A stress test may be done as part of a thallium scan because coronary perfusion may only decrease with a certain amount of exertion. Research has suggested that combining a thallium scintogram with a stress test improves the prognostic ability of the tests, particularly in clients who have multivessel disease (Smeets et al., 1981). If a stress test is done in conjunction with the thallium scan, nursing care after the test will include careful assessment of the cardiac status of the client. (See Chapter 26 for a complete description of stress testing.) Persantine, a vasodilator, may be used during the scan.

Other Types of Cardiac Imaging. Sophisticated studies of heart function, including wall motion studies and ejection fraction studies, can be done by tagging red blood cells or albumin with Tc-99m. For ejection fraction studies, the scanning is done as the radionuclide passes through the heart. The amount of radionuclide ejected with each heart beat can be calculated, and any shunting can be detected. The function of the valves can also be assessed with the first "pass through" of the radionuclide. Scans done continuously over 1 or 2 hours are done in conjunction with electrographic monitoring of cardiac function. Signals from the ECG trigger the scintillation camera to record the flow of blood at precise times in the cardiac cycle. The procedure is called gated-cardiac imaging because the series of images of blood flow through the heart can be studied in sequence. At precise times in the cardiac cycle the scintillator is turned on to record function.

These gated types of images are used to assess ventricular function. For example, a postinfarction client can be evaluated to determine if developing congestive failure is due to overall poor contractibility or to a regional abnormality, such as a ventricular aneurysm.

Another use of radionuclides for cardiac scanning is to screen asymptomatic children with murmurs of questionable significance. Cardiac scanning by nuclear imaging may help avoid the need for angiocardiography (Robinson, 1979). (See Chapter 26 for a discussion on cardiac catheterization, which may be a follow-up after nuclear scanning.) Note also that isotopes are used in conjunction with positron emission tomography (PET) scans to do cardiac evaluations. (See Chapter 21 for a discussion on PET or SPECT.)

NURSING IMPLICATIONS FOR THALLIUM SCAN WITH STRESS TEST

If a stress test is to be done with a thallium scan, there are very specific preparations for the stress test component (see Chapter 26 for stress tests). For other cardiac scans, there is no special preparation, except for the general nursing implications discussed in the beginning of this chapter. Nuclear cardiac studies may be done in specialized care units, such as coronary care settings, as well as outpatient settings.

■ RENAL SCANS

Scans of the kidneys evaluate both renal perfusion and function. Technetium-99m is tagged to a compound such as dimercaptosuccinic acid (DSMA). The tagged compound is administered intravenously, and a series of scans are taken to assess the dynamic perfusion of the kidneys. Static scans are taken from 20 minutes up to four hours to assess the structure of the kidneys. Another type of compound orthoiodohippurate (Hippuran) tagged with radioactive iodine can be given as a second intravenous injection so continuous images can be obtained over approximately an hour to measure the time it takes to travel through the cortex and pelvis of each kidney. The times of uptake, transient, and excretion of the radionuclide by each kidney can be plotted on a graph called an isotope renogram curve. Plotted curves are compared to normal reference curves to determine abnormalities in either kidney. The use of two intravenous injections to obtain the perfusion, structure, and excretory ability of the kidneys is sometimes called a triple renal study.

Intravenous pyelogram (IVP) involves the use of a radiopaque dye to evaluate the excretory ability of the renal system (see Chapter 20 for IVP). For clients allergic to the contrast medium used for IVP, renograms can be used as a substitute to assess the excretory pattern. The use of renal imaging to assess renal dysfunction is used in conjunction with various other diagnostic studies. Renal biopsies (Chapter 25) are sometimes done in conjunction with renal scans.

NURSING IMPLICATIONS FOR RENAL SCANS

See the general nursing diagnoses in the introduction. In addition, the client should be well hydrated. For aftercare, see the discussion on safety precautions for disposing of urine.

■ THYROID SCANS

Several different isotopes of iodine are used for thyroid scans. Iodine, such as I-123, can be given either orally or intravenously. Scans of the thyroid are done to assess nodules, which may be felt in the thyroid gland. Benign nodules appear as "warm" spots on the scan because they tend to take up the radionuclide. Conversely, malignant tumors appear as "cold" spots because they do not tend to take up the radionuclide. The actual presence of a malignancy must still be determined by a biopsy. (A special type of scanning of the thyroid called a radioactive iodine uptake (RAI) is discussed in a separate section because the RAI is different from organ scans in general.)

When screening someone with no symptoms of thyroid problems, thyroid scans can be done with Tc-99m because the screening can be done faster with less radiation exposure due to the short half-life of Tc-99m. Thyroid scans are also done on people who have no thyroid problems, but do have a history of x-ray radiation to the face and neck. Until the late 1950s, x-ray therapy was used in the treatment of acne and thymus gland disorders, and this past radiation may promote malignant growths in the thyroid gland (Guimond & Wilson, 1979).

See the next section on RAI for the restrictions on iodine uptake before thyroid scans with radioactive iodine.

■ RAI UPTAKE

For an RAI uptake, the client is given radioactive iodine either in an oral capsule or intravenously. The uptake by the thyroid gland is measured by a scanner at several time intervals, such as 1 hour, 6 hours, and in 24 and 48 hours. A person with hyperthyroidism will have an increased uptake of iodine, perhaps as high as 90%. Conversely, the person with hypothyroidism will have a decreased uptake of iodine by the thyroid gland. The values of the RAI uptake are expressed in percentages: the amount of thyroid uptake divided by the amount of the dose given. The reference values vary depending on the locality because normal iodine consumption varies in different locales (Brunner & Suddarth, 1984).

Reference Values for RAI	
Scan (uptake)	1–13% after 2 hr
	2–25% after 6 hr
	15–45% after 24 hr
Urine with I-123	37–75% excreted

PRETEST NURSING DIAGNOSIS

Knowledge Deficit Regarding Sources of Iodine

Because the amount of iodine consumption before the test affects the uptake of radioactive iodine, it is important that the client not have additional iodine uptake for several weeks before the test. A list of medications currently being taken by the client should be put on the laboratory request. Thyroid medications and amiodarone (Cordarone) interfere with the test.

As mentioned in Chapter 20, most contrast mediums used for x-ray studies have an iodine base. A client should have an RAI before studies that use iodine dye. Clients need to be instructed to avoid all sources of iodine. Certain foods, such as kelp and enriched breakfast cereals, are high in iodine. Vitamin preparations may contain iodine, as do most cough syrups. Even suntan lotion and nail polish can be sources of exogenous iodine. Such a small amount of iodine is used for the RAI that it does not cause any allergic problems, even in people who are allergic to iodine. (In contrast, x-ray dyes that contain iodine can cause anaphylactic shock in allergic individuals.)

POSTTEST NURSING IMPLICATIONS

For some RAI tests, urine samples may be saved for monitoring, but saving urine is not common. If saved, the urine does not need a preservative. The amount of iodine excreted in the urine will depend both on the thyroid uptake and the normalcy of renal function. Adequate fluids should be encouraged for the client. If urine is to be handled, the precautions discussed earlier should be noted (e.g., wearing rubber gloves).

■ OTHER ORGAN SCANS INCLUDING FIBRINOGEN UPTAKE

The salivary glands, adrenals, lacrimal ducts, and testes are some of the other structures that can be scanned when the appropriate carrying compound is tagged with a radionuclide. Radioactive cholesterol is used to get images of the adrenal gland. The scan of the adrenals is done in 2–4 days or 7–10 days, depending on the radionuclide used to tag the cholesterol (Robinson, 1979). Imaging of some glands, such as the pancreas or parathyroid, has been difficult to achieve (Brunner & Suddarth, 1984). A compound must be specific for the target area. For example, tagged fibrinogen will go to a venous clot and may help assess the presence of a thrombus. The radiofibrinogen uptake test (RFUT) for detection of deep vein thrombosis was used in a large research study on dihydroergotamine–heparin prophylaxis (Multicenter Trial Committee, 1984). For fibrinogen uptake, the I-125 fibrinogen is given intravenously and the first scan done 4 hours later. The uptake of the I-125 is blocked by potassium iodide, 100 mg orally, the evening before and for a few days afterwards. The reader must consult current literature to obtain data on the newest techniques developed for organ scanning—a dynamic and growing field.

■ IN VITRO SAMPLING: COMPATABILITY AND RBC SURVIVAL

Sodium chromate (Cr-51) readily binds with the protein of hemoglobin so red blood cells can be tagged to evaluate the rate of hemolysis or red blood cell survival in certain types of hemolytic diseases. A sample of blood is withdrawn from the client, tagged with the radioactive Cr-51, and injected back into the client. A collection of blood samples are drawn at various time intervals. One sample may be drawn within 1 hour to measure compatability and then 2–3 times a week to assess survival. The RBC survival should be at least 31–39 days (Pollycove, 1985). No special preparation of the client is required. No blood transfusions should be given 48 hours prior to the study.

■ BLOOD VOLUME STUDIES

Sodium chromate is also used to determine blood volume. The blood volume should be 8.5–9% of body weight in kilograms (Scully, 1986). It is used to tag the RBCs, and radioiodinate serum albumin (RISA) is used to tag plasma. A measured amount of blood is withdrawn from the client, tagged with radionuclides, and injected back into the client. After 30–60 minutes, samples of blood are drawn and the amount of dilution of the original sample is calculated. The total blood volume of a client can thus be estimated. It is very important that the hydration of the client be normal before the blood studies are done. Intravenous solutions will invalidate the test, as will a n.p.o. state. The nurse must record the height and weight of the client before the test is done.

■ SCHILLING TEST

The Schilling test is used to assess the ability of the small intestine to absorb vitamin B_{12}. (Clients with a deficiency in vitamin B_{12} develop a macrocytic anemia; see Chapter 2.) An oral preparation of vitamin B_{12} is tagged with cobalt-57. The test measures how much of the tagged B_{12} is eliminated in the urine. The client is given a loading dose of untagged vitamin B_{12} intramuscularly to saturate the cells with B_{12} so that much of the tagged B_{12} can be excreted. Nurses usually give the intramuscular dose. The oral cobalt-tagged vitamin B_{12} is given by the nuclear medicine department personnel. A dual isotope technique may be used so that tagged B_{12} and the intrinsic factor is given with tagged B_{12} without the intrinsic factor. Thus the Schilling test is done in one step. All urine is collected for 24 hours and should be kept on ice. No preservative is needed. If renal function is questionable, the test may last longer. The precautions for urine handling should be noted, as discussed earlier in this chapter. The client must be fasting before the test begins and for 2 hours after the oral B_{12} is given.

Reference Values for Schilling Test (24-Hour Urine Excretion)	
B_{12} without intrinsic factor	10–40%
B_{12} with intrinsic factor	10–40%

Clinical Significance. Intrinsic factor is found in the gastric mucosa and is essential for the proper absorption of vitamin B_{12}. If urine values increase when intrinsic factor is given with B_{12}, a diagnosis of pernicious anemia is likely. In pernicious anemia and certain gastric lesions, the 24-hour excretion of tagged B_{12} without the intrinsic factor is usually less than 7% and the excretion of tagged B_{12} with the intrinsic factor is significantly greater than 6–12% (Pollycove, 1985). If defective absorption is low both with and without the intrinsic factor, other types of intestinal malabsorption must be considered such as sprue. Some unusual and unexplained anemias may be assessed by bone marrow biopsies. If bone marrow studies are ordered, these are done before any injections of vitamin B_{12} because vitamins change the picture of the bone marrow (see Chapter 25 on bone marrow studies). See Chapter 2 for nursing diagnoses related to macrocytic anemias.

QUESTIONS

1. Technetium (Tc-99m) is useful as an agent for diagnostic testing because this radioactive element

   a. Has a half-life of only 2 days
   b. Can be tagged to go to the brain, bone, liver, or lung
   c. Is radioactive only when it reaches the target organ
   d. Is excreted only in the urine

2. Scintography involves taking the reading of radioactivity from a body organ and transforming the reading into

   a. Audible sounds (Geiger counter)
   b. Quantitative measurements
   c. A two-dimensional image of the organ
   d. A vertical graph

3. The radiation hazard from radionuclide diagnostic testing is much less than when radionuclides are used for therapy because the dose used for diagnostic testing is about

   a. Half as much as used in therapy
   b. 10 times less than therapy
   c. 100 times less than therapy
   d. 1000 times less than therapy

4. Which of the following would be a reason to postpone, if possible, radionuclide diagnostic studies? The woman who is

   a. Seven days past onset of menstrual period
   b. Pregnant in last trimester
   c. Menstruating
   d. Allergic to iodine

5. Which of the following nursing actions is appropriate in preparing a client for any organ scan with technetium (Tc-99m)?

   a. Explain to the client that all urine must be monitored after the test
   b. Keep the client on n.p.o. status
   c. Explain that the test involves intravenous administration of a very small dose of a radioactive substance
   d. Shave the area that will be viewed by the scan

6. The major use of a bone scan done with radionuclides is to detect

   a. Silent metastasis from the breast or prostate gland

    b. Silent metastasis from the liver or kidney

    c. Utilization of phosphorous by the body

    d. Fractures

7. Mrs. Lourdes is going to have a gallium scan done this morning because of a fever of undetermined origin (FUO). Gallium is useful as a radionuclide for scintography because gallium localizes in

    a. Inflamed tissue or certain types of tumors

    b. The lungs

    c. The brain and spinal column

    d. The hepatobiliary system

8. Mrs. Hunter is scheduled for a radioactive iodine uptake (RAI) in 4 weeks so she is to have no iodine intake. Which of the following is *not* a potential source of iodine?

    a. Suntan lotions

    b. Vitamin preparations

    c. Contrast medium for x-ray tests

    d. Soft drinks, such as colas

9. Mr. Langerdorf is having a Schilling test done today. Which of the following is *not* an appropriate nursing function in regard to this test?

    a. Saving all urine for 24 hours after the oral cobalt-tagged B_{12} is given

    b. Giving an ordered intramuscular injection of B_{12} as a loading dose before the oral cobalt-tagged B_{12} is given

    c. Keeping the client isolated from other clients because radioactive cobalt is used

    d. Using rubber gloves when collecting urine samples.

REFERENCES

Brunner, L., & Suddarth, D. (1984). *Textbook of medical-surgical nursing* (5th ed.). Philadelphia: J.B. Lippincott.

Chang, W., & Blau, M. (1979). Optimization of the gray scale for photo scanners. *Journal of Nuclear Medicine, 20,* 57–59.

Disch, J. (1980). *Diagnostic procedures for cardiovascular disease.* Norwalk, CT: Appleton-Century-Crofts.

Dump Slump. (1979, October 29). It hurts nuclear medicine. *Time Magazine, 114,* 102.

Eikman, E. (1979). Radionuclide hepatobiliary procedures: When can HIDA help? *Journal of Nuclear Medicine, 20*(4), 358–360.

Eymontt, M., & Eymontt, D. (1977). Preparing your patient for nuclear medicine. *Nursing 77, 7*(12), 46–49.

Guimond, J., & Wilson, S. (1979). Postirradiation thyroid disorders. *AJN, 79*(7), 1256–1258.

Hales, D. (1980). Imaging—beyond CT. *UCSF Magazine, 3,* 9–10.

Holum, J. (1983). *Elements of general and biological chemistry.* (6th ed.). New York: Wiley.

Jankowski, C. (1986). Radiation and pregnancy: Putting the risks in proportion. *AJN, 86*(3), 261–265.

Karl, R., et al. (1985). Dual isotope scanning with gallium-67 citrate and technetium-99m radiopharmaceuticals. *Clinical Nuclear Medicine, 10*(7), 507–512.

Multicenter Trial Committee. (1984). Dihydroergotamine–heparin prophylaxis of postoperative deep vein thrombosis. *JAMA, 251*(22), 2960–2966.

Myers, W., & Wagner, H. (1974). Nuclear medicine: How it began. *Hospital Practice, 9*(2), 103–113.

NCRP Report 48. (1976). *Radioactive nuclides in radiation protection for medical and allied health personnel.* Washington, DC: National Council on Radiation Protection and Measurements.

NCRP Report 54. (1977). *Medical radiation exposure of pregnant and potentially pregnant women.* Washington, DC: National Council on Radiation Protection and Measurements.

Pelosi, M., et al. (1980). Combined use of ultrasonography and gallium scanning in the diagnosis of pelvic pathology. *Surgery, Gynecology and Obstetrics, 150,* 331–336.

Pollycove, M. (1985). *Nuclear medicine manual.* San Francisco: San Francisco General Hospital.

Robinson, P.J. (1979). Clinical uses of isotope imaging. In L. Kreel (Ed.), *Medical Imaging.* Chicago: Year Book Medical.

Rummerfield, P., & Rummerfield, M. (1970). What you should know about radiation hazards. *AJN, 70,* 780–786.

San Francisco General Hospital (1980). *Safety advisory for nurses handling excreta from patients confined to bed and undergoing nuclear medicine diagnostic procedures.* San Francisco: San Francisco General Hospital.

Shore, R., & Hendee, W. (1986). Radiopharmaceutical dosage solution for pediatric nuclear medicine. *Journal of Nuclear Medicine, 27*(2), 287–297.

Silberstein, E. (1980). Nuclear medicine and the lung: Perfusion and ventilation. *Basics of Respiratory Disease, 9,* 5–6.

Smeets, J.P., et al. (1981). Prognostic value of thallium-201–stress myocardial scintography with exercise ECG after myocardial infarction. *Cardiology, 68* (Suppl. 2), 67–70.

Snow, J., et al. (1979). Comparison of scintology, sonography and computed tomography in the evaluation of hepatic neoplasms. *American Journal of Roentgenology, 132,* 915–917.

Thakur, M. (1981). New radionuclides in the diagnosis of obscure infections. *Connecticut Medicine, 45,* 302–304.

Valk, P., et al. (1976). Technetium radiopharmaceuticals as diagnostic organ imaging agents. *Journal of Chemical Education, 53,* 542–543.

Whalen, J. (1979). Newer imagery methods of the abdomen. *American Journal of Roentgenology, 133,* 587–615.

23

Diagnostic Ultrasonography

- Doppler Techniques
- Pelvic Sonograms: Ultrasound Scans in Pregnancy and Gynecological Conditions
- Abdominal Sonograms
- Echocardiograms
- Echoencephalograms
- Thoracic Sonograms

OBJECTIVES

1. Explain the differences between A mode, B scans, and "real-time" scans as methods of pulse–echo recordings of ultrasound.
2. Describe three clinical situations where the nurse uses the Doppler method of ultrasound for assessment.
3. Describe the necessary preparation of the client for pelvic and abdominal sonograms.
4. Explain the specific use of echocardiograms as diagnostic tests for cardiac problems.
5. Describe the responsibilities of the nurse when a young child has an echoencephalogram.
6. Explain why ultrasound examinations of the thorax are of limited usefulness.
7. Identify at least two nursing diagnoses for clients undergoing sonography.

Ultrasound, a noninvasive method of diagnostic testing, uses sound waves to detect physical changes in the client. Sound is a physical force, and thus sonograms are in no way related to x-rays (discussed in Chapter 20), computer axial tomography scans (discussed in Chapter 21), and the radionuclide scans (discussed in Chapter 22).

Ultrasound, first used in industry to detect flaws in metal, is used as a sonar system to locate objects in the water and for depth sounding of the ocean floor. In addition, it has become a very common diagnostic tool in pregnancy. Ultrasound has also become well established as a cardiac diagnostic test (echocardiogram) for certain cardiac problems. A newer and very rapidly growing use of ultrasound is to assess various pathologic conditions of the abdomen. Common tests using both the pulse–echo recordings and Doppler methods are covered in this chapter (Table 23–1). The Doppler method of assessment is often used by the nurse in obstetric settings, in medical–surgical units and in home care.

ULTRASOUND PRINCIPLES

Although this chapter focuses on the use of ultrasound as a diagnostic tool, ultrasound waves are also used as therapy. Ultrasound, in large and continuous doses, can generate heat in tissues; therefore, ultrasound treatments are used for various kinds of low back pain. Ultrasound has also been tried as a method to promote tissue regeneration and to generate heat to kill malignant growths (Research Roundup, 1980). A procedure called percutaneous ultrasonic lithotripsy (PUL) has become well established as a therapeutic use of ultrasound to pulverize kidney stones (Harwood, 1985; Ruge, 1986).

Description. Ultrasonics is part of the science of acoustics that deals with sound waves that are beyond the range of audible sound. The human ear can hear sounds that are of a frequency between 16,000 and 20,000 cycles per second. The unit of frequency is a hertz (Hz), which is equal to one cycle per second. Thus, ultrasound waves are of a frequency higher than 20,000 Hz (Wells, 1979). Sonograms are done with transducers, which produce sound waves of varying strength or intensity. Intensity is the measure of the strength of a sound wave and is measured as the amount of power per a cross-sectional area. However, more useful to the nurse than figures of frequencies and intensities is the comparison of dosages used in tests. Intensities employed for therapeutic treatment are at least 20 times the intensities used in diagnostic testing (Ziskin, 1980).

TABLE 23-1. ULTRASOUND METHODS USED FOR ASSESSMENT

Method	Examples of Use
Pulse–echo methods	
1. A mode (amplitude modulation)	Echocardiogram
2. B mode (brightness modulation)	Sonograms of fetus, pelvic and abdominal structures
Doppler method	
1. Doppler stethoscope	Monitoring of fetal heart rate
2. Doppler instrument	Monitoring of peripheral pulses
3. Pulse volume recorder	Assessing extent of peripheral vascular disease

For diagnostic purposes, ultrasound waves are sent into the body by a small transducer,* pressed against the skin. A transducer changes one form of energy into another. An electric signal from the machine is converted to ultrasound waves. Air almost completely impedes the transmission of the ultrasound waves into the body; thus the transducer must be in good contact with the skin as it is being moved. A lubricant, such as mineral oil, glycerin, or a water-based jelly, is used to ensure good contact with the skin. The lubricant is called the coupling agent. When it is difficult to evenly move the transducer over an area (e.g., ultrasound of the neck, scrotum, or breast), the transducer can be supported in a plastic bag of water (Pachaczevsk, 1979). The transducer not only sends the sound waves into the body, it also receives any returning sound waves, which are deflected back as they bounce off various structures. Some sound waves pass through the body. The transducer converts the returning sound waves into electric signals that can then be transformed by a computer into either scans or graphs (pulse–echo methods) or into audible sounds (Doppler method). Regarding sound waves that go through the body, research is just now beginning to look at the "through transmission" technique. One example is the measurement of pass through in lung conditions such as pulmonary embolism.

PULSE–ECHO METHOD OF DISPLAYING ULTRASOUND

All of the pulse–echo techniques measure the time it takes the sound waves to reach various structures and return to the transducer. There are various ways that the read out can be done. In the A mode (amplitude modulation) the echoes are displayed in a graphic form, for example, the graph done for an echocardiogram. In the B mode (brightness modulation) the echoes appear as different intensities of brightness. B scans use these dots of brightness to show a two-dimensional cross-sectional view of the various structures. Thus, with a B scan, one can actually see a "picture" of the fetus in the womb, for example. The B scans may be still (static scans) or motion may be added.

REAL-TIME IMAGING

The terms *real time* and *real-time imaging* are computer jargon for scanners that are capable of very rapid scanning so that motion can be displayed (Meire, 1977). A still picture with a B scan takes 20 seconds. For upper abdominal sonograms, the client must lie very still and hold his or her breath so the usual movement of the diaphragm will not interfere with the picture. A scan that has real-time imaging is capable of 30 frames per second. In other words, the real-time scanning is like a movie. A fetus can be seen moving around, sucking a thumb, or other motions. The use of the scanner with rapid sequencing is very valuable in observing heart action. For real-time imaging there is no need for the client to suspend respiration during the scan. Thus, real-time scanning is better suited for infants, children, or confused adults (James, 1980). Real-time scanning can survey the whole abdomen to detect suspicious areas that may be needed to be examined in detail. This scan is like a sophisticated physical assessment (Fields & Calvert-Hill, 1985).

---

*Technically, the transducer is just the piezoelectric crystal, which does the changing of electric energy to sound waves and vice versa. However, the unit that houses the crystal is also called the transducer in general terms.

GRAY SCALE AND MAGNIFICATION

The first sonograms were black and white. In 1979 the gray scale became available. The various shades of gray allow some distinctions among structures, but are still not precise for each type of tissue. Kreel & Steiner (1979) predicted that in a few years computer analysis would be able to specifically identify different tissues to make a very sophisticated scan. Now computerized sonographic machines are able to magnify a selected area 5 to 7 times and thus give a view as powerful as with low-power microscopic techniques (Birnholz, 1985). Also color-coded sonograms are available (Goldman, 1986).

POSSIBLE RISKS FROM ULTRASOUND

There are two known effects of ultrasound in tissue: the production of heat and cavitation (Taylor & Dyson, 1980). Cavitation is the appearance of gas-filled bubbles in a sound field. Ultrasound waves over 100,000 Hz cause formation of gas bubbles in bacterial cells, killing the bacteria. As far as is known, the low-intensity dose of ultrasound used for sonograms is harmless to humans; there is no heat formation or cavitation in the tissues. The sound waves are delivered intermittently for sonograms and not continuously as with therapy.

Sonograms have been used in pregnancy since the mid-1960s, and there have not been reports of damage to either the woman or the fetus (American College of Obstetricians and Gynecologists, 1979). Yet some authorities have questioned the possible risks of ultrasound for the developing fetus (Mendelsohn, 1983). Studies are continuing to determine if there are any possible long-term effects. One study is being planned which will involve 10,000 healthy women (Freiherr, 1986). The Doppler devices used in fetal monitoring are of low enough dosages to be free of adverse heating effects or cavitation in tissues. However, the Doppler instrument used in arterial studies does use intensities of sound that produce some heat in tissues; consequently, arterial Doppler monitors are not considered suitable for fetal investigation (Taylor & Dyson, 1980).

A consensus statement from the National Institute of Child Health and Human Development (1984) stressed that "routine" sonograms cannot be recommended. When sonograms are needed clients should be given information about the test and educational materials provided. Certainly sonograms do not pose the risk of radiation and any other risks seem unlikely now, but as research continues clients need the latest data.

■ DOPPLER TECHNIQUES

With the Doppler method, returning sound waves are transformed into audible sounds, which can be heard with earphones. Not only are sound waves produced by moving objects, but sound waves bounced off of different moving objects have slightly different frequencies. The sound produced by an artery is pulsatile and multiphasic, whereas the sound from a vein is intermittent and varies with respiration (Hudson, 1983). The Doppler technique is used to assess the movement of the opening and closing of the heart valves and the flow of blood. This technique is used for bedside assessments, as well as a laboratory diagnostic aid. The Doppler stethoscope can detect the presence of fetal heartbeats, even when the heartbeat is inaudible by the conventional stethoscope. The Doppler technique can be used as a type of fetal monitoring during labor and delivery. The Doppler technique is also used to monitor the fetus during the ocytocin challenge test (OCT) or the nonstress test (NST), which may be done during the last trimester of pregnancy. (See Chapter 28 for tests in pregnancy.)

In addition to the use of a Doppler stethoscope or monitor for evaluating fetal status, the nurse may also use a Doppler instrument to monitor blood flow in clients who have altered arterial circulation. A portable Doppler instrument is about the size of a tissue box. A small flat transducer is placed over the vessel to be assessed, and when the unit is turned on, transmitted sound waves are bounced off the moving blood, producing a pulse heard via earphones. The portable Doppler unit, useful in the first few days after an arterial graft to assess the continued patency of the graft, may also be used in a clinic setting to assess clients with chronic perfusion problems. Another type of Doppler unit is sometimes used to monitor the blood pressure in shock when the blood pressure is barely audible. Pulses can be detected with the Doppler unit when the pulse is too faint to be felt with the fingertips. Also, a Doppler unit with blood pressure cuffs can measure the pulse volume of both arteries and veins and obtain a pressure index by comparing leg and arm pressure readings.

■ PELVIC SONOGRAMS: ULTRASOUND SCANS IN PREGNANCY AND GYNECOLOGICAL CONDITIONS

Purposes. As mentioned earlier, sonograms were originally used for evaluating the position of the placenta and the status of the fetus. Before an amniocentesis (Chapter 28) is done the position of the placenta is determined by ultrasound. The fetal growth rate can also be determined by measurements of the pictures taken by ultrasound. Ectopic pregnancies, hydatidiform moles, or structural abnormalities in the fetus can all be detected by ultrasound, as can death of the fetus (Sanders, 1980). The presence of twins can almost always be detected, too. It is possible, however, for one twin to "hide" behind the other so that the two-dimensional scan does not show the second fetus. In questionable scans, several sonograms may be done. One of the great advantages of ultrasound is that repeated scans are not usually considered risky. If necessary, sonograms may be done several times during a pregnancy. Ultrasound scans may also be done after a delivery to check for any retained placenta. Pelvic sonograms are also used to evaluate pelvic inflammatory disease and abscess formation. Pelvic masses can also be detected with ultrasound.

PRETEST NURSING DIAGNOSES RELATED TO PELVIC SONOGRAMS

Anxiety Related to Well-being of Fetus
The movement of the transducer over the abdomen is not at all painful. The client can see the scan on the monitor. Most pregnant women are thrilled to be able to see a picture of the baby on the monitoring screen. The technician can point out the head, feet, and so on, of the baby as it moves about. The heart beat is seen as a blip of light. At many centers, any woman who wishes a picture of her baby is given a copy of the sonogram. Obviously, watching the monitor can be an unbelievable, chilling moment for the woman whose child is dead or if the ultrasound is being done to assess malformations.

Alteration in Comfort Related to Full Bladder and Positioning

Besides the anxiety of finding possible abnormalities with the sonogram, two other factors may make a sonogram slightly uncomfortable for the pregnant woman. One factor is the need for the woman to have a full bladder during the procedure. A full bladder is an "acoustical window" so that other structures can be seen in relation to the bladder. Sound waves travel well through liquid. The other factor is the need for the woman to lie in a flat position for 20 or so minutes. Some pregnant women can get hypotensive from the pressure on the vena cava. It may be necessary for the woman to turn on her left side to relieve this pressure.

Knowledge Deficit Regarding Physical Preparation

There is no need to restrict any medications nor alter the client's diet before the test. It is essential, however, that the client's bladder be full during the sonogram; thus, the client must drink about ¾ liter of water (750 ml) before the test. As noted above, a full bladder is an "acoustical window." If the client has an intravenous going, the nurse needs to check to see how much the IV rate should be increased. If the client has a Foley catheter, the catheter must be clamped so that the bladder is full for the pelvic sonogram (Table 23–2). As with the pregnant woman, but to a lesser degree, the discomfort of maintaining a full bladder for the time of the test is expected and should be explained to the client.

POSTTEST NURSING IMPLICATIONS

There are no special nursing implications after the client has had a pelvic sonogram. If the sonogram was done to assess for fetal abnormalities or fetal death (demise), the nurse must be sensitive to helping the woman find the needed support to cope with the distressing news. (See Chapter 28 for a discussion on the role of the nurse in helping couples deal with loss.)

■ ABDOMINAL SONOGRAMS

Purposes. Sonography of the abdomen is being used more and more as the equipment becomes more sophisticated and clinicians become more adept at identifying abdominal problems by sonogram. A sonogram of the abdomen may mean the client

TABLE 23-2. PREPARATION OF CLIENT FOR SONOGRAPHY

Test	n.p.o.?	Bowel Preparation?	Other
Pelvic sonograms	No	No	Must have full bladder
Abdominal sonograms	Usually but not always	Varies	See text for medication used and other prep
Echocardiograms	No	No	None
Echoencephalograms	No	No	Sedation for children?
Thoracic sonograms	No	No	None

does not need to have exposure to radiation or invasive procedures done to diagnose a problem.

Sometimes surgery can be avoided if sonograms are done. For example, sonograms of a dilated bilary tree can be used to differentiate between intrahepatic and extrahepatic obstruction with 96% accuracy (Taylor et al., 1979). An extrahepatic obstruction requires surgery, but an intrahepatic obstruction does not. Whalen (1979) contains a series of ten flow charts that show how ultrasound can be used to help diagnose ten common abdominal problems. These ten common abdominal problems are:

1. Retroperitoneal adenopathy
2. Aortic aneurysm
3. Renal mass
4. Nonfunctioning kidney
5. Adrenal mass
6. Pancreatic mass
7. Liver mass
8. Obstructive jaundice
9. Acute cholecystitis
10. Chronic cholecystitis or gallstones

For the diagnosis of some of these abdominal conditions, ultrasound may be the first test performed. In other clinical conditions, abdominal sonograms are complementary to other workups, such as radionuclide studies (Chapter 22), x-ray studies (Chapter 20), or CT and MRI scans (Chapter 21). Various studies, such as Snow et al. (1979), have compared the usefulness of scintigraphy (radionuclides), sonography, and CT for various types of abdominal pathology. In addition to no radiation hazard, sonography has the advantage of being less costly than CT or MRI scans.

PRETEST NURSING DIAGNOSIS RELATED TO ABDOMINAL SONOGRAMS

Knowledge Deficit Regarding Any Needed Preparations

The actual procedure for an abdominal sonogram is similar to that of a pelvic sonogram, discussed earlier. However, the client does *not* need to have a full bladder for an abdominal sonogram as for a pelvic sonogram. The client may be on n.p.o. status or may be allowed only liquids, depending on the exact nature of the abdominal sonogram. For example, if the gallbladder is the focus, the client will need to be on n.p.o. status for 12 hours and may have a fat-free diet the evening before the examination. If the client eats before the sonogram of the gallbladder, the gallbladder will be less full and thus not as easily visualized. For other scans, the purpose of allowing only liquids is to reduce gas formation in the colon because gas does interfere with the scan. Another way to reduce gas in the gastrointestinal tract is by administering drugs with simethicone (Mylicon). Smoking and gum chewing are prohibited because they increase gas formation. Sometimes an enema is needed to clear the bowel. Barium used for other tests interferes with the sonogram (see Chapter 20 for principles of bowel preparations). Abdominal scars and obesity make it difficult to obtain a good abdominal sonogram. Abdominal dressings must be removed before the sonogram. If the scan is a static scan, the client will need to hold his or her breath for 20 seconds at a time so the diaphragm will be static. (See the earlier discussion on use of real-time imaging versus static scans.)

Potential for Ineffective Coping of Child
Children should be given a chance to practice holding their breath before the scan is begun. Even young children can cooperate if they are not overly anxious and they are told to hold their breath while the assistant counts to 20. Also, the transducer can be first placed on a doll and the child allowed to see the shadows on the screen. (See Chapter 25 on preparing children for diagnostic procedures.)

POSTTEST NURSING IMPLICATIONS

The client may be ill from the underlying pathophysiology that necessitated the sonogram, but there is no concern over the direct effects of a sonogram. Occasionally, the sonogram may only be a preliminary test to some invasive procedure, such as a liver or renal biopsy. If so, the invasive procedure will have some nursing implications (see Chapter 25).

■ ECHOCARDIOGRAMS

Purposes. Ultrasound has become a well-established diagnostic tool for valvular defects. Ultrasound was first used to detect abnormalities in the mitral valve. The echocardiogram is also used to measure the diameters of the cardiac chambers and evaluate other structural abnormalities of the heart such as atrial septal defect and patent ductus arteriosus. Pleural effusion and cardiac tamponade are other abnormalities identified by ultrasound (Disch, 1980). An ECG is often run simultaneously therefore echographic findings can be correlated with the cardiac cycle (Haughey, 1984). Earlier echos used the M mode (motion) to do time motion studies of the heart. Newer types can also do cross-sectional scans, which can detect some changes in coronary vessels. Thallium scanning (Chapter 22) is used as a radionuclide scanning of the heart for infarcted areas. Echocardiograms, in combination with other tests, may eliminate the need for more invasive procedures such as a cardiac catheterization (Chapter 26). For neonates, echocardiography is recommended in place of angiography for assessing abnormalities of the aorta (Freiherr, 1986).

PRETEST NURSING DIAGNOSIS

Knowledge Deficit Regarding Procedure
The client needs no special preparation. The echocardiology technician will direct the beam of ultrasound at specific points on the client's chest to get pictures of the mitral valve and other structures. During the test the client may be asked

to do the Valsalva maneuver. Also, the client may be given a vasodilator, such as amyl nitrite, that can have a side effect of tachycardia. If an ECG is done, the client needs instruction about the procedure (see Chapter 24).

POSTTEST NURSING IMPLICATIONS

There is no specific care of the client after an echocardiogram because it is a noninvasive procedure.

■ ECHOENCEPHALOGRAMS

Purposes. Ultrasonic visualizations of the head may be used to evaluate certain head injuries but the adult brain cannot be well imaged because ultrasound cannot penetrate bone. Computerized tomography and MRI are more valuable in identifying masses and tumors because these scans give a three-dimensional cross section of the entire brain (see Chapter 21). Echoencephalograms are effective to monitor certain cerebral pathologies that cause shifts of cerebral midline structures. For example, ultrasound has been useful in monitoring the state of hydrocephalus in young infants. The size of the ventricles and the functions of the shunts are monitored by echoencephalograms or echoventriculograms (Babcock et al., 1980). Because the newborn's skull is not completely fused into a solid bony structure, ultrasound is a very useful tool for detecting intracranial hemorrhage.

PRETEST NURSING DIAGNOSIS

Knowledge Deficit Regarding Procedure
As with other ultrasound procedures, there is no pain or risk for the client. The head is placed on a foam sponge. If the echoencephalogram is done on a small child, the nurse may need to hold the child's head. Then, a water soluble gel is applied to the skull. Thick hair may make it difficult to do a sonogram, but any cutting of the hair must be done via hospital procedure. During the sonogram the client must remain motionless. If the client cannot lie still during the examination, the physician may order a sedative. Drugs, food, and fluids can be taken normally. Portable ultrasound units may be wheeled to neurological units or newborn nurseries to avoid transporting critically ill clients.

POSTTEST NURSING IMPLICATIONS

There is no special aftercare, but the nurse should be aware of underlying pathophysiology, which may indicate a need for frequent neurological assessments. The client may wish to wash his or her hair to remove the gel.

■ THORACIC SONOGRAMS

Purposes. Because ultrasound does not penetrate air, sonograms are not as useful for thoracic disease as for abdominal disease. For a lesion to be identified by ultrasound, there must be no air-filled lung between the chest wall and the lesion. Sonograms of the chest may be useful in identifying pleural fluid, abscess formation, or malposition of the diaphragm (Spitz, 1980). More recently, ultrasound in combination with scans and Doppler techniques has shown promise of being a reliable way to diagnose pulmonary embolism.

NURSING IMPLICATIONS

There is no special preparation of the client and no special care after the procedure.

QUESTIONS

1. Sonograms or ultrasound scans are done with ultrasound waves, which are
    a. Waves of energy closely related to the gamma rays of x-ray
    b. High frequency sound waves, which are beyond the range of audible sound
    c. Sound waves of very low frequency that are undetectable by the human ear
    d. Part of a still undefined physical force

2. The type of ultrasound scan that demonstrates motion, such as the movement of a fetus is
    a. A mode scan   b. B mode scan   c. Real-time scan   d. Doppler scan

3. The nurse may use the Doppler method of ultrasound to assess all these clients except
    a. Mrs. Jarvis, who is in the first stage of labor
    b. Mr. Bixby, who has had an aortic–femoral bypass
    c. Mr. Tucker, who had a pacemaker inserted yesterday
    d. Mrs. Horn, who is undergoing an oxytocin challenge test (OCT)

4. One of the known physical effects of *large continuous* doses of ultrasound is
    a. Decreased circulation to the body part
    b. Generation of heat in the body part
    c. Radiation burn in deep tissues
    d. Skin breakdown and redness in superficial layers

5. Which of the following is essential preparation before a *pelvic* sonogram? The client must

    a. Maintain n.p.o. status   **c.** Not take any medications

    b. Be given an enema or suppository   **d.** Have a full bladder

6. Which of the following preparations is *not* necessary when the client is having an *abdominal* sonogram?

    a. Removing abdominal dressings

    b. No smoking for several hours before the examination

    c. Use of drugs such as simethicone for antiflatulent activity

    d. Having the client drink two to three glasses of water before the examination

7. Echocardiograms are not very useful tools for detecting

    a. Valvular defects   **c.** Pleural effusion

    b. Cardiac tamponade   **d.** Myocardial infarction

8. Baby Dabney is having an echoencephalogram done to monitor a ventricular shunt that was inserted for hydrocephalus. The responsibilities of the nurse who accompanies the baby to the ultrasound department may include all *except*

    a. Explaining the results of the sonogram to the parents

    b. Reassuring the mother that the examination is not painful for the child

    c. Giving an ordered sedative before the examination

    d. Holding the baby's head while the sonogram is being done

9. The use of ultrasound in the thorax is severely limited because

    a. The transducer cannot be moved evenly on the chest wall

    b. Ultrasound does not penetrate air

    c. Thoracic tumors are solid masses

    d. The movement of the heart interferes with the sound waves

REFERENCES

American College of Obstetricians and Gynecologists, Committee on Patient Education. (1979). *Ultrasound examinations in OB-Gyn.* Chicago: American College of Obstetricians and Gynecologists.

Babcock, D., et al. (1980). B-Mode gray scale ultrasound of the head in the newborn and young infant. *American Journal of Roentgenology, 134,* 457–468.

Birnholz, J. (1985). Evolution of the ultrasonic exam. *Journal of Clinical Ultrasound, 13*(2), 83–84.

Disch, J. (1980). *Diagnostic procedures for cardiovascular disease.* Norwalk, CT: Appleton-Century-Crofts.

Fields, S., & Calvert-Hill, M. (1985). Clinical efficacy of screening the entire abdomen during real-time ultrasound examination. *Journal of Clinical Ultrasound, 13*(6), 411–413.

Freiherr, G. (1986). Tapping the medical potential of ultrasound. *Research Resources Reporter, 10*(1), 1–6.

Goldman, M. (1986). Real time two dimensional Doppler flow imaging: A word of caution. *Journal of American College of Cardiology, 7*(1), 89–90.

Harwood, C. (1985). Pulverizing kidney stones: What you should know about lithotripsy. *RN, 48*(7), 32–37.

Haughey, C. (1984). Preparing your patient for echocardiography. *Nursing 84, 14*(5), 68–71.

Hudson, B. (1983). Doppler ultrasound stethoscope. *Nursing 83, 13*(5), 55–57.

James, E. (1980). Future developments in ultrasound. In R. Sanders (Ed.), *Principles and practices of ultrasound in obstetrics and gynecology* (2nd ed.). Norwalk, CT: Appleton-Century-Crofts.

Kreel, L., & Steiner, R. (Eds.). (1979). Section 6, Ultrasonography. In *Medical imaging.* Chicago: Year Book Medical.

Meire, H.B. (1977). Ultrasound—Current status and prospects. *British Journal of Radiology, 50,* 379–380.

Mendelsohn, R. (1983). The risks of ultrasound. *RN, 46*(5), 101.

National Institute of Child Health and Human Development. (1984). *Consensus statement on the use of diagnostic ultrasound imaging in pregnancy.* Bethesda, MD: National Institute of Child Health and Human Development.

Pachaczevsk, R. (1979). Simple transducer supported water bath device for ultrasonography. *American Journal of Roentgenology, 133,* 553–555.

Research Roundup. (1980). *UCSF Magazine, 3,* 29.

Ruge, C. (1986). Shock(wave) treatment for kidney stones. *AJN, 86*(4), 400–401.

Sanders, R. (1980). Ultrasound in the diagnosis of fetal death. In R. Sanders (Ed.), *Principles and practices of ultrasonography in obstetrics and gynecology* (2nd ed.). Norwalk, CT: Appleton-Century-Crofts.

Snow, J., et al. (1979). Comparisons of scintigraphy, sonography and computed tomography in the evaluation of hepatic neoplasms. *American Journal of Roentgenology, 132,* 915–917.

Spitz, H. (1980). Use of ultrasound in the thorax. *Basics of Respiratory Disease, 9,* 5.

Taylor, K., et al. (1979). Diagnostic accuracy of gray scale ultrasonography for the jaundiced patient. *Archives of Internal Medicine, 139,* 60–63.

Taylor, K., & Dyson, M. (1980). Experimental insonation of animal tissues and fetuses. In R. Sanders (Ed.), *Principles and practices of ultrasonography in obstetrics and gynecology* (2nd ed.). Norwalk, CT: Appleton-Century-Crofts.

Whalen, J. (1979). Newer imaging methods of the abdomen. *American Journal of Roentgenology, 133,* 587–615.

Wells, P. (1979). Ultrasound limits, resolution and equipment. In K. Kreel (Ed.), *Medical imaging.* Chicago: Year Book Medical.

Ziskin, M. (1980). Basic principles of ultrasound. In R. Sanders (Ed.), *Principles and practices of ultrasonography in obstetrics and gynecology.* Norwalk, CT: Appleton-Century-Crofts.

24

Common Noninvasive Diagnostic Tests

- Electrocardiograms (ECG or EKG)
- Vectorcardiograms
- Telemetry and Cardiac Monitors
- Ambulatory ECG Recording
- Phonocardiograms
- Electroencephalograms (EEG)
- Electromyelographs (EMG)
- Pulmonary Function Tests: Spirometry
- Thermography

OBJECTIVES

1. Identify two general nursing diagnoses useful in preparing clients for non-invasive diagnostic testing.
2. Describe five basic characteristics of a normal sinus rhythm on a lead II ECG strip and how common arrhythmias change these characteristics.
3. Given an ECG of a normal sinus rhythm, calculate the heart rate of the client.
4. State what nursing assessments are useful in monitoring the mechanical events of the heart when the client has an abnormal ECG or is on telemetry.
5. State four important nursing functions to help prepare a client for an EEG.
6. Describe what a nurse should teach a client about an EMG.
7. Explain how the pulmonary function tests, FVC, FEV, MVV, and FEF are used in assessing lung ventilation defects that are obstructive or restrictive.
8. Describe how the measurement of heat is accomplished with diagnostic thermography.

The preceding four chapters covered specific types of noninvasive procedures, which use x-rays (Chapters 20 and 21), radionuclides (Chapter 22), and ultrasound (Chapter 23). This chapter covers several types of noninvasive tests, including measuring such diverse things as electric events (ECG, EEG, and EMG), audible sound (phonocardiogram), air flow (pulmonary function tests), and body surface heat (thermography) (Table 24–1). The unifying theme throughout all of these tests is: because they are noninvasive, there is little or no risk to the client. These tests give an indirect assessment of an organ and its structure or function. Most are fairly easy to perform (usually done by a skilled technician) and are relatively inexpensive.

Invasive diagnostic tests are those that utilize methods that invade the body, such as cardiac catheterization (Chapter 26) or an endoscopy procedure (Chapter 27). Other common invasive procedures are the subject of Chapter 25. The nurse must realize that this division of invasive and noninvasive tests is strictly from the professional's view. For the client, *any* test is an invasion of his or her personal space and privacy. Although the health professional considers an ECG noninvasive (because the body is not entered), the client may (because of the use of electrodes on his or her body) perceive it as being very invasive. The same holds true for the use of needles with an EMG, even though the invasion is under the skin and not into the body proper.

GENERAL NURSING DIAGNOSES FOR NONINVASIVE TESTS

Knowledge Deficit Regarding Test Procedures and Any Needed Preparation

It is the nurse's responsibility to see that the client is both physically and psychologically ready for the test. Preparation of the client should include reassurance that the test is neither painful nor harmful. Note that pain from the needles used for EMG (and sometimes EEG) is momentary and does not require a local anesthetic, as do the tests covered in the next chapter. Special consent forms are not needed because there is no anticipation of any complications from the test itself. There are very specific physical preparations for several of the tests, such as a shampoo before an EEG. Certain drugs affect the results of several of these tests; thus, the nurse must be aware of what information needs to be put on laboratory requests. Also, the nurse must make sure the client understands any restrictions on drugs, food, or liquids. Preparation for a child must take into account children's concepts of illness (Pidgeon, 1985). School age children are very receptive to teaching. (See Chapter 25 for more on children's reactions to procedures.)

Anxiety Related to Outcome of Test

The general focus of nursing care after a noninvasive test is to let the client rest once an assessment has been done. It is important for the nurse to validate that the client is physically stable and not psychologically upset by the test, which was done. The results of the test may not be known for a while, and this may be a source of anxiety for the client. (See the discussion in Chapter 20 on post-test anxiety.) With a few exceptions, there are no specific nursing implications after noninvasive testing. Although these tests are relatively simple to perform and there is practically no risk to the client, the client may be quite ill from the basic pathological problem. The aftercare of the client is therefore geared to the underlying problems.

TABLE 24–1. NONINVASIVE DIAGNOSTIC PROCEDURES USING VARIOUS TYPES OF MEASUREMENTS

	Electrical Event	Sound	Ultrasound	Magnetic Field	Air Flow	Heat	X-Rays
Heart	ECG Vectorgrams Telemetry Holter monitors	Phonocardiogram	Echocardiogram	Magnetic resonance imaging (MRI)			Chest x-rays
Brain	EEG		Encephalogram	MRI			Skull films CT scan
Muscles	EMG						
Lungs			Thoracic sonogram	MRI	Spirometry		Chest x-rays Tomogram CT scan
Tumors or inflammation			Abdominal and pelvic sonograms	MRI		Thermography	Flat plates of abdomen CT Scan

Note: See this chapter for nursing diagnoses for most noninvasive tests, Chapter 20 for x-rays, Chapter 21 for CT and MRI, and Chapter 23 for sonograms.

■ ELECTROCARDIOGRAMS (ECG or EKG)

Description. An electrocardiogram comprises the electrical impulses generated by the heart during its depolarization and repolarization that are picked up by electrodes and are displayed on a strip of graph paper. These electrodes are fastened to all four of the client's extremities by rubber straps. A jelly or paste is used under each electrode to help conduction of the electrical impulse. The electrodes on both arms and the left leg are used to record impulses. The electrode on the right leg is just a ground. A suction bulb is moved across the client's chest to obtain six different views of the heart (precordial leads).

The most common lead used for monitoring (and the one usually displayed in nursing textbooks) is lead II, which records the electrical activity of the heart by using the negative electrode on the right arm and the positive electrode on the left leg. As the heart's electrical current moves down through the heart, the current moving toward the positive electrode will show as a positive deflection on the graph (above the baseline). If the electrical current moves away from the positive electrode, the graph will show a negative deflection (below the baseline). In lead II, as the electrical current goes down through the atrium and the ventricles, there are two positive deflections: P-wave and QRS complex. In other leads, such as the augmented leads, the P-wave and QRS complex will be seen as negative deflections because of the placement of the electrodes. Lead I uses both arm electrodes and lead III uses the left arm and left leg electrodes. In addition to these three leads (I, II, and III) and the six precordial leads (V_1 through V_6), there are also three augmented unipolar leads (a VR, a VL, and a VF), which make up the standard 12-lead electrocardiogram. Six inches of each lead are taken. With all 12 leads of the ECG, a clinician can gain a great deal of knowledge about the total electrical activity of the heart. However, for basic monitoring of the client or for an assessment of an arrhythmia, Lead II may suffice.

Purposes. The ECG is a diagnostic tool used very frequently for clients with chest pain or other cardiac symptoms. Toxicity to certain drugs, such as tricyclic antidepressants, can be monitored by ECGs (Boehnert & Lovejoy, 1985). The ECG is the definitive way to diagnose the various arrhythmias. It is also very helpful in distinguishing myocardial infarction from myocardial ischemia. A cardiologist interprets the ECG and writes a formal summary of his or her findings. This summary is put in the chart with samples from the various leads of the ECG. Although a 12-lead ECG can tax the skill of even an experienced cardiologist, nurses in expanded roles may do an initial analysis. Purcell and Haynes (1984) describe a five-step analysis used to detect ischemia or necrosis.

Characteristics of a Normal Sinus Rhythm

Although the formal interpretation of the ECG is done by a cardiologist, the nurse should have some understanding of what a normal sinus rhythm (NSR) looks like (Figure 24–1) so arrhythmias can be detected on a monitor. The characteristics of a normal ECG are:

1. The heart rate is between 60 and 100 in an adult (two ways to calculate rates are discussed later)
2. The rhythm is regular
3. A P-wave precedes each QRS complex
4. The PR interval is between 0.12 and 0.20 seconds (shorter in children)
5. The QRS complex is normal and less than 0.12 seconds
6. The T-wave is normal

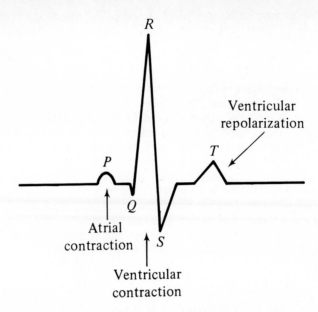

Figure 24–1. Basic components of an ECG tracing. (Note that atrial repolarization is hidden in QRS complex.) See text for definition of: P—Wave; PR interval; QRS complex; T—wave; QT intervals; ST segment.

Describing Arrhythmias

In describing arrhythmias, a normal *sinus* rhythm means that the heart rate is under the control of the sinoatrial node (SA node). A *sinus* tachycardia means that the rate is faster than 100, in the adult, but the SA node is still controlling the rate. On the other hand, *atrial* tachycardia means that the atrium is controlling the heart rate, whereas a *ventricular* tachycardia means that the ventricle is controlling the heart rate. In *nodal* or junctional arrhythmias, the AV node is controlling the rate. Thus, by just reading the name of the arrhythmia from the ECG report, the nurse can assess something about the origin of the arrhythmia.

Ectopic or Premature Beats

A premature ventricular contraction (PVC) occurs when the ventricle originates a beat before the normal conduction of the impulse from the SA node. In rhythms with an occasional premature beat, the cardiac rate is still being controlled by the SA node. Another name for premature beat is ectopic beats, which means displaced or malpositioned. (An ectopic pregnancy occurs outside the uterus.) Ectopic or premature contractions can arise from the atrial tissue (PAC), ventricular tissue (PVC), or from AV junctional tissue.

P-Wave

The P-wave occurs at the beginning of each contraction of the atria (depolarization). The rounded P-wave is the impulse spreading through muscle, not going down conductive tissue in a straight line. (In contrast, the QRS complex is a straight line with a peak because the impulse is traveling directly down conductive tissue.)

Abnormal P-Wave

In premature atrial contraction (PAC), the P-wave will look different, not the usual sequence seen with the normal sinus rhythm. In arrhythmias, such as atrial fibrillation, the P-waves cannot be distinguished on the ECG because the atria are quivering or fibrillating. In atrial enlargement, the P-wave will look different because the impulse travels through more tissue.

PR Interval
The PR interval is the time it takes the impulse to travel from the atrium to the ventricle through the AV node and the Bundle of His. Normally the PR interval is 0.12–0.20 seconds. (One large square on the ECG paper measures 0.20 seconds.)

A PR interval longer than 0.20 seconds indicates a slowing of the impulse through the AV node and Bundle of His. Drugs, such as digitalis, can cause a widening PR interval or first degree heart block. Other types of drugs may also prolong the PR interval. In one type of second degree heart block, the PR interval gets longer and longer until the ventricular beat is dropped. In a complete heart block, the PR interval cannot be measured because the ventricles are originating beats that are totally independent of the SA impulses, which generate the atrial beats. Thus, in complete heart block, the P-waves may be normal, but no QRS complex follows. The P-waves and QRS complexes will be totally independent of each other.

QRS Complex
The QRS complex reflects the contraction (depolarization) of the ventricles. Normally, the QRS complex is less than 0.12 seconds.

An ectopic beat, which arises from the ventricle (PVC), will cause a distorted and widened QRS complex. A PVC usually looks very different from the other QRS complexes in the strip. Often, the QRS complex will be a negative deflection rather than the positive deflection seen in lead II. All of these changes in the QRS complex are due to an impulse that originated in ventricular tissue and traveled through the ventricle differently than the normal impulse, which comes from the SA node.

In myocardial infarction, the appearance of the QRS complex is one part of the ECG that is changed. Abnormal Q-waves are characteristic of myocardial infarction, but other conditions can cause changes in the Q-waves, too.

In ventricular tachycardia, the ventricles have taken control of the heart rate, and the ECG shows only spikes of QRS complexes, which are wide and rather bizarre looking.

ECG Documentation of the Type of Cardiac Arrest
In ventricular fibrillation, there are only wavy lines on the ECG with nothing that resembles a P-wave or QRS complex. Ventricular fibrillation causes cardiac arrest—when the ventricles are fibrillating (quivering) there is no cardiac output—and the ECG shows chaotic electrical activity. For the other type of cardiac arrest, cardiac standstill or asystole, the ECG shows a straight line—even the quivering or fibrillation of the ventricle has stopped. Only the ECG can distinguish whether a cardiac arrest is due to asystole or fibrillation.

T-Wave
The T-wave occurs as the ventricles recover from the contraction period. This period of electrical recovery is called repolarization. (The repolarization of the atrium is not seen on the ECG graph because it is hidden in the larger electrical event of the QRS complex.)

Myocardial damage may cause inversion of the T-waves. High levels of serum potassium (hyperkalemia) cause tall, peaked T-waves. An ECG on an oscilloscope is sometimes used to monitor potassium replacement in severe cases of hypokalemia. Low levels of potassium (hypokalemia) cause inverted T-waves. A flattened T-wave means the ventricle is not able to repolarize normally. See Chapter 5 for a discussion on the effects of potassium on cardiac function.

QT Interval
The QT interval covers the period of both ventricular depolarization and repolarization. Its normal duration is 0.36–0.44 seconds.

The QT interval is useful in evaluating the effects of drugs on the heart such as quinidine. Ischemia or electrolyte changes may prolong or shorten the QT interval.

ST Segment
The ST segment is the time between completion of depolarization and the beginning of repolarization of the ventricles. One often interprets only a nonspecific ST abnormality on an ECG.

A decidedly depressed or downward slope of the ST segment is somewhat characteristic of myocardial ischemia. Digitalis will cause depression of the ST segment, as well. (See the "Stress Test" in Chapter 26 for more explanation about ST changes from exertion and other factors.) Conversely, an elevated ST segment is one of the characteristics of a myocardial infarction. As with all other changes in the ECG, the meaning of the changes may be open to several interpretations, depending on other clinical data.

DETERMINING PULSE RATE WITH AN ECG

Because the ECG paper is horizontally marked for time, pulse rate can be determined by looking at an ECG strip. (The vertical deflections reflect the amplitude of the voltage, but this is not of major usefulness to the nurse who is just beginning to learn about ECGs.) As seen in Figure 24-2, each tiny square of ECG strip measures 0.04 seconds, and each larger square (which consists of five tiny ones) is 0.20 seconds. By remembering that each large square signifies a time of 0.20 seconds, one can calculate the pulse rate by several different formulas. Two simple methods that a nurse can use to time a pulse rate by scanning an ECG strip are discussed below. Both of these methods assume a steady rate of impulses.

Method A: Counting the Squares between the Beats
The squares between each QRS complex can be counted to determine the time between each beat. For example, if there are three large squares between each beat (QRS complex), this implies a time interval of (3 squares times 0.2 seconds) 0.6 seconds between each beat. Thus, in 60 seconds, there would be (60 seconds divided by 0.6) 100 beats. If there were five large squares between each beat, this would mean (5 times 0.20 seconds) 1 second between each beat. In 60 seconds, there would be (60 seconds divided by 1 second per beat) 60 beats. Thus, when a client has a normal rhythm on an ECG strip, which has no fewer than three squares and no more than five squares between beats, the rate is within the normal adult range of 60–100 beats per minute, respectively. The formula for calculating pulse rate by this method is:

$$\frac{60 \text{ Seconds per Minute}}{\text{Number of Squares between Beats} \times 0.20 \text{ Seconds}} = \text{Beats per Minute}$$

Example:

$$\frac{60}{3 \text{ (Squares between Beats)} \times 0.20} = \frac{60}{0.6} = 100$$

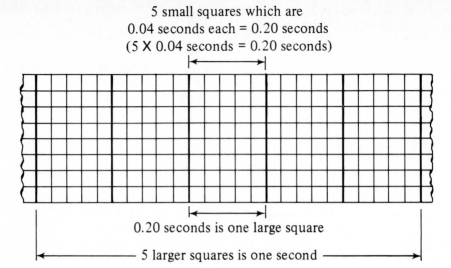

Method A: Count the number of large squares that occur between each QRS complex.

$$\textit{Formula:} \quad \frac{60 \text{ Seconds}}{\text{Number of Squares between Beats} \times 0.2 \text{ second}} = \text{Beats per Minute}$$

Method B: Count the number of beats in 30 large squares.
           Formula: Number of Beats in 30 Squares $\times$ 10 = Beats per Minute

Figure 24–2. Two methods to determine pulse rate from an ECG tracing. See text for examples of use.

Method B: Counting the Beats in 30 Squares

Another way to calculate the heart rate from an ECG strip is to count the number of QRS complexes in a certain number of squares. Recall that the large square measures 0.20 seconds in time. By counting the beats in 30 large squares, one has counted the number of beats occurring in 6 seconds because 30 squares times 0.20 seconds equals 6 seconds. The number obtained for 6 seconds is multiplied by 10 to obtain the number of beats per minute. The time markings on the ECG strip designate 3-second intervals and can also be used to determine 6-second segments. For example, if the total number of beats in 30 squares is 5, then the pulse rate is 50 (five beats in 0.6 seconds times 10). The formula for this method of calculating pulse rate is:

Number of Beats in 30 Squares (or 0.6 Seconds) $\times$ 10 = Number of Beats per Minute

Example:

5 Beats (in 30 Squares) $\times$ 10 = 50 Beats per Minute

PRETEST NURSING DIAGNOSES

Knowledge Deficit Regarding Needed Preparation for ECG
It is not necessary to withhold drugs or food from the client before an ECG. The client should not wear metal jewelry. Clothing must be loose so the elec-

trodes can be fastened on the arms and legs and the suction bulb moved across the chest. Women will need to remove hose because the electrode paste must be applied directly to the skin. The jelly or paste used with the electrodes is nonallergic, but it may feel messy to the client. Clients may be slightly skeptical about "being strapped to an electrical box," as a client once said. Therefore, the client may need reassurance that the machine only detects electrical signals *from* the client and not to the client. Because many drugs, such as quinidine or digitalis, affect certain aspects of the ECG, it is important that the cardiologist who interprets the test be aware of any cardiac drugs the client has received. Most ECG requests have a place to note the cardiac drugs that the client has received.

Potential for Injury Related to Malfunctioning Equipment

From a safety point of view, any electrical equipment does have the potential for an electrical hazard if the machine is defective and not properly grounded. As a general rule, all electrically operated appliances for a client should be plugged into the same wall outlet so there is no difference in ground points. Improperly grounded or defective equipment can cause a current leakage through the client if the two pieces of equipment are plugged into outlets more than 12 feet apart (Meth, 1980). The ECG technician has the responsibility of checking the machine to make sure that there are no frayed cords, and so on, and that the machine is properly grounded. Sumner and Grau (1985) note that with a changing economic climate, nurses may find that running a 12-lead ECG becomes a nursing task. The nurse needs to keep in mind that for very ill clients, such as those with electrodes placed into the ventricle, all electrical equipment must be checked and grounded properly, including ECG machines. The nurse should consult with the hospital's electrical engineer about any problems that occur and how to do safety checks of routine equipment.

POSTTEST NURSING DIAGNOSES

Potential for Alteration in Cardiac Output Related to Underlying Pathophysiology

The ECG technician or nurse helps the client wipe off the electrode paste or jelly. Aside from this, there is no other special client care related directly to the test in general. However, if the ECG was done to evaluate a possible myocardial infarction, cardiac precautions should be continued until other diagnostic tests, such as cardiac enzymes (Chapter 12), are interpreted by the client's physician. If the ECG was done to evaluate an arrhythmia, the nurse may need to inquire about any changes in medication orders. Usually the ECG technician scans the graph for blatant abnormalities and calls this to the attention of the physician. Also an experienced nurse can often distinguish between benign supraventricular abnormalities and potentially dangerous ectopic beats arising from the ventricle (Cudworth, 1986). Sometimes the ECG strip is kept with the client's chart; thus, the client's personal physician can immediately evaluate the strip. Otherwise the interpretation of the ECG will be done by a cardiologist, and a typed summary will later appear on the client's chart.

Heart rate, rhythm, and the presence or absence of a pulse deficit should be routinely monitored by the nurse if there is any question of arrhythmias.

The nurse must remember that the ECG is measuring only the electrical events in the heart and not the cardiac output. The quality of peripheral pulses, capillary filling time, and color of the client are all signs of adequacy or inadequacy of cardiac output. Noting any dyspnea, angina, abnormal heart or breath sounds, and a decrease in urine output are all determined by the nurse—not detected from an ECG reading. Therefore, even when the client is on a monitor of the ECG pattern, the nurse must still collect the above information to obtain a complete picture of the efficiency of the heart.

■ VECTORCARDIOGRAMS

A vectorgram and an ECG differ only in the type of instrument used to record and analyze the electrical events of the heart. A mathematical analysis of the different leads (usually six) is done to detect the direction and magnitude of electrical energy on a moment-to-moment basis (Disch, 1980). The vectorgram gives a three-dimensional picture of the heart, which comprises a P loop, QRS loop, and ST-T segment loop. A vectorcardiogram may be very helpful in evaluating conduction defects or abnormal impulse pathways, which are not as evident on the conventional ECG. The client can be told that a vectorgram is a "sophisticated" ECG. Otherwise, the nursing implications are the same as for the routine ECG.

DIAGNOSTIC MONITORING IN INTENSIVE CARE UNITS

Clients with the potential for serious cardiac arrhythmias may be connected to cardiac monitors, which provide continuous surveillance of the electrical impulses of the heart. The ECG pattern is displayed on an oscilloscope, and when needed, on graph paper for a permanent record. When the client is connected to a monitor in an intensive care unit or coronary care unit, the nurse must have special training on how to recognize those arrhythmias that need immediate medical attention. Coronary care units may have standardized orders that permit a nurse, who has had special training, to administer antiarrhythmia drugs (such as lidocaine [Xylocaine], when the client has certain patterns of premature ventricular contractions). Today's critical care nurse also focuses on early recognition of potentially lethal cardiac conduction defects by recognizing electrical axis deviations on the ECG (Alspach, 1979). The reader is encouraged to consult one of the many excellent textbooks that focus on critical care nursing.

■ TELEMETRY AND CARDIAC MONITORS

Telemetry is making measurements at a distance from the subject by the use of radio signals. Telemetry has been extensively used in assessing physiological functioning during space travels. In the hospital setting, telemetry is used to monitor an ECG of a client without the client having to be hooked up to a monitor. Nurses on general care units may take care of a client who is being monitored "long distance" by a monitor in the intensive care or coronary care unit. The critical care nurse monitors the monitor.

Small electrode discs are applied to the client's chest to obtain a good reading on the monitor. Disposable prelubricated discs can be kept on the client for several days unless skin irritation is noted. The wires from the electrodes are connected to a portable transmitter. The portable transmitter is about the size of a small tissue box, and can be left lying in bed by the client or can be strapped to the ambulatory client's waist. It should be reemphasized that telemetry, like a conventional ECG, only measures the rate and electrical events of the heart. The nurse is still needed to assess the mechanical events (i.e., cardiac output) of the client.

Telemetry by Telephone

Telephone recordings of ECGs originated in 1971. A special instrument is used with the telephone. The heart rhythm's graphic representation is fed into a computer and a duplicate is made for analysis by a cardiologist. The response time for emergency requests is from 10–15 minutes for a complete reading. Clients with pacemakers may be followed by telephone and thus eliminate more costly visits to clinics. They are also evaluated by a physician. One brand name for a telephone heart monitor is Cardio Beeper* (Survival Technology, Bethesda, MD).

■ AMBULATORY ECG RECORDING

In outpatient settings, clients may be given a portable recorder (sometimes referred to as Holter monitor) to wear, which records the ECG on magnetic tape. When the tapes are returned to the cardiology laboratory, a computer scans the tapes to pick out any specific points of interest. This method is costly, but it can be very helpful in pinpointing the type of arrhythmia that is causing the client's symptoms. It can reduce the number of costly ambulance trips to the hospital. Also, the ambulatory ECG can be used to evaluate the effects of certain treatments. Nurses may prepare the client for the test and scan the strips to see which clients need medical interventions.

NURSING DIAGNOSIS

Knowledge Deficit Regarding Procedure for Monitoring

The client is not to swim or bathe when the monitor is in place. Also the client must not have any x-rays while the monitor is being used—x-rays will erase the tape. Metal detectors, remote control TV, CB radios, microwave ovens, and even electric blankets may interfere with the readings. The client should be instructed to keep a diary of any events that cause such symptoms as shortness of breath, dizziness, or angina. The client should also keep a record of such activities as sleeping time, exercise, eating, bowel movements, cigarette smoking, sexual activity, and emotional stress, which may be related to the cardiac symptoms.

McNeal (1978), a nurse cardioscanalyst (the person inspecting the 24-hour strips), observed that clients are often unaware that symptoms, such as dizziness, are due to an arrhythmia. In addition to the usual cardiac symptoms, symptoms such a headache, indigestion, or "feeling weak" may be linked to the specific time of an arrhythmia. Thus, a 24-hour strip may elucidate the cause of vague client symptoms so that the symptoms can be treated.

Visiting nurses should instruct clients in the use of Holter monitors when it is necessary to evaluate arrhythmias related to physical reconditioning at home after cardiac surgery or postmyocardial infarction.

---

*See Streiff (1981) for a discussion on the usefulness of the Cardio Beeper for visiting nurses.

■ PHONOCARDIOGRAMS

Description. The phonocardiogram is a graphic recording of the sounds generated during the cardiac cycle. The phonocardiogram is a sophisticated way to evaluate abnormal heart sounds, detected with a standard stethoscope. A microphone is positioned on the chest wall and picks up the sounds that are transmitted to the graph paper. The phonocardiogram is usually recorded in conjunction with an ECG, which records the electrical events of the heart, and a pulse tracing, which records the mechanical events of the heart.

Purpose. By documenting the precise time of the abnormal heart sound, in relation to the mechanical and electrical events of the heart, the cardiologist can better interpret the abnormal heart sound. (See echocardiograms, Chapter 23, on how sound waves are used for diagnosing heart problems.)

NURSING DIAGNOSIS

Knowledge Deficit Regarding Procedure
The client can eat and have medications before the test. If the client has a lot of hair on his chest, a small area may be shaved so that the microphone will not pick up the sounds from hair movement. During the test, the client may be given vasodilating drugs, such as amyl nitrite, which can cause dizziness and light-headedness in some clients. Otherwise the test is not at all uncomfortable, and requires no special client care afterward.

■ ELECTROENCEPHALOGRAMS (EEG)

Description. The electroencephalogram (EEG) is a recording of the brain's electrical activity. The EEG primarily records activity of the superficial layers of the cerebral cortex.

If the client is comatose; the EEG can be done at his or her bedside. However, for routine diagnostic studies, the client is taken to the EEG laboratory, where the environment can be better controlled. The recording takes an hour or two and includes a nap. The first part of the recording is done with the client as relaxed as possible to obtain a baseline reading. The client is then asked to hyperventilate for several minutes, to see how this changes the patterns of the brain. The client may become a little light-headed from hyperventilating. The brain may also be stimulated by flickering lights. If the client cannot nap for the last part of the test, a sedative, such as chloral hydrate, may be given. Sleep may evoke abnormal patterns that are not present when the brain is more active.

Approximately 20 electrodes are applied to the client's scalp. The electrode wires are attached to the EEG machine, which records the electrical signals on a piece of graph paper. These electrodes may be surface electrodes or subdermal needle electrodes. The pain accompanying the subdermal needles is sometimes compared with the brief pain felt when one hair is pulled from the scalp. They are not very painful because the scalp is much less sensitive than other surface areas of the body. Most EEG laboratories use surface electrodes with a jelly to help conduction of the electrical signals. The skin is wiped with acetone, and the area is slightly abraded with an electrical paste. It has been found that in children, this slight abrasion may cause calcium nodules in the skin (Wiley & Eaglstein, 1979). Thus, EEG paste with calcium chloride probably should not be used with young children or infants, whose skin has a less effective barrier against absorption of the calcium from the jelly. The papules of calcium do, however, disappear with no apparent harmful effects.

Purposes. Although the EEG is nonspecific, it can help identify a focus of disturbance in the brain. The majority of clients with cerebral seizures will have abnormal EEGs, but a normal EEG does not rule out a seizure disorder. About 10% of the clients with epilepsy have normal EEGs. The EEG must be correlated with other clinical assessments of the client.

When the brain is dead, the electrical activity of the brain is absent, and the EEG is flat. The EEG is used as one of the ways to detect brain death in the comatose client. Studies done on comatose clients show that the findings of the EEG have a high correlation with the survival or death of the client in a coma (Taylor & Ballenger, 1980).

NURSING DIAGNOSIS

Knowledge Deficit Regarding Needed Preparation for EEG

For routine EEG testing, the client should have no medicines for 24 to 48 hours before the test, except those medicines particularly ordered by the physician. Tranquilizers, stimulants (including coffee, tea, colas, and cigarettes), and alcohol all cause changes in brain patterns. The client should have normal meals because hypoglycemia can also cause changes in brain patterns. The client's hair should be shampooed the day before the test, and no oils, sprays, or lotions should be applied to the hair. It may be desirable that the client not have much sleep before the EEG recording because sleep deprivation may evoke abnormal brain patterns. Also, as mentioned earlier, the last part of the EEG recording may be done with the client asleep, and the client may have trouble falling asleep if he or she has just had a lot of sleep. Therefore, the adult client may be instructed to go to bed late the night before the test and to awake early. Children and infants should not be allowed to nap before the scheduled test.

If an EEG is being done to evaluate the possibility of brain death, it is important that artifacts be kept to a minimum. Artifacts can be caused by manipulation of the electrodes or by electrical interference. The nurse will need to follow the specific guidelines of the institution when EEGs are done at the client's bedside (The electrical hazards covered for the ECG would also be pertinent here where several electrical appliances may be in use at once.)

POSTTEST NURSING DIAGNOSIS

Potential for Injury

The only specific care needed by the client after an EEG is a shampoo to remove electrode gel from his or her hair. Also, as mentioned earlier, the calcium chloride in the gel may irritate the skin of children; thus, any gel on the skin must be carefully removed. If seizure activity is a possibility, seizure precautions should be noted.

■ ELECTROMYELOGRAPHS (EMG)

Description. The electromyelograph (EMG) measures the electrical activity of muscles. Needle electrodes are inserted into selected skeletal muscles. (Although in one sense the test is somewhat invasive, it is discussed here because of the similarities between ECGs and EMGs.) This procedure does cause some pain. The skin is cleansed with alcohol or iodine, but no local anesthetic is used. The muscle activity is recorded at rest, during voluntary activity, and with electrical stimuli. The findings from the EMG are recorded and usually summarized in narrative form for use on the client's chart. An informed consent is needed for this test.

Purposes. In nerve atrophy, there may be a characteristic fibrillation, even in the resting muscle. Usually a resting muscle has no electrical activity. The test can be useful in determining the extent of peripheral nerve injuries and differentiating paralysis of psychological origin.

The EMG cannot diagnose specific neuromuscular diseases, but it can specifically differentiate between neuropathy and myopathy (Spiegel, 1978). All neuromuscular abnormalities are classified in two categories:

1. *Myopathy* is a disease or disturbance of striated muscle fibers or cell membranes. Myasthenia gravis or primary muscular dystrophy are examples of myopathies that produce abnormal EMGs.
2. *Neuropathy* is a disease or disorder of the lower motor neuron. Toxic effects of drugs, hypothyroidism, polio, and diabetes can all cause neuropathy.

NURSING DIAGNOSIS

Knowledge Deficit Regarding Procedure for EMG
No special physical preparation of the client is required before or after the test. Premedications for sedation or pain relief are avoided to assess a normal neuromuscular pattern (Ross, 1979). Muscle aches after the procedure may be relieved with mild analgesics. The procedure may take up to an hour or two if extensive testing is done. The nurse should prepare the client for the discomfort and sounds of an EMG. The client may feel pain on insertion of the needle electrodes and will hear audio amplification that sounds like firecrackers (Bubb, 1982). If nerve conduction studies are done, the feelings may be similar to static electricity.

Potential for Impaired Mobility
Before and after an EMG the nurse can be very useful in evaluating the functional capacity of the client with an unknown neuromuscular problem. Thus, the gait of the client, ability to do ROM exercises, and any motor–power–sensory deficits should be recorded. Clinical data are always used as part of the base for interpreting EMG reports.

■ PULMONARY FUNCTION TESTS: SPIROMETRY

Description. Pulmonary function tests (PFT) can be classified as (1) ventilation tests and (2) specialized pulmonary function tests of gaseous diffusion and distribution. Pulmonary function tests, done in the pulmonary function laboratory, cover the entire range of respiratory volume and capabilities. On the other hand, PFTs done on the unit or in ambulatory care settings are modified to ventilation tests of FEV, VC, and MVV measures. This section focuses only on the more common ventilation studies. Chapter 22 includes information about lung perfusion scans. The clinical significance of blood gas analysis, an important aspect of most pulmonary studies is discussed in Chapter 6.

For ventilation studies of lung volume and capacity, the client breathes into a machine called a spirometer. (The nurse sometimes uses a portable spirometer, the Wright spirometer, for clinical assessment of the client's ventilation status.)

Purposes. PFTs for lung volume and capacity help identify whether the client has an obstructive defect, a restrictive defect, or a combination of both (Boyce & King, 1980). When there is an increase in airway resistance, the defect in ventilation is called an *obstructive defect*. Asthma, bronchitis, and emphysema cause obstructive defects in ventilation. When the defect in ventilation is due to a limitation on chest expansion, the defect is called a *restrictive defect*. Pathological conditions that limit chest expansion are conditions, such as fibrosis of the lungs, muscle dystrophy, obesity, and abnormal curvature of the spine. Conditions, such as pulmonary congestion, may cause both obstruction and restriction of ventilation. The ventilation tests help delineate the type of defect present, and whether the defects are reversible with therapy, such as bronchodilators. Ventilation tests are often ordered before a client has surgery, so any respiratory problems can be anticipated and better treated or prevented. Nurses, in ambulatory settings, may be actively involved in actually doing the ventilation tests as one part of a nursing assessment. Nurse-directed clinics for clients with chronic lung disease have routinely done FEV, FEV_1 to VC ratios, and MVV for many years (Nield, 1974). Petty (1986) notes that measurement of volume and flow should be as common as measuring vital signs, as these pulmonary function tests are very helpful in assessing clients who have to be protected from developing acute problems. Home testing can even be done by clients. Sobel and Ferguson (1985) describe inexpensive peak flow monitors that can be used by asthmatics to assess a worsening of their status. More expensive hand-held spirometers can also be purchased by clients to do FVC, FEV, and MVV.

PRETEST NURSING DIAGNOSIS

Knowledge Deficit Regarding Procedure
The clinician conducting the pulmonary function test will give the client specific instructions for each step of the test. The client must breathe only through his or her mouth. A noseclip is used on the nose. The client needs to rest before the test so that he or she can perform as well as possible. The client should not have any bronchodilators or narcotics before the test because they can change breathing capabilities. Because the various breathing maneuvers require the maximal cooperation of the client, the test is not reliable in young children or confused adults. Food and fluids are not withheld.

POSTTEST NURSING DIAGNOSIS

Potential for Ineffective Breathing Patterns
The client may be discouraged if the tests showed less than optimal lung functioning. Poor test results may be an incentive for the client to stop smoking to prevent further damage. Also, the test results can help guide the clinician in determining what breathing exercises may be beneficial for the client and whether drugs such as bronchodilators are being effective. Clients with restrictive defects may need help to maximize respiration. Clients with obstructive defects need to learn how to get more air out (pursed lip breathing, etc.) Nurses skilled in teaching breathing techniques may foster positive changes in the client.

Summary of Findings from Ventilation Studies

VC and FVC. The vital capacity (VC) is the maximum amount of air that can be expired after a normal inspiration. The forced vital capacity (FVC) is the vital capacity when the breathing is forced.

Reference Values for VC and FVC

Must be determined by charts, which are specific for sex, age, and height. A
  value less than 75-80% the predicted value would be abnormal.

Clinical Significance. For most clients the results of VC and FVC are similar. Vital capacity increases with physical fitness. In fact, FVC may be a good indicator of overall good health. In restrictive diseases, the VC or FVC is always decreased—this test is the best assessment of restrictive defects. In obstructive defects, the VC may not be appreciably decreased. However, the more severe the obstruction, the more likely that the air trapping will reduce vital capacity.

FEV. The forced expiratory volume (FEV) is the percentage of vital capacity, which can be expressed in 1, 2, or 3 seconds. The figures are expressed as FEV_1, FEV_2, and FEV_3. The test is useful to evaluate the severity of airway obstruction and to evaluate the effectiveness of bronchodilators.

Reference Values for FEV

Normally 65-85% of the vital capacity can be expressed in the first second and
  up to 95-97% by 3 seconds. For FEV_1 less than 75% of the predicted value
  is considered abnormally low.

Clinical Significance. In obstructive disease, the FEV_1 is decreased. In restrictive disease, the FEV_1 is normal or can be decreased. In some restrictive diseases where there is an increase of elastic resistance, the FEV_1 may be normal or elevated.

Ratio of FEV₁ to FVC

Reference Values for FEV₁

Younger people can expel 75–85% of the VC in 1 second. Older people can normally expel about 65–75% in the first second. This is the only pulmonary function test where age is an important determinant and where increases as well as decreases may be abnormal (Boyce & King, 1980).

Clinical Significance. The ratio of the total FVC to FEV₁ is decreased with obstructive disease, and increased, normal, or sometimes decreased with restrictive disease.

VE, MVV, or MBC. These tests measure the volume exhaled in 1 minute. The volume exhaled per minute at rest is the VE. The volume exhaled in 1 minute when the person breathes as deeply and rapidly as possible is called the maximum voluntary ventilation (MVV) or the maximal breathing capacity (MBC). Usually the minute volume is 15–20 times the one time volume of the FVC.

Reference Values for VE, MVV, or MBC

Values are matched on a chart for age and weight. Less than 80% of predicted value is considered abnormally low.

Clinical Significance. Patients with obstructive defects have volumes less than 80% of the predicted values. In restrictive disease, the values will usually be normal. Very severe ventilation defects may show less than 35% of predicted value.

FEF. This test of forced expiratory flows (FEF) measures how fast a person can exhale a specific amount of air. This test is useful in screening clients for subclinical obstructive disease. The person breathes in as deeply as possible and then times how many seconds it takes to exhale through an open mouth. The test is done three times and the fastest time recorded. Most people can expel all the air in 2–5 seconds. If clients do a simple version of this test at home they should contact a doctor if it takes longer than 5 seconds to expel the air (Sobel & Ferguson 1985).

Reference Values for FEF

Values are matched on a chart for age and weight. Less than 75% of the predicted value is abnormally low.

Clinical Significance. A long-time smoker may have no symptoms of respiratory problems but the FEF will be less than 75% of the predicted values.

In summary, the test used most often for restrictive defects is the FVC. The tests used for obstructive defects are the FEV, FEV₁ to FVC ratio, MVV, and FEF for subclinical cases. For mixed types of defects, all of these tests will be helpful. The programmed instruction by Boyce and King (1980) is excellent for the reader who wishes detailed explanations about the use of the above pulmonary function tests. Perry (1986) is geared for the nurse practitioner.

■ THERMOGRAPHY

Description. Thermography is a technique that uses an infrared camera to photograph the surface temperature of the body. The pictures of the temperature of the skin's surface can show variations from cold blue to red hot. The body part to be photographed is exposed to air. The client is disrobed in a 68- to 70-degree environment for 15 minutes. Some methods involve spraying the area with 95% alcohol. Inflammation and malignant processes, where there is an accelerated local metabolism, generate additional heat, which may be detected on the body surface.

Purposes. Thermography has been researched as a possible diagnostic tool for cancer of the breast. Different patterns are found in premenopausal and postmenopausal women. For premenopausal women, the breast tissue is more thermally active. At the present time, thermography is not recommended as a screening device for breast cancer because the results are not conclusive and mammography is much more effective (See Chapter 20).

Some research has been done to see if thermography can help detect bone tumors, vascular disease, or conditions where inflammation is present. For example, thermography has been suggested as a possible way to measure reactions to skin tests and the change of skin temperature when there is nerve impairment. Thermography has been used to assess areas of pain in the body. The locus of pain is often cooler than the rest of the body (Friedman, 1981). Because thermography is noninvasive, with no risk to the client, it may be a diagnostic tool that will become more useful in clinical practice in the future. The reader is encouraged to consult current research literature.

QUESTIONS

1. Special consent forms for noninvasive diagnostic tests are
   a. Usually required and are obtained by the physician in charge
   b. Always required if the client has not had the test before
   c. Not usually required because there is no risk for the client
   d. Done if the client is fearful of the procedure

2. The repolarization of the ventricle is shown on the ECG as the
   a. QRS complex   c. ST segment
   b. QT interval   d. T-wave

3. The characteristics of a normal ECG for an adult include all but
   a. A PR interval less than 0.10 seconds

    b. A heart rate between 60 and 100

    c. A positive deflection of the QRS complex on lead II

    d. A P-wave before each QRS complex

4. Premature heart beats change the appearance of the ECG. Which of the following is a characteristic of a premature ventricular contraction?

    a. A P-wave precedes the QRS complex

    b. A T-wave is absent after the QRS complex

    c. The QRS complex is wider than normal

    d. The QRS complex is absent

5. Mr. Smiley has just had an ECG done. The nurse has noted that the rhythm is regular and that there are 8 QRS complexes in 30 large squares of the ECG graph. Therefore, Mr. Smiley's pulse rate is

    a. 50   **c.** 70

    b. 60   **d.** 80

6. Another way to figure Mr. Smiley's pulse rate on the ECG graph would be to count the large squares between each QRS complex. If there were 4 large squares between each QRS complex, Mr. Smiley's rate would be

    a. 55   **c.** 75

    b. 65   **d.** 85

7. Mr. Faber has a history of angina. He had some nonspecific changes on an ECG done today. He is now on telemetry. Which of the following measures of cardiac activity would *not* be necessary by the nurse because telemetry is being used? (Assume the telemetry has been checked and is functioning properly.)

    a. Counting the apical rate and noting the rhythm

    b. Noting any dyspnea, angina, or abnormal breath sounds

    c. Checking the quality of peripheral pulses

    d. Noting the amount of urinary output

8. Which of the following nursing actions is *inappropriate* when the client is to have an EEG?

    a. Allowing a child to nap before the procedure

    b. Seeing that the client has a shampoo

    c. Allowing regular meals but no coffee, tea, or colas

    d. Checking to see if tranquilizers and sedatives should be withheld

9. Mrs. Tooler is to have an EMG to assess a weakness in her left leg. Which of the following statements is correct to tell Mrs. Tooler when she asks about the test?

    a. There is no pain or discomfort during an EMG

    b. The test can specifically determine the type of muscular disorder present

    c. The client must remain on bedrest for a while after the test

    d. The test can help the physician determine whether the muscular problem is due to nerve or muscle dysfunction

10. Which one of the following pulmonary function tests is most useful for detecting subclinical cases of obstructive defects in ventilation?

    a. FVC (forced vital capacity)

    b. FEV_1 (forced expiratory volume in 1 second)

    c. MVV (maximum voluntary ventilation)

    d. FEF (forced expiratory flow)

11. Pulmonary function tests with a spirometer may be useful in all these clinical situations *except*

    a. Mr. Harris, who is going to surgery for an exploratory thoracotomy

    b. Mr. Warzyniak, who is a heavy smoker

    c. Mr. Leonard, who took an overdose of a narcotic and had respiratory depression for a few hours

    d. Sandy Blake, age 15, who has a history of severe asthmatic attacks

12. Thermography is based on the principle that inflammation and some malignant processes cause accelerated heat production. This increase in heat is measured by

    a. Rectal and oral thermometers

    b. Pictures with an infrared camera

    c. Heat-sensitive electrodes attached to the body

    d. Immersion in a water bath of a certain temperature

REFERENCES

Alspach, J. (1979). Electrical axis: How to recognize deviations on the ECG and interpret them. *AJN, 79*(11), 76–83.

Boehnert, M., & Lovejoy, F. (1985). Value of the QRS duration versus the serum drug level in predicting seizures and ventricular arrhythmias after an acute overdosage of tricyclic antidepressants. *NEJM, 313*(8), 474–477.

Boyce, B., & King, T. (1980). Pulmonary function tests in patient care. *AJN, 80*(6), 1135–1159.

Bubb, D. (1982). Helping your patient through two painful tests. *RN, 45*(1), 64–65.

Cudworth, K. (1986). Is that funny looking beat dangerous? *RN, 49*(5), 32–35.

Disch, J. (1980). *Diagnostic procedures for cardiovascular disease.* Norwalk, Ct: Appleton-Century-Crofts.

Friedman, E. (1981). Imaging technology approaches the frontiers of physics. *Hospital, 55*, 76–78.

McNeal, G. (1978). Twenty-four-hour ambulatory monitoring. *Nursing Clinics of North America, 13,* 437–447.

Meth, I. (1980). Electrical safety in the hospital. *AJN, 80*(7), 1344–1348.

Nield, M.A. (1974). A nurse directed chest clinic. *Nursing Clinics of North America, 9,* 147–155.

Perry, T. (1986). ABC's of simple pulmonary function assessment. *Nurse Practitioner, 11*(6), 50–60.

Pidgeon, V. (1985). Children's concepts of illness: Implications for health teaching. *Maternal-Child Nursing Journal, 14*(1), 23–33.

Purcell, J., & Haynes, L. (1984). Using the ECG to detect MI. *AJN, 84*(5), 628–642.

Ross, A. (1979). Neuromuscular diagnostic procedures. *Nursing Clinics of North America, 14*(3), 107–121.

Sobel, D., & Ferguson, T. (1985). *The people's book of medical tests.* New York: Summit Books.

Spiegel, M. (1978). Electromyoneurography. *American Family Practice, 18,* 119–130.

Streiff, L. (1981). Need to track your patient's heart? Try telephones and tape recorders. *Nursing 81, 11,* 74–77.

Sumner, S., & Grau, P. (1985). Guidelines for running a 12-lead EKG. *Nursing 85, 15*(12), 30–33.

Taylor, J., & Ballenger, S. (1980). *Neurological dysfunction and nursing intervention.* New York: McGraw-Hill.

Wiley, H., & Eaglstein, W. (1979). Calcinosis cutis in children following electroencephalography. *JAMA, 242,* 455–457.

25

Common Invasive Tests

- Lumbar Puncture (LP)
- Bone Marrow Aspiration or Biopsy
- Thoracentesis (Pleural Tap)
- Paracentesis (Abdominal Tap)
- Gastric Analysis
- Papanicolaou Smears or Exfoliative Cytological Studies
  Papanicolaou Smears of the Uterus
- Cervigram
- Colposcopy, Cervical Biopsy, and Edometrial Biopsy
- Breast Biopsy and Needle Aspiration
- Liver Biopsy
- Renal Biopsy

OBJECTIVES

1. Identify nursing diagnoses related to preparing adults and children for invasive diagnostic procedures done at their bedsides, in a treatment room, or outpatient department.
2. Identify the key nursing implications for clients having bone marrow aspirations.
3. Describe the usual procedure for the collection of spinal fluid and the normal characteristics of CSF as demonstrated by routine laboratory analysis.
4. Compare and contrast the pre- and postcare of clients having a thoracentesis or paracentesis.
5. Describe the procedures needed for a gastric analysis, including the use of medications, which may be given by the nurse.
6. Identify the key nursing diagnoses for clients having breast and cervical biopsies for potential malignancies.

7. Compare and contrast the pre- and postcare of clients having renal and liver biopsies.
8. Identify what is important in informing consumers about the Papanicolaou smear as a cancer detection tool.

As discussed in Chapter 24, the division of diagnostic tests into invasive and noninvasive testing is somewhat artificial because all testing may be considered as an invasion of the person to some degree. The term invasive is usually used to describe diagnostic tests that entail the use of needles or instruments inserted inside the body to directly record or assess the structure and function of an organ. Some invasive diagnostic procedures are done at the client's bedside, such as a thoracentesis or pleural tap. Others are done in specially equipped treatment rooms, radiology suites, or even in a very specialized laboratory, such as the cardiac catheterization laboratory. Invasive tests require specialized equipment and highly skilled clinicians. When invasive procedures are done by experienced, skilled clinicians, the incidence of serious side effects is low. But there is always the possibility of complications when the body is invaded by needles and other types of probes. The possibility of complications ranges from minor problems to severe injury and even death. After the physician explains the possible risks to the client and the expected benefits of the test, the client or guardian must sign a specific consent form for a particular test. Hogue (1986) notes that a tape recording of the discussion with the client or a witness can substitute for a written document. However, institutions almost always use written forms. *The policy of an informed consent is essential for all invasive tests.* A general form used at admission is not acceptable.

The invasive tests covered in this chapter are those that are usually done in the hospital unit or in an outpatient clinic. A nurse is often present during these procedures and actively assists the physician and supports the client. These tests include needle aspirations or taps and various kinds of biopsies done under local anesthesia. Nurse practitioners may actually perform selected procedures for stable clients.

The second broad type of invasive procedures are those done in a special laboratory or specially equipped procedure room, such as endoscopic procedures or cardiac catheterizations. The role of the staff nurse for these very specialized procedures is to prepare the client for the test and to care for the client afterward. If a nurse wants to be an assistant with endoscopic procedures or cardiac catheterization, some special clinical training is required. Cardiac catheterizations are discussed in Chapter 26 and endoscopic procedures in Chapter 27.

GENERAL PRETEST NURSING DIAGNOSES

Potential for Injury Related to Risks of Procedure
As mentioned earlier, the physician must have the client or guardian sign a specific consent form for any invasive procedure. The usual risks are mentioned on the form. The nurse must be aware of the specific policy of the institution. Most institutions require one or more routine laboratory tests before invasive procedures. The nurse coordinates the collection of any samples needed for laboratory analysis such as hematocrit (Hct) and urinalysis (UA). The nurse

also assesses the physical and mental status of the client before the test; these are baseline assessments, which are referred to after the test. One of the most critical baseline assessments is the client's normal blood pressure and pulse rate. For some of these tests, the blood pressure cuff is left on the client's arm during the procedure so the nurse can take readings throughout the procedure.

Alteration in Comfort Related to Pain of Procedure

All of the invasive procedures are to some degree uncomfortable for the client, and most cause a certain amount of pain. At the very least, the pain is confined to the prick accompanying the injection of the local anesthetic. Some procedures also cause momentary pain or unpleasantness during the test. If the nurse is with the client during the procedure, he or she can be very valuable in assisting the client to deal with any expected momentary pain. For example, various breathing techniques or pain distractors can be taught to the client. Sometimes just squeezing the nurse's hand will help the client cope. Depending on the interest of the client and the skill of the nurse, the client may be taught techniques, such as imaging or other ways, to divert his or her attention from the present situation. For example, if the client has learned the LaMaze breathing technique to reduce discomfort during labor, this technique could be used to lessen the discomfort during a painful procedure. The nurse should find out what the client thinks will be a help to ease discomfort. For some clients sedatives may be needed, but accurate information about the test may alleviate anxiety and make sedatives unnecessary. The key points to emphasize are that (1) the duration of pain will be very brief and (2) local anesthetics will be used. Pretest information should include what the person will see, smell, taste, or feel to lessen the dread of the unknown. Some clients may want a lot of technical information. Others may want to know *only* how much it will hurt. Research studies have demonstrated that adult clients who receive information about the "sensations" of a procedure appear to have less anxiety than clients who receive no information or only procedural information (Johnson & Rice, 1974; Johnson, 1978).

Anxiety and Fear of Children

Preparing children for invasive tests means preparing the parents, too. The use of a booklet designed for children is also a helpful tool (Waidley, 1985). It is sometimes better to let the parents do the explaining to the child. It has been suggested that is is better to tell the adolescent when he or she is alone (Pidgeon, 1977). The nurse's assessment of the child's growth and developmental stage is essential for appropriate health teaching. For example, school-age children are usually very receptive to teaching (Pidgeon, 1985). Encouraging a young child to play with some of the equipment may help alleviate anxiety. Research studies have suggested that, as with adults, telling the child about the "sensations" he will feel may lower distress (Johnson et al., 1975). Adolescents may be particularly interested in seeing what equipment will be used during the test. Children, as well as adults, need to know how they can help during the test. Young children may have to be restrained; thus, they deserve explanations. By age three, it may be possible to do procedures without the use of a restraint if (1) the parent holds the child, (2) the child is allowed to participate, and (3) acceptable behavior is rewarded (Beckemeyer & Bahr, 1980). Keeping a security blanket or favorite toy nearby may also help relieve the child's anxiety.

Knowledge Deficit Regarding Test Procedure

Some of the tests require the client to maintain n.p.o. status, whereas others do not. Medications may or may not be withheld; specific medications may be part of the test. The client should be physically comfortable; thus, he or she should be given a chance to void before the procedure begins. (For some of the procedures, such as a paracentesis, an empty bladder is essential.) The specific physical preparation for the client is covered under the discussion for each individual test. (Table 25–1 lists key points about the tests.) The nurse also needs to explain what aftercare will be needed. Thus, children and parents will not be concerned because the child is being carefully watched after the test. By the same token, the adolescent or adult needs to be told before the test that his or her blood pressure will be taken, say, every 15 minutes so there is no misconception that something is amiss.

Preparation of Equipment

For all of these procedures, special trays are used. For example, the basic equipment for a lumbar puncture (LP) is sterilized on one tray. A check must be done to see if the necessary slides, chemistry tubes, culture tubes, and so on, are included on a special procedure tray. Someone may need to check with the laboratory to determine what tubes are necessary to collect.

In some institutions, the nurse may be responsible for setting up equipment for a procedure. In other settings, the person who performs the procedure is responsible for acquiring all needed equipment. Many procedure trays are now packaged commercially with all disposable items. The nurse must check with the particular institutions to see exactly what procedures are followed in that setting. Most prepared trays contain packets of skin antiseptics, such as povidone–iodine (Betadine), which has broad-spectrum microbicidal action.

Preparing for Local Anesthesia

The syringes and needles used for the local anesthetic are included on the various trays. These routine types of needles on a procedure tray are: (1) 25-gauge ⅝-inch needles for local skin infiltration, (2) 22-gauge 1½-inch needles for deeper structures, and (3) spinal needles, which are various gauges and extra long (over 3 inches) for very deep injections. (Note that specific trays, such as a bone marrow or paracentesis tray, will also include specific cutting needles or trocars for different test procedures.) Sterile towels are also on prepared procedure trays. Usually the vial of anesthetic is not included on the equipment tray and must be added.

Types of Local Anesthetics

The two most common local anesthetics used for invasive diagnostic testing are procaine (Novocaine) and lidocaine (Xylocaine). Procaine lasts about ¾ to 1½ hours; lidocaine lasts for 1½ to 2 hours. Sometimes a very small amount of epinephrine (adrenalin) is combined with a local anesthetic agent to promote local vasoconstriction. Two reasons why some local vasoconstriction may be desirable are: (1) the vasoconstriction slows down the absorption of the drug to lengthen its duration and (2) the vasoconstriction may cause decreased bleeding at the injection site. Note that epinephrine is not used in areas of the body supplied by end-arteries, such as "fingers, toes, penis, or nose." Epinephrine is never used with a local anesthetic if tissue circulation is compromised. Also, epinephrine is not used if a client is on beta blockers.

TABLE 25–1. COMMON INVASIVE TESTS: SUMMARY OF KEY POINTS FOR NURSING CARE[a]

Test	n.p.o. Status Pretest?	Local Anesthetic Used?	Restricted Activity Posttest?	Assess for Complications?
Lumbar puncture	Varies	Yes	Varies, usually several hours	Spinal headache; nerve damage to legs or bladder
Bone marrow biopsy	No	Yes	No	None likely; infection possible
Thoracentesis	No	Yes	1 hour on affected side	Pneumothorax; subcutaneous emphysema
Paracentesis	No	Yes	No	Hypovolemia; peritonitis
Gastric analysis	Yes	No	No	Possible allergic reaction to histamine-type drugs
Papanicolaou smears of uterus	No	No	No	None likely
Cervical biopsy—endometrial biopsy	No	No	No	Bleeding from biopsy site
Breast biopsy	No	Yes	No	None likely; infection at site or bleeding possible
Liver biopsy	Yes	Yes	Up to 24 hr	Internal bleeding; bile peritonitis
Renal biopsy	Yes	Yes	Up to 24 hr	Hematuria and internal bleeding; urinary tract infection

[a]See text for more detailed discussions about all preparations before and after each test and for possible nursing diagnoses.

Adverse Reactions to Local Anesthetics

Systemic effects can arise from local injections containing epinephrine. Nurses should assess for any skin flush or increased pulse when epinephrine is used. Anaphylaxis can occur from lidocaine or procaine if the client is allergic to local anesthetics. Nurses must assess for allergies before any drugs are given. Emergency drugs and equipment for resuscitation should always be available when an invasive test is performed. Preparation for the unexpected is as important in an outpatient setting as in a hospital setting.

Arranging Environment for the Test

The nurse or clinician doing the procedure must check the lighting in the area. Most hospitals have a treatment room, which ensures adequate lighting and privacy. If the procedure is done at the client's bedside, a treatment light should be brought to the room. A good light is needed so doors do not have to open—closed doors ensure privacy for the client. In a multiple bed unit, it is better to take the client to a treatment room, otherwise, the bed should be screened and perhaps the other client can go to a waiting room, if possible. Clients should not be exposed to another client's invasive procedure.

Nurse's Role During Procedure

The nurse may remain with the client to offer support. It has already been stressed that the nurse can help prepare the client for the procedure by exploring, with the client, the best way to cope with any pain or discomfort. The nurse can explain that the antiseptic will feel cold to the skin and the injection of the local anesthetic will cause a stinging sensation. The nurse can offer to hold the client's hand or let the client squeeze his or her hand. Hand holding also helps remind the client not to put his or her hands on the sterile field. For a child, special restraining procedures may be required to ensure the safety of the child and the sterility of the procedure. The parent may help hold the child. If the parent is not present, the nurse can hold the child. The nurse may be essential in helping the client maintain a certain position, such as with an LP. The nurse also assists the physician or the clinician, who is actually doing the procedure. This may require pouring an antiseptic into a basin, opening extra gauze packages, or holding collection tubes. The nurse must make sure all collected samples are clearly marked in the order collected. Also, the nurse is needed to observe any untoward effects of the procedure, e.g., check the blood pressure several times during a procedure.

With the expanding role of the nurse, a nurse-practitioner may actually perform the test (Markus, 1981). Nurse-practitioners do bone marrow aspirations on clients as part of their caseloads. However, the focus of this chapter is for the nurse in general practice, who is, usually the assistant during invasive diagnostic procedures. Guarriello (1984), a nurse and a lawyer, cautions nurses to (1) never perform any act that is beyond the established scope of nursing and (2) never attempt procedures they have not been trained to do. No one else, including the physician, can assume responsibility for an error because the nurse was told to go ahead and do a procedure.

GENERAL POSTTEST NURSING DIAGNOSES

Potential for Injury Related to Adverse Reactions

One of the nursing implications for any invasive test is to carefully check vital signs before, during, and after the procedure. Typical orders after an invasive procedure would be vital signs every 15 minutes for 1 hour, then every hour for 4 hours, and then routine if stable. Routines may vary for different procedures, depending on the policy of the specific institution and the exact procedure done. The nurse should take the vital signs more often if there is any apparent instability. Regardless of the stability of the vital signs, they should be taken at regular intervals as long as there is any possibility of the client bleeding or having other complications. Vital signs after an invasive test include blood pressure, pulse, and respiration. (The client's temperature is *not* taken every 15 minutes. The client's temperature may become more important later if there is any possibility that the procedure caused an infection.) If there is any indication of possible febrile reactions, then temperature should be checked routinely every 4 hours. All vital signs must be documented on the client's record and should be graphed so trends (i.e., decreasing blood pressure and increasing pulse rate) are readily apparent. Hematocrits may be done a few hours after the procedure. (See Chapter 2 for an explanation of why hematocrits are done several hours after any bleeding has occurred.)

The time and the name of the clinician, who performed the procedure, should be recorded. The amount of any fluid withdrawn and its color and characteristics (i.e., cloudy or bloody) should be noted. The number of specimens sent to the laboratory should also be documented.

In addition to the specific items, such as the vital signs and other items discussed later, the nurse should record the general condition of the client after the test. For example, if there were no untoward reactions, this should be noted as "client tolerated procedure well with no complications noted at present." *Specific* assessments for the client's condition depend on the test. These are emphasized in the discussion about each test.

Potential for Activity Intolerance Related to Need for Bedrest

The positioning of the client after the procedure may be important. If the client is to remain in a certain position or on bedrest for a specified amount of time, the client needs to know this information. Also a sign can be placed at the foot of the bed. For example, the sign may say "Keep flat in bed until 7 P.M." Information about positioning should also be recorded in the kardex. Clients may be dizzy when first allowed to walk. Also ambulatory care clients often need someone to drive them home.

Alteration in Comfort Related to Pain and Possible Complications

The nurse must know what type of pain is usual after a procedure so ordered analgesics can be used for relief without masking what could be a symptom of a complication. The nurse must also know any specific complications associated with a procedure so the posttest assessment is appropriate. For example, listening for breath sounds after a pleural tap or thoracentesis is necessary to detect a pneumothorax. There may be a need for a medical follow-up if pain persists after the use of mild analgesics.

Potential for Infection

The dressing over the site of an invasive procedure should remain sterile. The nurse must use sterile technique if the dressing becomes wet and needs to be changed. Some procedures may require a pressure dressing with a sandbag, whereas others only require a small adhesive dressing.

Alterations in Fluid or Nutritional Requirements
Any limitations on eating after the procedure will be discussed for the specific tests. For some tests, encouraging fluids is beneficial.

■ LUMBAR PUNCTURE (LP)

Description. Positioning of the client for an LP is very important. Clients are turned on their sides and told to curl up into a ball with head and feet as close to each other as possible (fetal position). This position allows for the maximum separation of the vertebrae. An LP can be done with the client in a sitting position, but pressure readings cannot be obtained. The usual preparation of the skin with antiseptic and local anesthetic is done. The clinician inserts a spinal needle into a lumbar space, which is below the end of the spinal cord. The spinal cord usually terminates at the second lumbar vertebra. Thus, the spinal cord is not touched by the needle. Sometimes the needle does graze a spinal root causing a sharp pain, which radiates down the client's leg (Taylor & Ballenger, 1980). If the client has pain in one of the legs, the clinician needs to know which leg, so the needle position can be slightly readjusted. Once the needle is positioned in the subarachnoid space, a pressure reading is taken with a three-way stopcock and a manometer (standard equipment on an LP tray). The client must relax and straighten out his or her legs before the opening pressure is done because intra-abdominal pressure will increase cerebrospinal fluid (CSF) pressure. After a baseline pressure has been obtained, the physician may want the client to strain slightly (Valsalva's maneuver) to see if the increased abdominal pressure causes an increase in CSF pressure. If there is a blockage in the spinal canal, the CSF pressure may not change. The Queckenstedt test is also used to see if there is a block in the flow of CSF. The physician may ask an assistant to apply finger pressure to both internal jugular veins of the client. Obstruction of these veins will cause a rise in CSF pressure, unless there is a block somewhere in the spinal column. The Queckenstedt test can be dangerous if too much pressure is put on the carotid receptors. The assistant must know exactly how and where to apply the pressure. After the pressure readings are done, a few milliliters of CSF are obtained in tubes for (1) chemistry, (2) cell counts, and (3) microbiology. A closing pressure may be obtained. The CSF pressure drops 5 to 10 mm of water pressure for each milliliter of fluid removed. Usually only about 10 ml are removed, but this can reduce pressure by 50 to 100 mm. The needle is withdrawn and a dry sterile dressing is placed over the site.

Contraindications for LP
A measurement of the CSF pressure will help detect any obstruction in the normal flow of the CSF. However, if increased intracranial pressure is suspected, an LP is *not* attempted because a quick reduction in the pressure in the spinal column can cause a herniation of the brainstem into the foramen magnum. This downward shift of the brain can put lethal pressure on the vital centers in the medulla (Bullock & Rosendahl, 1984).

Purposes. An LP or spinal tap measures CSF pressure and is used to obtain CSF for laboratory examination. An LP is also done to inject dye into the spinal column (see myelograms, Chapter 20). The LP done for a spinal tap is similar in type of procedure to that done for spinal anesthetics.

Spinal fluid is formed in the lateral ventricles in the brain. The fluid bathes the brain and spinal cord and protects the central nervous system from injury. Measurements of the various CSF components helps in the diagnosis of various conditions of the central nervous system. A special summary about the clinical significance of CSF changes is covered at the end of this section. Nurses should be aware of the normal characteristics of CSF because the laboratory results are usually sent to the unit.

PRETEST NURSING IMPLICATIONS

Note the general nursing diagnoses for all invasive testing; e.g., consent forms and other policies. The client does not need to maintain n.p.o. status for LP. Sedation is usually not used, but may be necessary for children or confused adults. A blood glucose sample must be drawn about ½–1 hour before the test to be used as a comparison for the CSF glucose level. A serum chloride level may be used for comparison too, but this is not routine.

POSTTEST NURSING DIAGNOSES

Potential for Alterations in Sensory Perceptions
See the general guidelines about vital signs, assessing for pain, and so on. Special attention should be paid to any change in the level of consciousness, particularly if increased intracranial pressure is suspected. The client may have a temporary problem in voiding due to the effect on nerves to the bladder. Also damage to nerves may affect the legs.

Potential Alteration in Comfort Related to Development of Spinal Headache
The exact reason for a spinal headache is not known, but it is assumed to be related to the loss of CSF. The use of a large needle (18-gauge) or other trauma during the procedure may cause more loss of spinal fluid, and thus, there is less fluid to bathe the meninges of the brain. Petito and Plum (1974) advocate that a client lie prone for only 3 hours after an LP because they believe it is the size of the needle that causes the headache, more than the position afterward. If a headache does begin, the client is maintained on bedrest with an icecap and mild analgesics given as ordered. The spinal headache usually goes away in 24 hours, but it may persist longer, sometimes for weeks. Commonly, the client may be instructed to stay flat in bed for several hours to prevent any spinal headaches. If the LP is done on an outpatient basis, the client may be allowed to go home without being prone for a period.

Alteration in Fluid Requirements
After an LP, the client can eat and drink as soon as he or she desires. Unless otherwise contraindicated, drinking plenty of fluids should be encouraged because this helps the body replace any lost CSF and this may decrease the chance of a headache developing.

Reference Values for CSF

Bilirubin	negative
Cell count	0–5 mononuclear cells—infants and young children up to 20
Chloride	120–130 mEq/L—compare with serum, would be 10 mEq higher
Glucose	50–75 mg/dl—compare with serum glucose, should be 20 mg less
Protein	15–45 mg/dl
Albumin	29.5 mg/dl
IgG	4.3 mg/dl
Oligoclonal bands absent	
Pressure	70–180 mm H_2O—infants and young children, 50–100 mm H_2O
LDH	About 10% of serum level

Note: Values from Sculley (1986).

General Significance of Abnormal Findings in CSF

Blood in the Fluid. Normally, the fluid should be very clear in color. Bleeding from the tap itself will usually not make all the tubes bloody. The collection of samples should be marked as #1, #2, and #3, so it is possible to see if the blood is less in the last tube than in the first tube. If the CSF is grossly bloody, this is a sign of hemorrhage somewhere in the central nervous system. It may not be possible to do any other tests on the CSF when a great deal of blood is present.

Bilirubin. Bilirubin (the indirect portion) can cross the blood–brain barrier in infants. (Note that bilirubin in the spinal fluid of the newborn [kernicterus] can cause brain damage; see Chapter 11).

Cell Counts. Normally there are fewer than five cells per milliliter in CSF, all are lymphocytes. In bacterial infections there may be enough neutrophils to make the CSF cloudy. In tuberculosis and some viral diseases lymphocytes may be increased. Tumor cells can also be identified by a Papanicolaou smear.

Chlorides. Chlorides are decreased in some bacterial infections, including tuberculosis. This test is not specific enough to be of much use and is not done anymore unless specifically requested.

Glucose. The glucose level is lowered in bacterial infections because the bacteria use sugar. Some types of tumors may also cause a lowered CSF sugar. The blood glucose sample is needed for a comparison. Ideally the blood glucose sample is drawn about 30 minutes before the LP because it takes glucose about 30 minutes to an hour to diffuse into the CSF.

Proteins. Degenerative diseases and brain tumors tend to cause increased protein in the CSF. Structural lesions that interrupt the blood–brain barrier cause increased total protein in the CSF because there is increased diffusion from the blood to the brain tissue. In general, an increase in the total protein of the CSF is a sign of a serious neurological disorder. Because various diseases cause elevations in only certain types of proteins, much research is directed toward identifying exactly what types of proteins are elevated in various diseases of the central nervous system. Demyelinating diseases of the central nervous system are those in which the myelin sheath covering the neurons is lost (Taylor & Ballenger, 1980). During active demyelination a basic protein is present in the serum, as well as the CSF (Cohen et al., 1976). Immunoelectrophoresis can be done on CSF. IgG and an abnormal type of protein band called oligoclonal bands are often present in multiple sclerosis and neurosyphilis (Wallach, 1986).

Gram Stains and Cultures
Cultures are done to identify any organisms found in the CSF. If a preliminary Gram stain identifies any organisms, the physician is notified immediately so treatment can begin at once (see Chapter 17 on C&S tests).

Serological Tests
The laboratory may do various types of serological tests to determine the presence of neurosyphilis. See Chapter 14 for examples of serological tests for syphilis (STS).

LDH
An elevated LDH level is usually associated with inflammatory processes and bacterial meningitis. LDH isoenzymes (see Chapter 12) give more detailed information on the origin of the LDH.

■ BONE MARROW ASPIRATION OR BIOPSY

Description. Common sites used for the adult are posterior iliac crest, anterior iliac crest, and sternum. The tibia may be used in a small child. If a biopsy, rather than just an aspiration, is planned, the iliac crest is used. The area is prepped and a local anesthetic is used. Hair may have to be shaved from the site. The physician or nurse-practitioner inserts the needle through the bone until the marrow is reached. For an aspiration, the plunger of the syringe is pulled back to withdraw a little bit of the marrow into the syringe. When the plunger is pulled back, the client often feels sharp pain. The client should be prepared for this momentary pain. Normal bone marrow is soft and semifluid, and thus, a sample can often be obtained by aspiration with a syringe. Otherwise, a bone marrow biopsy can be done with a large-size needle, which has a cutting blade. The specimen obtained must be carefully placed in the correct container. A smear may be microscopically examined immediately to make sure tiny bone particles, called spicules, are present (Markus, 1981). Six or more slides may be done. A culture tube may also be necessary. Usually only a Band-Aid or small adhesive dressing is placed over the site because there is minimal bleeding or drainage. A small pressure dressing is used if a biopsy was done.

Purposes. Bone marrow studies are done when there are abnormal types of cells on a peripheral blood smear. They are used to confirm the presence of metastatic tumors or diseases such as leukemia or various types of anemias. Bone marrow studies may be done periodically to evaluate the response to treatment.

PRETEST NURSING DIAGNOSIS

Knowledge Deficit Regarding Procedure Requirements
The client is usually not given sedation, but if sedation is deemed necessary, it does not interfere with the test. The client can eat and drink before the test. The procedure, including the momentary pain, should be explained to the client. The client is positioned with pillows under the thoracic spine if the sternum is used. The iliac crest is done with the client in a side-lying position or on his or her abdomen. The nurse needs to help the client get into as comfortable position as possible, so the client can remain still during the procedure.

POSTTEST NURSING IMPLICATIONS

Vital signs and other routines are done as for other invasive tests although the risk of bleeding is very slight. The client may stay in bed for an hour or so to rest, but then can resume normal daily activities. There may be a slight aching or pain, which requires the use of a mild analgesic. Chapter 2 discusses nursing diagnoses related to decreased RBC and abnormal WBC counts, which are often present when a bone marrow is required.

■ THORACENTESIS (PLEURAL TAP)

Description. The site usually used for a thoracentesis (pleural tap) is the seventh or eighth intercostal space. The clinician determines the exact site to put the needle by studying the client's chest x-ray and by percussion and auscultation of the chest. The client is usually in a sitting position so fluid will pool in the base of the pleural space. If the client cannot sit up, he or she may be turned toward the unaffected side and placed in a high Fowler's position. The area is prepped and anesthetized. After the needle is positioned in the pleural space, fluid is withdrawn with a syringe and a three-way stopcock. (If the tap is therapeutic, 1000 ml or more may be withdrawn.) The client may feel some pain as the pleural space is entered, but the withdrawing of fluid is not uncomfortable. Once the fluid is withdrawn, a small bandage is placed over the site. Some clinicians may spray the site with a collodian seal. The thoracentesis is usually done at the client's bedside or in the procedure room on the unit. Thoracentesis can also be done in an office or clinic setting.

Purposes. A thoracentesis is an insertion of a needle into the pleural space with aspiration of air, pleural fluid, or blood from the pleural cavity. A thoracentesis is often done for therapy as well as for diagnosis. Inflammatory diseases of the lungs and neoplasms are common reasons for a large collection of pleural fluid. Blood in the pleural space (hemothorax) is usually from a traumatic injury.

Laboratory Examination of Pleural Fluid
The fluid collected for the laboratory may include (1) chemistry, (2) bacteria, and (3) histopathology. Tumor cells can be identified as well as various organisms. *Ex-*

udates, found in inflammation and tissue destruction, have a specific gravity above 1.017 with a high concentration of protein and LDH. *Transudates,* found in congestive heart failure, have a protein count no higher than in the serum and do not clot (Bullock & Rosendahl, 1984).

PRETEST NURSING IMPLICATIONS

The general pretest nursing diagnoses for bedside examinations are considered. An extra bedside table may be necessary to help position the client in a comfortable sitting position. The client can lean over the table with his or her feet on a chair for support. Chest x-rays are needed. The nurse should listen to the client's breath sounds to be used as a baseline for a posttest assessment. The nurse should also note any breathing difficulty and the color of the client's skin before the test is begun. Sedation, although not usually used, will not interfere with the procedure if needed. Food, fluids, and medicines do not need to be withheld.

POSTTEST NURSING DIAGNOSES

Potential for Injury Related to Fluid Loss
The client is usually turned on the *unaffected* side for 1 hour to allow the pleural puncture to seal. Vital signs are recorded as per hospital routine. The amount of fluid withdrawn for diagnosis, if more than a few milliliters, should be recorded as part of the intake and output record and the client should be assessed for potential hypovolemia. There is no restriction on food or fluids following the procedure. If the client has no respiratory or other problems within an hour after the test, all normal activity can be resumed.

Potential for Ineffective Breathing Patterns
Careful note should be made of the respiratory rate and the character of the respirations. The nurse should listen for any diminished breath sounds, which could be a sign of a pneumothorax. Any dyspnea or shortness of breath should be carefully compared with the respiratory status before the test. If a large amount of fluid was withdrawn as therapy, the client should be able to breathe with less effort. A chest x-ray is done to evaluate the amount of fluid that was removed and to check for any pneumothorax.

Subcutaneous emphysema is leakage of air into the subcutaneous tissues. The tissues feel like rolled up tissue paper and crackle when touched (crepitus). The air in the tissues is from a leak in the pleural cavity. If the client has no respiratory problems associated with the crepitus, this air will gradually be reabsorbed without treatment.

Clients with pleural effusion due to malignancies may have cytotoxic or antibiotic drugs injected into the pleural space after the fluid is withdrawn. The nurse must be aware of possible reactions to the particular drug injected into the pleural space.

■ PARACENTESIS (ABDOMINAL TAP)

Description. The word *paracentesis* actually means puncture of any cavity for the aspiration of fluid. An abdominal paracentesis is used for the removal of fluid from a peritoneal cavity. In general practice, the abdominal paracentesis is usually just called a paracentesis because withdrawals of fluids from other cavities have specific names (i.e., thoracentesis, amniocentesis).

A paracentesis is done at the client's bedside or in an outpatient setting. The client must sit up with the feet supported. A bedside table may be used to support the arms in a comfortable position. The physician inserts a large-gauge needle or trocar through the abdominal wall. (It is essential that the bladder be empty so there is no accidental puncture of the bladder.) Once the needle is in the peritoneal cavity, the fluid is withdrawn by a syringe if just a small amount is needed for diagnosis. If the tap is also needed to relieve pressure from ascites, the needle may be connected to a tubing and a large collection bottle is used, which is much like the set-up used to withdraw blood. Up to 1000 ml may be withdrawn at one time. Another technique is to do a slow continuous drainage of ascites and take out as much as nine liters in eight hours (Fisher, 1979). The major concern when a large amount of fluid is removed is there may be a shift of fluid from the vascular space to the now-empty peritoneal cavity. Intravenous fluid or albumin may be used to prevent hypotension when large amounts of fluid are withdrawn. Once the needle or trocar is withdrawn, a small sterile dressing is placed over the site. If the client has a great deal of ascites, and only a small amount of fluid was removed, the pressure of the remaining fluid may cause a continued leakage from the puncture site. The dressing may need to be changed frequently and extra fluff gauze used to absorb the leakage. The use of Montgomery straps eliminates the need to change the tape every time the dressing is changed.

Purposes. A paracentesis may be done to assess for peritonitis. If the client has had peritoneal dialysis, the specimen may be aspirated from the peritoneal catheter. The nurse may collect this specimen by withdrawing a small amount of fluid via a syringe (Shetler & Bartos, 1981), using sterile technique.

An abnormal collection of fluid in the peritoneal cavity is called *ascites*. Ascites is most often seen in clients with advanced cirrhosis or widespread abdominal malignancies. For these conditions, a paracentesis is done for therapeutic rather than diagnostic reasons. The major drawback of doing a paracentesis for therapeutic reasons is that ascitic fluid contains a significant amount of protein. Because paracentesis causes a loss of protein, other measures, such as diuretics, are used before a paracentesis is done for therapy.

In addition to diagnostic aids or therapeutic relief in cirrhosis and malignancies, paracentesis is also done as a diagnostic procedure for traumatic injuries to the abdomen. A peritoneal tap, or a peritoneal lavage with Ringer's lactate solution, is done to see if there is any bleeding into the peritoneal cavity.

Laboratory Examinations of Peritoneal Fluid

Laboratory examination of the peritoneal fluid may include RBC, WBC, cultures, fecal content, bilirubin, and amylase (if pancreatitis is suspected). Normally peritoneal fluid is clear and yellowish. If there is any blood in the fluid, this is abnormal. If the blood is intraperitoneal blood, it will not clot, but if it is venous blood (which was accidentally withdrawn from a vessel), the blood will clot. The amount of protein in the fluid helps distinguish a transudate from an exudate. Exudates, which usually result from inflammation, contain more protein than transudates, which are usually due to pressure changes from mechanical factors.

PRETEST NURSING IMPLICATIONS

In addition to the general nursing diagnoses for invasive testing, the client should be weighed before and after the procedure to assess the fluid loss. (Recall that 1 liter of fluid weighs 1 kilogram or 2.2 pounds.) The client *must have* an empty bladder so it is not pricked by the needle. If the client cannot void, a catheter may be necessary. The client needs to be in a comfortable sitting position with the feet supported on a bedside stool or chair.

POSTTEST NURSING DIAGNOSES

Potential for Fluid Volume Deficit and Electrolyte Imbalance
When a large amount of fluid is being withdrawn, the client's blood pressure needs to be taken several times during the procedure. Intravenous equipment should be readily available in case of hypotension from shifts of fluid out of the vascular space. Intravenous albumin is sometimes given immediately after the procedure (see Chapter 10 on albumin levels). Vital signs are checked after the paracentesis is completed and other routine aftercare for invasive procedures is done. The client's pre- and postweight should be compared. The exact amount, color, and character of the removed fluid should be noted on the nurse's notes and as part of the intake and output record. The client should be on I&O for a period of 24 hours. Depending on the reasons for the ascites, the client may be on a restricted fluid or sodium diet. Electrolytes must be closely monitored (see Chapter 5).

Potential for Infection and Injury from Other Complications
As noted above, if any excess fluid was left in the peritoneal cavity, there may be a problem with leakage from the site. The dressing may need to be changed frequently. Sterile techniques must be used. The client's temperature should be taken every four hours for 24 hours. The nurse should carefully observe the client for other signs or symptoms of a developing peritonitis, such as abdominal pain and tense, rigid abdominal muscles. For the client with cirrhosis, a paracentesis may precipitate hepatic coma (see Chapter 10 on ammonia levels).

■ GASTRIC ANALYSIS

Description. A gastric analysis is usually done at the client's bedside, in a treatment room, or in an office or clinic. The nurse or physician may insert the tube, which should be well lubricated with a water-soluble jelly. The client is seated in an upright position. The nasogastric tube is passed into the stomach and left for the duration of the test. Either nostril may be used. The client may know that one side of his nose is more patent than the other side. The client's head should be hyperextended for the passage of the tube to the back of the throat. Once the tube reaches the posterior pharynx, the client can put his or her head back in a normal position or slightly forward. Sips of water, unless contraindicated, are given to help the tube go down the esophagus. A slight pulling back on the tube and a slight downward thrust are needed when the tube is felt to touch the posterior pharynx. Passing of a nasogastric tube is an unpleasant experience for the client. It may be necessary to stop for a moment to let the client relax. Once the tube is going down the esophagus easily, it should be passed rapidly so that the client does not gag. (It is possible to stimulate a vagal response by gagging and this can cause bradycardia, which can be dangerous to some clients.) If the nasogastric tube is inadvertently put into the trachea of an alert client, this mistake will be very obvious because the client will cough violently and will very actively resist the tube, which is suddenly blocking the air passage. Once the tube is in the stomach, a fasting specimen is obtained by aspiration with a large syringe. Obtaining gastric contents is the best evidence the tube is indeed in the stomach. Proper placement of the gastric tube is critical. Many authorities recommend assistance by fluoroscopy (Ravel, 1984).

Use of Drugs in Gastric Analysis

A drug is given subcutaneously to stimulate gastric secretions. A histamine analogue, betazole hydrochloride (Histologue), is used but a newer drug, pentagastrin, has fewer side effects (Jacobs et al., 1984). The client should be observed for an increased pulse rate and a decreased blood pressure because of the vasodilating properties of histamine and histaminelike drugs. Some clients may experience a warm, flushed feeling or more severe symptoms of an allergic response. Antihistamine drugs and epinephrine should be readily available in the event that the client does have a severe allergic reaction to the drug. After the drug has been given to stimulate gastric secretions, gastric secretions are taken at certain time intervals. The time of each specimen is marked on each collection tube, and all of the specimens are sent to the laboratory for acidity analysis.

Reference Values for Gastric Analysis

Basal
    Male 3.0 ± 2.0 mEq/h
    Female 2.0 ± 1.8 mEq/h
Maximal (after histalog or gastrin)
    Male 23 ± 5 mEq/h
    Female 16 ± 5 mEq/h

(Sculley, 1986)

Purposes. A gastric analysis is most commonly done to measure the acidity of the gastric contents. The response of the gastric glands to drug stimulation with histamine or histaminelike drugs is helpful in diagnosing a peptic ulcer, gastric carcinoma, and pernicious anemia. Gastric acidity is usually increased with a peptic ulcer and decreased or totally absent (anacidity or achlorhydria) in pernicious anemia and gastric carcinoma (See Chapter 22 on the Schilling test for pernicious anemia). An analysis of gastric contents may also be done to detect acid-fast bacillus in the client with undiagnosed tuberculosis. The client with tuberculosis usually swallows some sputum containing the organism that causes tuberculosis, which is acid-fast so it is not destroyed by the gastric juices. The gastric contents can also be examined for the presence of malignant cells by doing a Papanicolaou smear. Test for occult blood may also be done (see Chapter 13).

Insulin may be given to test the stomach's response to vagal stimulation. The vagus nerve causes increased production of hydrochloric acid by the stomach. Hypoglycemia, caused by the insulin, is a stimulus to the vagus. The response of the stomach may be used to evaluate the effect of a vagotomy or to diagnose other problems of gastric acidity. The use of insulin with a gastric analysis is called the Hollander test.

PRETEST NURSING IMPLICATIONS

It is important that the client be checked for any history of allergic reactions. (See the general nursing diagnoses discussed at the beginning of this chapter.) If the client is known to be highly allergic, a small test dose of betazole hydrochloride (Histalogue) may be given before the test. The client must maintain n.p.o. status for 6–8 hours before the test. The client should not smoke because it increases the secretion of gastric acid. Also, the client should not receive anticholinergic drugs, such as atropine, because they markedly decrease gastric secretions by blocking the action of the vagus nerve.

POSTTEST NURSING IMPLICATIONS

Once all specimens are obtained, the nasogastric tube can be removed. The client should be told that the tube will be removed quickly. The nurse can remove the tube by pinching it and quickly pulling it out. Paper towels should be handy to catch the tube, and the the client will need tissues to blow his or her nose. The client may want to close his or her eyes or concentrate on something else while the tube is pulled out.

There are no restrictions on activity after a gastric analysis. Vital signs are only necessary once or twice to ensure the continued stable condition of the client. The client can eat as soon as he or she wishes. A sip of water or some weak, warm tea may be offered first as the client may prefer to rest for a while.

■ PAPANICOLAOU SMEARS OR EXFOLIATIVE CYTOLOGICAL STUDIES

The Papanicolaou smear usually refers to a test for malignant cells from the uterus, but the test can be done of many body secretions. The Papanicolaou smear was named after Dr. George Papanicolaou who, in the 1940s, developed a technique for identifying malignant cells in body secretions. Malignant cells slough off (exfoliate) more readily than do normal cells. The field that involves Papanicolaou smears is sometimes called *exfoliative cytology*. In addition to uteral or cervical secretions, exfoliative cytology studies are done on sputum, pleural fluid, bronchial washings from a bronchoscope, gastric contents, bladder secretions, peritoneal fluid, and even secretions from the mammary glands. The collection of a sample for exfoliative cytology is often part of an invasive study. The laboratory will tell the nurse exactly how the specimen should be prepared. The results of a Papanicolaou smear used to be reported as:

- Grade I: Normal appearing cells
- Grade II: Atypical cytology, but no evidence of malignancy
- Grade III: Suggestion of malignancy, but not conclusive
- Grade IV: Strongly suggestive of malignancy
- Grade V: Conclusive of malignancy

A newer system labels the grades as:

- Normal
- Inflammatory
- Mild—cervical intraepithelial neoplasia (CIN)
- Severe CIN
- Cancer

It must be remembered that all reports of exfoliative cytology are used for screening, not for a final diagnosis. Thus, the presence of a malignancy is always confirmed with a biopsy (Bullock & Rosendahl, 1984).

PAPANICOLAOU SMEARS OF THE UTERUS

Description. A small amount of secretion is obtained from the cervix by swabbing the exterior of the cervix with an applicator. A Gravlee jet washer may be used to get cells from the endometrium. Most sources suggest that two smears should be taken to increase the chance of obtaining any atypical cells, which may be present. The smears are put on dry slides and immediately sprayed with a commercial fixative. It is important that the cells not dry up before they are fixed on the slide.

Purposes. The American Cancer Society used to recommend annual Papanicolaou smears for all women over age 20, or for those under age 20 who were sexually active. The recommendation of the American Cancer Society (1981) is that a Papanicolaou smear be done at least every 3 years, after two initial smears done a year apart are negative. This applies to all women age 20 and over, as well as sexually active women under age 20. The American College of Obstetricians and Gynecologists (1980) has taken the stand that *yearly* examination of a Papanicolaou smear be done on all adult women regardless of age. They cite that the annual smear is not only useful for detecting cancer but also other problems, which can be detected by a yearly visit to a gynecologist.

PRETEST NURSING IMPLICATIONS

The Papanicolaou smear is usually done 5–6 days after the menses. The client should not have intercourse or douche for 48 hours before the smear. If the client has used antibiotic vaginal creams, the examination should be delayed a month. The use of any medications, particularly birth control pills, should be noted on the request slip. For some women, a pelvic examination is an unpleasant and embarrassing procedure, and the nurse must be sensitive to the need to respect the privacy of the client by draping procedures and so on. There are do-it-yourself-type kits for Papanicolaou tests. If the woman is to collect the sample herself, she must be taught how deep in the vagina she must go to get the specimen and how to fix it in the proper preservative. As a guide, the woman can be told that the cervical os feels like the tip of the nose. Nurses may also do Papanicolaou smears as part of a health screening program. Fisher et al. (1977) describes the role of the nurse in doing Papanicolaou smears in the general hospital setting and Austin (1983) describes the role of the nurse with the Gravlee method in a public health setting.

POSTTEST NURSING IMPLICATIONS

There are no client restrictions after a Papanicolaou smear. If the cytology report shows atypical cells, the client may have a colposcopy and cervical biopsy done. See the general nursing diagnosis on anxiety related to tests.

■ CERVIGRAM

Description. Another way to screen for CIN is the use of photographs to record a colposcopic image of the cervix. After applications of 5% acetic acid, photographs of the whole cervix are taken with a specially designed camera. The slide (cervigram) is then magnificed times 16 to assess any changes in the cervix.

■ COLPOSCOPY, CERVICAL BIOPSY, AND ENDOMETRIAL BIOPSY

Description and Purposes. The colposcope or colpomicroscope is a binocular microscope with a magnifying glass and a high-intensity light source, and is used to examine the vagina and cervix and take a biopsy if needed. Nurses, as primary care practitioners, do colposcopic examinations. The biopsy is planned for about a week after the client's menses because the cervix is more vascular before and after the menses. The biopsy is done after the menstrual period so there is no possibility of pregnancy. (See the 10- to 14-day rule discussed in Chapter 20, for x-ray procedures for women of childbearing age.) The client is prepared for a pelvic examination as described earlier. The client is not given any local anesthetic because the cervix is sensitive to pressure but not to burning or cutting, as is the skin. The momentary pressure will be slightly uncomfortable for some clients. The biopsy site may be sealed with a silver nitrate stick or cauterized. A packing will probably be put in the vagina.

With the colposcope, the clinician can identify areas of the cervix that appear atypical and thus, perform direct punch biopsies. It takes about 10 minutes to view the cervical epithelium and note suspicious areas. Normally, the cervix is pink. During pregnancy, the cervix becomes dusky in color. After menopause the cervix is light pink. Any secretions should be odorless and clear. The stickiness of the secretions is related to ovulation time. If abnormal areas are seen in the cervix, or if there are abnormal secretions, a cervical biopsy and/or an endocervical curettage should be done. Endometrial biopsies may be done as part of an infertility work-up (see Chapter 28). An endometrial biopsy is done with a special instrument inserted through the cervix. Usually no anesthetic is used. The pain is momentary, but sharp. Some bleeding may be expected, so a tampon or pad is needed.

POSTTEST NURSING IMPLICATIONS

Often a cervical or endometrial biopsy is done on an outpatient basis. (If a cone biopsy is needed, the patient must be given general anesthesia.) The client should be told that she will feel some pressure and that slight bleeding is normal. The vaginal packing or tampon is left in place for several hours. Any unusual bleeding or severe abdominal pain should be reported immediately. Some spotting is expected. The client needs to be given instructions about when intercourse can be resumed.

■ BREAST BIOPSY AND NEEDLE ASPIRATION

Description and Purposes. A breast biopsy or needle aspiration as diagnostic procedures for malignancies are being done more often in an outpatient setting. In the past, surgeons did a breast biopsy with the client under a general anesthetic so that a mastectomy could be immediately done if the frozen section was positive for cancer. However, the newer trend is to wait and perform the more extensive surgery at a later date. Several reports demonstrated that a short delay between biopsy and mastectomy did not adversely affect survival (Townsend, 1980). This delay gives the client and family more time to adjust to the surgery or to the other treatment options such as radiation implants or chemotherapy. Estrogen receptor assay is widely used as an aid in selection of the therapy for breast cancer (Ravel, 1984). For a breast biopsy, the skin is prepped and anesthetized in the usual manner. A small amount of tissue is incised. Either a biopsy or needle aspiration takes only a few minutes to complete. A probe may be placed when a mammogram is done (see Chapter 20) to identify the exact site for the biopsy.

PRETEST NURSING IMPLICATIONS

The setup for the procedure is similar to that of any other local biopsy—sterile drapes and local anesthetic. The physical discomfort is minimal, but the anxiety level of the woman, or, less frequently, the man, is likely to be quite high. Although the majority of breast lumps are *not* malignant, there is always the possibility that this one may be. Roughly 80% of breast lumps are benign. Hall (1986) has noted that the increase of mammograms may increase the number of unneeded biopsies.

POSTTEST NURSING DIAGNOSIS

Knowledge Deficit Related to Health Maintenance
The client should be told exactly when the results will be available because the waiting time can be very difficult. If a biopsy was done, there may be a few stitches, which need to be removed. The woman should wear a supportive bra 24 hours a day until healing is completed. The nipple may have numbness for a couple of months, which can interfere with sexual arousal (Wiley, 1981).

The nurse can also make sure that the client does know how to do self-breast examinations. (See Chapter 20 for information on mammograms as screening devices for high-risk women.) The American Cancer Society has excellent material for client teaching on breast cancer. The Department of Health and Human Services also publishes a pamphlet on breast self-examination, which can be obtained free for client teaching.

■ LIVER BIOPSY

Description. A liver biopsy can be done at the client's bedside or in a special treatment room. The skin is prepped and anesthetized. Before the biopsy needle is inserted into the liver, the client is asked to take a deep breath and then hold the breath after an expiration. Not breathing keeps the diaphragm motionless. Also, holding the breath after an expiration leaves the diaphragm further up in the thoracic cavity than after an inspiration. (For a renal biopsy, the client is asked to hold his or her breath after inspiration, which is a little easier to do.) For children or confused adults, the nose can be momentarily blocked at the end of an expiration. At the end of a cry, the child with have maximal expiration. Obviously it is much more desirable to have a quiet, cooperative client because jerking or thrashing about can cause a tear in the liver. An uncooperative client usually makes the procedure unsafe. The actual insertion of the needle and a collection of tissue only takes a minute or two. The entire procedure can be done in 10 or 15 minutes. When the needle is withdrawn, a pressure dressing is applied to the area.

Purposes. A liver biopsy may be useful in determining the exact nature of liver pathology, such as tumors, cysts, or cirrhosis. A sonogram (Chapter 23) or a liver scan (Chapter 22) gives the physician valuable information about the exact area to biopsy.

PRETEST NURSING IMPLICATIONS

The client must have coagulation tests (PT, PTT, and platelet counts) done before the liver biopsy. A hematocrit (Hct) will also be done as a baseline assessment. For a liver biopsy, the general rule is that the prothrombin time (PT) activity should be over 50% and not more than 3 seconds over the control in time. The platelets should be above 100,000 mm³. Because a diseased liver may be unable to manufacture prothrombin in normal amounts, vitamin K may be ordered in an attempt to raise the PT percentage and decrease the time in seconds. See Chapter 13 for a discussion on laboratory tests for prothrombin and the relationship to liver disease and vitamin K.

The client is usually kept on n.p.o. status for about 6 hours before the test. Fasting makes the liver less congested and the biliary ducts less turgid. Fasting also prevents any vomiting if complications occur. The client is usually not given any sedation, but some sedation may be needed in selected cases. Baseline vital signs are taken, and the client is given a chance to practice holding the breath after an expiration.

POSTTEST NURSING DIAGNOSES

Potential for Injury Related to Internal Bleeding

The client is turned on his or her right side for 1 to 4 hours. Bed rest may continue for 8–12 hours or longer. A sandbag may be used to apply pressure to the area. It is important to check the dressing for any bleeding, but a pressure dressing should *not* be removed to look for bleeding. Usually serious bleeding will be internal, and thus, it is not detected by visual inspection. Clients can bleed to death from a liver biopsy; therefore, vital signs are checked frequently, as with any invasive procedure. Food may be withheld until it is certain that the client is not having any immediate complications. An 8-hour posttest Hct may be done to assess for any blood loss. Even a slight drop in the Hct should be called to the physician's attention immediately.

Potential for Injury from Other Complications

In addition to hemorrhage and shock, other complications that can occur from a liver biopsy include bile peritonitis, pneumothorax, or perforation of an abdominal organ (e.g., the colon). Any pain in the abdomen or any dyspnea calls for a thorough physical assessment of the thorax and abdomen. Slight pain at the biopsy site and right shoulder pain can be expected as the local anesthetic wears off. The client may be kept on bedrest for an entire 24 hours or longer if there are any complications. The client should be cautioned not to cough or strain because this can increase intra-abdominal pressure. The day after the biopsy, the client can resume most activities, but should not do strenuous activities or heavy lifting for a week or two.

■ RENAL BIOPSY

Description. The renal biopsy is usually done in a treatment room close to the ultrasound or x-ray department because the insertion of the needle is monitored by fluoroscopy or scanning. Renal biopsies can also be done with a cystoscope, using a brush inserted up into the ureter to get a fragment of renal tissue (Gittes, 1978). The brush technique with a cystoscope requires general anesthesia, therefore is done in the operating room as is an open biopsy when a wedge of renal tissue is obtained. A renal biopsy, under local anesthesia, is done through a skin puncture or through a small skin incision. The skin is prepped and anesthetized as usual. The client is usually not given any sedation, but the use of drugs will not interfere with the procedure. The client is asked to take a breath and hold it while the needle is being inserted to obtain the biopsy. Only a very small piece of tissue is obtained. When the needle is withdrawn a pressure dressing is applied to the area, and the client is transported back to the nursing unit.

Purposes. Renal biopsies are most helpful in diagnosing diseases that alter the structure of the glomeruli. Only the cortex is biopsied, not the medulla. Renal biopsies may also determine the exact nature of a mass, which could be a tumor, clot, or stone. Renal biopsies may be done periodically to evaluate and monitor the course of chronic renal disease, such as the nephrotic syndome.

PRETEST NURSING IMPLICATIONS

Preparation is similar to that for a liver biopsy in that coagulation studies (PT, PTT, and platelet count) must be done, vital signs taken for a baseline, and Hct done. In addition, the client should have a urinalysis and an intravenous pyelogram done (Chapter 20) to determine that there are two functioning kidneys. Food and fluids are withheld before the procedure. As mentioned before, sedation does not affect the test and might be needed if the client is very anxious even after optimal preparation. The client should be told approximately how long he or she will be in the radiology or ultrasound department and what the aftercare will be.

POSTTEST NURSING DIAGNOSIS

Potential for Injury Related to Bleeding
The client is usually instructed to remain motionless for 4 hours. A sandbag may be placed on the biopsy site. Bedrest may be continued for 24 hours. If a piece of artery is discovered in the biopsy tissue, the bedrest may be prolonged. Vital signs and dressing check routines are done. An Hct is usually ordered 8 hours after the procedure. During the first 24 hours, urine is collected in separate cups and left in the bathroom so any hematuria can be monitored. The timing of each specimen should be marked on the cup. Some urine may also be sent to the laboratory for microscopic examination. Microscopic hematuria occurs in about half of the cases, and a few cases will show some gross hematuria. There are dipsticks for detecting occult hematuria, but these are not as sensitive as a microscopic examination. (See Chapter 13 on guaiac tests and Chapter 2 on urinalysis.) Any severe jolt to the retroperitoneal area can cause bleeding, even several days after the biopsy. The client should be instructed to avoid strenuous activities or heavy lifting for several days. The client should also be told to report any flank pain, gross hematuria, or signs of dizziness or weakness.

Potential Alteration in Urinary Patterns
Clients should have a large intake of fluids if permissible. Infection can occur after a biopsy so the client's temperature should be routinely checked for a few days after the biopsy. The client should report any burning on urination or frequency.

QUESTIONS

1. Which of the following nursing interventions is usually the *least useful* in alleviating the client's anxiety before a painful diagnostic procedure?

   a. Emphasizing the technical details of the procedure
   b. Preparing the client on ways to cope with painful sensations
   c. Explaining the purpose of any pretest preparations
   d. Providing privacy to maintain self-esteem

2. Epinephrine may be added to a local anesthetic, such as lidocaine (Xylocaine), to

   a. Increase the duration of the local anesthetic and decrease bleeding
   b. Decrease the allergic effects of the anesthetic
   c. Maintain the blood pressure
   d. Cause vasodilation and better blood flow

3. Timmy, age 7, must have a bone marrow aspiration done. Which of the following actions by the nurse would be the *least* helpful in preparing Timmy for this invasive procedure?

   a. Letting Timmy play with replicas of some of the equipment
   b. Telling Timmy how he can help during the procedure
   c. Explaining the reason for the procedure
   d. Telling briefly about how the procedure will feel (i.e., some pain)

4. Mr. Fox has just had a lumbar puncture done. Which of these factors seems to be the most significant in preventing Mr. Fox from developing a "spinal headache"?

   a. Keeping him flat in bed for 24 hours after the procedure
   b. Maintaining n.p.o. status for 2–3 hours before and after the procedure
   c. Encouraging fluids after the lumbar puncture
   d. Using prophylactic analgesics after the procedure

5. Which of the following nursing actions is least appropriate for Mrs. Sangria who just had a thoracentesis done? Four hundred milliliters of clear fluid was obtained from the right pleural space.

   a. Encouraging extra fluids orally to rehydrate Mrs. Sangria
   b. Assessing the thorax for diminished breath sounds
   c. Positioning Mrs. Sangria on her left side for 1 hour after the thoracentesis
   d. Reporting any symptoms of blood in the sputum (hemoptysis) or shortness of breath (dyspnea)

6. Mr. Heppy is to have an abdominal paracentesis done this morning. Which of the following nursing actions is *not* routine for this diagnostic procedure?

   a. Making sure that the client's bladder is empty
   b. Using sterile equipment for the procedure

    c. Helping the client assume a comfortable side-lying position for the procedure

    d. Letting the client eat as tolerated

7. Procedures done for a gastric analysis would *not* include:

    a. Administration of atropine to dry up secretions before the test

    b. Insertion of a nasogastric tube that stays in the stomach for the duration of the test

    c. Administration of a drug to stimulate gastric secretions

    d. Collection of several samples for determining gastric acidity

8. The American Cancer Society recommendation (1981) on the frequency of Papanicolaou smears for women age 20–40 is that after two yearly Papanicolaou smears are negative, the Papanicolaou smear should be done at least:

    a. Annually

    b. Every 2 years

    c. Every 3 years

    d. Every 4 years

9. Mr. Cronkite is to have a liver biopsy done today. Which of the following nursing actions is appropriate in preparing Mr. Cronkite for the liver biopsy?

    a. Have him practice holding his breath after an inspiration

    b. Encourage fluids to keep him well hydrated

    c. Explain that a local anesthetic will be used to eliminate the pain

    d. Explain that he can resume normal activities as soon as the biopsy is finished and his vital signs are stable

10. Mr. Ralph has just returned from the radiology department where he had a closed-renal biopsy done with a local anesthetic. Which of the nursing actions is most appropriate?

    a. Keep Mr. Ralph as motionless as possible on bedrest for 30 minutes to 1 hour

    b. Save all urine in one container for a 24-hour urine sample

    c. Administer the ordered analgesic for pain at the biopsy site

    d. Restrict fluid intake to no more than 1000 ml per day

REFERENCES

American Cancer Society. (1981). *Most often asked questions concerning ACS guidelines on the cancer related checkup.* New York: American Cancer Society.

American College of Obstetricians and Gynecologists. (1980). Cancer test controversy in *Maternal Child Nursing, 5,* 430.

Austin, J., et al. (1983). The Gravlee method. An alternative to the Pap smear. *AJN, 83*(7), 1057–1058.

Beckemeyer, P., & Bahr, J. (1980). Helping toddlers and pre-schoolers cope while suturing their minor lacerations. *Maternal Child Nursing, 5,* 326–330.

Bullock, B., & Rosendahl, P. (1984). *Pathophysiology.* Boston: Little, Brown.

Cohen, S., et al. (1976). Radioimmunoassay of myelin basic protein in spinal fluid. *NEJM, 295,* 1455–1457.

Fisher, D., et al. (1977). Nurse-run Pap smear as hospital screening. *Connecticut Medicine, 41,* 143–145.

Fisher, D. (1979). Abdominal paracentesis for malignant ascites. *Archives Internal Medicine, 139,* 235.

Gittes, R. (1978). Retrograde renal and ureteral brush biopsy. *AJN, 78*(3), 410–412.

Guarrielo, D. (1984). When doctor's orders are not the best medicine. *RN, 47,* 19–20.

Hall, F. (1986). Screening mammography. Potential problems on the horizon. *NEJM, 314*(1), 53–55.

Hogue, E. (1986). Informed consent. *Nursing 86, 16*(6), 47–48.

Jacobs, D., Kasten, B., DeMott, W., & Wolfson, W. (1984). *Laboratory test handbook with DRG index.* St. Louis: Mosby/Lexi.

Johnson, J., et al. (1975). Altering children's distress behavior during cast removal. *Nursing Research, 24,* 404–410.

Johnson, J. (1978). Sensory information, instruction in a coping strategy and recovery from surgery. *Research in Nursing and Health, 1,* 4–17.

Johnson, J., & Rice, V. H. (1974). Sensory and distress components of pain: Implications for study of clinical pain. *Nursing Research, 23,* 203–209.

Markus, S. (1981). Taking the fear out of bone marrow examinations. *Nursing 81, 4,* 64–67.

Petito, F., & Plum, F. (1974). The lumbar puncture. *NEJM, 290,* 225–226.

Pidgeon, V. (1977). Characteristics of children's thinking and implications for health teaching. *American Journal of Maternal–Child Nursing, 6,* 1–7.

Pidgeon, V. (1985). Children's concepts of illness: Implications for health teaching. *Maternal–Child Nursing Journal, 14*(1), 23–33.

Ravel R. (1984). *Clinical laboratory medicine.* Chicago: Year Book.

Sculley, R. (Ed.). (1986). Normal reference laboratory values. *NEJM, 314*(1), 47, 49.

Shetler, M., & Bartos, H. (1981). Spinal and peritoneal taps. *RN, 44*(1), 50–53.

Taylor, J., & Ballenger, S. (1980). *Neurological dysfunctions and nursing intervention.* New York: McGraw-Hill.

Townsend, C. (1980). Breast lumps: Diagnostic techniques. *Ciba Clinical Symposia, 32,* 22–24.

Waidley, E. (1985). Preparing children for invasive procedures. *AJN, 85*(7), 811–812.

Wallach, J. (1986). Interpretation of diagnostic tests. Boston: Little, Brown.

Wiley, K. (1981). Post-biopsy care. *AJN, 81*(9), 1553–1662.

26

Stress Tests and Cardiac Catheterizations

- Stress Tests: ECG Treadmill Test and Exercise Tolerance Test
- Cardiac Catheterization

OBJECTIVES

1. Describe the general purposes of stress testing (exercise treadmill electrocardiographs) for healthy persons and for those with some degree of heart disease.
2. Explain what nurses should teach clients about stress testing.
3. Describe appropriate nursing interventions before and after stress tests.
4. Explain how stress test results are used to plan activity levels.
5. Compare the purposes and procedures of right-sided and left-sided cardiac catheterizations.
6. Describe appropriate nursing interventions before and after cardiac catheterization.
7. Identify expected effects of medications used before and during cardiac catheterizations.

Chapters 24 and 25 have given basic information about noninvasive and invasive testing, respectively. This chapter discusses stress testing, a noninvasive test, which, unlike other noninvasive tests, is not risk free. Although stress testing is fairly common, it is not always well understood by nurses or the general community. Even if nurses are not involved in stress testing procedures, they should be able to explain the test and the needed precautions to clients and their families. Stress tests can be very dangerous if not conducted properly. Nurses help prepare clients for the tests, sometimes help administer the test, and more often are involved in follow-up programs for cardiac rehabilitation.

The second test covered in this chapter, cardiac catheterization, is a sophisticated invasive cardiac procedure. In the past few years, as cardiac catheterization has become a common practice in most medical centers, many nurses have become involved in preparing clients for cardiac catheterizations and caring for clients during the recovery phase.

The cardiac catheterization laboratory not only requires elaborate equipment, it also requires a team of highly skilled clinicians. A cardiologist, trained to do cardiac catheterizations, heads a team comprised of various technicians, who are highly skilled in using the laboratory's monitoring equipment. Registered nurses are sometimes part of a cardiac catheterization team. In addition to being an assistant during the procedure, the nurse may also help prepare the client for the procedure and do a follow-up assessment. (Several of the references used in this chapter were written by nurses who function as part of a cardiac catheterization team.)

■ STRESS TESTS: ECG TREADMILL TEST AND EXERCISE TOLERANCE TEST

Description. The forerunner of the modern heart stress test was the Master's two-step test, which involved stepping up and down on a 20-cm platform 30 times a minute while an ECG recorded the effect of the stress on the heart. The more modern stress test is done in a cardiology laboratory, which is set up to monitor blood pressure, ECG, and sometimes oxygen consumption while the client exercises by walking on a treadmill. The treadmill is speeded up at intervals and the pitch is changed to determine the exercise tolerance of the person. The test is continued until a predetermined end-point has been obtained or the client shows signs of undue fatigue. A stationary exercise bicycle called a bicycle ergometer, which is portable and cheaper than a treadmill can be used. However, it is not as easy to standardize the results because many people develop thigh muscle fatigue before they reach their maximum heart rate. The bicycle ergometer is more common in Europe.

When assessing exercise tolerance in cardiac clients, a physician must be present so the test can be stopped if certain clinical symptoms or dangerous arrhythmias develop. For a healthy person undergoing exercise tolerance testing, a physician or qualified delegate can observe the client's response while on the treadmill. A certification examination for stress exercise testing is given by the American College of Sports Medicine (Sivarajan & Halpenny, 1979). Nurses must realize that stress testing can be a dangerous procedure if not handled properly. Only qualified people should conduct the tests. The American Heart Association (1979) has excellent information on quality control for operation of an exercise tolerance laboratory.

Before beginning the test, the client must be told exactly what to expect and that he or she can stop the test at any time, but the test is of greater value if the exercise is continued until a certain predetermined level is obtained. The predetermined levels are arbitrarily set, based on the client's age and expected response to a certain level of exercise. Tables show the usual maximal heart rate for different ages. The target heart rate to be achieved may be up to 85% of the estimate for the maximal heart rate for a certain age. For example, an untrained person age 40 may have a maximal heart rate of 189; thus, the recommended target heart rate would be 161 (American Heart Association, 1979).

The client is connected to the apparatus necessary to monitor ECG, blood pressure readings, and if oxygen consumption is done, a mouthpiece is used. Baseline measurements are taken in advance, and the physician does a brief physical assessment to clear the client for the test.

After the client has a chance to practice walking on the treadmill, the test is begun. The ECG is constantly monitored, blood pressure, heart rate, and sometimes oxygen consumption are recorded every 3 minutes.

During the test, clinicians assess for symptoms, such as vertigo, extreme dyspnea, pallor, or signs of exhaustion. Depending on the ECG reading and other circumstances, the client may be allowed to continue with mild or moderate angina, but severe angina necessitates an abrupt end of the test. Leg fatigue or severe pain in the calves of the leg (claudication) may also necessitate a halt of the test.

Other reasons to stop the test would be (Janz & Lampman, 1981):

1. Fall of systolic blood pressure of 22 mm Hg
2. Marked ST segment depression
3. Ventricular tachycardia (VT)
4. Heart block, second or third degree
5. Atrial fibrillation (AF)
6. Paroxysmal atrial tachycardia (PAT)

Some people do have occasional ectopic beats with exercise so a few premature atrial contractions (PACs) or even premature ventricular contractions (PVCs) are not indications to stop the test if there is no clinical evidence of a change in cardiac output. (See Chapter 24 for a detailed discussion on common types of arrhythmias and clinical assessment for changes in cardiac output.)

Note that a thallium scan may be done in conjunction with a stress test. Thallium scans may be particularly useful for a client with multivessel coronary disease (Smeets et al., 1981). (See Chapter 22 for a discussion on cardiac imaging with thallium. The client receives thallium intravenously.)

Assessing Exercise Tolerance

When planning exercise programs, stress tests are done to evaluate the exercise tolerance of the person. The information from a stress test is useful in planning a graduated exercise program for the person. Even for people without cardiac disease, a stress test may be used to evaluate cardiovascular function to help a person train effectively.

Stress tests are even more necessary in presumably healthy persons with risk factors for coronary disease, such as hypertension, hyperlipidemia, or cigarette smoking. Persons with known heart disease are also evaluated for exercise tolerance. For example, a client with an uncomplicated myocardial infarction may have a stress test 10 days to 2 weeks after the infarction (Janz & Lampman, 1981). Stress testing may also be used to assess the exercise capacity of a client with pulmonary disease.

Computation of Energy Units: Metabolic Equivalent Levels. Metabolic equivalent level (MET) is the energy expenditure at rest, equivalent to approximately 3.5 ml O_2 per kg body weight per minute. The MET is determined by dividing the client's exercise oxygen consumption by the resting oxygen consumption. Tables can be used to determine the person's total capability in terms of METs. The American Heart Association (1975) has published charts that show the metabolic equivalent of various activities. For example, level walking at 2 miles an hour, takes about 2–3 METs, walking 4 miles an hour takes 5–6 METs, and running 6 miles per hour takes 10 METs. The charts also show the approximate metabolic cost of many occupational and recreational activities in terms of METs.

Assessing Coronary Ischemia and Arrhythmias

Stress testing is also used to help assess chest pain or arrhythmias triggered by physical stress. The stress test may allow diagnosis of early ischemia heart disease, undetected by a resting ECG. (The test can also demonstrate if there is a correlation between clinical symptoms and certain arrhythmias.)

The characteristic sign of myocardial ischemia is a depressed ST segment. The changes in the ST segment must be carefully analyzed by a cardiologist. Some clients have a drop in the ST segment when standing or hyperventilating; thus, these factors and others must be considered so as not to make a false diagnosis of coronary artery insufficiency (Wenger et al., 1980). A cardiac catheterization, discussed later in this chapter, may be needed to determine the extent and exact location of atherosclerotic plaques in the coronary arteries. Sobel and Ferguson (1985) note that many people (20–30%) who have normal stress tests still have significant heart disease and that 20–50% of the persons who have an abnormal exercise test have essentially normal coronary arteries. A new computer-aided method for analyzing treadmill exercise tests may eliminate the chance of false-positive results (Hollenberg et al., 1985).

Drugs, such as nitroglycerin, may be given during the test to evaluate their effectiveness for angina. Nitroglycerin can cause considerable improvement in exercise tolerance. Nitroglycerin causes some venous pooling and thus a reduction of left ventricular volume and some reduction of arterial pressure (Simoons, 1981).

PRETEST NURSING IMPLICATIONS

Obtaining Informed Consent. Although a stress test can yield valuable information, it is not risk free, even when clients have been carefully screened. The exercise, which is equal in stress to walking briskly or running up a steep hill, can cause severe arrhythmias, a myocardial infarction, or a stroke in susceptible persons. Most authorities quote a mortality rate of about 0.01% or one death in every 10,000 clients tested. Because of the risk of morbidity and even mortality, the client must sign an informed consent after the physician explains the benefits versus the risks. The nurse can reassure the client that trained personnel and emergency equipment will be available in the laboratory to deal with any complications that may occur.

Many institutions have written information about stress tests, including the risks and benefits of the test. One such client information sheet stresses, "You should not feel that you are being pressured or persuaded to have the test if you feel at all uncomfortable about it" (Kaiser Permanente Medical Center, 1981). People should be given *time* to digest verbal and written information and then make an informed decision. (See Chapter 25 for more about the role of the nurse as the advocate for the client who is having invasive tests or tests that can cause complications.)

Limiting Food and Fluid Intake. The client should eat a light meal a couple of hours before the test. Some clinicians prefer that the person have no beverages containing caffeine whereas others allow one cup of coffee or tea before the test. Milk or other foods, which may cause nausea during exercise, should be avoided. The person should be adequately hydrated before the test.

Administering Medications. If the client is on diuretics, assessment of the serum potassium level is done before the exercise test. Hypokalemia, often a side effect of diuretics, predisposes the person to arrhythmias. If clients are taking digitalis, they are usually not considered candidates for stress testing, but this is an individual medical decision. Nitroglycerin or other vasodilators are not given before the test, unless the test is being done to evaluate the efficiency of the medications. Pain medications, even aspirin, may invalidate the test. The nurse must confer with the physician to see what medications are permissible before the test. Clients need clear instructions on which routine medications are to be continued and which are to be withheld.

Clothing Needs. Comfortable *walking* shoes are a must for the test. Bedroom slippers, sandals, or high-heeled shoes are unsatisfactory. Rubber-soled shoes provide the best grip on the treadmill.

Men strip to the waist so electrodes can be applied to the chest area. Women can wear a bra and a hospital gown or blouse, which opens in the front. Pants, skirts, or trousers should be loose and comfortable. Constricting clothing and nylon fabrics are to be avoided. Hair should be arranged off the face, and any bothersome jewelry should be removed.

Resting before the Test. A good night's sleep before the test is essential so undue fatigue is not a factor in the results. Relaxation exercises before the test may be beneficial. The client goes through some warming up exercises and cooling down exercises in the laboratory. No other diagnostic procedures or tests should be scheduled on the same day.

POSTTEST NURSING IMPLICATIONS

Assessing Vital Signs. The client remains in the cardiology laboratory until vital signs are normal. To ensure that baseline levels have returned, ECG tracings are taken at various intervals. Very rarely, the client may need to be monitored for several hours because of an arrhythmia or other complication. If the client returns to a nursing unit, vital signs are checked at certain intervals to assess the client's stability.

Promoting Rest and Relaxation. An outpatient may be allowed to drive home, depending on the circumstances. After the test, the client should rest for the remainder of the day. A shower should not be taken for a few hours because the warm water and standing may cause vasodilation. If the client's performance level was low, the nurse can help the person ventilate his or her feelings of dejection.

Resuming Food and Fluids. Depending on the level of exertion, the person may be thirsty, and fluids should be provided. As with other exercise, hunger may be abated for a while, but diet can be normally resumed.

Planning Follow-ups. The MET levels, discussed earlier, can be helpful in gauging the expected exercise capability of the person. An individualized exercise program is planned on the basis of the various results of the stress testing. An ideal exercise plan is one which helps the person achieve the target heart rate for 30 minutes three times a week. Target heart rates may be up to 85% of the person's maximum heart rate. The American Heart Association has detailed guidelines for exercise prescriptions. Whatever the length and type of exercise prescribed by the physician, it is important that the client also understand the importance of warm-up and cooling-down exercises. Janz and Lampman (1981) and Sivarjan and Halpenny (1979) discuss the role of the nurse in conducting exercise programs.

If the stress test was done to evaluate angina and possible coronary ischemia, more diagnostic tests may be ordered by the physician. For example, the client may need instructions about cardiac catheterizations, discussed next.

■ CARDIAC CATHETERIZATION

Description. A cardiac catheterization is done under local anesthetic because the client needs to cooperate by doing some deep breathing and coughing maneuvers. (Coughing helps clear the dye from the coronary arteries.) The client may also be asked to do bicycle-type leg exercises to see the effect of stress on cardiac function and coronary blood flow. (Small children are catheterized under general anesthesia.) Depending on the information needed, a catheter may be inserted into a vein for a study of the right side of the heart or into an artery (usually the femoral artery) for a study of the left side of the heart. The catheter for cardiac catheterization is a flexible hollow tube about 2 mm wide—the thickness of a ballpoint pen refill. The tube is 100 cm, or 40 inches, long. For a left-sided catheterization, an artery is punctured by a short stubby needle and a guide wire is inserted. The catheter slides over the guide wire into the artery. The guide wire makes it possible to guide the catheter through the left atrium into the left ventricle. Fluoroscopy is used to view the catheter; the room must be darkened. (See Chapter 20 for a discussion on fluoroscopy.) For a right-sided catheterization, a vein is used, and the catheter is threaded via the vena cava into the right atrium and right ventricle.

A transseptal technique uses a small needle inserted in the right side of the heart, which is gently maneuvered through the septum to get pressure readings and blood samples from the left side of the heart. In some cases of aortic stenosis, the heart's valve cannot be crossed in the usual manner, and a transseptal technique is needed.

After the pressures and readings and blood samples are obtained, a catheter is threaded into the coronary artery and a radiopaque dye is inserted to outline the coronary arteries. This dye (Diatrizoate or Hypaque) contains iodine (see Chapter 20 for the precautions when dye with iodine is used for a diagnostic procedure). During the passage of the dye, the room is darkened so that the motion can be observed on the fluoroscope screen. Movies (cineography) may also be taken of the flow of the dye. The table is tilted to help with dye flow.

The entire procedure of a left-sided and right-sided cardiac catheterization takes about 1–2 hours, depending on the findings. However, clients may not need all the different aspects done. For example, an adolescent with a valve defect may not have studies done of the coronary arteries.

Because cardiac catheterization is an elaborate procedure requiring a specialized laboratory setup, it is not done in small hospitals or clinics.

Purposes. As mentioned earlier in this chapter, the stress test may be a preliminary test before cardiac catheterization. Cardiac catheterization is used when noninvasive forms of cardiac diagnostic tests—such as echocardiograms (Chapter 23), ECG, phonocardiograms (Chapter 24), and radionuclide scans (Chapter 22)—have not provided enough diagnostic information. As with any invasive procedure, there is a certain amount of risk for the client, and if less complicated, less risky, and less costly procedures will suffice, they are preferred.

Cardiac catheterization is often needed to confirm the need for heart surgery. For example, the need for a coronary bypass procedure is assessed by cardiac catheterization, which demonstrates the lack of coronary perfusion. Cardiac catheterization also defines the exact type of other cardiac problems, especially congenital heart defects. Cardiac catheterization can also determine the severity of the heart disease and evaluate the progress of the client after medical or surgical interventions.

Conventional cardiac catheterization measures the pressures and calculates the flows in the various chambers of the heart and "great" vessels. Blood samples are obtained to measure dilutions of dye and oxygen and carbon dioxide values. Radiopaque dye is used to take x-rays and fluoroscopy of the heart and vessels. More advanced procedures such as the His-bundle ECG or coronary sinus lactate determination are discussed in specialty texts, such as Wenger et al. (1980).

PRETEST NURSING IMPLICATIONS

Checking the Chart. The client's chart will contain the results of other diagnostic tests, such as coagulation studies and hematocrit. In addition, vital signs and other baseline data are charted as for other invasive procedures (Chapter 25). The precatheterization physical stability of the client must be assessed and documented.

Although the risks of major complications, such as a myocardial infarction or cerebral vascular accident, are slight, they sometimes occur with a catheterization. Thus, the client must sign a consent form that lists the possible complications, including such things as the possibility of a loss of a limb or cardiac arrest. Obviously, the client's physician must explain the possibility of such risks in relationship to the potential greater benefits of the procedure.

PRETEST NURSING DIAGNOSES

Anxiety Related to Lack of Knowledge about Procedure

A nurse from the cardiac catheterization laboratory or from the general unit should reinforce the explanation of the cardiac catheterization procedure. Most cardiac catheterization laboratories have client information booklets, which describe the procedure and answer common questions that clients may have about the preparation for the test. For example, Kaiser Permanente Medical Centers in Northern California have a booklet that explains not only the catheterization procedure, but also why the client must come to the San Francisco facility and be admitted to the hospital for the procedure. The booklet even contains a map of the medical center to help the referred client find the hospital and parking lot. The client checks in the night before or arrives the day of the procedure. Some institutions use audiovisual material to explain the cardiac catheterization procedure. This can be done the morning of the examination. Past studies have not shown whether it is more or less effective to have clients actually visit the cardiac laboratory before the procedure (Edwards & Payton, 1976). Without adequate preparation, viewing the "cath lab" may be anxiety-producing. Teasley (1982) has suggested a check list for teaching the client about the procedure, followed by viewing the laboratory, if feasible.

Rice et al. (1986), in a pilot study, found relaxation training did not significantly decrease anxiety before cardiac catheterization but suggest the effects need to be explored with a larger sample.

Potential for Pain and Discomfort from Cardiac Catheterization

Disch (1980) has found some clients experience much discomfort during a cardiac catheterization, whereas others do not. The anxiety level of the client seems to be an important factor. Certainly, the idea of a catheter entering one's heart is a frightening idea. The nurse should explain to the client that he or she may experience a little discomfort so that he or she does not imagine the worst. Because the positioning of the catheter may cause a rapid or irregular pulse, the client may feel his or her heart "flip-flop" or race. Therefore, it may be comforting for the client to know that arrhythmias are rather common during the threading of the catheter and usually disappear without treatment. The client should be told that there will be constant monitoring for serious arrhythmias and that emergency equipment and drugs will be present for immediate use.

Another discomfort is a venous or, even more so, an arterial puncture. A local anesthetic is used before the arterial puncture, but there is usually some pain associated with the procedure. Needles in general are very unpleasant for some people. (See Chapter 25 on ways nurses can help prepare clients for momentary pain.) The injection of the dye may be a source of pain or discomfort for some clients, because of a metallic taste, a warm feeling, or a more intense "rush" from the dye. (The symptoms of an allergic reaction can occur, but this is not common, see Chapter 20.) Another discomfort may be the length of time the client must lie relatively still on the table—this may be very taxing for some clients. Nevertheless, the discomforts should be explained to the client.

Physical Preparation of Client. The client's groin, used for the femoral puncture, should be shaved. This may be done on the unit or in the laboratory. Depending on the policy of the institution, the client may be allowed clear liquids or kept on n.p.o. status. Fluids may be withheld because of the danger of aspiration if an emergency occurs (Finesilver, 1980). The client should void and empty his or her bowels, if possible, because the procedure is a long one. The client is transported to the laboratory by stretcher. A hospital gown is worn. Glasses can be worn, as well as a watch because the client will be awake. Dentures are left in place because they may be needed if the client is to do any breathing exercises with a mouthpiece. Hearing aides should be worn if needed. The client's chart should note the presence of a hearing difficulty or any communication problems.

Use of Medications Before and During the Procedure. Routine medications are usually not withheld, but this should be checked with the cardiologist. Certain drugs, such as long-term anticoagulants, are usually contraindicated before the procedure because of the risk of bleeding. Thus, if a client has been on coumarin (Coumadin), this must be evaluated by the physician. The premedications differ from institution to institution. Atropine may be given to prevent bradycardia. Atropine is an anticholinergic drug so it decreases the vagal effect from the manipulation of the catheter. Some cardiologists prefer no sedation for clients. Others routinely order a sedative such as hydroxine (Vistaril). Antihistamines or a cortisone preparation may be ordered for clients who are allergy-prone. Some institutions have a policy to give cortisone 1–2 days before cardiac catheterization (Ventura, 1984). Test doses of the contrast medium or dye may be done, too. During the procedure the client may be given vasodilators, such as nitroglycerin, to promote arterial dilation or ergonovine to constrict the arteries. Pain medications, other than a local anesthetic, are not routine before or during the procedure. An intravenous is usually started in the laboratory, not before. Protamine is given at the end of the procedure to neutralize the effect of heparin. Clients who are on NPH insulin may have antibodies to protamine and thus have an allergic reaction (Stewart et al., 1984).

POSTTEST NURSING DIAGNOSES

Potential for Alteration in Cardiac Output
Vital signs are checked the same as for other invasive procedures. Arrhythmias usually occur during the procedure, not afterward, but an *apical* pulse should be part of the assessment each time the client's vital signs are taken. If there is any arrhythmia, the client may need to be monitored for a time (see Chapter 24 on monitoring). An intravenous line will be kept open (k/o rate) if arrhythmias have persisted. See Chapter 20 on anaphylactic reactions from contrast medium which could also cause an alteration in cardiac output.

Potential for Alteration in Tissue Perfusion
Because more than one entry site may be used, the nurse needs to check for more than one bandaged area, postcatheterization. Occasionally, a cutdown may be done to find the vessel for the catheter. If so, the client will have skin sutures at the cutdown site.

A sandbag may be kept on the arterial puncture site. The outside of the pressure dressing should be checked for any bleeding or hematoma formation. The pulse distal to the arterial puncture site should be checked and compared with the uninvolved site for a thrombus in the artery. Spasms of the artery can also cause diminished arterial flow. The venous site is less likely to have any serious complications. Phlebitis (inflammation of the vein) can develop later and may be relieved by warm compresses.

The length of bedrest will depend on whether the procedure was left-sided, right-sided, or both. Bedrest for an arterial entry may be 6–8 hours or longer. Some institutions routinely require strict bedrest until the next day (Teasley, 1982). With a venous entry bedrest may be only a few hours. The client can turn from side to side while on bedrest, but the extremity used for the arterial puncture should not be moved for several hours.

Alteration in Fluid Needs
The client can eat and drink as soon as he or she desires. An adequate intake of fluids is needed to help with the excretion of the dye. The dye, a hypertonic

solution, can create a fluid volume deficit. Clients can have delayed allergic reactions to the iodine dye so the nurse must keep this in mind when assessing any pain or discomfort (see Chapter 20 on radiopaque dyes).

Alteration in Comfort

Back pain from the positioning is common, and a backrub may be very helpful. Mild analgesics may be needed for pain at the puncture site. Pain distal to the puncture site is not expected and could mean an embolus to the extremity.

Clients undergoing catheterization usually exhibit some of the following symptoms: fatigue, dyspnea on exertion, edema, paroxysmal nocturnal dyspnea (PND), or angina. Nurses need to know what symptoms were present before catheterization so new symptoms can be noted and called to the physician's attention. New symptoms should not be masked by pain medication.

Potential for Injury Related to Cardiac Tamponade and Other Complications

In addition to arrhythmias, embolisms, and infarctions, cardiac tamponade can occur after a cardiac catheterization. Bleeding into the pericardial sac causes reduced cardiac output, as the heart is compressed in the pericardial sac. Symptoms of cardiac tamponade include anxiety, tachypnea, distended neck veins (when the client sits forward), muffled heart sounds, narrowing pulse pressure, and a paradoxic pulse. To detect a paradoxic pulse, the nurse must take the systolic blood pressure during inspiration and expiration, noting if the systolic is less during inspiration. A difference of more than 10 mm Hg in the two is evidence of a paradoxic pulse. One easy way to detect a paradoxic pulse is to ask the client to hold his or her breath after you take the first systolic reading (Kinnebrew, 1981). Any questionable symptoms or significant change in vital signs should be immediately called to the attention of the physician. Although cardiac tamponade and other complications are unlikely after a cardiac catheterization, they can occur, and the prudent nurse is always alert for adverse reactions after all invasive tests.

QUESTIONS

1. Stress tests are not useful for:

   a. Assessing the location of partially obstructed coronary arteries
   b. Evaluating postmyocardial infarction exercise tolerance
   c. Evaluating effectiveness of vasodilators for myocardial ischemia
   d. Assessing the relationship of arrhythmias to stress level

2. Mrs. Dunbar, age 48, is scheduled for a stress test tomorrow because she has had some heart palpitations while exercising. She asks the clinic nurse about the procedure. The nurse would be correct in informing Mrs. Dunbar that

   a. Blood pressure cuff and electrocardiogram leads will be used during the test
   b. A treadmill will be adjusted to decreasing and increasing speeds during the test

    c. If Mrs. Dunbar has any angina, the test will stop

    d. Clients must be admitted to the hospital in preparation for the test

3. Mr. Faber has been scheduled for a stress test in the cardiology laboratory for tomorrow morning. He had an uncomplicated myocardial infarction 2 weeks ago. Which of the following nursing interventions is most appropriate in preparing Mr. Faber for the test?

    a. Reassuring him that there are no risks from the test

    b. Keeping him on n.p.o. status before the test

    c. Giving him nitroglycerin tablets, if needed before the test

    d. Asking his family to bring him walking shoes for the test

4. Mr. Faber's stress test demonstrated that his metabolic equivalent level (MET) was 7–8. The MET is useful in determining

    a. Surgical procedures needed   **c.** Type of medications needed

    b. Activity programs   **d.** Dietary needs

5. Regina, age 16, is going for a cardiac catheterization, right-sided and left-sided, this morning. She is on digitalis and a no-added-salt (NAS) diet. Which of the following is *not* an appropriate nursing action in preparing Regina for the cardiac catheterization?

    a. Checking to see if all ordered laboratory reports are on the chart, such as PT, PTT, and Hct

    b. Allowing liquids but withholding all oral medicines

    c. Explaining that she will be awake and that she will be asked to do such maneuvers as coughing and deep breathing during the procedure

    d. Allowing Regina to wear her glasses and a watch to the cardiac catheterization laboratory

6. Regina was given 50 mg of hydroxine (Vistaril) and 0.6 mg (gr. 1/100) of atropine sulfate intramuscular (IM) before the cardiac catheterization procedure. The desired effect of atropine in relation to cardiac catheterization is to

    a. Promote sedation   **c.** Prevent bradycardia

    b. Decrease respiratory secretions   **d.** Eliminate gastrointestinal spasms

7. Regina, age 16, has just returned from the cardiac catheterization laboratory. She had a right-sided and left-sided (left femoral artery was used) catheterization with no complications, except a minor arrhythmia during the procedure. Her vital signs are stable. Which nursing action is unnecessary for the first hour that Regina is back on the unit?

    a. Keeping her left leg immobilized

    b. Offering her something to drink and telling her fluids help eliminate the dye

    c. Checking the pulses distal to the left femoral artery and comparing these with the pulses in the right foot

    d. Taking her temperature every 15 minutes for three times

REFERENCES

American Heart Association, Committee on Exercise. (1975). *Exercise testing and training of individuals with heart disease or at high risk for development. A handbook for physicians.* Dallas: National Center American Heart Association.

American Heart Association Subcommittee on Rehabilitation Target Activity Group. (1979). *Standards for adult exercise testing laboratories.* Dallas: National Center American Heart Association.

Disch, J. (1980). *Diagnostic procedures for cardiovascular diseases.* Norwalk, CT: Appleton-Century-Crofts.

Edwards, M., & Payton, V. (1976). Cardiac catheterization, technique and teaching. *Nursing Clinics of North America, 11,* 271–281.

Finesilver, C. (1980). Reducing stress in patients having cardiac catheterizations. *AJN, 80*(10), 1805–1807.

Hollenberg, M., et al. (1985). Comparison of a quantitative treadmill exercise score with standard electrocardiographic criteria in screening asymptomatic young men for coronary artery disease. *NEJM, 313*(10), 600–606.

Janz, N., & Lampman, R. (1981). The treadmill stress test. *Nursing 81, 11*(12), 37–41.

Kaiser Permanente Medical Center. (1981). *Instructions for Exercise Treadmill Electrocardiogram: Patient Information Sheet.* San Francisco: Kaiser Medical Center.

Kinnebrew, M. (1981). Add paradoxical pulse to your assessment routine. *RN, 44*(11), 32–33.

Rice, V., Caldwell, M., Butler, S., & Robinson, J. (1986). Relaxation training and response to cardiac catheterization: A pilot study. *Nursing Research, 35*(1), 39–43.

Simoons, M. (1981). The effects of drugs on the exercise electrocardiogram. *Cardiology, 68*(Suppl. 2), 124–131.

Sivarajan, E., & Halpenny, J. (1979). Exercise testing. *AJN, 79*(12), 2163–2170.

Smeets, J. P., et al. (1981). Prognostic value of thallium-201-stress myocardial scintography with exercise ECG after myocardial infarction. *Cardiology, 68*(Suppl. 2), 67–70.

Sobel, D., & Ferguson, T. (1985). *The people's book of medical tests.* New York: Summit Books.

Stewart, W. J., et al. (1984). Increased risk of severe protamine reactions in NPH insulin-dependent diabetics undergoing cardiac catheterization. *Circulation, 70*(5), 788.

Teasley, D. (1982). Don't let cardiac catheterization strike fear in your patient's heart. *Nursing 82, 12*(3), 52–56.

Ventura, B. (1984). What you need to know about cardiac catheterization. *RN, 47*(9), 24–30.

Wenger, N., et al. (1980). *Cardiology for Nurses.* New York: McGraw-Hill.

27

Endoscopic Procedures

- Bronchoscopy
- Gastroscopy
- Esophagogastroduodenoscopy (EGD)
- Endoscopic Retrograde Choledochopancreatography (ERCP)
- Sigmoidoscopy or Proctoscopy (Proctosigmoidoscopy)
- Colonoscopy and Enteroscopy
- Cystoscopy
- Laparoscopy and Culdoscopy
- Arthroscopy

OBJECTIVES

1. Describe nursing assessments for seven possible complications, which may occur after endoscopic procedures.
2. Identify at least five general nursing diagnoses for clients undergoing endoscopic procedures.
3. Compare and contrast the nursing interventions before and after clients have bronchoscopies, gastroscopies, or other endoscopic procedures involving the upper airway.
4. Identify areas for client teaching about sigmoidoscopy and other endoscopic procedures of the lower gastrointestinal tract.
5. Identify endoscopic procedures requiring standard pre- and postoperative care due to general anesthesia.
6. Describe nursing interventions for a client after a cystoscopy, under local anesthesia.

Endoscopes are used for direct visualization of hollow organs or body cavities. Specifically designed endoscopes are named for the cavity that is being viewed, such as a gastroscope, bronchoscope, or sigmoidoscope. See Table 27-1 for a complete list of endoscopic procedures. The scopes contain lights so that the interior or cavity of the organ can be seen. The scopes are hollow instruments with suction tips, biopsy forceps, and other accessories for obtaining tissue samples. Electrodes for cauterization may also be an accessory. Photocoagulation can be used to actually control gastrointestinal bleeding and gallstones can be removed with a special adaptor. Endoscopes are also used with lasers to vaporize small tumors and cysts and to cut more precisely than a scalpel (Freeman, 1986). Cameras can be used to record the findings for later reference.

Earlier scopes were all rigid instruments, but newer models are flexible nylon tubes, which can more easily be advanced into a body cavity, such as the intestinal tract. Fiberscopes or fiberoptic scopes are made of strands of glass fibers that reflect light and actually make it possible to see around corners. A flexible fiberscope can be threaded from the mouth into the duodenum (duodenoscopy) or from the rectum through the ileocecal valve into the small bowel (enteroscopy). The first fiberscopes were used in the early 1960s and much improvement has been made since then (Salmon, 1974). Industry also uses fiberoptic instruments to peer into cavities, such as automobile engines, so that the engine does not have to be dismantled (Hirschowitz, 1979).

POSSIBLE COMPLICATIONS FROM ENDOSCOPIC PROCEDURES

Although endoscopic procedures cause some pain and discomfort, topical anesthetics make the procedure tolerable for an alert, cooperative client. An endoscopic procedure may save the client the risk and expense of a surgical procedure, under general anesthesia. Specific complications for the different types of endoscopic procedures

TABLE 27-1. AREAS VISUALIZED BY ENDOSCOPIC PROCEDURES

Name of Procedure	Area Visualized[a]
Arthroscopy	Knee joint
Bronchoscopy	Bronchial tree
Colposcopy	Vagina and cervix (see Chapter 25)
Culdoscopy	Female pelvic organs
Cystoscopy	Urinary bladder
Endoscopic retrograde choledocho-pancreatography (ERCP or ECPG)	Common bile duct and pancreatic duct
Enteroscopy	Upper colon and small intestine
Esophagoscopy	Esophagus
Esophagogastroduodenoscopy (EGD)	Esophagus to small intestine
Fetoscopy	In amniotic sac to view fetus (see Chapter 28)
Gastroscopy	Stomach
Laparoscopy	Abdominal cavity
Proctoscopy	Anus and rectum
Sigmoidoscopy	Sigmoid colon

[a]Preparation discussed in this chapter unless noted.

will be covered later, but there are at least seven possible risks from any type of endoscopic procedure. These major risks are:

1. The possibility of perforation of the organ or cavity being scoped.
2. Aspiration of saliva or gastric contents when the upper airway or esophagus is being scoped.
3. Untoward reactions to the drugs used, which include topical anesthetics and medications such as meperidine (Demerol) and diazepam (Valium). Narcotics, tranquilizers, or other sedatives may be used both before the test and during the test to help relax the client. The major side effects of the above drugs are respiratory depression and hypotension. Other specific drugs may also be used during the scope and can cause other side effects.
4. Cardiovascular problems, such as arrythmias and even myocardial infarction, can occur due to the psychological and physical stress of the procedure. A vasovagal effect can be stimulated. The vagus can cause bradycardia because the effect of the vagus is to slow the heart.
5. Hemorrhage can occur, particularly if a biopsy has been done as part of the diagnostic scope.
6. Infections may develop. Transient bacteremia may also occur. The danger of this bacteremia is further explored in the section on cystoscopes.
7. In a survey of 10,000 endoscopic procedures in which iodinated contrast medium was locally instilled, the incidence of hypersensitivity was 0.3% compared with 10% for IV delivery (Sable et al., 1983). Because locally instilled dye reaches peak serum levels after the endoscopy is completed, clients should be monitored for delayed reactions (see Chapter 20 on contrast medium).

The risks of these complications are low and the exact rates of occurrence depend on the skill of the clinician doing the procedure, the physical status of the client and the type of instrumentation used. Because of the possible risks mentioned, the physician has the client sign a special consent form (see Chapter 25 on consent forms). This form should be on the client's chart before any sedative medications are given. Baseline studies, hematocrit and urinalysis are routine in most clinic and inpatient settings. Coagulation studies (i.e., partial thromboplastin time (PTT) and platelet studies) are needed if bleeding is a potential problem. If the client has had any other diagnostic tests before the endoscopy, those results should be available on the chart.

GENERAL PRETEST NURSING DIAGNOSES

Anxiety Related to Unknowns about Procedure
Because the client will usually be awake during the procedure, he or she should understand the general procedure. As emphasized in Chapter 25 most clients particularly want to know how the procedure "feels" (Johnson & Rice, 1974). Some clients may want a detailed explanation of the technical aspects, others do not. Clients should also be told what causes the sensations—if they know what to expect they are less likely to misinterpret the experience. Physical sensations should be described but not evaluated by the nurse because this may create more anxiety (McHugh et al., 1982).

Because the endoscopy is done in a specialized procedure room or operating room, the nurse is usually not present during the actual procedure. Thus, the nurse performs his or her anxiety relieving function well before the client goes for the examination. As with other diagnostic tests, the nurse can reinforce the information given by the physician and try to find out answers to those questions that continue to bother the client about the test. Nurses who work in the procedure rooms will have specific functions during the test, but can also focus on helping clients deal with anxious feelings.

Knowledge Deficit Regarding Needed Physical Preparation

With the exception of sigmoidoscopy and culdoscopy (vagina visualization), all the endoscopic procedures discussed in this chapter require that the client maintain n.p.o. status. Vital signs must be taken as baseline data, and a notation should be made of the client's general physical status before the examination, e.g., a client may have abdominal cramps before the examination or shortness of breath. Any preprocedural complaints should be documented in the nurse's notes. The client should be informed of the frequency of routine vital signs after the procedure so that he or she will not be alarmed by the frequency of the assessments done after the procedure. The client should void before the procedure so he or she will not have to urinate during the procedure. The client should be told that the premedications used may cause drowsiness, euphoria or a feeling of "not self." If general anesthesia is planned, the client should be instructed on deep breathing and coughing exercises and other standard postoperative care. The nurse must protect the client from injury by keeping the client on bedrest, with side rails up after the premedications are given.

GENERAL POSTTEST NURSING DIAGNOSES

Potential for Injury due to Adverse Reactions or Complications

The frequency with which to record the client's vital signs is determined by the routine practices discussed for other invasive procedures in Chapter 25. The client may want to rest, because the procedures are somewhat of an ordeal. The nurse should check for specific complications each time vital signs are taken. The nurse should particularly assess for bleeding if a biopsy was part of the procedure. The nurse needs to know what medicines were used both pretest and during the test so that untoward reactions can be noted. See the earlier discussion on seven possible complications.

Alteration in Comfort due to Pain

Mild analgesics may be needed when local anesthetics wear off. Because severe pain could be due to a perforation, any severe or persistent pain should be carefully assessed. The risk of perforation increases if laser therapy was part of an endoscopic procedure (Zettel, 1986).

Potential for Ineffective Airway Clearance

For scopes that involve entry via the throat, the gag reflex can be abolished by administration of a topical anesthetic. With flexible scopes, a topical anesthetic may not be needed. The nurse must check to see if a local anesthetic was used. Even though the client can swallow, he or she may still not have a gag reflex. The return of the gag reflex can be checked by gently touching a tongue blade to the back of the throat. Once the gag reflex returns, the client is allowed to resume whatever diet is tolerated.

Knowledge Deficit Regarding Home Care

Any specific instructions for follow-ups, such as sitz baths or warm gargles, should be explained to the client. If the client is going home after the diagnostic procedure, he or she needs explicit instructions on symptoms that should be reported immediately to the physician or clinic. The client should be accompanied by a friend or family member who in addition to driving the client home, can also be taught what to look for because the drugs used during the procedure can produce some amnesia in the client.

■ BRONCHOSCOPY

Description and Purposes. For a bronchoscopy, a lighted bronchoscope is passed into the bronchial tree. A local anesthetic may be sprayed or swabbed on the throat. The client lies on his or her back with the head hyperextended. The bronchoscope is inserted via the nose or mouth into the trachea and main stem bronchi. The client must breathe around the tube. This can cause a fear of suffocation. It is very important that the client be relaxed and not fight the tube. Oxygen may be administered to assist respirations. A visualization of the mucosa of the bronchi shows the surgeon what area needs to be biopsied when cancer is suspected. Bronchial washings or brush biopsies can be obtained for culturing fungi, acid-fast bacilli, *Pneumocystis carinii,* and *Legionella pneumophila.* (Immune deficient clients are prone to parasitic infections such as *Pneumocystis carinii* and simple sputum cultures do not identify the organism.) Bronchoscopy is also used therapeutically to remove foreign objects or to do deep suctioning. For suctioning, the bronchoscopy may be done at the client's bedside, but is usually done in the operating room or a specially equipped room. The bronchoscopy is usually done under a topical anesthetic or with some parenteral sedation. Sometimes general anesthesia is used. Bronchograms (Chapter 20) are sometimes done as part of a bronchoscopy when it is necessary to see the outline of the bronchial tree by x-ray.

PRETEST NURSING IMPLICATIONS

Completing Routine Preoperative Care. Most institutions have a routine preoperative check list, which is completed before a bronchoscopy. The consent form must be signed. Hematocrit and urinalysis must be done. The client is kept on n.p.o. status for about 6–8 hours before the procedure. The client may be on expectorants a few days before the bronchoscopy to clear the respiratory tract. Good mouth care is important before the procedure, so that less bacteria are present in the mouth. Dentures must be removed, and the physician must be warned of any loose teeth.

Patient Teaching. During the procedure, breathing is done through the nose with the mouth open. The client may need time to practice this. The client will not be able to talk while the bronchoscope is in his or her throat; therefore, the nurse should explain that the client will have to communicate by hand signals.

Administering Medications. The pretest medications given parenterally usually include atropine (to dry up respiratory secretions), a narcotic—

meperidine (Demerol), and a sedative or minor tranquilizer such as diazepam (Valium). Diazepam is also a muscle relaxant, which helps with the passage of the tube. As noted in the general nursing diagnoses respiratory depression can occur.

POSTTEST NURSING DIAGNOSES

Potential for Ineffective Airway Clearance
The client is kept in a semi-Fowler's position, but may be turned to either side. The client should not smoke. Tissues and a paper bag are needed for the expectorations. An emesis basin, lined with tissue, may be useful for copious secretions. (Lining the basin makes it much easier to empty.) Once the gag reflex has returned, encouraging fluids to keep the client well hydrated makes secretions less viscous and easier to expectorate. Vigorous coughing after a biopsy could loosen a clot. A suction machine should be available. Some institutions have routine orders for oxygen for 4 hours postbronchoscopy (Cameron, 1981). Arterial blood gases are used to assess any persistent hypoxemia. Because severe respiratory embarrassment can occur, a tracheostomy set should also be nearby. An absence of breath sounds may indicate a pneumothorax. Subcutaneous emphysema (a collection of air in tissues) can occur if there is a leak in the pleural space. (See the discussion on thoracentesis or pleural taps in Chapter 25.) Some pink-tinged mucus or small amounts of blood in the sputum are not unusual after the bronchoscope, but hemoptysis can signal hemorrhage from a biopsy site.

Alteration in Comfort
The client should not do much talking. A pad and pencil can be used for communication. Fluids, particularly warm fluids which are soothing, are encouraged once the gag reflex has returned. A gargle with warm saline may help relieve throat discomfort. Throat lozenges may be used, too. A soft diet may be better tolerated if swallowing is painful. The client may be very anxious to hear the results of the biopsy because this test is often the determinant of whether malignancy of the lung is operable.

Knowledge Deficit Related to Bronchogram
If a bronchogram was done (Chapter 20) the client may be instructed on postural drainage. If dye was used, this is another reason to force as much fluid as is tolerated so the dye can be eliminated quickly. The dye will cause a fever as a result of the chemical irritation to the lungs. The physician should be notified if the fever persists more than 2 days (Sobel & Ferguson, 1985).

■ GASTROSCOPY

Description and Purposes. A gastroscopy may include viewing the esophagus (esophagoscopy), as well as the interior of the stomach. The presence of any ulcers can be verified and a biopsy taken. If the client has a gastrointestinal bleed, it may be possible to actually control the bleeding with photocoagulation so early endoscopic treatment may be advisable.

All endoscopic examinations of the upper gastrointestinal tract are performed with the client in the left lateral recumbent position. The client can easily swallow the newer flexible instruments and will not gag if relaxed and properly sedated (Grossman, 1980).

There is sometimes retching as the tube is passed, but usually not vomiting. Most physicians give a small dose of diazepam (Valium 5 mg) and meperidine (Demerol 50 mg) intravenously just prior to the procedure to help relax the client. A gastroscopy is done in a specially equipped procedure room or operating room. Note that the older nonflexible gastroscopes required an anesthetic to be sprayed on the throat to prevent gagging and to reduce discomfort (Salmon, 1974). With the newer flexible scopes, even a local anesthetic may not be used unless laser therapy is planned. There is, therefore, less danger of aspiration of secretions into the lung. General anesthesia is not routinely used.

PRETEST NURSING IMPLICATIONS

The general preoperative preparation is done, including consent forms and laboratory work. As with a bronchoscopy, it is very important that dentures be removed and the client checked for any loose teeth. The client is kept on n.p.o. status for 6–8 hours before the procedure. The usual sedatives and narcotics may be given before the procedure, or sedation may be given intravenously in the procedure room. Studies have shown clients require less analgesia and have less tension if they are given sensory information about the procedure (Stiklorius, 1982b). Mouthcare is important, but not as critical as with a bronchoscopy because the stomach normally receives bacteria from the mouth area.

POSTTEST NURSING IMPLICATIONS

The client may be kept in a semi-Fowler's position or turned to the side to help expectorate any fluids. The standard vital sign routine is followed, as well as careful checking for any signs of gastric bleeding. If a local anesthetic was used, no liquids are allowed until the gag reflex returns (see bronchoscopy care). Warm saline gargles may be used to relieve a sore throat or throat lozenges can be used. The client may prefer to rest, rather than eat anything even after the gag reflex has returned. Liquids and soft bland food may be needed until the soreness disappears. As with other procedures, the use of drugs may cause specific posttest reactions.

■ ESOPHAGOGASTRODUODENOSCOPY (EGD)

Description and Purposes. A special fiberscope may be passed down into the duodenum. The client may have his or her throat sprayed with a local anesthetic or given an oral lidocaine (Xylocaine) solution. The drugs used for sedation are usually those described in the introduction to this chapter, meperidine (Demerol) and diazepam (Valium). In addition to these two drugs for sedation, atropine may also be given intravenously. Atropine, an anticholinergic drug, controls gastrointestinal spasms because it blocks the vagal effect on the bowel. (Gastrointestinal motility is stimulated by the vagus.) Two side effects of atropine are a dry mouth and possible tachycardia. Atropine can produce tachycardia because it blocks the slowing effect of the vagus on the heart. Glucagon may also be given to slow peristalsis. The nurse needs to be aware of the drugs used before and *during* the procedure so that side effects can be quickly noted. The pre- and postcare of the client with an EGD is similar to the care for gastroscopy discussed above. The client may burp large amounts of air after the procedure (Beck, 1981).

■ ENDOSCOPIC RETROGRADE CHOLEDOCHOPANCREATOGRAPHY (ERCP)

Description and Purposes. Endoscopic retrograde choledochopancreatography is usually referred to by the initials ERCP or ECPG. The procedure involves the passage of a flexible fiberscope through the mouth, stomach, and into the duodenum, as for a EGD discussed above. When the endoscope reaches the ampulla of Vater, dye is injected to outline the common bile duct and the pancreatic ducts. X-rays are taken of the biliary tree (cholangiogram). ERCP is an important diagnostic tool for the client with ·cholestatic jaundice (Scharschmidt et al., 1983). The usual precautions before and after an esophagoscopy or gastroscopy are applicable to the scope of the upper gastrointestinal tract. The additional concerns related to the injection of dye into the biliary system are covered in the section on cholangiograms (Chapter 20). Possible complications from ERCP are acute pancreatitis, cholangitis, pancreatic abscess, drug reactions, and instrument injury (Burdick, 1978). Serum amylase and lipase levels are useful in assessing for pancreatitis (see Chapter 12). ERCP can be combined with a surgical procedure, (sphincterotomy) to actually remove a gallstone from the common bile duct. Transient pancreatitis after sphincterotomy is considered normal and the client has an elevated amylase for a few days (Peternel, 1985).

■ SIGMOIDOSCOPY OR PROCTOSCOPY (PROCTOSIGMOIDOSCOPY)

Description and Purposes. Sigmoidoscopes are used to view the lower colon or sigmoid, and proctoscopes are used to view the anus and rectal areas. When the scope is put through the rectal sphincter, the client has a strong sensation of a need to defecate. The client is usually in a knee–chest position or lying on the left side with the knees bent (Sim's position). The knee–chest position is not needed with the newer flexible sigmoidoscope. The flexible sigmoidoscope also causes little discomfort so no sedation is required. Warming the instrument may make the insertion less uncomfortable. Examination by an experienced endoscopist can take less than 5 minutes (Grossman, 1980).

Scopes of the lower colon are used to detect and biopsy polyps and tumors. The clinician can sometimes see the exact site of bleeding or the extent of an inflammatory process. Because most of the cancer of the large intestine is in the lower colon, the sigmoidoscopy is a useful detection tool for cancer.

The American Cancer Society used to recommend a yearly sigmoidoscopy for all people after age 40. The latest recommendation (American Cancer Society, 1980) is an examination every 3–5 years after age 50, once the person has had two negative sigmoidoscopies a year apart. A digital rectal exam is still recommended as a yearly examination for clients over age 40. Guaiacs of stool are recommended yearly after age 50. (See Chapter 13 for tests for occult blood and cancer detection.) Nurses should help educate the public on the usefulness of rectal examinations to detect cancer of the lower colon.

PRETEST NURSING IMPLICATIONS

If the client has been taking iron pills, these are usually discontinued several days before the examination. The client may have a light meal the evening before the examination and clear liquids the day of the examination. Bowel preparation usually includes two cleansing enemas an hour or two before the examination. A laxative is not given because this may move stool down into the sigmoid area. As a general rule, the client is not given sedation. The client may take enemas at home if the sigmoidoscopy is done on an outpatient basis. As with other diagnostic tests, stress reduction is an important nursing function to ensure maximum cooperation (Stiklorius 1982a).

POSTTEST NURSING IMPLICATIONS

The standard routines for vital signs and checking for bleeding are followed. The client will probably need to rest for awhile. A warm sitz bath may be relaxing if the condition permits. The client may have some mild abdominal cramping because of the air instilled for the test.

■ COLONOSCOPY AND ENTEROSCOPY

Description and Purposes. These procedures use flexible fiberscopes to view the upper colon and small intestine. Sedation is required but not general anesthesia. Glucagon is given intravenously to decrease any intestinal spasms. Food is withheld for 6–8 hours and the bowel preparation must be extensive. Sometimes polyps are biopsied and cauterized during a colonoscopy. There is a rare risk of a fatal explosion of colonic gases if electrocautery is used in a poorly prepared colon (Grossman, 1980). In a well-prepared colon, there is little danger from electrocautery.

PRETEST NURSING IMPLICATIONS

The client may be on a clear liquid diet for a day or two before the examination. Laxatives and suppositories will be used as well as cleansing enemas just before the examination. Other nursing implications are similar to those for other endoscopic procedures.

POSTTEST NURSING DIAGNOSIS

Alteration in Comfort Related to Flatus
The client may have abdominal cramps after the procedure because of the air injected during the examination. Lower endoscopic laser treatments with colonoscopy and flexible sigmoidoscopy also creates distention and cramps. A rectal tube may be used, depending upon the site of treatment (Zettel, 1986). Changing positions or walking, if permissible, can also relieve gas pains.

■ CYSTOSCOPY

Description and Purposes. The cystoscope is passed through the urethra into the bladder so the interior of the bladder can be examined for inflammation, tumors, stones, or structural abnormalities. For some diagnostic workups, such as for interstitial cystitis, it is necessary that the bladder be distended during examination to assess for changes in the mucosal lining of the bladder. Small stones may be removed via the cystoscope. Ureteral catheters may be passed into each ureter to obtain samples of urine from the pelvis of each kidney. A radiopaque dye may be injected to do a retrograde pyelogram (see Chapter 20). A cystoscope can be done with topical anesthesia, but more extensive procedures require the use of general or spinal anesthesia. The topical anesthetic is in jelly form and is put into the urethra. The discomfort may be similar to that of a catheterization.

PRETEST NURSING IMPLICATIONS

Routine preparations are done in relation to consent forms, vital sign checks, laboratory work, and so on. If the client is to have general anesthesia, he or she should be instructed on routine deep breathing and coughing and other routines for postgeneral anesthesia. The client is allowed a full liquid diet if the procedure is to be done under a local anesthetic. The client may be started on prophylactic antibacterials.

POSTTEST NURSING DIAGNOSES

Potential for Bleeding
The standard vital sign routine is followed. Some hematuria is not uncommon, but the client should be carefully watched for hemorrhage if a biopsy was done. The client may be on bedrest for up to 4 hours. If the procedure was done in a urology clinic, the client and the client's family should be instructed on these routine assessments and the other pertinent aftercare.

Potential for Urinary Retention
The client's intake and output should be monitored for at least 24 hours. The adult client should have an intake of 2500–3000 ml, unless contraindicated. If

the client does not have a Foley catheter, the nurse must check for the possibility of urinary retention with overflow. Small amounts, 50–100 ml frequently, may be a sign of urinary retention with overflow. Cholinergic drugs, such as beth-anechol chloride (Urecholine), may be needed to stimulate bladder contraction. If the client has a Foley catheter, it must be kept connected to a sterile drainage system.

The client may have a ureteral catheter. These catheters are very tiny and are usually fastened on a splint. It is important that there not be any tension on the catheter or any kinking. Nurses do not routinely irrigate ureteral catheters. If the catheter is to be irrigated, only a few cubic centimeters of sterile normal saline are used because the kidney pelvis holds only about 5 cc of urine. Because the kidney pelvis does not have room for much collection of urine, it is very important that the physician be notified if a ureteral catheter is not draining properly.

Potential for Infection

Clients are sometimes given antibacterials after a cystoscope because of the high possibility of urinary tract infections from the instrumentation. Any break in the tissue of the bladder may let bacteria into the bloodstream; consequently, the client may have chills and fever from a transient bacteremia. This transient bacteremia may be dangerous for the client with mitral valve disease because bacterial endocarditis can occur. The client should be instructed about the signs of urinary tract infection, such as burning on urination or cloudy, foul-smelling urine. Some burning after urination is expected the first day after instrumenta-tion. A urinalysis is usually obtained as part of the posttest procedure. (See Chapter 3 for interpretation of routine urinalysis and Chapter 16 for culture and sensitivity tests.)

Alteration in Comfort Related to Bladder Spasms

The client may have some pain when urinating (dysuria) and bladder spasms. Sometimes anticholinergic drugs, such as methantheline bromide (Banthine), are given for bladder spasms. Mild analgesics may also be needed such as phenazopyridine (Pyridium). If permitted, warm tub baths may be soothing. Clients with interstitial cystitis may need instructions on foods and drugs which irritate the bladder wall.

■ LAPAROSCOPY AND CULDOSCOPY

Description and Purposes. An instrument can be used to inspect the pelvic viscera. If the instrument is inserted into the abdomen through a small incision in the lower abdominal wall, the procedure is called a laparoscopy. The procedure may be done under general anesthesia. Laparoscopic examination is sometimes done to help diagnose infertility (see Chapter 28). Minor surgical procedures and tubal ligations are also done by laparoscopy. Surgery done via the laparoscope is sometimes called "Band-Aid" surgery, because the incision, only 1 or 2 cm long, requires a very small dressing.

The culdoscope is an instrument similar to the laparoscope and also permits direct visual examination of the female viscera. The culdoscope is introduced into the pelvic cavity through a very small incision in the vaginal posterior fornix. The woman is placed in a knee–chest position. Culdoscopy may be done under general anesthesia. Culdoscopy has been largely replaced by laparoscopy (Sobel & Ferguson, 1985) (see Chapter 24 on colposcopy).

NURSING IMPLICATIONS

If a laparoscopy is done under light, general anesthesia the client needs routine preoperative preparation. A Foley catheter is usually inserted to keep the bladder deflated. Aftercare is the standard care discussed in the beginning of this chapter. If a culdoscopy was done, the woman should not douche or have sexual intercourse until the incision heals, which takes about a week.

Gas injected into the abdominal cavity during the laparoscopy can irritate the diaphragm and cause referred pain in the shoulder area. Clients can be assured the pain disappears in a day or two. Mild analgesics may be needed.

■ ARTHROSCOPY

Description and Purposes. An arthroscope is a fiberoptic endoscope used to examine the interior of joints. Although other joints can be visualized, the common arthroscopic procedure involves the knee joint. Arthroscopy of the interior of the knee joint can directly reveal injuries to the meniscus as well as other abnormalities. Normal saline is used to flush the knee and to remove loose bodies and allow easier scope management. Minor surgical repairs can also be done by the use of the arthroscope. General anesthesia is used if surgical repair is anticipated or if the client has a lot of pain. Arthroscopic surgery is another of the "Band-Aid" surgeries, made possible by fiberoptic endoscopes and microscopic surgical instruments.

NURSING IMPLICATIONS

Pre- and postprocedure care depend on whether the client has had local or general anesthesia. Nursing diagnoses discussed in the beginning of this chapter are pertinent. In addition, the nurse should assess for any possible infection, which can be serious in a joint. Some clients may be given prophylactic antibiotics when joints are entered to prevent osteomyelitis. Ice bags may be used to reduce postprocedure swelling. Any limitations on weight bearing are related to the procedure done. See Chapter 20 on arthrograms, which may be done with an arthroscopy.

QUESTIONS

1. The nurse should assess for all these potential complications from endoscopic procedures *except*

   a. Shock due to perforation of a body organ

   b. Hemorrhage due to bleeding from a biopsy site

    c. Oversedation due to the use of sedatives before or during the procedure

    d. Burns from the light on the end of the instrument

2. Mr. Kent is scheduled for a bronchoscopy today. Which of the following preparations is not part of the routine before a client has a bronchoscopy done under a local anesthetic?

    a. Administration of atropine and a sedative

    b. Special emphasis on mouth care

    c. Explaining to the client that he should not talk much after the procedure

    d. Teaching the client how to breathe in and out through the mouth with a noseclip on the nose

3. When a client has had an anesthetic sprayed on the throat, the assessment that determines the client can have fluids is

    a. Ability to swallow without discomfort

    b. Presence of gag reflex when a tongue blade touches the back of throat

    c. Absence of nausea or abdominal distention

    d. Presence of active bowel sounds

4. Clients should be taught that the American Cancer Society's latest recommendation (1980) for routine sigmoidoscopies after two negative examinations a year apart is

    a. Annually for all people over 40   **c.** Every 3–5 years after age 40

    b. Annually for all people over 50   **d.** Every 3–5 years after age 50

5. Standard nursing care following general anesthesia is most often necessary for a client having a (an):

    a. Laparoscopy   **c.** Gastroscopy

    b. Enteroscopy   **d.** Proctoscopy

6. Nursing interventions after a client has had a cystoscopy under local anesthesia would include all *except;*

    a. Putting the client on I&O for at least 24 hours

    b. Checking for urinary retention with overflow

    c. Keeping the patient on n.p.o. status for 4–6 hours after the procedure

    d. Assessing for bladder spasms and giving ordered analgesics PRN

REFERENCES

American Cancer Society. (1980). *Report on the cancer-related health checkup.* New York: American Cancer Society, Inc.

Beck, M. (1981). Preparing your patient physically for an esophagogastroduodenoscopy. *Nursing 81, 11*(2), 88–96.

Burdick, G. (1978). Endoscopic retrograde cholangiopancreatography. *Arizona Medicine, 35,* 655–656.

Cameron, T. (1981). Fiberoptic bronchoscopy. *AJN, 81*(9), 1462–1464.

Grossman, M. (1980). Gastrointestinal endoscopy. *Ciba Clinical Symposia, 32*(3).

Freeman, D. (1986). Lasers in the OR. *AJN, 86*(3), 278–282.

Hirschowitz, B. (1979). A personal history of the fiberscope. *Gastroenterology, 76,* 864–869.

Johnson, J.E., & Rice, V.H. (1974). Sensory and distress components of pain: Implications for study of clinical pain. *Nursing Research, 23,* 203–209.

McHugh, N., et al. (1982). Preparatory information: What helps and why. *AJN, 82*(5), 780–782.

Peternel, E. (1985). A high-tech approach to a GI problem. *RN, 48*(6), 44–47.

Sable, R., et al. (1983). Absorption of contrast medium during ERCP. *Digestive Diseases and Science, 28,* 801–806.

Salmon, P. (1974). *Fibre-optic endoscopy.* London, England: Pitman Medical.

Scharschmidt, R., et al. (1983). Current concepts in diagnostic approach to the patient with cholestatic jaundice. *NEJM, 308,* 1515–1519.

Sobel, D., & Ferguson, D. (1985). *The people's book of medical tests.* New York: Summit.

Stiklorius, C. (1982a). Large bowel diagnostics challenge your stress-reduction skills. *RN, 45*(5), 56.

Stiklorius, C. (1982b). Fair warning for patients facing esophagoscopy and gastroscopy. *RN, 45*(6), 64–65.

Zettel, E. (1986). Beaming in on the G.I. tract. *AJN, 86*(3), 280–282.

28

Diagnostic Procedures Related to Childbearing Years

- Basal Body Temperature (BBT) and Ovulation Tests
- Semen Analysis
- Postcoital Examination: Sims–Huhner Test (Huhner Test)
- Tubal Patency Tests, Hysterosalpingogram, and Tubal Insufflation (Rubin's Test)
- Amniocentesis

  Amniocentesis for Prenatal Diagnosis of Genetic Defects: Three Major Assessments, Alpha-Fetoprotein in the Serum, Amniocentesis in Isoimmune Disease (Rh Factor), Amniocentesis for Assessing Fetal Maturity, and Other Tests on Amniotic Fluid for Fetal Maturity
- Chorionic Villi Biopsy (CVB)
- Fetoscopy
- Fetal Monitoring Nonstress Test (NST)
- Oxytocin Challenge Test (OCT)

OBJECTIVES

1. Identify appropriate nursing diagnoses for clients undergoing tests related to reproduction.
2. Explain client instruction needed for each of the five basic infertility tests.
3. Describe some basic facts about amniocentesis and chorionic villi biopsy that are helpful in planning nursing care for a couple, where the woman is to have a procedure for prenatal genetic diagnosis.
4. Name some common genetic diseases that are detected by three types of tests of amniotic fluid or chorionic villi biopsy.
5. Explain the therapeutic value of amniocentesis in assessment of iso-immune disease (Rh factor).
6. Explain the clinical significance of determining lecithin-sphingomyelin ratio (L/S ratio) and creatinine levels in amniotic fluid.

7. Describe the routine preparation, including client teaching, for a client who is to have an amniocentesis done in the last trimester.

8. Compare and contrast the oxytocin challenge test (OCT) and the nonstress test (NST) for antepartal monitoring.

Even the nurse who is not a specialist in maternal–child health nursing may at times be called on to assist with diagnostic procedures commonly done during the child-bearing years. The intent of this chapter is to give the reader an overview of the diagnostic procedures used to assess the ability to conceive or to carry a fetus to term. The chapter begins with the five basic tests of fertility because the inability to become pregnant is a common problem. The new and rapidly developing technique of chorionic villi biopsy for prenatal diagnosis is discussed. Amniocentesis is discussed in regards to tests for chromosome defects, inborn errors of metabolism, and neural tube defects. Two other uses of amniocentesis, evaluation of the severity of hemolysis from the Rh factor and assessment of fetal maturity, are also explained. Some basic information about fetal monitoring is presented at the end of the chapter.

GENERAL NURSING DIAGNOSES

Family Coping, Potential for Growth

During the childbearing years, many couples suffer disappointments because of the inability to have the longed for "perfect" child. In recent years, nurses have become very involved in helping families deal with unexpected or crisis situation. Leavitt (1982) describes the impact of nurses who do primary prevention for high-risk families. Nurses who contract with the couples for follow-up visits after a family crisis can actually help strengthen the adaptive capacity of a family. The key point is for the nurse to focus on the family as a unit. Whether it is the crisis of infertility, an unhappy report from an amniocentesis test, or the stress of fetal monitoring, the professional nurse can be instrumental in helping the family cope and even grow from the experience.

Anxiety Related to Test Procedures and Impact on Self-concept

The nurse's sensitivity to the needs of the client undergoing a diagnostic test is important for short-term care as well as for follow-up. For example, when clients are connected to monitors, or undergoing technical procedures, they may begin to feel depersonalized. However, in one study of 50 mothers who had been monitored during labor, none found the monitor depersonalizing. The investigators noted that the nurses did not walk in the room and look at the monitor first—a normal tendency when machines are being used. Rather, the nurse first spoke with the woman and asked her how she was doing. After the personal interaction and after feeling the woman's contractions, the nurse correlated the clinical findings with the readouts from the monitors (McDonough et al., 1981). As more and more diagnostic procedures are used to assess the natural events of child-bearing, the nurse can continue to supply the essential human element of caring. She Chapter 25 for more discussion on relieving anxiety about diagnostic procedures.

FERTILITY TESTING

A growing number of couples in the United States (estimated as 15–20% of all married couples) seek medical help for infertility (Pfeffer, 1980). Birnbaum (1980) gives three possible reasons for an increased focus on infertility tests: (1) the diminished number of children available for adoption because of legalized abortions: (2) a rising incidence of gonorrhea, which can cause pelvic inflammatory disease (PID) and sterility; and (3) the fact that more women are opting to delay pregnancy until they are in their thirties, when reproduction may not be as easy.

Infertility is defined as the inability of a couple to achieve pregnancy after 1 year of unprotected intercourse. For some couples, such circumstances as past pelvic inflammatory disease, suspected hormone imbalances, or other physical problems indicate sterility may be a problem. If there are no obvious reasons why a couple should not be able to conceive, fertility tests are not advocated until after a year of unprotected intercourse. For women over 35, tests may be done sooner than a year. A nurse can reassure a couple, who seem healthy, that the failure to get pregnant after only a few months is not an indication to too quickly seek medical help.

For some couples, who have tried for much longer than a year to get pregnant, the decision to begin fertility testing may be a difficult one to make. The tests may be costly. They are an invasion into an area that is usually very private. And beginning the tests is, in a way, an acknowledgment of failure to do something that is thought of as being "natural." Clients may discuss with nurses the frustration in not being able to get pregnant. The nurse can assess if the couple needs a referral for fertility testing. The nurse can stress that infertility may be due to a problem with the man, woman, or both: therefore, both people need to be tested, once the couple has decided they need help. A brief explanation of the five basic tests for fertility are summarized in Table 28–1.

■ BASAL BODY TEMPERATURE (BBT) AND OVULATION TESTS

The term basal refers to the lowest possible level of a physiologic measurement (i.e., baseline). The BBT is taken early in the morning before the woman gets out of bed. Because this test requires only a thermometer and a graphic chart, women may do

TABLE 28–1. FIVE BASIC TESTS FOR INFERTILITY

Test	Purpose
Basal body temperature recordings	Gives presumptive evidence of ovulation.
Semen analysis	Assessment of number and characteristics of sperm in one ejaculation.
Hormone analysis	Assessment of hormonal imbalances, which may be primary or secondary hypofunction (see Chap. 15). Some physicians use the endometrial biopsy (see Chap. 25).
Postcoital examination (Sims–Huhner)	Assessment of mobility and number of sperm in cervical mucus after intercourse. Also checks characteristics of mucus at time of ovulation.
Hysterosalpingogram	Assessment of tubal patency and any structural defects in uterus or tubes (Rubin's test only tests tubal patency). (See Chap. 20 on hysterosalpingogram.)

See text for explanation of tests and client teaching.

this test before they seek medical advice. There are special BBT or ovulation thermometers that are measured in tenths of degrees rather than the two tenths on standard thermometers. An electronic thermometer linked to a microcomputer can also
be purchased. Also see the discussion on the newer urine tests that predict ovulation.
If the woman can determine her ovulatory pattern, the couple can plan intercourse
to take advantage of her fertile period. (Using a temperature chart to avoid concep-
tion is not always reliable because the change in temperature is associated with ovulation, not before.)

In women who have a normal menstrual cycle, the basal temperature is usually
below 98 °F (36.7 °C) in the preovulatory phase. Before ovulation occurs, an increasing production of estrogen may cause a slight downward trend in the basal
temperature. Then with ovulation, the "other female hormone," progesterone, is
secreted by the corpus luteum. Progesterone affects the hypothalamus so there is up
to a degree rise in the basal temperature. The increase in temperature at ovulation
usually makes the woman's basal temperature above 98 °F (36.7 °C). If the woman
accurately keeps a graphic recording for a few months, a physician can interpret the
charts and note if there is presumptive evidence that ovulation is occurring. The client
needs to note on the chart any colds or infections, which would disrupt the normal
temperature pattern.

Preparation of Client for Basal Temperature Recordings

The client should be instructed on exactly when to take the temperatures and how
to record them on the graph. (Nurses seem to forget that shaking down a thermometer,
reading the results in tenths, and plotting the number on a graph are skills that may
need to be learned.) The woman should be given the chance to practice any of the
necessary skills of which she is unsure. Each morning as soon as she wakes up, she
should take and record her temperature. The woman should be instructed to take
the temperature before she goes to the bathroom or does any physical activity, including sex. Oral temperatures are usually sufficient. The client is given a special chart
to record the temperatures, which is brought back to the physician's office or infertility clinic to be analyzed. The newer electronic thermometers will keep a daily record.

■ SEMEN ANALYSIS

An investigation of semen is the most important initial diagnostic study of the man.
If the analysis seems normal, more intensive investigation of the woman is in order.
In the laboratory a sperm count is done as well as an examination of the form of
the sperm, its mobility, and the amount and characteristics of the semen. If any abnormalities are noted or if the count is low, a second specimen will be examined because there are variations with each ejaculation. Semen analysis is also done after
a vasectomy to determine that surgery has been successful.

Preparation of Client and Collection of Sample

The client needs specific instructions on how to collect the specimen. Semen is collected after two or more days of sexual abstinence. The client may be given privacy
in a bathroom to collect the specimen in a jar by masturbation. Obviously, this is
a highly intimate matter and creates tension and anxiety in the man. Some men, for
psychological or religious reasons, prefer to collect semen at home by using a condom during intercourse. The condom should not contain lubricants or substances
that may interfere with the analysis. The client may be given a plastic sheath to use
as the condom. (Religious practices may necessitate a small puncture in the sheath.)

All of the semen is put into a clean jar. It must be sent to the laboratory within two hours after ejaculation.

Reference Values for Semen Analysis

20–40 million sperm per ml
Semen volume of 2–5 ml
Sperm motility 60% (within 2 hr of collection)

■ POSTCOITAL EXAMINATION: SIMS–HUHNER TEST (HUHNER TEST)

The Sims-Huhner test is an examination of the number and motility of the sperm found in the cervical mucus of the woman after intercourse. The test is done a day or two before expected ovulation because an increased secretion of estrogen causes certain characteristic changes in the mucus. Estrogen increases the elasticity and sodium content of the cervical mucus. The elasticity of the mucus is called spinnbarkeit. Normally, these mucus changes enhance sperm survival. (Learning the mucus changes for ovulation is the basis for a form of contraception called the Billings method.) Ferning refers to the pattern created when cervical mucus dries under the influence of estrogen. The postcoital examination of the mucus and the sperm can help determine if there is any immunological or hormonal problem contributing to the infertility.

Preparation of Client and Collection of Sample
The test is planned for a day or two before the woman's expected time of ovulation. The couple has intercourse, and the woman then goes to the clinic or office for a pelvic examination. The woman may be told to stay in bed for about half an hour after intercourse. The sample of cervical mucus needs to be obtained 2–4 hours after intercourse. The couple should not use any lubricants, and the woman should not douche. (These instructions may seem obvious, but the health professional must make sure that the patient really understands the test.)

Reference Values for Sims-Huhner Test

The microscopic examination shows the quality of the mucus, including the pattern it makes on a slide. Certain patterns such as ferning discussed above are considered normal. The number and motility of the sperm are observed. Ten or more sperm found per high power field is considered a normal count.

■ TUBAL PATENCY TESTS, HYSTEROSALPINGOGRAM, AND TUBAL INSUFFLATION (RUBIN'S TEST)

The tubes can be insufflated with carbon dioxide (Rubin's test) or radiopaque dye (hysterosalpingogram) to see if the tubes are patent. Instillation of carbon dioxide can be done in the physician's office, but it does not give the detailed information that the dye does. Hysterosalpingogram is very useful for observing any structural defects in the uterus or tubes. A hysterosalpingogram is done in the radiology department. (See Chapter 20 for the discussion on nursing implications of a hysterosalpingogram.)

Hysterosalpingogram or the Rubin's test may also have a therapeutic effect because they break up adhesions in a tube or remove debris that was blocking the tube.

MEASUREMENT OF HORMONES

The levels of FSH and LH, as well as testosterone, progesterone, and estrogen, may be assessed by laboratory tests to determine normal hormonal balance in both the man and the woman (see Chapter 15 for detailed information). Some physicians prefer an endometrial biopsy to determine the quantity of progesterone rather than serum levels of the hormone (Pfeffer, 1980). Others consider an endometrial biopsy part of a second phase (Sobel & Ferguson, 1985). An endometrial biopsy can be done as part of a cervical examination (see Chapter 25).

Commercial kits are available that detect the hormonal changes in the urine that signal ovulation. Clients may do these tests, which take about 20 minutes, as a self-test for fertility awareness. The color change means ovulation will occur in 12–24 hours. A specially trained nurse can be consulted at a toll-free number listed in the kit.

OTHER FERTILITY TESTS AND TREATMENT OPTIONS

Laboratory tests may or may not be sufficient to identify the cause of infertility. Depending on the results of the basic tests, the physician may order other tests, such as laparotomy, to examine the female reproductive organs in more detail (see Chapter 27). Surgical reconstruction may be needed. For women who are not ovulating, medications such as clomiphene (Clomid) may be prescribed by the physician. The nurse's role will depend on the particular treatments tried (Friedman, 1981). The reader is encouraged to consult current literature on some of the available options.

NURSING DIAGNOSES RELATED TO FERTILITY TESTS

Potential for Ineffective Coping Related to Inability to Conceive
Although treatment can help many infertile clients, the success rate for all infertility clients, irrespective of etiology, is approximately 50% in most centers. These statistics mean little or nothing to the individual couple, but they do have implications for counseling because for many couples infertility cannot be presently treated. The final pronouncement of it being highly unlikely that a couple can have a biological child is a difficult fact for many couples to accept. Adoption may or may not be the answer for a couple. Unusual solutions such as "surrogate mothers" are being tried by some couples when the man is fertile. Couples may benefit from talking to other couples who have been unable to conceive. There are various support groups for infertile couples. The nurse can find out if there is a support group in a local area. The individual who has an infertility problem may feel guilt over the perceived "inadequacy." If the couple does not remain a couple, the individual may have problems explaining this infertility to a new partner.

Anticipatory Grieving Related to Loss of a Desired Goal

The loss of a child, either real or desired, does cause a period of grieving. Wong (1980) has written about the empty-mother syndrome. Although Wong's work has been with mothers who have lost children after a lengthy illness, the four interventions she has used to help resolve grief may be applied to several situations discussed in this chapter, including infertility, the birth of a defective child, or the termination of a pregnancy. Interventions to help relieve grief can include (1) preparing the couple for anticipating *normal* feelings of emptiness, loneliness, and failure; (2) helping the couple reevaluate their roles in a childless family (or in a family that does not have the perfect or longed-for child); (3) encouraging the couple to explore fulfilling activities, which utilize their special talents and abilities; and (4) supporting the couple by helping them to communicate with each other and with other family members who have been affected by the loss of a child (Wong, 1980, p. 389). For example, potential grandparents can be very hurt by the lack of a grandchild so they too need help to express their feelings of loss. Obviously the meaning of the loss is very individualized and varies tremendously from situation to situation. Devore and Baldwin (1986) give excellent guidelines for counseling clients who have lost a fetus due to an ectopic pregnancy.

SCREENING TESTS DONE DURING PREGNANCY

The introduction of "the Pill" gave women more control deciding when or whether to have a child. Also, as women's roles have changed in America, more women are opting to have children at a later age—after a career is established. The media is full of stories about women who postpone babies until their thirties. For example, in *McCall's* magazine, the question, "How old is too old to have a baby?" is answered with a quote from a physician who says, "When you quit menstruating" (Pines, 1980). The use of amniocentesis and chorionic villi biopsy have increased the probability of healthy normal babies for what used to be called elderly (over age 35) primigravidas. These two screening techniques have also made it possible for couples, who may be at high risk for genetic defects, to undergo a pregnancy knowing that certain defects can be detected by laboratory testing. Nurses need to be aware of some of the basic tests genetic counseling can offer prospective parents because people often ask nurses for referrals and information on newer trends in health care. Genetic counseling is recommended for (1) women over age 35, (2) couples who already have one child with a genetic defect, (3) couples with a family history of genetic defects, and (4) couples from ethnic or racial groups at high risk for genetic disease. Note that the Department of Health and Human Services has up-to-date information on genetic tests via the National Center for Education in Maternal and Child Health (formerly the National Clearinghouse for Human Genetic Diseases).

■ AMNIOCENTESIS

Purposes. Amniocentesis is the removal of some amniotic fluid for diagnostic purposes. (Amniocentesis can also be done to introduce urea or another hypertonic solution into the amniotic fluid in order to cause an abortion.) The three major reasons for doing amniocentesis for diagnostic purposes include (1) prenatal detection of genetic disorders, (2) follow-up and possible treatment of isoimmune disease with the Rh factor, and (3) assessment of fetal maturity. Much more rare is the use of amniocentesis when other children in the family have Wilms' tumor (Wallach, 1983). See Table 28-2 for a summary about the different purposes of amniocentesis.

AMNIOCENTESIS FOR PRENATAL DIAGNOSIS OF GENETIC DEFECTS: THREE MAJOR ASSESSMENTS

Karyotyping for Chromosome Study

A variety of diseases can be detected through a study of the cells and chemicals in the amniotic fluid. Identification of the chromosomes is called karyotyping. A karyotyping of chromosomes is a pattern of the 22 pairs of autosomal chromosomes and one pair of sex chromosomes: XX of the female or the XY of the male. All the severe chromosomal abnormalities can be detected by fetal karyotypes. Trisomy of chromosome 21 (Down's syndrome) is the most common abnormality found and the most common genetic birth defect (March of Dimes, 1984). Widmann (1983) notes that the risk of Down's syndrome is 1:100 in women over age 35. Although other sources may give various statistical rates for Down's syndrome, most centers routinely offer genetic counseling services to any woman over the age of 35 because there is general agreement that the incidence of Down's syndrome continues to increase with increasing maternal age. Amniocentesis is also offered to women who have had one child with a defect or have a family history of chromosomal defects.

If there is a possibility of a sex-linked defect such as hemophilia, the sex of the baby may be important. Some diseases, such as hemophilia, are linked to the X chromosome; therefore, if the fetus is a female, there is little if any possibility of the disease. The hemophilia trait is transmitted by the female and occurs in males. A female must have two defective X chromosomes, which is a very rare possibility. Although the sex of the baby is always determined with the chromosomal study, the parents may prefer to not know the results unless there is a possibility of a sex-linked disease. Centers inform the prospective parents that they can know the sex if they so desire.

Biochemical Defects

Numerous enzyme or biochemical abnormalities can be detected by amniocentesis as research finds more and more gene markers for diseases such as Huntington's chorea and muscular dystrophy (Walton, 1986). Some of the metabolic diseases tested for are galactosemia, maple syrup urine disease. Gaucher's disease, and Tay–Sachs disease. Some of these diseases will only be tested if it is known that both parents are carriers. For example, Tay–Sachs can be detected in the carrier state in parents and because the disease is caused by a recessive gene, both parents must be carriers for the fetus to be at risk. Some of the common genetic metabolic defects, such as cystic fibrosis and PKU cannot be tested currently by study of the cells in amniotic fluid. (See Chapter 18 for laboratory tests of carrier states for biochemical defects.)

Alpha-Fetoprotein Levels to Detect Neural Tube Defects

Alpha-fetoprotein (AFP) is manufactured by the fetal liver. Normally, there is a low level of this protein in the amniotic fluid, but if the neural tube does not close properly, large amounts of AFP leak into the amniotic fluid (Kimball et al., 1977). If the neural tube does not enclose at the top, the fetus fails to develop a normal brain (anencephaly). If the defect in the neural tube is lower, the fetus has spina bifida. A

TABLE 28-2. THREE MAJOR PURPOSES OF AMNIOCENTESIS

Purposes	Timing	Results	Usual Follow-up
1. Assessment of genetic defects	15th–18th week of gestation		
a. Karyotyping of chromosomes		Can identify Down's syndrome and other chromosomal abnormalities	Takes 3–6 weeks to get all[a] results
			Couple may opt for abortion if serious genetic defect found
b. Biochemical defects		Over 60 defects can be identified	
c. Alpha-fetoprotein levels		May indicate improper closure of neural tube	
2. Assessment of isoimmune disease (RH factor)	After 24–25 weeks' gestation	Level of bilirubin in amniotic fluid indicates severity of hemolysis	Increasing levels of bilirubin may indicate need for intrauterine transfusions or induced labor
3. Assessment of fetal maturity	Near end of gestation		
a. Lecithin/sphingomyelin ratio		Ratio of 2:1 is usually evidence of lung maturity	Labor may be induced if tests indicate mature fetus
b. Creatinine levels		Level of 2 mg/dl is evidence of maturity of kidneys	
c. Staining of fat cells		Evaluate fetal maturity by fat cells	

[a]*Note*: A newer test, chorionic villi biopsy (CVB), is also used to test for genetic defects (Davis, 1986). Results are obtained much sooner. CVB cannot test for AFP, but can detect sickle cell anemia (Goossens, 1983).

meningocele or myelomeningocele may be associated with the spina bifida. The more involvement of the spinal cord, the more severe the handicap. The child may be paralyzed from the waist down, have the lack of bowel and bladder control, or the damage may be slight and amenable to therapy. Severe omphalocele (protrusion of intestines) or congenital nephrosis can also cause increased levels of AFP. If the amniotic fluid is contaminated with fetal or maternal blood, the AFP level may be falsely high because the protein is normaly high in the blood. Twins will also cause increased levels of AFP in amniotic fluid. As with other tests of amniotic fluid, the physician must make interpretations cautiously based on as much data as possible. Some of these structural defects may also be identified by ultrasound tests (see Chapter 23).

ALPHA-FETOPROTEIN IN THE SERUM

By about 16–18 weeks of pregnancy, AFP can also be measured in the mother's blood. Note that currently a maternal blood test for AFP is the *only* screening test that can be done of the pregnant woman's blood as a check for genetic defects in the child. (Several defects can be tested by fetal blood samples, as will be discussed later.)

Unfortunately, high levels of AFP in pregnant women do not always indicate a problem with neural tube defects because there may be an incorrect estimation of the fetal age, twins, or other reasons for an increase, which are not well understood yet. Still, even with these drawbacks, AFP blood screening must by law be offered to pregnant women in certain states in the United States. Alpha-fetoprotein screening is already being routinely done in other countries, such as England and Australia. If the AFP blood screening test is elevated, a repeat is done. If the test is positive on a second blood sample, the woman has an ultrasonogram (Chapter 23). If there is still doubt about the possibility of a defect, an amniocentesis is done.

Because AFP blood testing is the first large-scale screening test offered to any woman, there are concerns about how the test will be conducted and if the couple will have the benefit of informed advice. Originally the sale of AFP materials to laboratories was available only when physicians were participating in comprehensive screening programs (Chedd, 1981). Opponents of mass screening say that testing of all pregnant women causes a great deal of unnecessary anxiety, particularly if one is opposed to terminating the pregnancy. See Chapter 18 for reference values for the serum levels and for information on Down's syndrome which may be associated with low levels of AFP.

Counseling Before an Amniocentesis for Prenatal Diagnosis

Although the technical preparation of the client for amniocentesis is very simple, the psychological care of the client may be very complex. Tischler (1981) described in detail the psychological aspects of genetic counseling. If amniocentesis is being done for genetic counseling, the bottom line is "what action will be taken if there is an abnormality found?" Counseling is done before the amniocentesis to help the couple fully understand the ramifications of the test so they can make an informed decision. If the couple has no desire to terminate the pregnancy, most centers advise against having an amniocentesis because it does not change the course of events. (At the present time, treatment or correction is not usually feasible in utero. The exception is for isoimmune problems, which will be discussed later.)

Although amniocentesis is considered to have very little risk for the mother and less than 1% risk for the fetus, the couple must be aware of the possibility of damage or death to the fetus. The physician in a particular center or a genetic counselor, who may be a nurse or other health professional, can explain the statistics of a particular center.

Although a couple may not want to agree to terminate a pregnancy if the results show a defect, they may desire the amniocentesis to better plan for the birth of a defective child. The nurse who works in a setting where amniocentesis is done must be aware of the hard decisions couples must make about whether the findings from an amniocentesis are reason for an abortion. Pressures from family and friends, and society in general, may make it difficult for the couple to choose what is right for them.

A genetic counselor can be invaluable in supplying the couple with correct data to help them make their own decision. Obviously, there are several bioethical issues that are raised when prenatal diagnosing is done. Chedd (1981) discusses not only the broad ethical issues of genetic screening but also the legal problems that can arise. Surely this is an area that will spark even more legal and ethical arguments in the future as more women take advantage of amniocentesis or the newer procedure, chorionic villi biopsy.

NURSING DIAGNOSIS

Anxiety Related to Waiting for Results

An amniocentesis for prenatal diagnosis is usually done between 14 and 18 weeks of gestation. Before this time, there is not enough fluid and cells for a culture. The results of the test take 3–6 weeks because of the need to culture cells to do chromosome patterns (karyotyping) and metabolic studies. This waiting period is a time of extreme anxiety for most couples. The woman may be trying to conceal the pregnancy until she knows the fetus is all right. (A pregnancy of 20 or more weeks is difficult to conceal.) The couple tend to have very ambivalent feelings about the fetus because it is possible that it may be aborted. Crying and indecision about the pregnancy are common. If the results indicate a serious defect and an abortion is done, the abortion must be by induction because the client is in the second trimester. Happily, the most common result of an amniocentesis is a *prediction* of normality (Hogan & Tcheng, 1978). It is important that couples understand not all possible defects are tested by amniocentesis and there is always a possibility of error. The fact is stressed that no test can *guarantee* a healthy baby. But for a couple with reason to fear one of the defects that can be identified by amniocentesis, a report of no defect is joyous news. The woman who does not have the support of the father of the child may have an even more difficult time awaiting the report of the amniocentesis.

AMNIOCENTESIS IN ISOIMMUNE DISEASE (Rh FACTOR)

If the mother has a rising titer of Rh antibodies, the amniocentesis may be done several times during the pregnancy to monitor the welfare of the fetus. (A rising bilirubin level in the amniotic fluid indicates hemolysis of fetal red blood cells.) Usually the first amniocentesis is done as early as 18 weeks if the mother has a high antibody titer and a history of previously affected fetuses, and as late as 24 weeks if there is a low fixed antibody titer and no history of an affected fetus (Perry et al., 1986).

Elevated or rising Rh antibody titers in the mother indicate that the fetus may have hemolytic disease of the newborn (HDN). This disease, formerly called erthyroblastosis fetalis, was even more common before the introduction of immunoglobulins of Rh antibodies (RhoGam), which can be given in certain cases to prevent the mother from making antibodies against the Rh factor of the fetal cells. (RhoGAM is used within 72 hours after each pregnancy of an Rh negative mother with an Rh positive infant.) Other isoimmune factors, such as ABO incompatibility, can cause some hemolytic reactions, but it is the Rh factor that causes the severe increase in bilirubin due to massive hemolysis of the red blood cells of the fetus (see Chapter 14 for a discussion on Rh testing).

Reference Values for Bilirubin in Amniotic Fluid

The amount of bilirubin in the amniotic fluid is measured by how it changes patterns of light at a certain wave length (spectrophotometry). Charts are available to compare the concentration of bile pigments at different gestational ages.

Clinical Significance

If there is an abnormal amount of bilirubin for the gestational age, the obstetrician must decide whether to do intrauterine transfusions of the fetus or to induce labor. One of the considerations for inducing labor is the maturity of the fetus. (See the L/S test discussed next.) Perry et al. (1986) discuss the role of the nurse in helping with exchange transfusions for the fetus.

AMNIOCENTESIS FOR ASSESSING FETAL MATURITY

Lecithin/Sphingomyelin Ratio

The lecithin/sphingomyelin ratio (L/S ratio) is a test for fetal lung maturity. Lecithin and sphingomyelin are two phospholipids found in amniotic fluids, as well as serum. Sphingomyelin, which is associated with nervous tissue, remains at about the same level in the amniotic fluid throughout the pregnancy. Lecithin is a major component of alveolar surfactant. If there is sufficient surfactant to lubricate the alveolar surfaces, the lungs can inflate normally at birth. Without sufficient surfactant, the newborn infant is very prone to develop hyaline membrane disease or respiratory distress syndrome (RDS). Lecithin begins to rise in the amniotic fluid at about 35 weeks' gestation. This rise parallels the development of lung maturity. When the lecithin ratio is about double the sphingomyelin level in the amniotic fluid, the lungs are usually mature.

Reference Values for Lecithin/Sphingomyelin Ratio

A ratio of 2:1 is strong evidence that the fetus has mature lungs.

Shake Test for L/S Ratio. A quick way to check if there is sufficient lecithin present is to mix equal parts of alcohol and saline with a sample of amniotic fluid and shake the test tube for 15 seconds. If bubbles persist in the sample, it is presumed that adequate lecithin is present. Certain factors may interfere with this test, such as dirty. glassware. The laboratory can also do a quantitative measurement of the L/S ratio.

OTHER TESTS ON AMNIOTIC FLUID FOR FETAL MATURITY

The obstetrician may use various data to assess if it is relatively safe to induce labor. The L/S ratio mentioned above is the most heavily used indicator because if there is evidence of mature lung function the risk of respiratory distress syndrome (RDS) is much decreased. The laboratory can also stain fetal fat cells to assess the maturity of the fetus (Widmann, 1983). Creatinine levels are an indication of maturity of the kidneys. The creatinine level usually begins to rise at about 34 weeks of gestation. By 37 weeks' gestation the level is 2 mg/dl or above. The interpretation of all the data from amniocentesis requires the skilled judgment of the obstetrician because no one test can be viewed in isolation of the overall clinical picture of the mother and the fetus.

PRETEST NURSING DIAGNOSES

Anxiety Related to Unknowns about Procedure
The actual physical preparation of the client for amniocentesis is the same whether the collection of fluid is for prenatal diagnosis of a genetic defect, to assess isoimmune disease, or to determine if the fetus is mature enough for an induced labor. As noted earlier, detailed counseling is very important if the couple are having the amniocentesis done because of possible genetic defects. Even at the time of the procedure, the couple may need last minute reassurance. Sammons (1985) found that clients undergoing prenatal amniocentesis identified as helpful (1) ongoing physician explanation, (2) use of Lamaze relaxation techniques, and (3) presence of a trusted support person, be it husband, mother, or nurse. If the amniocentesis is being done to determine if transfusions are needed or if labor should be induced, the mother will also need on the spot reassurance of the purpose of the test and how the physician will use the results to make a decision about care. The client will need to sign a special consent form that indicates that she understands the purposes of the procedure and the potential complications that can occur (see Chapter 25 on consents for invasive tests).

Potential for Injury to Fetus
The nurse should take baseline vital signs. If the amniocentesis is being done in late pregnancy, the fetal heart rate should also be monitored for a baseline reading. No premedications are given. Depending on the timing of the procedure, the client may or may not need a full bladder for visualization by ultrasound. (See Chapter 23 for a detailed explanation of the use of ultrasound in pregnancy.) Ultrasound is used to visualize the placenta and the position of the fetus to avoid injury.

Procedure. The client lies in a recumbant position throughout the sonogram process and actual withdrawal of the fluid. The skin of the abdomen is prepped with an iodine solution (Betadine or Iodophor). Because only one needle puncture is used to remove the fluid the physician does not usually use a local anesthetic. (Chapter 25 describes the medications that are used for local anesthesia.) The physician inserts a long needle through the abdominal wall into the amniotic sac and withdraws 20–30 ml of amniotic fluid. The client will feel the stick, but the aspiration is not painful. The fluid sample is placed in clearly marked test tubes. If the specimen is to be tested for bilirubin, the fluid should be collected in a dark tube and protected from the light because light will change the composition of indirect bilirubin. (Light is actually used as a therapy, phototherapy, for high indirect bilirubin in the newborn.) After the needle is withdrawn, a Band-Aid is put over the puncture site in the abdomen.

POSTTEST NURSING DIAGNOSIS

Knowledge Deficit Regarding Follow-up Care
If the amniocentesis was done in early pregnancy, for prenatal diagnosis, the client can go home after the test is completed. The client is told she may have some mild cramps for a short time and is given instructions to notify the physician or clinic if severe cramps develop or if bleeding occurs. The genetic counselor will have already impressed on the couple that the results of the test will not be available for several weeks, but the couple should be reminded again that they will be called as soon as the results are known. (See the earlier discussion on the anxiety of waiting for results.)

If the amniocentesis is done in late pregnancy, to assess the status of the fetus, the client may or may not be hospitalized. The fetal heart rate is monitored for 30 minutes after the test to assess for any difficulty. The pregnant woman's vital signs will also be assessed.

■ CHORIONIC VILLI BIOPSY (CVB)

This test of a chorion sample is a test of cells similar to those of the fetus. The physician inserts a small catheter through the vagina and cervix into the uterus. Suction is applied to obtain some cells. The great advantage of the CVB over amniocentesis is that it can be performed earlier in pregnancy (eighth to ninth week) and results are obtained in a few days rather than 3–6 weeks. CVB cannot detect neural tube defects (Davis, 1986).

■ FETOSCOPY

By using a fiberoptic lens, physicians can actually view the fetus while it is still in the uterus. (See Chapter 25 for a discussion on the use of fiberscopes.) This visualization can allow the physician to take samples of blood and skin tissues from the fetus. At the present time, fetoscopy is still in its infancy. When fetoscopy becomes more widely available, this will broaden not only the detection of defects but will also make it routine to do treatments to the fetus. The reader is encouraged to consult recent literature for the latest advances in fetoscopy.

■ FETAL MONITORING NONSTRESS TEST (NST)

Fetal monitoring, a noninvasive technique to evaluate the status of the fetus, is called the nonstress test (NST) to distinguish it from the oxytocin challenge test (OCT), which does put stress on the fetus. The mother is attached to a fetal monitor and the fetal heart rate (FHR) is recorded. The specific patterns of fetal heart rate acceleration and deceleration are classified as abnormal or normal responses to stimuli.

PRETEST NURSING IMPLICATIONS

The test may be done in a clinic, office, or in a quiet room in an obstetrical unit. The client is put in a recliner chair or a comfortable bed. The client should void before the procedure so she will remain comfortable. It is also advisable for the client to eat before the test because the active bowel sounds of an empty stomach may interfere with the test. The nurse should take a baseline blood pressure. The monitors are applied per hospital routine. The sleep–awake pattern of the fetus is observed for about 40 minutes because a rest–activity pattern of the fetus is usually in a 20–40 minute pattern (Lieber, 1980). Some women may have to be monitored longer to obtain a reactive pattern. If the mother is on any sedative drugs, the fetus may be less active.

Experienced maternal child health nurses may do the entire monitoring procedure. The interpretation of the reading will be done by a physician experienced in antepartal monitoring. During labor, nurses do monitor the readings and base nursing interventions on the findings (Aukamp, 1984).

Although the nonstress method of antepartal monitoring does not cause any pain or physical discomfort for the woman, most women are highly anxious about the results. Fetal monitoring is done on clients where there is a probability of fetal jeopardy such as a mother with diabetes or hypertension or other risk factors. The false-positive rate is high, so questionable cases may need further studies such as fetal acid–base studies to document if the fetus is truly at risk (Dierker et al., 1986). The nurse should allow the woman to ventilate her concerns and anxieties. The nurse can get answers for any questions the woman may have about her prenatal care or the process of labor and delivery. The nurse can also help the client use some of the relaxation techniques that she may be learning in childbirth classes. A study of maternal reactions to fetal monitoring revealed that the women wanted the nurse with them much or most of the time. The women in the study wanted "someone to hold onto, someone who cares" (Shields, 1978).

■ OXYTOCIN CHALLENGE TEST (OCT)

The oxytocin challenge test (OCT) is used to determine the ability of the fetus to withstand contractions prior to labor. Because contractions produce a transient decrease in the uteroplacental blood flow, some infants may be stressed by labor. The challenge test may indicate which fetus would be in less jeopardy if a cesarean delivery were initiated. Because there is some risk of inducing labor with this test, the test must be done close to a delivery suite. In a study of 800 OCTs on 300 patients, the complication of induced labor was rare, unless the client was postmaturity (Diamond, 1978). Oxytocin challenge test is definitely contraindicated with rupture of membranes or a previous classical cesarean delivery and usually contraindicated with multiple pregnancy, previous premature labor, placenta previa, hydramnios, and previous low transverse cesarean delivery (Boback & Jensen, 1984). The OCT is not done in a pregnancy less than 33 or 34 weeks. Because OCT does have some risks, more qualified personnel are needed to give the test. The OCT takes longer and is more costly than the nonstress method (NST) of antepartal monitoring.

Reference Values for Oxytocin Challenge Test

The specific patterns must be carefully evaluated by the physician in conjunction with other clinical data. A negative OCT would show no late deceleration in the fetal heart rate after a contraction. In essence, a negative test is evidence that the fetus is not in jeopardy at the present time and the pregnancy may be allowed to progress normally because the fetus can withstand the stress of labor contractions.

PRETEST NURSING IMPLICATIONS

The test is given near a delivery suite. The general preparation of the client is the same as with the NST except the client will be asked to sign a special consent form, which explains the possible risks of the procedure. (See Chapter 25 on informed consent.) The usual procedure is to give oxytocin intravenously at a specific dilution ordered by the physician. The drip rate is increased until the mother is having three contractions in 10 minutes. The fetus is monitored for at least 30 minutes. The nurse must carefully monitor the client during the test. The client can be helped to go with the contractions by using the techniques she is learning in her childbirth class.

QUESTIONS

1. John and Mary Menendez (both age 27) have been married a little over 2 years. Although they have used no form of birth control for the past 16 months, pregnancy has not occurred. The couple desire a child so they have asked a nurse in a clinic about fertility testing. Which statement contains appropriate information?

   a. Infertility is most likely not a problem because they have only been having unprotected intercourse for a little over a year
   b. Infertility is usually due to female problems so only Mary needs to be tested initially
   c. Most all infertility problems are easily treated with new drugs such as clomiphene (Clomid) or minor surgery
   d. Basic infertility tests include semen analysis, postcoital examinations, and tubal patency tests such as the hysterosalpingogram

2. As part of an infertility workup, Mary is to keep a record of her basal body temperature on a daily basis. The nurse is assessing to see if Mary can accurately read the thermometer. In addition, the nurse should stress

   a. The temperature should be taken before Mary gets out of bed in the morning
   b. An increase in temperature is expected before ovulation occurs
   c. Rectal temperatures are the only way to obtain a basal reading
   d. A one month's graph of temperatures will usually suffice

3. Which of the following statements about amniocentesis is an important fact when planning care for the client who is to undergo an amniocentesis for prenatal diagnosis of genetic defects?

   a. The amniocentesis must be done as early as possible, usually before the eighth week of gestation
   b. The test is a guarantee of a healthy baby
   c. The results take 3–6 weeks so this is a period of great anxiety for the couple who may decide to terminate the pregnancy
   d. There is a significant risk of 5–10% for the fetus

4. Mrs. Sanders is a 39-year-old primigravida who has elected to have a chorionic villi biopsy (CVB) for prenatal diagnosis. The major advantage of the CVB over the amniocentesis is that the CVB is

   a. Less hazardous to the fetus
   b. Less expensive
   c. Detects a greater number of defects
   d. Done earlier in the pregnancy

5. One of the tests done on amniotic fluid is a test for fetal alpha protein because an elevation of this protein is suggestive of:

   a. Fetal lung immaturity   c. Neural tube defects
   b. Immunologic deficiencies   d. Phenylketonuria

6. Mrs. Ragella is 34 weeks pregnant. An amniocentesis revealed an increased bilirubin level as compared to levels done a week ago. This rising bilirubin level is indicative of

   a. Possible fetal jeopardy due to hemolytic disease
   b. Normal liver functioning
   c. Renal immaturity
   d. Fetal distress due to hypoxia

7. The physician is concerned because a too early cesarean delivery may predispose Mrs. Ragella's infant to respiratory distress syndrome (RDS). Which of these tests of amniotic fluid is used to assess lung maturity in the fetus?

   a. Lecithin–sphingomyelin ratio
   b. Creatinine levels
   c. Karyotyping of chromosomes
   d. Spectrophotometric analysis of bilirubin levels

8. Mrs. Foster is a diabetic who is near term with her second pregnancy. Her other pregnancy was a stillbirth. She has been admitted to the obstetric unit for a possible early delivery. She is scheduled for an amniocentesis this afternoon to assess fetal maturity. Mrs. Foster asks the nurse about the procedure. The nurse should explain to Mrs. Foster that

    a. Premedication will be used to relax her

    b. Local anesthesia must be used to eliminate pain

    c. Ultrasound will be done to visualize the placenta and fetus

    d. X-ray of the abdomen is routine after the procedure is completed

9. Mrs. Foster is scheduled for more tests. She asks the nurse if an OCT is the same as the routine fetal monitoring she had with her last pregnancy. The nurse should explain that the oxytocin challenge test (OCT) *differs* from the nonstress technique (NST) of antepartal monitoring in that the OCT

    a. Requires the fetal heart rate be assessed with internal fetal monitors to detect any abnormal patterns

    b. Uses a drug to cause contractions

    c. Is used for women who have high-risk pregnancies

    d. Causes anxiety while the NST is anxiety-free for the mother

REFERENCES

Aukamp, V. (1984). *Nursing care plans for the childbearing family*. Norwalk, CT: Appleton-Century-Crofts.

Birnbaum, S. (1980). Procedures and prognosis for the infertile couple. *Mother's Manual, 16,* 14–22.

Bobak, I., & Jensen, M. (1984). *Essentials of Maternity Nursing*. St. Louis: Mosby.

Chedd, G. (1981). The new age of genetic engineering. *Science, 81,* 32–40.

Davis, R. (1986). New methods of prenatal diagnosis. Chorionic biopsy and AFP screening. *Alabama Journal of Medical Sciences, 23.*

Devore, N., & Baldwin, N. (1986). Ectopic pregnancy on the rise. *AJN, 86*(6), 674–678.

Diamond, F. (1978). High-risk pregnancy screening techniques. *JOGN, 7,* 15–19.

Dierker, P., et al. (1986). The role of fetal monitoring today. *Patient Care, 20*(3), 91–114.

Friedman, B. (1981). Infertility workup. *AJN, 81*(11), 2040–2046.

Goossens, M., et al. (1983). Prenatal diagnosis of sickle cell anemia in the first trimester of pregnancy. *NEJM, 309*(14), 831–833.

Hogan, K., & Tcheng, D. (1978). The role of the nurse during amniocentesis. *JOGN, 7,* 24–27.

Kimball, M., et al. (1977). Prenatal diagnosis of neural tube defects: A reevaluation of the alpha fetoprotein assay. *Obstetrics and Gynecology, 49,* 532–536.

Leavitt, M. (1982). *Families at risk: Primary prevention in nursing practice*. Boston: Little, Brown.

Lieber, M. (1980). Nonstress antepartal monitoring. *Maternal Child Health Nursing, 5,* 335–339.

McDonough, M., et al. (1981). Parents' response to fetal monitoring. *MCN, 6,* 32–34.

March of Dimes. (1984). *Down syndrome. Public health education information sheet*. West Plains, NY: Birth Defects Foundation.

Perry, S., Parer, J., & Inturrisi, M. (1986). Intrauterine transfusion for severe isoimmunization. *Journal of Maternal Child Nursing, 11*(3), 182–189.

Pfeffer, W. (1980). An approach to the diagnosis and treatment of the infertile female. *Medical Aspects of Human Sexuality, 14,* 121–122.

Pines, M. (1980, June). How old is too old to have a baby? *McCalls,* p. 107.

Sammons, L. (1985). Effects of preparation for amniocentesis on anxiety. (Abstract) *California Nurse, 81*(10), 8.

Shields, D. (1978). Maternal reactions to fetal monitoring. *AJN, 78*(12), 2110–2112.

Sobel, D., & Ferguson, T. (1985). *The people's book of medical tests.* New York: Summit Books.

Tischler, C. (1981). The psychological aspects of genetic counseling. *AJN, 81*(4), 733–734.

Wallach, J. (1983). *Interpretation of pediatric tests.* Boston: Little, Brown.

Walton, J. (1986). Change, challenge and responsibility in medicine. *Clinical Radiology, 37*(1), 1.

Widmann, F. (1983). *Clinical interpretation of laboratory tests.* Philadelphia: Davis.

Wong, D. (1980). Bereavement: The empty-mother syndrome. *Maternal Child Nursing, 5,* 385–389.

Appendices

Reference Values
And Other Information

As stressed in Chapter 1, laboratory books such as this one cannot provide a table of *normal* values for laboratory tests because each laboratory must provide its own normal range for the particular technique that it uses and for the unique population it serves. Values that are listed in a book are only *reference* values, and they must be adapted to a particular setting. The primary source for reference values used in this text are those printed periodically in the *New England Journal of Medicine,* with whose permission the tables in Appendix A are reprinted. Reprints and updates of the normal reference values are available (at $2.50 each) by ordering from:

Normal Reference Values
New England Journal of Medicine
1440 Main Street
Waltham, MA 02254

In addition to the specific reference values listed in Appendix A, Appendix B contains a summary of the changes in newborns and in children. Appendix D presents the changes in pregnancy, and Appendix C, those in the elderly. Documentations for the changes in various populations are included with the tables and throughout the text.

The collection of blood is most often done with the Vacutainer or other commercial system, which has different colored tops on the collection tubes to note the additive present. Table 1–3 in Chapter 1 lists the meaning of the color-coded tops. The type of additive needed is listed in the third column of these tables. The vast majority of serum blood samples require no additives, so blood is collected in a red-top tube.

The tables of reference values also contain the values in SI units, which are explained in Chapter 1. Because reference tables contain many abbreviations and measurement terms, there is a list of common abbreviations included in Appendix E and measurements to help the reader decipher laboratory reports in Appendix G.

APPENDIX A, TABLE 1. BLOOD, PLASMA, OR SERUM VALUES

Determination	Reference Range		Minimal ML Required	Note	Explanation of Test and Possible Nursing Diagnoses
	Conventional	SI			
Aldolase	1.3–8.2 U/L	22–137 nmol·s⁻¹/L	2-S	Use fresh, unhemolyzed serum	Chap. 12
Ammonia	12–55 µmol/L	12–55 µmol/L	2-B	Collect in heparinized tube; deliver *immediately* packed in ice	Chap. 10
Amylase	4–25 U/ml	4–25 arb. unit	1-S		Chap. 12
Bilirubin (van den Bergh test)	One minute: 0.4 mg/100 ml — Total: 1.0 mg/100 ml — Indirect is total minus direct	Up to 7 µmol/L — Up to 17 µmol/L	1-S		Chap. 11
Blood volume	8.5–9.0% of body weight in kg			Isotope dilution technique with I-131 albumin	Chap. 22
Bromide	0 — Toxic level: 17 mEq/L	0 mmol/L	3-S		Chap. 17
Calcium	8.5–10.5 mg/100 ml (slightly higher in children)	2.1–2.6 mmol/L	1-S		Chap. 7
Carbon dioxide content	20–30 mEq/L — 20–26 mEq/L in infants (as HCO_3)	24–30 mmol/L	1-S	Draw without stasis under oil or fill tube to top	Chap. 6
Chloride	100–106 mEq/L	100–106 mmol/L	1-S		Chap. 5
Creatine kinase (CK)	Female 10–79 U/L — Male 17–148 U/L	167–1317 nmol·s⁻¹/L — 283–2467 nmol·s⁻¹/L	3-S	Immediately separate and freeze serum	Chap. 12
Creatinine	0.6–1.5 mg/100 ml	53–133 µmol/L	1-S		Chap. 4

Analyte	Conventional value	SI value	Specimen	Comments	Reference
Ethanol	0.3–0.4%, marked intoxication; 0.4–0.5%, alcoholic stupor; 0.5% or over, alcoholic coma	65–87 mmol/L 87–109 mmol/L > 109 mmol/L	2-B	Collect in oxalate and refrigerate	Chap. 17
Glucose	Fasting: 70–110 mg/100 ml	3.9–5.6 mmol/L	1-P	Collect with EDTA-fluoride mixture	Chap. 8
Iron	50–150 μg/100 ml (higher in males)	9.0–26.9 μmol/L	1-S	Shows diurnal variation higher in A.M.	Chap. 2
Iron-binding capacity	250–410 μg/100 ml	44.8–73.4 μmol/L	1-S		Chap. 2
Lactic acid	0.6–1.8 mEq/L	0.6–1.8 mmol/L	2-B	Collect with oxalate-fluoride: Deliver immediately packed in ice	Chap. 6
Lactic dehydrogenase	45–90 U/L	750–1500 nmol·s⁻¹/L	1-S	Unsuitable if hemolyzed	Chap. 12
Lead	50 μg/100 ml or less	Up to 2.4 μmol/L	2-B	Collect with oxalate fluoride mixture	Chap. 17
Lipase	2 U/ml or less	Up to 2 arb. unit	1-S		Chap. 12
Lipids					
Cholesterol	120–220 mg/100 ml	3.10–5.69 mmol/L	1-S	Fasting	Chap. 9
Triglycerides	40–150 mg/100 ml	0.4–1.5 g/L	1-S	Fasting	Chap. 9
Lipoprotein electrophoresis (LEP)			2-S	Fasting; do not freeze serum	Chap. 9
Lithium	0.5–1.5 mEq/L	0.5–1.5 mmol/L	1-S		Chap. 17
Magnesium	1.5–2.0 mEq/L	0.8–1.3 mmol/L	1-S		Chap. 7
Methanol	0		5-B	May be fatal as low as 115 mg per 100 ml; collect in oxalate	Chap. 17
5′ Nucleotidase	1–11 U/L	17–183 nmol·sec⁻¹/L	1-S		Chap. 12
Osmolality	280–295 mOsm/kg water	280–296 mmol/kg	1-S	Using freezing point depression	Chap. 4

(Continued)

APPENDIX A, TABLE 1. (Continued)

Determination	Reference Range Conventional	Reference Range SI	Minimal ML Required	Note	Explanation of Test and Possible Nursing Diagnoses
Oxygen saturation (arterial)	96–100%	0.96–1.00	3-B	Deliver in sealed heparinized syringe packed in ice	Chap. 6
P_{CO_2}	35–45 mm Hg	4.7–6.0 kPa	2-B	Collect and deliver in sealed heparinized syringe	Chap. 6
pH	7.35–7.45	Same	2-B	Collect without stasis in sealed heparinized syringe; deliver packed in ice	Chap. 6
P_{O_2}	75–100 mm Hg (dependent on age) while breathing room air Above 500 mm Hg while on 100% O_2	10.0–13.3 kPa	2-B	See above for other ABGs	Chap. 6
Phenobarbital	15–50 µg/ml	62–215 µmol/L	1-S		Chap. 17
Phenytoin (Dilantin)	Therapeutic level, 5–20 µg/ml	20–80 µmol/L	1-S		Chap. 17
Phosphatase (acid)	Male—Total: 0.13– 0.63 Sigma U/ml Female—Total: 0.01– 0.56 Sigma U/ml Prostatic: 0–0.7 Fishman-Lerner U/100 ml	36–175 nmol·s^{-1}/L 2.8–156 nmol·s^{-1}/L	1-S	Must always be drawn just before analysis or stored as frozen serum; avoid hemolysis	Chap. 12
Phosphatase (alkaline)	13–39 IU/L; infants and adolescents up to 104 IU/L	217–650 nmol·s^{-1}/L up to 1.26 µmol·s^{-1}/L	1-S	BSP dye interferes; for Bodansky U multiply IU/L by 0.15 up to 90 U; 0.13 to 256 U	Chap. 12

Test	Reference (conventional)	Reference (SI)	Specimen	Comments	Chapter
Phosphorus (inorganic)	3.0–4.5 mg/100 ml (infants in 1st year up to 6.0 mg/100 ml)	1.0–1.5 mmol/L	1-S		Chap. 7
Potassium	3.5–5.0 mEq/L	3.5–5.0 mmol/L	1-S	Serum must be separated promptly from cells (within 1 hr)	Chap. 5
Primidone (Mysoline)	Therapeutic level 4–12 µg/ml	18–55 µmol/L	1-S		Chap. 17
Procainamide	Therapeutic level 4–10 µg/ml	17–42 µmol/L	1-S		Chap. 10
Protein: Total	6.0–8.4 g/100 ml	60–84 g/L	1-S	Client should be fasting; avoid BSP dye	Chap. 10
Albumin	3.5–5.0 g/100 ml	35–50 g/L	1-S	Globulin equals total protein minus albumin	
Globulin	2.3–3.5 g/100 ml	23–35 g/L			
Electrophoresis	% of total protein		1-S	Quantitation by densitometry	Chap. 10
Albumin	52–68	0.52–0.68 L			
Globulin:					
Alpha$_1$	4.2–7.2	0.042–0.072 L			
Alpha$_2$	6.8–12	0.068–0.12 L			
Beta	9.3–15	0.093–0.15 L			
Gamma	13–23	0.13–0.23 L			
Quinidine	Therapeutic: 1.2–4.0 µg/ml Toxic: 5–6 µg/ml	3.7–12.3 µmol/L 15.4–18.5 µmol/L	1-S		Chap. 17
Salicylate	20–25 mg/100 ml; 25–30 mg/100 ml to age 10 yr, 3 h post dose Therapeutic	1.4–1.8 mmol/L 1.8–2.2 mmol/L	2-P	Collect in heparin or EDTA (check with laboratory)	Chap. 17

(Continued)

APPENDIX A, TABLE 1. (Continued)

| Determination | Reference Range | | Minimal ML Required | Note | Explanation of Test and Possible Nursing Diagnoses |
	Conventional	SI			
Sodium	Toxic Over 20 mg/100 ml after age 60	Over 1.4 mmol/L			Chap. 5
Sulfonamide	135–145 mEq/L	135–145 mmol/L	1-S		Chap. 16
	Therapeutic: 5–15 mg/ 100 ml		2-P	Value given as unconjugated unless total is requested	
Transaminase (SGOT) (aspartate aminotransferase)	7–27 U/L	117–450 nmol·s^{-1}/L	1-S		Chap. 12
Transaminase (SGPT) alanine aminotransferase)	1–21 U/L	17–350 nmol·s^{-1}/L	1-S		Chap. 12
Urea nitrogen (BUN)	8–25 mg/100 ml	2.9–8.9 mmol/L	1-S	Urea = BUN × 2.14. Use oxalate as anticoagulant	Chap. 4
Uric acid	3.0–7.0 mg/100 ml	0.18–0.42 mmol/L	1-S	Serum must be separated from cells at once and refrigerated	Chap. 4

These values are in common use in the laboratories at the Massachusetts General Hospital and were compiled by Scully, R. (Ed); Mark, E. (Assoc. Ed.); and McNeely, B., (Assist. Ed.) with the aid of James G. Flood, Ph.D., the Chemistry Laboratory, Leonard Ellman, M.D., the Clinical Laboratories, Bernard Kliman, M.D., the Endocrine Laboratories and Kurt J. Bloch, M.D., the Clinical Immunology Laboratory.
The SI for the Health Professions. World Health Organization: Office of Publications, Geneva, Switzerland, 1977.
Abbreviations used: SI, Systeme International d'Unites; d, 24 hours; P, plasma; S, serum; B, blood; U, urine; L, liter; h, hour; and s, second.
(Reprinted from the New England Journal of Medicine, (1986) 314(1), 39–41, with permission.)

APPENDIX A, TABLE 2. URINE VALUES

Determination	Reference Range		Minimal Quantity Required	Note	Explanation of Test and Possible Nursing Diagnoses
	Conventional	SI			
Acetone plus acetoacetate (quantitative)	0	0 mg/l	2 ml	Keep cold	Chap. 3
Amylase	24–76 U/ml	24–76 arb. unit			Chap. 12
Calcium	300 mg/d or less	7.5 or less mmol/d	24-h specimen	Collect in special bottle with 10 ml of concentrated HCl	Chap. 7
Catecholamines	Epinephrine: under 20 μg/d Norepinephrine: under 100 μg/d	<109 nmol/d <590 nmol/d	24-h specimen	Should be collected with 10 ml of concentrated HCl (pH should be between 2.0–3.0)	Chap. 15
Chorionic gonadotropin	0	0 arb. unit	1st morning voiding	Specific gravity should be at least 1.015	Chap. 18
Coproporphyrin	50–250 μg/d Children under 80 lb 0–75 μg/d	80–380 nmol/d 0–115 nmol/d	24-h specimen	Collect with 5 g of sodium carbonate	Chap. 3
Creatinine	15–25 mg/kg of body weight/d	0.13–0.22 mmol·kg^{-1}/d	24-h specimen		Chap. 4
Creatinine clearance	150–180 L/d (104–125 ml/min) per 1.73 m^2 of body surface	1.7–2.1 ml/s	24-h specimen	Order serum creatinine also	Chap. 4
Hemoglobin and myoglobin	0		Freshly voided sample	Chemical examination with benzidine	Chap. 2

(Continued)

APPENDIX A, TABLE 2. (Continued)

| Determination | Reference Range | | Minimal Quantity Required | Note | Explanation of Test and Possible Nursing Diagnoses |
	Conventional	SI			
5-Hydroxyindole acetic acid	2–9 mg/d (women lower than men)	10–45 μmol/L	24-h specimen	Collect in special bottle with 10 ml of concentrated HCl	Chap. 3
Lead	0.08 μg/ml of 120 μg or less/d	0.39 μmol/L or less	24-h specimen		Chap. 17
Phosphorus (inorganic)	Varies with intake; average 1 g/d	32 mmol/d	24-h specimen	Collect in special bottle with 10 ml of concentrated HCl	Chap. 7
Porphobilinogen	0	0	10 ml	Use freshly voided urine	Chap. 3
Protein: Quantitative	<150 mg/24 h	<0.15 g/d	24-h specimen		Chap. 3

	Age	Male (mg)	Female	Male (µmol/d)	Female (µmol/d)			
Steroids: 17-Ketosteroids (per day)	10	1–4	1–4	3–14	3–14	24-h specimen	Not valid if patient is receiving meprobamate	Chap. 15
	20	6–21	4–16	21–73	14–56			
	30	8–26	4–14	28–90	14–49			
	50	5–18	3–9	17–62	10–31			
	70	2–10	1–7	7–35	3–24			
17-Hydroxysteroids		3–8 mg/d (women lower than men)		8–22 µmol/d as tetrahydrocortisol		24-h specimen	Keep cold; chlorpromazine and related drugs interfere with assay	Chap. 15
Urobilinogen		Up to 1.0 Ehrlich U		To 1.0 arb. unit		2-h sample (1–3 P.M.)		Chap. 11
Uroporphyrin		0–30 µg/d		Less than 36 nmol/d		See Coproporphyrin		Chap. 3
Vanillylmandelic acid (VMA)		Up to 9 mg/d		Up to 45 µmol/d		24-h specimen	Collect as for catecholamines	Chap. 15

Reprinted from the New England Journal of Medicine, *(1986) 314(1), 41–42, with permission.*

APPENDIX A, TABLE 3. SPECIAL ENDOCRINE TESTS

Determination	Reference Range		Minimal ML Required	Note	Explanation of Test and Possible Nursing Diagnoses
	Conventional	SI			
A. Steroid Hormones					
Aldosterone	Excretion: 5–19 µg/24h	14–53 nmol/d	5/d	Keep specimen cold	Chap. 15
	Supine: 48 ± 29 pg/ml	133 ± 80 pmol/L	3-S,P	Fasting, at rest, 210 mEq sodium diet	
	Upright: (2h) 65 ± 23 pg/ml	180 ± 64 pmol/l		Upright, 2h, 210 mEq sodium diet	
	Supine: 107 ± 45 pg/ml	279 ± 125 pmol/L		Fasting, at rest, 110 mEq sodium diet	
	Upright: (2h) 239 ± 123 pg/ml	663 ± 341 pmol/L		Upright, 2 h, 110 mEq sodium diet	
	Supine: 175 ± 75 pg/ml	485 ± 208 pmol/L		Fasting, at rest, 10 mEq sodium diet	
	Upright: (2h) 532 ± 228 pg/ml	1476 ± 632 pmol/L		Upright, 2 h, 10 mEq sodium diet	
Cortisol	8 P.M.: 5–25 µg/100 ml	0.14–0.69 µmol/L	1-P	Fasting	Chap. 15
	8 P.M.: Below 10 µg/100 ml	0–0.28 µmol/L	1-P	At rest	
	4 h ACTH test: 30–45 µg/100 ml	0.83–1.24 µmol/L	1-P	20 U ACTH, IV per 4 h	
	Overnight suppression test: Below 5 µg/100 ml	<0.14 nmol/L	1-P	8 A.M. sample after 0.5 mg dexamethasone p.o. at midnight	

Test	Reference Value (Conventional)	Reference Value (SI)	Specimen	Special Instructions	Reference
11-Deoxycortisol	Excretion: 20–70 µg/24h	55–193 nmol/d	2-d	Keep specimen cold	
	Responsive: Over 7.5 µg/100 ml	> 0.22 µmol/L	1-P	8 A.M. sample, preceded by 4.5 g of metyrapone p.o. per 24 h or by single dose of 2.5 g p.o. at midnight	Chap. 15
Estradiol	Male: <50 pg/ml Female: 23–361 pg/ml	<184 pmol/L 84–1325 pmol/L	5-S,P	Female varies with cycle	Chap. 15
Progesterone	Male: <1.0 ng/ml Female: 0.2–32.2 ng/ml	<3.2 nmol/L 0.6–102 nmol/L	5-S,P	Female varies with cycle	Chap. 15
Testosterone	Adult male: 300–1100 ng/100 ml Adolescent male: Over 100 ng/100 ml Female: 25–90 ng/100 ml	10.4–38.1 nmol/L > 3.5 nmol/L 0.87–3.12 nmol/L	1-P	A.M. sample	Chap. 15
Unbound testosterone	Adult male: 3.06–24.0 ng/100 ml Adult female: 0.09–1.28 ng/100 ml	106–832 pmol/L 3.1–44.4 pmol/L	2-P	A.M. sample	Chap. 15
B. Polypeptide Hormones Adrenocorticotropin (ACTH)	15–70 pg/ml	3.3–15.4 pmol/L	5-P	Place specimen on ice and send promptly to laboratory. Use EDTA tube only.	Chap. 15

(Continued)

APPENDIX A, TABLE 3. (Continued)

Determination	Reference Range		Minimal ML Required	Note	Explanation of Test and Possible Nursing Diagnoses
	Conventional	SI			
Calcitonin	Male: 0–14 pg/ml Female: 0–28 pg/ml > 100 pg/ml in medullary carcinoma	0–4.1 pmol/L 0–8.2 pmol/L >29.3 pmol/L	5-S	Test done only on known or suspected cases of medullary carcinoma of the thyroid	Chap. 7, 15
Follicle-stimulating hormone (FSH)	Male: 3–18 mU/ml Female: 4.6–170 mU/ml	3–18 arb. unit 4.6–170 arb. unit	5-S,P	Same sample may be used for LH Female varies with cycle	Chap. 15
Growth hormone	Below 5 ng/ml Children: Over 10 ng/ml Male: Below 5 ng/ml Female: Up to 30 ng/ml Male: Below 5 ng/ml Female: Below 10 ng/ml	<233 pmol/L >465 pmol/L ><233 pmol/L 0–1395 pmol/L ><233 pmol/L 0–465 pmol/L	1-S	Fasting, at rest After exercise After glucose load	Chap. 15

Insulin	6–26 µU/ml Below 20 µU/ml Up to 150 µU/ml	43–187 pmol/L <144 pmol/L 0–1078 pmol/L	1-S	Fasting During hypoglycemia After glucose load	Chap. 8
Luteinizing hormone	Male: 3–18 mU/ml Female: 2.4–34.5 mU/ml 30–50 mU/ml	3–18 U/L 2.4–34.5 U/L 30–50 U/L	5-S,P	Same sample may be used for FSH Pre- or postovulatory Postmenopausal	Chap. 15
Parathyroid hormone	<25 pg/ml	<2.94 pmol/L	5-P	Keep blood on ice, or plasma must be frozen if it is to be sent any distance; A.M. sample	Chap. 7
Prolactin	2–15 ng/ml	0.08–6.0 nmol/L	2-S		Chap. 15
Renin activity	Supine: 1.1 ± 0.8 ng/ml/h Upright: 1.9 ± 1.7 ng/ml/h Supine: 2.7 ± 1.8 ng/ml/h Upright: 6.6 ± 2.5 ng/ml/h Diuretics: 10.0 ± 3.7 ng/ml/h	0.9 ± 0.6 (nmol/L)h 1.5 ± 1.3 (nmol/L)h 2.1 ± 1.4 (nmol/L)h 5.1 ± 1.9 (nmol/L)h 7.7 ± 2.9 (nmol/L)h	4-P	EDTA tubes, on ice; normal diet Low sodium diet Low sodium diet Low sodium diet	Chap. 15

(Continued)

APPENDIX A, TABLE 3. (Continued)

Determination	Reference Range		Minimal ML Required	Note	Explanation of Test and Possible Nursing Diagnoses
	Conventional	SI			
C. Thyroid Hormones					
Thyroid-stimulating-hormone (TSH)	0.5–5.0 μU/ml	0.5–5.0 mU/L	2-S		Chap. 15
Thyroxine-binding globulin capacity	15–25 μg T₄/100 ml	193–322 nmol/L	2-S		Chap. 15
Total tri-iodothyronine by radioimmunoassay (T₃)	75–195 ng/100 ml	1.16–3.00 nmol/L	2-S		Chap. 15
Total thyroxine by RIA (T₄)	4–12 μg/100 ml	52–154 nmol/L	1-S		Chap. 15
T₄ resin uptake	25–35%	0.25–0.35	2-S		Chap. 15
Free thyroxine index (FT₄I)	1–4	12.8–51.2 pmol/L	2-S		Chap. 15

Reprinted from the New England Journal of Medicine (1986), 314(11), 42-45, with permission.

APPENDIX A, TABLE 4. HEMATOLOGICAL VALUES

Determination	Reference Range		Minimal ML Required	Note	Explanation of Test and Possible Nursing Diagnoses
	Conventional	SI			
Coagulation factors:					
Factor I (fibrinogen)	0.15–0.35 g/100 ml	4.0–10.0 µmol/L	4.5-P	Collect in Vacutainer containing sodium citrate	Chap. 13
Factor II (prothrombin)	60–140%	0.60–1.40	4.5-P	Collect in plastic tubes with 3.8% sodium citrate	Chap. 13
Factor V (accelerator globulin)	60–140%	0.60–1.40	4.5-P	Collect as in factor II determination	Chap. 13
Factor VII-X (proconvertin-Stuart)	70–130%	0.70–1.30	4.5-P	Collect as in factor II determination	Chap. 13
Factor X (Stuart factor)	70–130%	0.70–1.30	4.5-P	Collect as in factor II determination	Chap. 13
Factor VIII (antihemophilic globulin)	50–200%	0.50–2.0	4.5-P	Collect as in factor II determination	Chap. 13
Factor IX (plasma thrombo-plastic cofactor)	60–140%	0.60–1.40	4.5-P	Collect as in factor II determination	Chap. 13
Factor XI (plasma thrombo-c plastic antecedent)	60–140%	0.60–1.40	4.5-P	Collect as in factor II determination	Chap. 13
Factor XII (Hageman factor)	60–140%	0.60–1.40	4.5-P	Collect as in factor II determination	Chap. 13

(Continued)

APPENDIX A, TABLE 4. (Continued)

Determination	Reference Range		Minimal ML Required	Note	Explanation of Test and Possible Nursing Diagnoses
	Conventional	SI			
Coagulation screening tests:					
Bleeding time (Simplate)	3–9.5 min	180–570 s		Simplate bleeding time device (General Diagnostics)	Chap. 13
Prothrombin time	Less than 2-s deviation from control	Less than 2-s deviation from control	4.5-P	Collect in Vacutainer containing 3.8% sodium citrate	Chap. 13
Partial thromboplastin time (activated)	25–38 s	25–38 s	4.5-P	Collect in Vacutainer containing 3.8% sodium citrate	Chap. 13
Fibrinolytic studies:					
Euglobin lysis	No lysis in 2 h	0 (in 2 h)	4.5-P	Collect as in factor II determination	Chap. 13
Fibrinogen split products:	Negative reaction at greater than 1:4 dilution	0 (at>1:4 dilution)	4.5-S	Collect in special tube containing thrombin and epsilon amino caproic acid	Chap. 13
"Complete" blood count:					
Hematocrit	Male: 45–52% Female: 37–48%	Male: 0.42–0.52 Female: 0.37–0.48	1-B	Use EDTA as anticoagulant; the seven listed tests are performed automatically on the ortho ELT 800,	Chap. 2
Hemoglobin	Male: 13–18 g/100 ml Female: 12–16 g/100 ml	Male: 8.1–11.2 mmol/L Female: 7.4–9.9 mmol/L			

Leukocyte count	4300–10,800/mm³	$4.3–10.8 \times 10^9/L$			
Erythrocyte count	4.2–5.9 million/mm³	$4.2–5.9 \times 10^{12}/L$			
Mean corpuscular volume (MCV)	86–98 μm³	86–98 fl		which directly determines cell counts, hemoglobin (as the cyanmethemoglobin derivative), and MCV and computes MCH, MCHC, and hematocrit	
Mean corpuscular hemoglobin (MCH)	27–32 pg	1.7–2.0 fmol			
Mean corpuscular hemoglobin concentration (MCHC)	32–36%	0.32–0.36 mmol/L			
Erythrocyte sedimentation rate	Male :1–13 mm/h Female: 1–20 mm/h	Male: 1–13 mm/h Female: 1–20 mm/h	5-B	Use EDTA as anticoagulant	Chap. 2
Erythrocyte enzymes:					
Glucose-6-phosphate dehydrogenase	5–15 U/g Hb	5–15 U/g	9-B	Use special anticoagulant (ACD solution)	Chap. 2
Ferritin (serum)					
Iron deficiency	0–12 ng/ml	0–4.8 nmol/L			Chap. 2
Iron excess	Greater than 400 ng/L	>160 nmol/L			
Folic acid					
Normal	Greater than 3.3 ng/ml	>7.3 nmol/L	1-S		Chap. 2
Haptoglobin	40–336 mg/100 ml	0.4–3.36 g/L	1-S		Chap. 14
Hemoglobin studies:					
Electrophoresis for abnormal hemoglobin			5-B	Collect with anticoagulant	Chap. 2
Electrophoresis for A₂ hemoglobin	3%	0.015–0.035	5-B	Use oxalate as anticoagulant	Chap. 2
Hemoglobin F (fetal hemoglobin)	Less than 2%	<0.02	5-B	Collect with anticoagulant	Chap. 18

(Continued)

663

APPENDIX A, TABLE 4. (Continued)

Determination	Reference Range		Minimal ML Required	Note	Explanation of Test and Possible Nursing Diagnoses
	Conventional	SI			
L.E. (lupus erythematosus) preparation:					
Method I	0	0	5-B	Use heparin as anti-coagulant	Chap. 14
Method II	0	0	5-B	Use defibrinated bloood	Chap. 13
Platelet count	150,000–350,000/ mm³	150–350 × 10⁹/L	0.5-B	Use EDTA as anticoagulant; counts are performed on Clay Adams Ultraflow; when counts are low, results are confirmed by hand counting	
Platelet function tests:					
Clot retraction	50–100%/2h	0.50–1.00/2h	4.5-P	Collect as in factor II determination	Chap. 13
Platelet aggregation	Full response to ADP, epinephrine and collagen	1.0	18-P	Collect as in factor II determination	Chap. 13
Reticulocyte count	0.5–2.5% red cells	0.005–0.025	0.1-B		Chap. 2
Vitamin B₁₂	205–876 pg/ml		12-S		Chap. 2

(Reprinted from the New England Journal of Medicine, (1986), 314(1), 45–47, with permission.)

APPENDIX A, TABLE 5. MISCELLANEOUS VALUES

Determination	Reference Range		Minimal ML Required	Note	Explanation of Test and Possible Nursing Diagnoses
	Conventional	SI			
Autoantibodies					
Thyroid colloid and microsomal antigens	Negative at a 1:10 dilution of serum		2-S	Low titers in some elderly normal women	Chap. 14
Carcinoembryonic antigen (CEA)	0–2.5 ng/ml, 97% healthy nonsmokers	0–2.5 µg/L, 97% healthy nonsmokers	20-P	Must be sent on ice	Chap. 10
Digitoxin	17 ± 6 ng/ml	22 ± 7.8 nmol/L	1-S	Medication with digitoxin or digitalis	Chap. 17
Digoxin	1.2 ± 0.4 ng/ml	1.54 ± 0.5 nmol/L	1-S	Medication with digoxin 0.25 mg per day	Chap. 17
	1.5 ± 0.4 ng/ml	1.92 ± 0.5 nmol/L	1-S	Medication with digoxin 0.5 mg per day	
Rheumatoid factor (RF)	<60 IU/ml	10 ml clotted blood		Fasting sample preferred	Chap. 14
Other immunological tests:					
Alpha-feto-globulin	Abnormal if present		2-S		Chap. 14
Alpha 1-Antitrypsin	85–213 mg/100 ml	0.85–2.13 g/L	10-B		Chap. 10
Antinuclear antibodies	Negative at a 1:8 dilution of serum		2-S	Send to laboratory promptly	Chap. 14
Anti-DNA antibodies	Negative at a 1:10 dilution of serum		2-S		Chap. 14
Bence-Jones protein	Abnormal if present		50-U		Chap. 10
Complement, total hemolytic	150–250 U/ml		10-B	Must be sent on ice	Chap. 14
C_3	Range 83–177 mg/100 ml	0.83–1.77 g/L	2-S		Chap. 14
C_4	Range 15–45 mg/100 ml	0.15–0.45 g/L	2-S		Chap. 14
C_1 esterase inhibitor	13.2–24 mg/100 ml			5 ml clotted blood	Chap. 14

(Continued)

APPENDIX A, TABLE 5. (Continued)

| Determination | Reference Range | | Minimal ML Required | Note | Explanation of Test and Possible Nursing Diagnoses |
	Conventional	SI			
Hemoglobin A$_{1c}$	3.8–6.4%	0.038–0.064	5-P	Send EDTA tube on ice promptly to laboratory	Chap. 8
Immunoglobulins: IgG IgA IgM	639–1349 mg/100 ml 70–312 mg/100 ml 86–352 mg/100 ml	6.39–13.49 g/L 0.7–3.12 0.86–3.52			Chap. 10
Viscosity	1.4–1.8		10-B	Expressed as the relative viscosity of serum compared to water	Chap. 10
Propranolol (includes bio-active 4-OH metabolite)	100–300 ng/ml	386–1158 nmol/L	1-S	Obtain blood sample 4 h after last dose of beta blocking agent	Chap. 17
Stool fat	Less than 5 g in 24 hr or less than 4% of measured fat intake in 3-d period	<5 g/d	24-hr or 3-d specimen, preferably with markers		Chap. 16

Reprinted from the New England Journal of Medicine, *(1986), 314(1), 48–49, with permission.*

APPENDIX B: REFERENCE VALUES FOR NEWBORNS AND CHILDREN COMPARED TO ADULT VALUES

Name of Test	Change in Value	Explanation for Change Found in
Acid phosphatase	Higher in newborns and children	Chap. 12
Aldolase	Higher in newborns and children	Chap. 12
Alkaline phosphatase	Higher until puberty	Chap. 12
ALT (SGPT)	Higher in newborns	Chap. 12
Ammonia	Higher in newborns, particularly prematures. Also higher in children	Chap. 10
Amylase	Low or absent in newborns	Chap. 12
AST (SGOT)	Higher in newborns and children	Chap. 12
Bicarbonate	Lower in newborns and slightly lower in children	Chaps. 5–6
Bilirubin	Higher until 1 month old	Chap. 11
BUN	Slightly lower in newborns and infants	Chap. 4
C_3, C_4	Lower at birth	Chap. 14
Calcium	Lower in newborns first few days. Slightly higher in children	Chap. 7
Carbon dioxide content	Lower in infants and children	Chap. 6
Cholesterol	Lower in children	Chap. 9
Creatinine	Lower in children. Increases with age. Higher in males after puberty	Chap. 4
Creatine kinase	Higher in newborns	Chap. 12
Fibrinogen	Lower in newborns	Chap. 13
GGTP	5 × higher in newborns	Chap. 12
Gonadotropins (FSH and LH)	Lower in children	Chap. 15
Glucose	Lower in newborns and slightly lower in children	Chap. 8
Growth hormone (GH)	Higher in newborns and children	Chap. 15
Hemoglobin, hematocrit, and RBC	High in newborns, lower by age 1 and adult levels by 8–13 years. Infants have some fetal hemoglobin	Chap. 2
Immunoglobulins—IgG, IgA, etc.	Newborns contain some from mother, varies with age	Chap. 10
17-ketogenic steroids	Low in newborns and increases with age	Chap. 15
LDH	Very high in newborn, child 1–2 × adult	Chap. 12
Magnesium	Slightly lower?	Chap. 7
Metanephrines (urine)	Higher in infants	Chap. 15
pH	Lower in newborns	Chap. 6
Po_2	Lower in newborns	Chap. 6
Phosphorus	Highest in newborns, levels decline by puberty	Chap. 7
Potassium	Slightly higher in newborns	Chap. 5
Pregnanediol	Lower in children	Chap. 15
Pregnantriol	Lower in children	Chap. 15
PT (prothrombin time)	Higher in newborns	Chap. 13
PTT (partial thromboplastin time)	Higher in newborns	Chap. 13
Platelets	Slightly lower in newborns	Chap. 13

APPENDIX B: (Continued)

Name of Test	Change in Value	Explanation for Change Found in
Reticulocytes	Higher in newborns	Chap. 2
Sedimentation rate	Slower in newborns and children	Chap. 2
Specific gravity	Lower until age 2	Chap. 3
Testosterone	Much lower in children	Chap. 15
Total protein	Slightly lower in children	Chap. 10
Triglycerides	Lower in children	Chap. 9
T_4	Higher in children and especially newborns	Chap. 15
Uric acid	Lower values until puberty	Chap. 4
Urine osmolality	Lower in newborns	Chap. 4
WBC	Extremely high in newborns, differential also different in children	Chap. 2

Also see other references for specific tests in each chapter. Note that the values for premature infants are not the same as for newborns at term. Consult a speciality text for high-risk neonate care.

References for Appendix B

Cherian, G., & Hill, G. (1978). Percentile estimates of 14 chemical constituents in sera of children and adolescents," *American Journal of Clinical Pathology, 69,* 24–31.

Jacobs, D., et al. (1984). *Laboratory test handbook with DRG index.* St. Louis: Mosby/Lexi.

Meites, S. (1977). *Pediatric clinical chemistry. A survey of normals, methods and instrumentation with commentary.* Washington, D.C.: American Association for Clinical Chemistry, Inc.

"Pediatric Values," Children's Hospital, San Francisco, California, 1986.

"Pediatric Values," Kaiser Hospital, San Francisco, California, 1986.

Tietz, N. (Ed.). (1983). *Clinical guide to laboratory tests.* Philadelphia: Saunders.

Wallach, J. (1983). *Interpretation of pediatric tests.* Boston: Little, Brown.

APPENDIX C: POSSIBLE ALTERATIONS IN REFERENCE VALUES FOR THE AGED

Name of Test	Possible Change in Value	Explanation for Change Found in
Alkaline phosphatase	Increase	Chap. 12
Amylase	Increase	Chap. 12
Antinuclear antibodies (ANA)	May be present	Chap. 14
Blood sugar, fasting and 2 hr pc	Increase	Chap. 8
BUN	Increase	Chap. 4
C_3C_4	Increase	Chap. 14
Calcium	May lower, but this not well documented?	Chap. 7
Cholesterol	Increase until after 70	Chap. 9
Cold agglutinins	Increase	Chap. 14
Creatinine clearance	Decrease	Chap. 4
Glucose tolerance test (GTT)	Change in curve	Chap. 8
Gonadotropins (LH, FSH)	Eventually decrease, but increase postmenopausal	Chap. 15
Immunoglobulins	Decreases and alterations	Chap. 10
Lymphocytes	May decrease	Chap. 2
17-ketosteroids	Decrease	Chap. 15
Po_2	Decrease	Chap. 6
Phosphorus	May lower with age	Chap. 7
Pregnanediol	Decrease in woman	Chap. 15
Rheumatic factor (RF)	May be present	Chap. 14
Sedimentation rate (ESR)	Increase	Chap. 2
T_3 RIA	Decrease?	Chap. 15
Triglycerides	Increase except very elderly	Chap. 9
Transaminases (SGOT, SGPT)	Slight increase	Chap. 12
Uric acid	Slightly higher values	Chap. 4
VDRL	May become reactive?	Chap. 14

Also see the reference values for specific tests in each chapter. Note that the effect of age on many tests is not known. The figures used for normals may sometimes be more reflective of the common underlying chronic diseases of the elderly rather than of a normal healthy stage. For example, hypertension affects many elderly clients, and it can cause some renal changes that in turn can change the values of various laboratory tests.

References for Appendix C

Gerboes, K., et al. (1979). Is the elderly patient accurately diagnosed? *Geriatrics, 34,* 91–96.
Gioiella, E., & Bevil, C. (1985). *Nursing care of the aging client.* Norwalk, CT: Appleton-Century-Crofts.
Harnes, J. (1980). Normal values with increasing age, *Journal of Chronic Diseases, 33,* 593–594.
Jacobs, D., et al. (1984). *Laboratory test handbook with DRG index.* St. Louis: Mosby/Lexi.
Ravel, R. (1984). *Clinical laboratory medicine.* Chicago: Year Book.
Tietz, N. (Ed). (1983). *Clinical guide to laboratory tests.* Philadelphia: Saunders.

APPENDIX D: ALTERED REFERENCE VALUES FOR COMMON LABORATORY TESTS IN NORMAL PREGNANCIES[a] AND WITH ORAL CONTRACEPTIVES[b]

Name of Test	Change in Value	Explanation for Change Found in
ACTH	Decrease	Chap. 15
Aldosterone[b]	Increase	Chap. 15
Alkaline phosphatase[b]	Marked increase	Chap. 12
Albumin[b]	Decrease	Chap. 10
B_{12}	Decrease	Chap. 2
Bilirubin[b]	Occasional increase	Chap. 11
Bicarbonate	Decrease	Chap. 6
Blood glucose[b]	Variations in trimesters	Chap. 8
BUN	Decrease	Chap. 4
C-reactive protein	Increase	Chap. 14
Calcium	Decreases with albumin levels	Chap. 7
Pco_2	Decrease	Chap. 6
Cholesterol[b]	Increase	Chap. 9
Cortisol	Increase	Chap. 15
Creatinine clearance	Increase	Chap. 4
Creatinine (serum)	Decrease	Chap. 4
Fibrinogen levels[b]	Increase	Chap. 13
Folic acid levels[b]	Decrease	Chap. 2
GGTP[b]	Increase	Chap. 12
Hemoglobin, hematocrit	Decrease	Chap. 2
Iron	Decrease	Chap. 2
LAP[b]	Increase	Chap. 12
Lipase	Increase	Chap. 12
Magnesium[b]	May decrease	Chap. 7
5′ Nucleotidase[b]	Increase	Chap. 12
Phosphorus	May decrease	Chap. 7
Protein electrophoresis	Change in pattern	Chap. 10
PT	May decrease	Chap. 13
PTT	May decrease	Chap. 13
Platelets[b]	Increase after delivery	Chap. 13
Retic	Increase	Chap. 2
Sed rate	Increase	Chap. 2
T_3-T_4 and thyroid-binding[b] globulin	Altered values	Chap. 15
Triglycerides[b]	Increase	Chap. 9
Uric acid	Decrease in early pregnancy	Chap. 4
WBC[b]	Increase in total and in neutrophils	Chap. 2

Increases or decreases are in relation to the woman's prepregnancy values.

[a]Also see references for specific tests discussed in each chapter.

[b]Note that many of the effects of oral contraceptives on laboratory tests are similar to those found in pregnancy. See the Medical Letter on Drugs and Therapeutics 21: 55–56, June 29, 1979 for 32 references about the effects of oral contraceptives. Also see Phipps et al. (1983), *Medical-Surgical Nursing,* for a list of laboratory tests affected by birth control pills. Consult current literature for specific effects for low dose pills.

References for Appendix D

Bobak, I., & Jensen. (1984). *Essentials of maternity nursing.* St. Louis: Mosby.

Hytten, F., & Lind, T. (1975). *Diagnostic indices in pregnancy.* Summit, NJ: Ciba-Geigy Corp.

Jacobs, K. (1984). *Laboratory test handbook with DRG index.* St. Louis: Mosby/Lexi.

Milne, J. A., (Ed.). (1979). Physiological response to pregnancy in health and disease. *Post Graduate Medical Journal, 55,* 293–367.

Tietz, N. (Ed.). (1983). *Clinical guide to laboratory tests.* Philadelphia: Saunders.

Wallach, J. (1983). *Interpretation of diagnostic tests.* Boston: Little, Brown.

Widmann, F. (1983). *Clinical interpretation of laboratory tests.* Philadelphia: Davis.

ABG	Arterial blood gases
ABO	Blood types
ACD	Acid citrate dextrose (anticoagulant)
ACT	Activated coagulation time
ACTH	Adrenocorticotropic hormone
ADH	Antidiuretic hormone
AFB	Acid-fast bacillus
AHG	Antihemophilia globulin
AFP	Alpha-fetoprotein
A/G ratio	Albumin/globulin ration (outdated)
ALA	(delta) aminolevulinic acid
ALT	Alanine amino transferase (new term for SGPT)
APPT	Activated partial thromboplastin time (also PTT)
ANA	Antinuclear antibodies
ASO	Antistreptolysin O titer
AST	Asparate amino transferase (new name for SGOT)
BC	Blood culture
BCP	Biochemical profile; also, birth control pills
BMR	Basal metabolic rate
Br	Bromide
BS	Blood sugar
BSP	Bromsulphalein (dye for liver function test)
BUN	Blood urea nitrogen
C_3 C_4	Complement factors
C&S	Culture and sensitivity
Ca^{++}	Calcium
CBC	Complete blood count
CEA	Carcinoembryonic antigen
CF	Complement fixation
Cl^-	Chloride
CO_2	Carbon dioxide (Pco_2 = partial pressure)
CPK or CK	Creatine phosphokinase
Cr	Chromium
CRP	C-reactive protein
Crit	Hematocrit
CSF	Cerebrospinal fluid
Cu	Copper
CUA	Clean urinalysis
Diff	Differential (white blood cell count)
EDTA	Ethylenediaminotetracetate (anticoagulant for blood samples)
ESR	Erythrocyte sedimentation rate
Fe	Iron
FBS	Fasting blood sugar
FEP	Free erythrocyte porphyrins
FSH	Follicle-stimulating hormone
FTA	Fluorescent treponemal antibodies
GC	Gonococcus
GFR	Glomerular filtration rate
GGTP	Gamma glutomyl transferase
GH	Growth hormone
GHB	Glycosylated hemoglobin (A_{1c})
G-6-PD	Glucose-6-phosphatase dehydrogenase

(Continued)

GTT	Glucose tolerance test
HAA	Hepatitis-associated antigen
HAT	Heterophile antibody titer
Hb (Hgb)	Hemoglobin
HBD	Hydroxybutyric dehydrogenase
HB$_s$ Ag	Hepatitis B surface antigen
HCG	Human chorionic gonadotropin
Hct	Hematocrit
Hg	Mercury
5HIAA	5-hydroxyindoleacetic acid
ICSH	Interstitial cell-stimulating hormone (LH in female)
IFA	Immunofluorescence antibody test (may be direct or indirect)
Ig	Immunoglobulin (such as IgA, IgM, etc.)
IEP	Immunoelectrophoresis
K^{++}	Potassium
17-KGS	17-ketogenic steroids
17-KS	17-ketosteroids
LAP	Leucine aminopeptidase
LDH	Lactic dehydrogenase
LDL	Low-density lipoprotein
LE Prep	Lupus erythematosus test
LE (urine)	Leukocyte esterase
LEP	Lipoprotein electrophoresis
LFT	Liver function tests
LH	Luteinizing hormone (ICSH in male)
Li	Lithium
lytes	Electrolytes (Na, K, Cl, bicarbonate)
MCH	Mean corpuscular hemoglobin (erythrocyte indices)
MCHC	Mean corpuscular hemoglobin concentration (erythrocyte indices)
MCV	Mean corpuscular volume (erythrocyte indices)
MHA	Microhemagglutination test
Mg	Magnesium
MIC	Minimal inhibitory concentration
N	Nitrogen
Na^{++}	Sodium
NBT	Nitro blue tetrazolium test
NC	Normal color
NL	Normal
NPN	Nonprotein nitrogen
O$_2$	Oxygen (Po$_2$ = partial pressure)
O&P	Ova and parasites
17-OH	17-hydroxysteroids
OTC	Over-the-counter (drugs)
P	Phosphorus
Pb	Lead
PBI	Protein-bound iodine (outdated)
PCV	Packed cell volume (hematocrit)
pH	Hydrogen-ion concentration
PKU	Phenylketonuria
Pl.ct.	Platelet count
PMNs	Polymorphonuclear (type of WBC)
PMV	Platelet mean volume

PSP	Phenolsulfonphthalein (dye for renal excretion test)
PPLO	Pleuropneumonia-like organism (has characteristics between virus and bacteria)
PT	Prothrombin time
PTH	Parathyroid hormone or parathormone
PTT	Partial thromboplastin time (*see also* APTT)
PP or PC	Postprandial (or after meals)
QNS	Quantity not sufficient
RAST	Radioallergosorbent test
RAI	Radioactive iodine
RBC	Red blood cell
RDW	Red cell distribution width
Retic	Reticulocyte count
RF	Rheumatoid factor (also called RA factor)
Rh	Rhesus; Rh factor in blood
RIA	Radioimmunoassay
R/O	Rule out
RPR	Rapid plasma reagin
segs	Segmented neutrophils of WBC
S&A	Sugar and acetone
SG	Specific gravity
SGOT	Serum glutamic-oxaloacetic transaminase (newer name is AST)
SGPT	Serum glutamic-pyruvic transaminase (newer name is ALT)
SMA	Sequential multiple analyzer (SMA-6 does 6 tests, SMA-12, 12 tests)
SPEP	Serum protein electrophoresis
Stat	Immediately
STS	Serologic test for syphilis
T-C	Type and cross match
T&S	Type and screen
T_3	Triiodothyronine
T_4	Thyroxine
TPI	Treponema pallidum immobilization
TBG	Thyroid-binding globulin
TIBC	Total iron-binding capacity
TP	Total protein
TRH	Thyroid-releasing hormone
TSH	Thyroid-stimulating hormone (thyrotropin)
TSP	Total serum proteins
UA	Urinalysis
UC	Urine culture
UrAc	Uric acid
VDRL	Venereal Disease Research Laboratory (test for syphilis)
VLDL	Very low-density lipoprotein
VMA	Vanillylmandelic acid
WBC	White blood cell; white blood count
WNL	Within normal limits
WNR	Within normal range
X match	Cross match (of blood)
X	Female chromosome
Y	Male chromosome

Compiled from various sources. Same abbreviations are common in Canada. See Watson, E. M. (1974). Clinical Laboratory Procedures. *Canadian Nurse*, 70, 25–44.

APPENDIX F: COMMON ABBREVIATIONS FOR DIAGNOSTIC PROCEDURES (PART III)

ABG	Arterial blood gases
AFP	Alpha-fetoprotein
BE	Barium enema
BMR	Basal metabolic rate
CT scan	Computerized axial tomography (*also* CAT)
CSF	Cerebrospinal fluid
CVB	Chorionic villi biopsy
ECG	Electrocardiogram (*also* EKG)
ECHO	Echocardiogram
EEG	Electroencephalogram
EGD	Esophogastroduodenoscopy
EKG	Electrocardiogram (*also* ECG)
EMG	Electromyelogram
ERCP	Endoscopic retrograde choledochopancreatography or cholangiopancreatography (*also* ECPG)
FEF	Forced expiratory flow
FEV$_1$	Forced expiratory volume in one second
FVC	Forced vital capacity
GA	Gastric analysis
GB series	Gallbladder series
GFR	Glomerular filtration rate
GI series	Gastrointestinal series
I-131, I-123, etc.	Radioactive iodine
IVC	Intravenous cholangiogram
IVP	Intravenous pyelogram
KUB	Kidneys, ureters, bladder (flat plate of abdomen)
LP	Lumbar puncture
L/S ratio	Lecithin/spingomyelin ratio
MBC	Maximal breathing capacity (*also* MVV)
MRI	Magnetic resonance imaging (*see* NMR)
MVV	Maximum voluntary ventilation (*also* MBC)
NMR	Nuclear magnetic resonance (*see* MRI)
NSR	Normal sinus rhythm
NST	Nonstress test (for fetus)
OCG	Oral cholecystogram
OCT	Oxytocin challenge test
PEG	Pneumoencephalogram
PET	Positron emission tomography
PFT	Pulmonary function tests
RAI	Radioactive iodine
RISA	Radio-iodinated serum albumin (for blood volume)
Tc-99	Technetium (radionuclide)
TV	Tidal volume
UGI	Upper gastrointestinal
VC	Vital capacity
VE	Volume exhaled per minute at rest

cc	cubic centimeter (same as ml, 1/1,000 liter, which is the preferred term)
cm	centimeter
cu mm or mm³	cubic millimeter
d or dl	deciliter (1/10 of a liter)
g or gm	gram (1/1000 of a kilogram, 15 grains)
hpf	high power field microscope
G%	grams in 100 ml
IU	international unit
kg, K, or k	kilogram (1000 grams, or 2.2 pounds)
L	liter (1000 ml or 1000 cc)
lpf	low power field microscope
mcg or μg	micrograms (1/1000 milligram)
mc	millicurie
mEq or meq	milliequivalent (see Chapter 5 for formula)
mg or mgm	milligram (1/1000 gram)
mg%	milligrams in 100 milliliters (same as dl)
mIU	milliinternational unit (1/1000 IU)
ml	milliliter (1/1000 liter, same as cc)
mm	millimeter (1/10 centimeter)
mm³ or cu mm	cubic millimeter (see RBC count, Chap. 2)
mm Hg	millimeters of mercury (see blood gases, Chap. 6)
mmol	millimoles (see Chap. 1 on SI units)
mOsm	milliosmoles (see Chap. 4)
ng	nanogram (1/1000 microgram, see Chap. 15)
pg	picogram (1/1000 nanogram, see Chap. 15)
QNS	quantity not sufficient
SI	international system, see Chap. 1
u	international enzyme unit
μ	micro
μg (mcg)	microgram (1/1000 milligram)
w/v	weight/volume
μc	microcurie (1/1000 of a millicurie)
WNL	within normal limits
WNR	within normal range
<	less than
>	greater than

APPENDIX H: ANSWERS TO QUESTIONS FOR PART I (LABORATORY TESTS)

Chapter 1	Chapter 2	Chapter 3	Chapter 4
1. c	1. d	1. c	1. c
2. d	2. c	2. d	2. a
3. b	3. b	3. c	3. b
4. c	4. a	4. a	4. d
5. d	5. c	5. d	5. c
6. b	6. c	6. c	6. b
7. c	7. d	7. d	7. b
8. a	8. a	8. b	8. c
9. d	9. d	9. d	9. b
	10. b	10. c	10. b
	11. a	11. b	11. a
	12. d		
	13. a		
	14. c		
	15. d		
	16. a		

Chapter 5	Chapter 6	Chapter 7	Chapter 8
1. d	1. b	1. a	1. c
2. a	2. a	2. a	2. d
3. b	3. c	3. a	3. d
4. b	4. d	4. c	4. c
5. b	5. d	5. d	5. d
6. c	6. d	6. b	6. a
7. a	7. b	7. c	7. c
8. a	8. b	8. c	8. c
9. c	9. d	9. b	9. b
10. c	10. b	10. d	10. c
11. c	11. a	11. a	11. c
12. d	12. b	12. a	12. a
13. b	13. d	13. d	13. a
14. c	14. c	14. c	14. b
15. c	15. a	15. b	15. d
16. b	16. a		16. d
17. d	17. b		
18. c	18. d		
	19. d		
	20. b		
	21. c		

Chapter 9	Chapter 10	Chapter 11	Chapter 12
1. b	1. b	1. d	1. a
2. c	2. c	2. d	2. a
3. a	3. d	3. c	3. a
4. d	4. b	4. c	4. c
5. c	5. d	5. b	5. a
6. b	6. b	6. a	6. a
7. d	7. a	7. a	7. a
8. a	8. b	8. d	8. c
	9. c	9. d	9. d
	10. a	10. d	10. a
	11. c	11. c	11. b
	12. c	12. d	
	13. d		

Chapter 13	Chapter 14	Chapter 15	Chapter 16
1. d	1. c	1. c	1. c
2. a	2. b	2. a	2. d
3. a	3. a	3. b	3. b
4. b	4. b	4. b	4. d
5. d	5. d	5. d	5. c
6. d	6. c	6. b	6. a
7. d	7. d	7. d	7. b
8. b	8. b	8. b	8. d
9. d	9. d	9. b	9. a
10. d	10. a	10. d	10. b
11. c	11. d	11. a	11. d
12. d	12. c	12. b	12. b
13. b	13. d		13. b
14. b	14. b		14. a
15. b			
16. a			
17. c			

Chapter 17	Chapter 18
1. d	1. b
2. c	2. a
3. d	3. d
4. b	4. c
5. a	5. a
6. b	6. c
7. c	7. c
8. b	8. c
9. a	9. c
10. b	
11. d	
12. b	

APPENDIX I: ANSWERS TO QUESTIONS FOR PART III (DIAGNOSTIC PROCEDURES)

Chapter 20	Chapter 21	Chapter 22	Chapter 23
1. a	1. c	1. b	1. b
2. c	2. b	2. c	2. c
3. d	3. a	3. d	3. c
4. b	4. d	4. b	4. b
5. d	5. b	5. c	5. d
6. d	6. b	6. a	6. d
7. a	7. b	7. a	7. d
8. d		8. d	8. a
9. c		9. c	9. b
10. d			
11. c			
12. a			
13. a			

Chapter 24	Chapter 25	Chapter 26	Chapter 27
1. c	1. a	1. a	1. d
2. d	2. a	2. a	2. d
3. a	3. c	3. d	3. b
4. c	4. c	4. b	4. d
5. d	5. a	5. b	5. a
6. c	6. c	6. c	6. c
7. a	7. a	7. d	
8. a	8. c		
9. d	9. c		
10. d	10. c		
11. c			
12. b			

Chapter 28

1. d
2. a
3. c
4. d
5. c
6. a
7. a
8. c
9. b

INDEX